OBSTETRICS AND GYNECOLOGY FOR POSTGRADUATES

Volume 2

OBSTETRICS AND GYNECOLOGY FOR POSTGRADUATES

Volume 2

Third Edition

General Editors

SABARATNAM ARULKUMARAN PhD, FRCOG, FRCS
Professor and Head of Obstetrics and Gynecology
St George's University of London
London, United Kingdom

SARALA GOPALAN FRCOG, PhD, FAMS
Formerly Professor and Head, Department of Obstetrics and Gynecology
Postgraduate Institute of Medical Education and Research
Chandigarh, India

PRATAP KUMAR MD, DGO, FIMCH
Professor and Head, Department of Obstetrics and Gynecology
Kasturba Medical College
Manipal, India

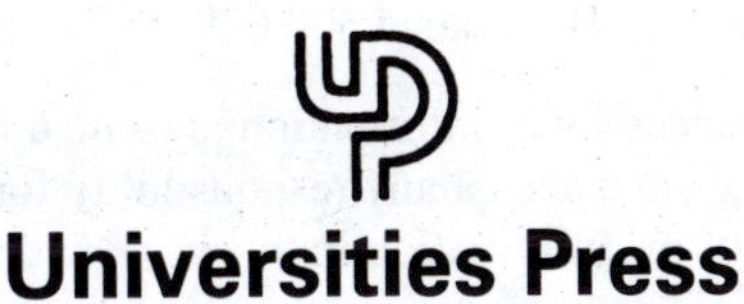

UNIVERSITIES PRESS (INDIA) PRIVATE LIMITED

Registered Office
3-6-747/1/A & 3-6-754/1, Himayatnagar, Hyderabad 500 029, India
email: info@universitiespress.com, www.universitiespress.com

Distributed by
Orient Blackswan Private Limited

Registered Office
3-6-752 Himayatnagar, Hyderabad 500 029, India

Other Offices
Bengaluru / Bhopal / Bhubaneshwar / Chennai / Ernakulam / Guwahati
Hyderabad / Jaipur / Kolkata / Lucknow / Mumbai / New Delhi / Noida / Patna

First published 1994
Reprinted 1995, 1996, 1999, 2001
Second Edition 2003, Reprinted 2006
Third edition 2009
Reprinted 2011, 2013, 2014

ISBN 978 81 7371 691 1

Cover design
Binita Desai

Cover and book design:
© Universities Press (India) Private Limited 2009

Typeset by
Trinity Designers and Typesetters
Chennai 600 041

Printed at
Baba Barkha Nath Printers
New Delhi

Published by
Universities Press (India) Private Limited
3-6-747/1/A & 3-6-754/1, Himayatnagar, Hyderabad 500 029, India

Preface to the third edition

The first two editions of *Obstetrics and Gynecology for Postgraduates* were brought out under the distinguished editorship of Professor SS Ratnam from Singapore, Professor K Bhasker Rao from Chennai and one of the current editors, Professor Sabaratnam Arulkumaran who then worked in Singapore but is currently Head of Obstetrics and Gynecology at St. George's Medical School, University of London. With the passing away of Professor SS Ratnam and the retirement of Professor K Bhasker Rao, a decision was taken to bring in two new editors with distinguished careers in obstetrics and gynecology. Professor Sarala Gopalan, formerly Head of the Postgraduate Institute of Obstetrics and Gynecology, Chandigarh and Professor Pratap Kumar, Head of the Department of Obstetrics and Gynecology from the Manipal University kindly agreed to help.

A distinct difference from the previous editions is that the chapters on obstetrics are in the first volume and those on gynecology in the second. This is a deviation from the past 16 years, where we had both obstetrics and gynecology in the two volumes, with 20 chapters in obstetrics and 20 in gynecology in each volume. We have maintained the number of chapters in each volume at 40.

The other major difference has been for the editors to divide the chapters based on their expertise. We commissioned well known authors and edited their respective chapters with the help of the authors. This provided more freedom to the authors to express their views, backing it with strong evidence. This approach has expanded the contents of each chapter compared to the previous editions; they are much richer in quality and quantity.

The field of obstetrics and gynecology has seen major advances starting from obstetric and gynecological ultrasound by Ian Donald in the 1960s and in vitro fertilisation in the 1970s by Steptoe and Edwards. In addition to these there have been major advances in developing new hormones and new types of operative procedures. Not only have new medicine and new technology advanced the field, but also the culture of evidence-based medicine has added greatly to it. Having protocols and guidelines have unified our views and have enhanced safe practice in this specialty. It is not an easy task to be up to date with all the current literature. These two volumes have made an attempt to synthesise recently available, acceptable and appropriate management in different settings. We believe that these volumes will enable postgraduates and clinicians to provide the best care possible in women's health.

Needless to say, there might be questions on best or acceptable practice. The editors and the publishers welcome comments so that errors, if any, can be rectified in the subsequent reprints or edition. Since the editorial work was divided amongst the three editors, there may be some overlap of the contents in different chapters. This is deliberately left as it is to provide continuity of the subject in each individual chapter.

The publishers have taken great pains to bring these two volumes with a new format, more pictures, readable type, and new layout. We are most grateful to them. We hope that readers will benefit from these two volumes.

2009

SABARATNAM ARULKUMARAN
SARALA GOPALAN
PRATAP KUMAR

Preface to the second edition

It has been a source of great satisfaction and pleasure to the editors that the first edition of this book was extensively used by postgraduates not only in India but also in many parts of Asia. We are also happy that the book has been particularly useful to students preparing for examinations. The book has undergone several reprints and we are happy to present this revised edition.

While the editors recognise that it would not be possible to cover all aspects of obstetrics and gynecology, and women's health in a comprehensive manner, we have attempted to cover all the major aspects of the discipline in the two volumes of the book. Most of the chapters in this volume have been extensively revised and new chapters on operative vaginal deliveries, tropical diseases and thyroid disorders have been included to make the volume more complete and to assist postgraduate students and practising clinicians in updating their knowledge and keeping pace with current advances.

The editors have made special efforts to identify contributors with interest in a particular subject area so as to make their chapter authoritative. The contributors belong to different parts of Asia. Every chapter of the book has been edited, independently and jointly by the editors and despite all efforts to make the book as comprehensive as possible we do recognise that the reader will need to refer to published articles to further update their knowledge in a particular subject area.

We hope to deal with the advances in reproductive health, obstetrics and gynecology, and in awareness of women's health, particularly with relevance to socioeconomic status, in the new edition of the second volume.

We hope that this edition of volume 1, will be as relevant to and popular among postgraduate students and practising clinicians as the earlier edition.

1999

SS RATNAM
K BHASKER RAO
S ARULKUMARAN

Preface to the first edition

Although many books have been written on obstetrics and gynecology and a number of monographs appear regularly, there is a dearth of books for postgraduates with particular reference to Asian countries. This book does not attempt to cover basic information that is available in standard textbooks but aims to address current topics with emphasis on issues of controversy and advances that have taken place in recent times.

The editors have made a special effort to identify contributors with interest in the particular subject so as to make it authoritative. With this in mind, the editors have looked beyond India for contributors and fifty per cent of the contributions have come from outside. Every chapter has been edited by the three General Editors independently and jointly, and it is hoped that the book will serve as a textbook for postgraduates preparing for the higher examinations as well as serve as a reference book for practising obstetricians and gynecologists.

This volume covers a wider range of subjects spanning obstetrics and gynecology. It is not possible to cover all aspects of the discipline in one volume and the editors hope to bring out the second volume soon to address subjects of interest that have not been included in this volume and where advances have taken place and where controversies still persist.

1992

SS RATNAM
K BHASKER RAO
S ARULKUMARAN

Contents

Contributors

Aditi Tayade
Senior Resident,
KJ Somaiya Medical College,
Mumbai, India

Ajita Mandlekar MD, DFP
Consultant Obstetrician and Gynecologist
Mumbai, India

Alka Kriplani MD, MAMS, FICOG, FICMCH, FIMSA
Professor and Head of Unit II
Department of Obstetrics and Gynaecology
All India Institute of Medical Sciences
New Delhi, India

Barun Sarkar MS, FICOG, FICMCH
Formerly Professor in Obstetrics and Gynaecology
SN Medical College
Agra, India

K Bhasker Rao MD, FAMS
Formerly Director, Institute of Obstetrics and Gynaecology, Chennai and
Consultant Obstetrician and Gynecologist,
Vijaya Hospitals
Chennai, India

BN Chakravarty
Formerly Director
Institute of Reproductive Medicine
Kolkata, India

Edwin Chandraharan MS, DFFP, MRCOG
Consultant Obstetrician and Gynecologist,
Department of Obstetrics and Gynaecology,
St George's Hospital NHS Trust,
London, United Kingdom

Fauzia Haq Nawaz MRCOG, FCPS
Assistant Professor, Department of Obstetrics and Gynecology
Aga Khan University Hospital
Karachi, Pakistan

Firuza D Patel MD
Professor, Department of Radiotherapy
Postgraduate Institute of Medical Education and Research
Chandigarh, India

S Girija
Lecturer cum Research Associate, Department of Obstetrics and Gynecology
Kasturba Medical College
Manipal, India

Gita Arjun FACOG
Director and Obstetrician and Gynecologist,
EV Kalyani Medical Centre
Chennai, India

PM Gopinath MD, DGO
Assistant Professor of Obstetrics and Gynecology
Madras Medical College
Chennai, India

Gowri Ramanathan MRCOG
Specialist Registrar, Department of Obstetrics and Gynecology
St George's Hospital Medical School
London, United Kingdom

NJ Gupta
Institute Of Reproductive Medicine
Kolkata, India

Indu Gupta MD, PhD, FAMS, FNASc
Formerly Professor, Department of Obstetrics and Gynecology
Postgraduate Institute of Medical Education and Research
Chandigarh, India

Javed H Rizvi FACS, FRCOG
Professor and Chairman, Department of Obstetrics and Gynecology
Aga Khan University Hospital
Karachi, Pakistan

Jayita Chakrabarti MD, DNB
RMO cum Clinical Tutor, Depament of Obstetrics and Gyencology
Calcutta National Medical College, Kolkata University
Kolkata, India

Kamal Ojha MD, MRCOG
Consultant Obstetrician and Gynecologist
St Georges Hospital and Medical School
London, United Kingdom

RCM Kaza
Professor, Department of Surgery
Maulana Azad Medical College
New Delhi, India

Kurian Joseph MD
Director, Joseph Nursing Home, Chennai and Consultant Gynecologist, Southern Railway Headquarters Hospital and Vijaya Hospital
Chennai, India.

Kusagradhi Ghosh MD, DNB, FRCOG
Associate Professor, Department of Obstetrics and Gynecology
Vivekananda Institute of Medical Sciences, Kolkata University
Kolkata, India

Lee Hsueh Ni MD (Radiotherapy)
Senior Resident, Department of Radiotherapy
Postgraduate Institute of Medical Education and Research
Chandigarh, India

Mahalakshmi Gorti MD, MRCOG
Specialist Registrar, Department of Obstetrics and Gynaecology
St. Richard's Hospital
Chichester, United Kingdom

AP Manjunath MD
Associate Professor, Department of Obstetrics and Gynecology
Kasturba Medical College
Manipal, India

Mala Vijayakrishnan MD, DGO
Consultant Obstetrician and Gynecologist
Vijaya Hospital
Chennai, India

Mandakini Parihar
Director, Mandakini IVF Centre and Associate Honorary Professor,
KJ Somaiya Medical College
Mumbai, India

Mandakini Pradhan MD, DNB, DM
Additional Professor, Maternal and Reproductive Health
Sanjay Gandhi Postgraduate Institute of Medical Studies
Lucknow, India

Mandeep Singh MD
Specialist Registrar (East of England Deanery)
Basildon and Thurrock NHS Foundation Hospital,
Basildon, United Kingdom

Neelanjana Mukhopadhaya DGO, MRCOG
Specialist Registrar in Obstetrics and Gynecology
St George's Hospital
London, United Kingdom

Nutan Agarwal MD, FICMCH
Associate Professor, Department of Obstetrics and Gynecology
All India Institute of Medical Sciences
New Delhi, India

A Padma Rao MD, DGO
Emeritus Professor, Department of Obstetrics and Gynecology
Kasturba Medical College
Manipal, India

Pankaj Desai
Associate Professor and Unit Chief, Department of Obstetrics and Gynecology
Medical College,
Baroda, India

Poonam Goel MD MAMS
Professor, Department of Obstetrics and Gynecology
Govt. Medical College and Hospital
Chandigarh, India.

Pralhad Kushtagi
Professor in Obstetrics and Gynecology
District Maternity and Children Hospital
Udupi, India

Pranathi Reddy MD, DGO, DNB, MRCOG
Consultant Obstetrician and Urogynecologist and Clinical Director, Maternal-Fetal Medicine
Rainbow Hospital for Women and Children
Hyderabad, India

GRV Prasad MD, DNB
Associate Professor, Department of Obstetrics and Gynecology
Postgraduate Institute of Medical Education and Research
Chandigarh, India

Pratap Kumar MD, DGO, FIMCH
Professor and Head, Department of Obstetrics and Gynecology
Kasturba Medical College
Manipal, India

Rajesh Bhakta MD
Associate Professor, Department of Obstetrics and Gynecology
Kasturba Medical College,
Manipal, India

Rakesh Kapoor MD
Associate Professor, Department of Radiotherapy, Regional Cancer Centre,
Postgraduate Institute of Medical Education and Research
Chandigarh, India

Rekha Kurian MD, MRCOG
Consultant Obstetrician and Gynecologist
Joseph Nursing Home
Chennai, India

Reva Tripathi
Professor, Department of Obstetrics and Gynecology
Maulana Azad Medical College
New Delhi, India

Rupinder Kaur Ruprai MD
Associate Professor, Department of Obstetrics and Gynecology
Kasturba Medical College
Manipal, India

Sabaratnam Arulkumaran PhD, FRCOG, FRCS
Professor and Head of Obstetrics and Gynecology
St George's University of London
London, United Kingdom

PK Saha MD, MAMS
Senior Lecturer, Department of Obstetrics and Gynecology
Government Medical College and Hospital
Chandigarh, India

Sarala Gopalan FRCOG, PhD, FAMS
Formerly Professor and Head, Department of Obstetrics and Gynecology
Postgraduate Institute of Medical Education and Research
Chandigarh, India

Sarbani Ghosh
Consultant Gynecologist
Bhagirathi Neotia Hospital for Women and Children
Kolkota, India

PK Sekharan MD
Former Professor and Head, Department of Obstetrics and Gynecology
Medical College
Calicut, India

S Sevellaraja MBBS, FRCOG, FICS, Master of Reproductive Medicine
Consultant Obstetrician and Gynecologist
Specialist in Infertility, Mahkota Medical Centre and Visiting Lecturer, Melaka Manipal Medical College
Melaka, Malaysia

Siya S Sharma MD, DNB, DGO, MRCOG
Department of Obstetrics and Gynecology
Cambridge (Eastern) Deanery Hospitals
United Kingdom

C Soundaram
Specialist Registrar
St Georges Hospital and Medical School
London, United Kingdom

Sucheta Jindal MD, MRCOG
Department of Obstetrics and Gynecology
Cambridge (Eastern) Deanery Hospitals
United Kingdom

Suresh C Sharma MD
Professor, Department of Radiotherapy
Postgraduate Institute of Medical Education and Research
Chandigarh, India

Suresh Kumarasamy MObGyn, MRCOG, AM
Consultant Obstetrician and Gynecologist/ Gynecological Oncologist,
Gleneagles Medical Centre and
Adjunct Senior Lecturer, Penang Medical College
Penang, Malaysia

Thankam Rama Varma PhD, FRCS, FRCOG
Medical Director, Institute Of Reproductive Medicine and Women's Health
Madras Medical Mission
Chennai, India

Usha Krishna MD, DGO, FICS, FICOG
Director, Clinic for Women
Mumbai, India

Vanita Jain MD, DNB
Professor, Department of Obstetrics and Gynecology
Postgraduate Institute of Medical Education and Research
Chandigarh, India

MS Vidyasagar DMRT, MD
Professor and Head, Department of Radiology and Oncology
Shirdi Sai Baba Cancer Hospital,
Kasturba Medical College
Manipal, India

Virochana Kaul MD
Assistant Professor, Department of Obstetrics and Gynecology
Kasturba Medical College
Manipal, India

1

Malformations of the Female Genital System

Mandakini Parihar | Aditi Tayade

The true incidence and prevalence of genitourinary tract anomalies are difficult to assess. Examinations of different patient populations, non-standardised classification systems, and differences in data acquisition have resulted in widely disparate estimates, with a reported prevalence that ranges from 0.16% to 10%. In a selected population with patient selection bias, a prevalence of 0.4% has been reported in women being evaluated with ultrasonography (USG) for non-obstetric indications (Maneschi et al 1995; Byrne et al 2000); this incidence increased to 8%–10% in women being evaluated with hysterosalpingography (HSG) because of recurrent pregnancy loss. The overall data suggest that the prevalence both in women with normal fertility and in women with infertility approximates 1%, and the prevalence in women with repeated pregnancy loss is about 3% (Maneshi et al 1995; Stampe 1998; Byrne et al 2000).

Primary infertility in these women usually has an extrauterine cause and is not attributable to müllerian duct anomalies. However, there is a higher incidence of poor obstetric outcomes in this group of patients. This is usually because of associated cervical incompetence, higher associated rates of spontaneous abortion, premature delivery, and abnormal fetal lie and dystocia at delivery. Most studies report an approximate frequency of 25% for associated reproductive problems, compared with 10% in the general population (Green and Harris 1976; Harger et al 1983; Golan et al 1989; Raga et al 1997; Troiano and McCarthy 2004).

The majority of müllerian duct anomalies are considered to be multifactorial in nature; however, polygenic and genetic patterns of inheritance are also suggested in some of these anomalies. Extrauterine and intrauterine environmental factors, such as exposure to ionising radiation, intrauterine infections, and drugs with teratogenic effects such as thalidomide and diethylstilbestrol (DES), can also cause defects of the developing fetal genital tracts (Harger et al 1983; Golan et al 1989; Maneschi et al 1995; Stampe 1998; Byrne et al 2000).

Embryology: A wide spectrum of reproductive tract abnormalities can result when the series of complex interactions leading to the differentiation of müllerian ducts and urogenital sinus is interrupted; this ultimately leads to defects in development of the uterus, cervix, vagina and fallopian tubes. The urinary and genital systems both arise from a common ridge of mesoderm arising along the dorsal body wall, and both rely on normal development of the mesonephric system. As the developing urinary system is closely related to the reproductive tract, the kidney and other urinary tract anomalies are often associated with anomalies of the müllerian system.

The ovaries arise from the mesenchyme and epithelium of the gonadal ridge and are not influenced by the formation of the mesonephric or paramesonephric ducts. The ovarian development is a separate process from the formation of the uterovaginal canal and is not usually associated with müllerian duct anomalies (Larsen 1993; Byrne et al 2000).

At six weeks of development, the male and female genital systems are indistinguishable in appearance, constituting two sets of paired ducts—the paramesonephric (müllerian) ducts and the mesonephric (wolffian) ducts. In the absence of the testis-determining factor of the Y chromosome, the mesonephric ducts begin to degenerate and form a matrix for the developing paramesonephric ducts. Synchronously, the paramesonephric ducts develop bidirectionally along the lateral aspect of the gonads.

The female genital tract is formed from the müllerian ducts and the urogenital sinus.

Müllerian ducts are derived from the mesoderm and the urogenital sinus is derived from the endoderm. Initially separated by a septum, at nine weeks the paramesonephric ducts fuse at their inferior margin forming the single lumen of the uterovaginal canal. The proximal segments of the uterovaginal canal, derived from the coelomic epithelium, remain unfused and open into the peritoneal cavity to form the fallopian tubes. The distal segments induced by or derived from the adjacent mesonephric ducts, progress caudomedially and join each other before contacting the posterior aspect of the pelvic urethra at the level of the sinusal tubercle. These distal segments of the uterovaginal canal give rise to the uterus and upper four-fifths of the vagina (Lindenman et al 1997; Moore and Persaud 1998).

The formation of the female reproductive organs is by a process of fusion, canalisation and regression. Abnormalities during any one of these stages leads to abnormalities of the müllerian system.

By 12 weeks, the uterus has attained its normal fused external uterine contour of the myometrium and a triangular-shaped endometrial cavity. Because the fallopian tubes are derived from a different cellular origin than the uterus and mid-vagina, they are rarely involved in müllerian duct anomalies. Isolated congenital anomalies of the fallopian tubes are rare, although agenesis, hypoplasia, and segmental narrowing have been reported.

Regression of the uterine septum has been proposed to be a result of apoptosis, mediated by the bcl-2 gene (Lee et al 1998). Absence of this gene has been implicated in persistence of the septum. However, an alternative bidirectional theory has been proposed in which it is hypothesised that the process proceeds simultaneously in both the cranial and the caudal directions. This would explain anomalies such as a complete septum with a duplicated cervix or isolated vertical upper vaginal septum in an otherwise unremarkable uterus (Persaud 1993; Lee et al 1998).

For normal vaginal development, the mesodermal müllerian ducts and endodermal urogenital sinus have to fuse. The caudal tip of the uterovaginal primordium fuses with the dorsal wall of the urogenital sinus. There is a formation of sino-vaginal bulbs at the distal aspect of the sinus tubercle, which gives rise to the lower fifth of the vagina. These sino-vaginal bulbs fuse to form the vaginal plate where they canalise and progress downwards to form the vaginal canal. The uterovaginal canal remains separated from the sino-vaginal bulbs by the horizontal vaginal plate. The failure of canalisation will result in transverse vaginal septum. The vaginal plate elongates in the third to fifth months, and its interface with the urogenital sinus forms the hymen, which usually ruptures in the perinatal period (Rock 1992; Lee et al 1998; Speroff et al 1998).

The ureters, renal calyces and collecting tubules are formed from the ureteral bud, which arises from the mesonephric ducts: the last also induce formation of the kidneys. Hence, abnormal differentiation of the mesonephric and paramesonephric ducts may also be associated with anomalies of the kidneys. Renal agenesis is the most common associated anomaly, although crossed renal ectopy, cystic renal dysplasia, and duplicated collecting systems have all been described (Rock 1992; Fedele et al 1996a; Moore and Persaud 1998).

The aim of this chapter is to address the issue of management of müllerian anomalies, the different options available for the same, and represent the current modes of treatment.

Classifications: Müllerian structural anomalies are grouped according to the failed developmental mechanism responsible, such as, agenesis or hypoplasia, lateral fusion defects, vertical fusion and diethyl stiboestrol-related abnormalities. In 1979, Buttram and Gibbons proposed a classification of müllerian duct anomalies that was based on the degree of failure of normal development; they separated these anomalies into classes that demonstrate similar clinical manifestations, treatment and prognosis for fetal salvage. This was later modified in 1988 by a subcommittee of the American Fertility Society and remains the most widely accepted schematisation and addresses all uterovaginal anomalies. However, the most notable inherent deficiency of the classification is the description of anomalies that include features of two or more classes. These anomalies should be described according to their component parts and should not be categorised into the class that most closely approximates the dominant feature. It also fails to address disorders of an obstructive nature like the transverse vaginal septum or an imperforate hymen (Buttram and Gibbons 1979; American Fertility Society 1988) (Table 1.1 and Fig. 1.1).

ANOMALIES AND THEIR MANAGEMENT

Class I: Vaginal Agenesis

Vaginal and uterine agenesis and hypoplasia result from variable degrees of early failure of the paramesonephric ducts to develop prior to fusion; they compose approximately 5%–10% of müllerian duct anomalies. Mayer–Rokitansky–Kuster–Hauser syndrome is the most common manifestation. This is characterised by an absent or hypoplastic uterus, proximal vagina and, in a few cases, fallopian tubes.

Table 1.1: AFS classification of müllerian anomalies

Class I: Anomalies consist of segmental agenesis and variable degrees of uterovaginal hypoplasia.
Class II: Anomalies are unicornuate uteri that represent partial or complete unilateral hypoplasia.
Class III: is composed of uterus didelphys in which duplication of the uterus results from complete nonfusion of the müllerian ducts.
Class IV: Anomalies are bicornuate uteri that demonstrate incomplete fusion of the superior segments of the uterovaginal canal.
Class V: Anomalies are septate uteri that represent partial or complete nonresorption of the uterovaginal septum.
Class VI: Anomalies are arcuate uteri that result from near complete resorption of the septum.
Class VII: Anomalies comprise sequelae of in utero DES exposure

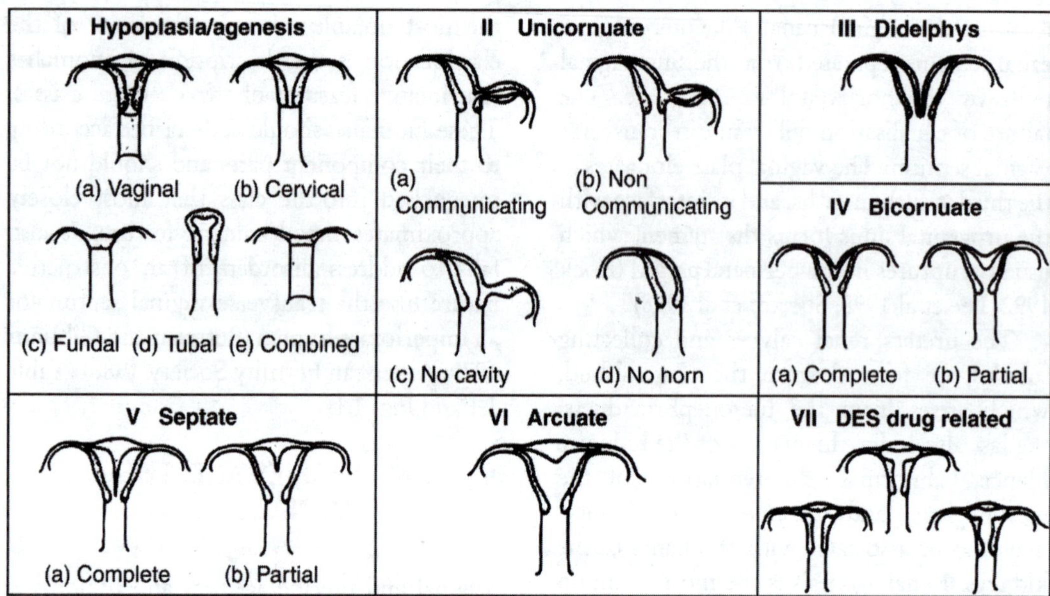

FIGURE 1.1: AFS CLASSIFICATION OF MÜLLERIAN ANOMALIES

The cause is unknown, but about 4% of the reported cases are familial and affect siblings. It is associated with variants of galactose-1-phosphate uridyl-transferase enzyme. Presence of persistent müllerian inhibitory substance is also implicated in the presence of this complex disorder. This and the fact that it is associated with other anomalies points to a polygenic mode of inheritance for this disorder. (Table 1.2) (American Fertility Society 1988; Cramer et al 1988; Aughton 1993; Lyons 1997).

Vaginal agenesis may be of two types:

- Partial agenesis: This is rare and is characterised by a normal uterus and small vaginal pouch, distal to the cervix. In about 10% of women, a normal but obstructed uterus or a rudimentary uterus with functional endometrium is present.
- Complete vaginal agenesis (Mayer–Rokitansky–Kuster–Hauser syndrome): There is complete absence of vagina and uterus. In most cases, the fallopian tubes are normal and ovaries demonstrate normal endocrine function (Griffin et al 1976; Baramki 1984; Aughton 1993).

Diagnosis: Presenting symptoms depend on the presence or absence of functioning endometrium. Complete agenesis and hypoplasia without functioning endometrium manifests in puberty with primary amenorrhea. Primary amenorrhea with severe cyclic pelvic pain may reflect isolated vaginal agenesis with a uterus that contains functional endometrium that is secondarily obstructed, resulting in hematometra. Patients usually present at puberty with primary amenorrhea, but may present at a later stage. Physical examination reveals normal growth and development of secondary sexual characteristics. On examination, the external genitalia are normal, but may reveal a patulous urethra in sexually active individuals. The vagina is usually felt as a dimple, is absent or is short. The uterus is not palpable per rectum.

The diagnosis is confirmed with

TABLE 1.2: ASSOCIATED ANOMALIES IN VAGINAL AGENESIS

- Urologic abnormalities 15%–40%
- Congenital fusion or absence of vertebrae 12%–50%
- Klippel–Feil syndrome
- MURCS association (that is, müllerian, renal, cervicothoracic, somite abnormalities) has also been associated with MRKH syndrome

ultrasonography which shows an absent uterus and normal ovaries. Additional study with magnetic resonance imaging (MRI) and intravenous pyelography (IVP) is important for detection of associated renal anomalies (Coney 1992; Doyle 1992; Mitchell 1992; Lyons 1997).

Preoperative evaluation: Psychological support and counselling form an important aspect of management. The counsellor should explain the need for surgical intervention if the patient wishes to be sexually active; however, she will never be able to become pregnant. Options of third-party reproduction should also be mentioned at this stage (adoption, foster child). Non-surgical methods rely on the use of graduated dilators; it takes several months to form a neovagina and the depth may still not be the same as in a normal vagina. Hence, surgery remains the most effective method of treatment. However, the timing of the surgery is very important: it should be undertaken only when the patient wishes to become sexually active and is motivated to use a vaginal prosthesis for several months continuously (Griffin et al 1976; Doyle 1992; Mitchell 1992).

Surgical methods: The aim of surgery is to create a neovagina by creating a space between the bladder and the rectum. The most common procedure is Abbe–McIndoe vaginoplasy. The procedure was described by Abbe in 1898, and modified by McIndoe in 1938. The essential steps are:

- Split-thickness skin graft
- Creation of vaginal space
- Assembly of prosthesis
- Graft attachment to prosthesis

Other tissue for graft include large and small intestine, human amnion, peritoneum and myocutaneous flaps. In place of skin graft, Interceed Absorbable Adhesion Barrier has also been used. Full-thickness skin grafts may also be used—these give better results than split-thickness grafts (fewer graft contractures and stenosis) (David et al 1975; Coney 1992; Jackson and Rosenblatt 1994; Sadove and Horton 1998).

Postoperative management: Patient compliance during rehabilitation is extremely important. The patient is given antibiotics and a low-residue diet. Early ambulation should be instituted to prevent contractures and promote healing. The labial stitches and prosthesis are removed after a week and the new mould is inserted. The patient is educated about the insertion and its continuous use. The prosthesis is to be worn continuously for six weeks and the patient is taught to give herself low-pressure douches with warm water daily. After six weeks, a silicone prosthesis is inserted nightly for 12 months. The new vagina is functional 6–10 weeks postoperatively. The results are satisfactory in over 80% of cases (Buss and Lee 1989; Goerzen et al 1994; Sadove and Horton 1998). Postoperative complications could be fistula, infection, hemorrhage and graft failure.

CLASS II: UNICORNUATE UTERUS

In this condition, the müllerian ducts fail

to elongate, while in others it develops normally. It can occur in the presence or absence of a rudimentary horn, with or without a functioning endometrium within it. Associated urological anomalies are seen in almost 40% of cases (Fedele et al 1996a). The anomaly is always ipsilateral to the rudimentary horn. Renal agenesis is the most commonly reported abnormality, occurring in 67% of cases. Ectopic kidney, horseshoe kidney, pelvic kidney, cystic renal dysplasia and duplicated collecting systems have also been described. A unicornuate uterus may be isolated in 35% of patients, in 33% there is a non-cavitary rudimentary horn and in 32% there is a cavitary rudimentary horn with an endometrial segment (Andrews and Jones 1982; Michalas 1991; Fedele et al 1996a; Heinonen 1997).

Without rudimentary horn: The patient has no symptoms and the anomaly is usually diagnosed because of poor obstetric outcome. Spontaneous abortion rates are reported to range from 41% to 62%. Reported premature birth rates range from 10% to 20% and fetal survival rates, from 38% to 57%. Common obstetric complications include abnormal fetal lie and intrauterine growth retardation (Rolen et al 1966; Donnez and Nisolle 1997; Heinonen 1997; Brody et al 1998).

Non-communicating rudimentary horn: Dysmenorrhea with hematometra may manifest at menarche in this subgroup. A cavitary rudimentary horn is designated 'communicating', if there is communication with the endometrium of the contralateral horn (10% of cases) and 'non-communicating' if there is no such communication (22% of cases). The obstetric complications are the same in both cases, but there are higher chances of an ectopic pregnancy lodging in the rudimentary horn. Resection of the non-communicating horn is indicated, not only for symptomatic relief but also because ectopic pregnancy may occur in the horn by means of transperitoneal sperm migration. About 89% of pregnancies that arise in a non-communicating uterine horn end in rupture. In addition, the incidence of endometriosis is increased in this subgroup (David et al 1975; Coney 1992; Jackson and Rosenblatt 1994; Sadove and Horton 1998).

Diagnosis: Speculum inspection of the cervix reveals a small cervix and a poorly developed contralateral vaginal fornix. On hysterosalpingogram, the endometrial cavity assumes a fusiform shape, tapering at the apex and draining into a solitary fallopian tube. The uterus is generally shifted away from the midline; HSG cannot delineate non-cavitary and non-communicating rudimentary horns (Fig. 1.2a, b).

Ultrasonography will show the rudimentary horn if present and the presence of hematometra if there is a functioning endometrium.

On MR imaging, the unicornuate uterus will appear curved and elongated, with the external uterine contour assuming a banana shape. The endometrium may be uniformly narrow or may assume a bullet shape, tapering at the apex. The endometrial-to-myometrial width and ratio are reported to be normal (Rolen et al 1966; Donnez and Nisolle 1997; Heinonen 1997; Brody et al 1998).

Surgical treatment: Surgical management involves laparoscopic hemi-hysterectomy of the associated rudimentary horn when an endometrial cavity is present. In the absence of functioning endometrium, there is no

necessity to remove the rudimentary horn. Counselling regarding obstetric outcome and complications form an integral part of the treatment.

Class III: Uterus Didelphys

Uterus didelphys, which constitutes approximately 5% of müllerian duct anomalies, is the result of nearly complete failure of fusion of the müllerian ducts. This müllerian defect is composed of two separate, normal-sized uteri and endocervical canals with cervices that are fused at the lower uterine segment. Vaginal duplication is usually present in 75% of the cases and is characterised by a longitudinal septum, either complete or partial. No communication is present between the duplicated endometrial cavities. Non-obstructive uterus didelphys is usually asymptomatic, while uterus didelphys with unilateral vaginal obstruction may become symptomatic at menarche and manifest as dysmenorrhea. Longitudinal vaginal septa may be complicated by defects in vertical fusion that result in a transverse vaginal septum and subsequent hematometrocolpos (Gray et al 1984; Pellerito et al 1992; Ott et al 1998; Propst and Hill 2000; Troiano and McCarthy 2004).

Diagnosis: On ultrasound, separate divergent uterine horns are identified, with a large fundal cleft. Endometrial cavities are uniformly separate, with no evidence of communication. Two separate cervices need to be documented.

Hysterosalpingography demonstrates two separate endocervical canals that open into separate fusiform endometrial cavities, with no communication between the two horns. Each endometrial cavity ends in a solitary fallopian tube. In cases of associated disorders of vertical fusion, USG and MRI imaging will be needed to demonstrate two separate uteri (Fig. 1.3a) with widely divergent apices, two separate cervices (Fig. 1.3b), and usually an upper vaginal longitudinal septum (Stampe 1988; Pellerito et al 1992; Propst and Hill 2000; Troiano and McCarthy 2004).

Preoperative evaluation: Spontaneous abortion rates are reported to range from 32% to 52%, premature birth rates range from 20% to 45% and fetal survival rates from 41% to 64%. Strassman's metroplasty, leaving the duplicated cervix intact in an attempt to prevent cervical incompetence, may be considered for select patients with recurrent spontaneous abortions and premature deliveries. However, the benefits of intervention remain unclear because no controlled trials have been performed (Strassman 1966; Harger et al 1983; Gray et al 1984; Rock 1992; Propst and Hill 2000; Troiano and McCarthy 2004).

Surgical techniques

- For uterus didelphys with obstructed unilateral vagina: Excision of obstructing vaginal septum with marsupialisation
- For uterus didelphys with non-obstructed vagina: If dyspareunia is present, excise vaginal septum.

Only select patients benefit from surgery. In cases of repeated pregnancy losses, the recommended procedure is Strassman metroplasty where both uterine cavities are unified at the fundus while the cervices are left intact (Strassman 1966; Gray et al 1984; Pellerito et al 1992; Fedele et al 1996a).

Class IV: Bicornuate Uterus

A bicornuate uterus consists of two symmetric cornua that are fused caudally, with communication of the endometrial

cavities, most often at the level of the uterine isthmus with a single cervix and vagina. A muscular uterine septum is present which further classifies it as complete or partial. It accounts for approximately 10% of müllerian duct anomalies. Patients with a bicornuate uterus and no extrauterine infertility issues usually have little difficulty conceiving (Rock and Jones 1977; Tulandi et al 1980; Forstner and Hricak 1994; Raga et al 1996; Troiano and McCarthy 2004).

Diagnosis: On HSG, the horns of the endometrial cavity are seen to be widely separated, at an inter-cornual angle greater than 105°. Each horn has a fusiform appearance, with apices that taper and end in a single fallopian tube (Fig. 1.4a,b).

On ultrasound, a large fundal cleft is seen with divergence of the uterine horns and associated echogenic endometrial complexes. On MR images, the bicornuate uterus demonstrates a cleft of at least 1 cm of the external fundal uterine contour. The horns demonstrate normal uterine zonal anatomy (Rock and Jones 1977; Tulandi et al 1980; Forstner and Hricak 1994; Raga et al 1996; Troiano and McCarthy 2004).

Preoperative evaluation: Spontaneous abortion rates are reported to range from 28% to 35%. Premature birth rates range from 14% to 23%; and fetal survival rates, from 57% to 63%. The bicornuate uterus seldom requires surgical correction. Metroplasty may be considered for women who experience recurrent spontaneous abortion, mid-trimester loss and premature birth (Michalas 1991; Propst and Hill 2000).

Surgical techniques: Surgical intervention is usually not indicated, and the length of subsequent gestations often increases with increasing parity. Strassman metroplasty has been advocated in women with a history of recurrent pregnancy loss. However, the benefits of metroplasty have never been formally studied in a prospective trial. The bicornuate uterus has been reported to have the highest associated prevalence (38%) of cervical incompetence among müllerian duct anomalies. Prophylactic placement of a cervical cerclage in selected patients has been reported to increase fetal survival rates (Strassman 1966; Golan et al 1990).

Class V: Septate Uterus

The septate uterus is the most common müllerian duct anomaly (about 55%) and results from partial or complete failure of resorption of the uterovaginal septum after fusion of the paramesonephric ducts (Acien 1997; Homer et al 2000; Troiano and McCarthy 2004).

The septum, which arises in the midline fundus, is considered to be complete when it extends to the external cervical os (Goldberg et al 1997; Kupesic and Kurjak 1998). Extension of the septum to the upper vagina is seen in approximately 25% of cases. A partial septum is variable in length. The external uterine contour may be convex, flat or mildly concave (<1 cm). It has been generally recommended that any septum which is more than 1 cm in size should be removed as it is associated with poor reproductive outcome (Fedele et al 1996b). Whether a septum found incidentally during routine evaluation for infertility is to be removed is debatable. The general consensus today favours its removal as it is proven to be associated with poor reproductive outcome, though some experts believe it should only be incised when there is a history of repeated pregnancy losses (Valle 1996; Kupesic and Kurjak 2000;).

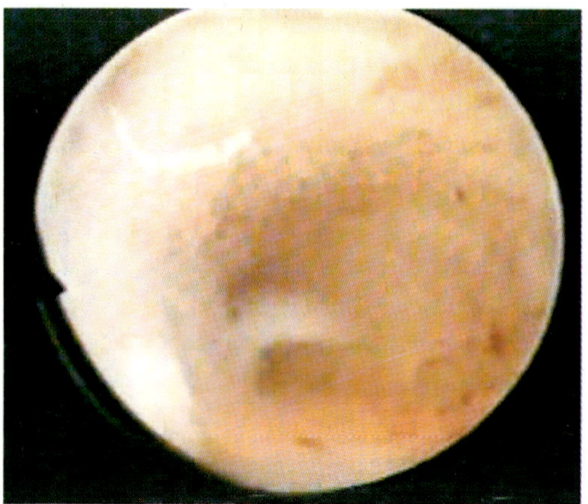

Figure 1.2a: Hysteroscopic view of a unicornuate uterus (Courtesy: Rakesh Sinha)

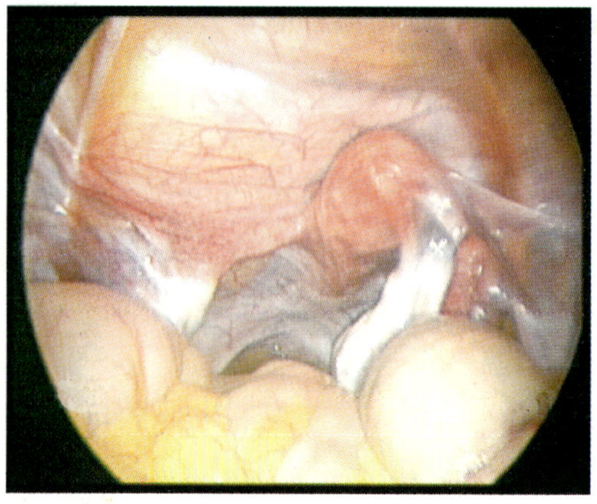

Figure 1.2b: Laparoscopic view of unicornuate uterus

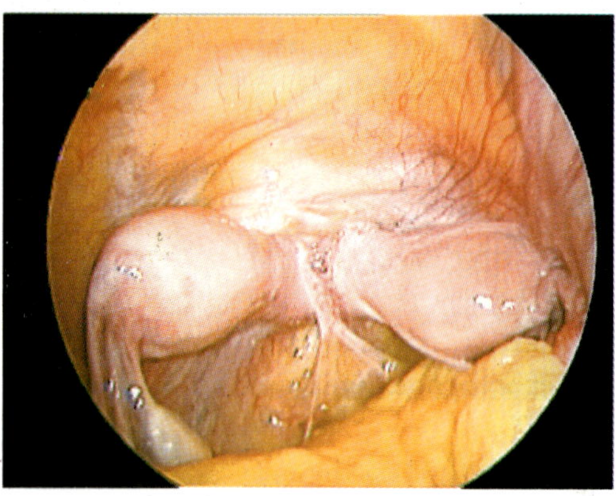

Figure 1.3a: laparoscopic view of uterus didelphys. Note the complete separation of the uteri (Courtesy: Rakesh Sinha)

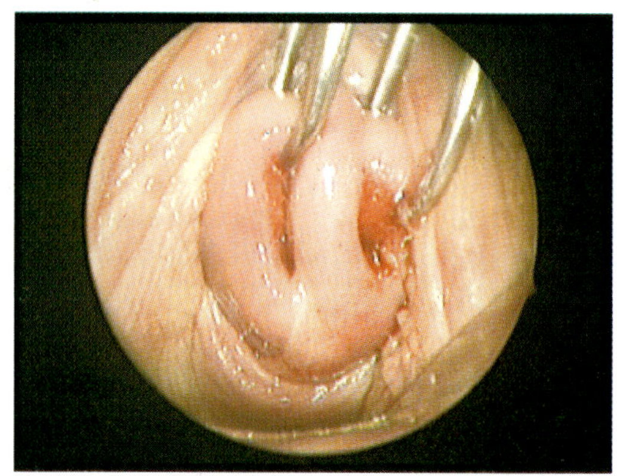

Figure 1.3b: note the double cervix in the same patient (Courtesy: Rakesh Sinha)

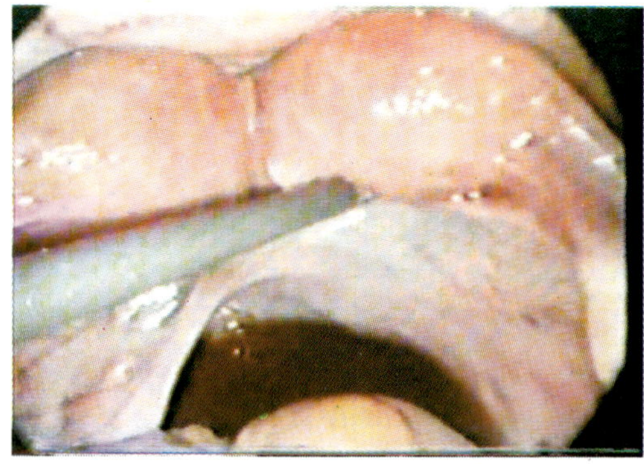

Figure 1.4a: Laparoscopic image of a bicornuate uterus

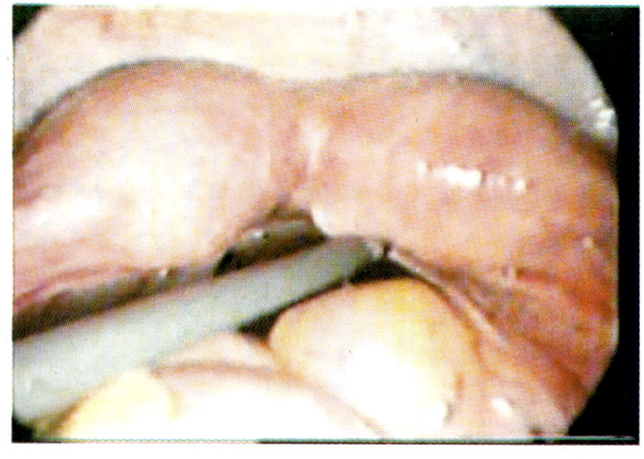

Figure 1.4b: Laparoscopic view of a bicornuate uterus

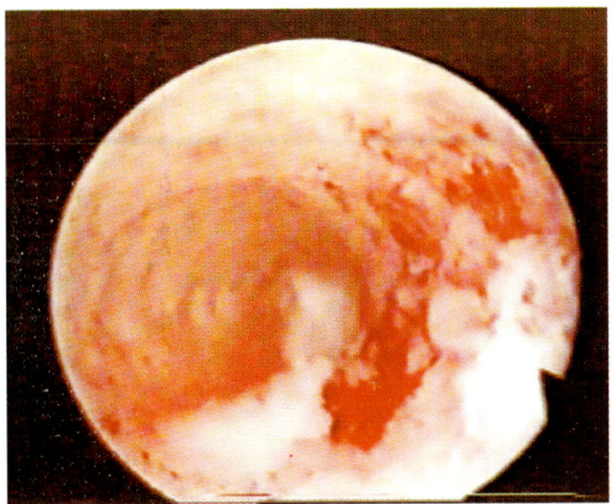

Figure 1.4c: Hysteroscopic view of a bicornuate uterus: one horn is seen

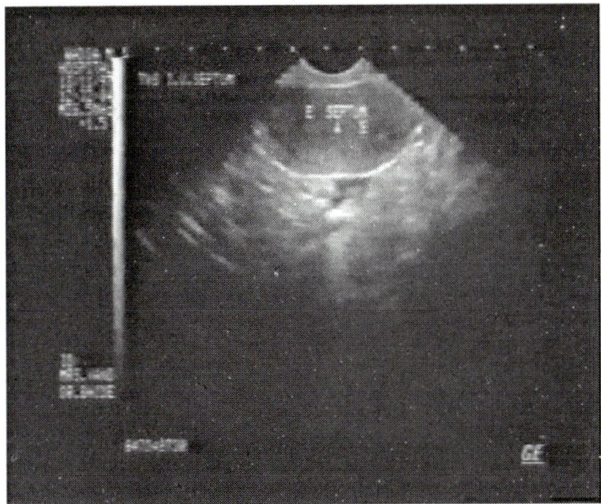

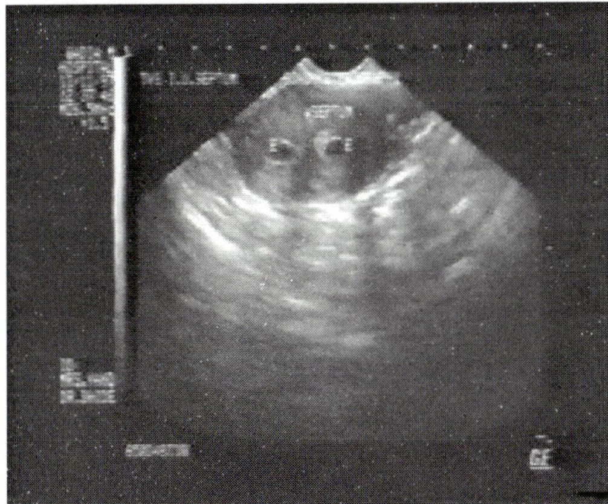

Figure 1.5: Ultrasound image of a septate uterus. Note the two separate endometrial echoes seen.

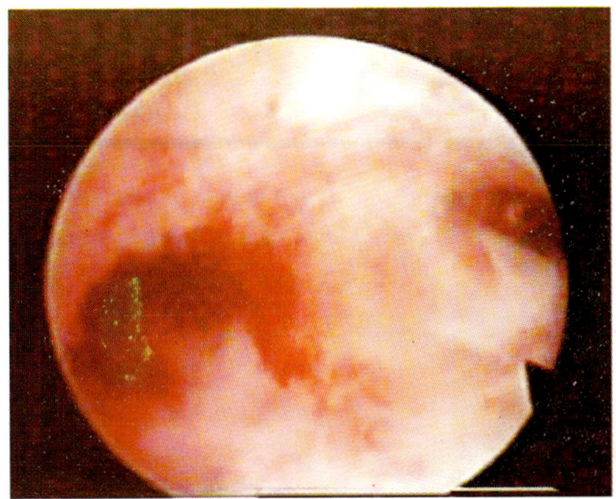

Figure 1.6: Hysteroscopic view of a septate uterus

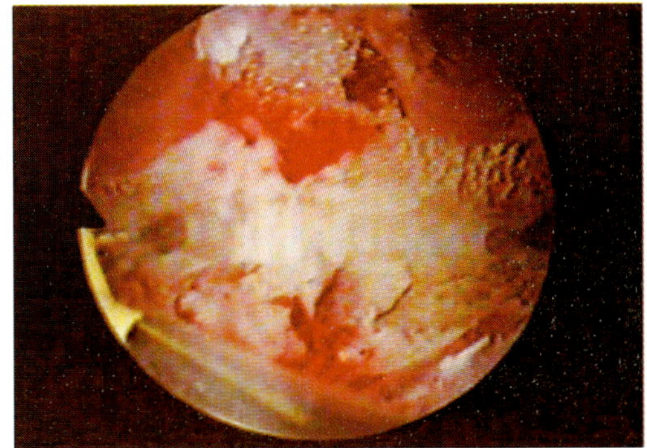

Figure 1.7: Hysteroscopic resection of a septate uterus

Diagnosis of septate uterus: Hysterosalpingography of a septate uterus may be used to evaluate the size, length, thickness and extent of septa. However, the diagnostic accuracy of HSG alone is only 55% for differentiation of septate uteri from bicornuate uteri. An angle of less than 75° between the uterine horns is suggestive of a septate uterus, and an angle of more than 105° is more consistent with bicornuate uteri (Michalas 1991; Ott et al 1998; Homer et al 2000; Troiano and McCarthy 2004).

Hysteroscopic visualisation of the septum (Fig. 1.6) and its removal is the recommended, gold standard for treatment and diagnosis (Fig. 1.7). It has been reported that when

USG is used in conjunction with HSG, an accurate diagnosis can be made in 90% of cases (Daly et al 1983; Fedele and Bianchi 1995; Valle 1996).

On ultrasonography, the echogenic endometrial cavities are separated at the fundus by the intermediate echogenicity of the myometrium (Fig. 1.5). The external uterine contour must demonstrate a convex, flat or mildly concave configuration and may best be appreciated on transverse images of the uterus.

On MR imaging, the septate uterus is generally normal in size; however, each endometrial cavity appears smaller than normal (Michalas 1991; Rock 1992; Troiano and McCarthy 2004).

As many of the müllerian anomalies are associated with anomalies of the urinary tract, an IVP is indicated to help identify renal defects (Fedele et al 1996a).

Preoperative evaluation: The septate uterus is also associated with the worst obstetric outcome of all müllerian duct anomalies—overall premature birth rates range from 9% to 33% and fetal survival rates from 10% to 75% (Rock 1992; Speroff et al 1998; Troiano and McCarthy 2004). Recurrent pregnancy loss in these patients was traditionally attributed to the fibrous and avascular nature of the septum, despite the lack of histologic data (Goldberg et al 1997; Kupesic and Kurjak 1998; Homer et al 2000). It is theorised that the decreased connective tissue may result in poor decidualisation and implantation, while increased muscular tissue may result in increased contractility of the tissue, thereby predisposing the patient to spontaneous abortion. In addition to the inherent deficiencies of the composition of the septum, the overlying endometrium has been shown to be defective. The length of the septum does not appear to correlate with differences in obstetric outcome (Kupesic and Kurjak 2000). Reproductive outcome has been shown to improve after resection of the septum, with reported decreases in the spontaneous abortion rate from 88% to 5.9% after hysteroscopic metroplasty (Daly et al 1983; Fedele and Bianchi 1995; Valle 1996).

Surgical technique: Currently, septate uterus is surgically corrected by hysterscopic division of the septum. Some surgeons prefer to use concurrent laparoscopy and hysteroscopy. The preferred procedure is operative hysteroscopic metroplasty using micro-scissors, electro-surgery or laser. Conjugated estrogens and progesterone are given in the postoperative period to assist epithelialisation. The follow-up examination is done after a month. In the case of very large septa, the procedure may be carried out in two stages. Residual septa may persist, but residual septum less than 1 cm will not affect the reproductive outcome adversely (Daly et al 1983; Fedele and Bianchi 1995; Valle 1996; Fedele et al 1996b; Homer et al 2000).

Class VI: Arcuate Uterus

Arcuate uterus has a small septate indentation at the superior aspect of the uterine cavity in the fundal region. The arcuate uterus is characterised by a mild indentation of the endometrium at the uterine fundus as a result of near-complete resorption of the uterovaginal septum, with complete fundal unification (Clifford et al 1994; Raziel et al 1994; Maneschi et al 1995).

Diagnosis: On ultrasonography, a normal external uterine contour is noted, with a broad smooth indentation on the fundal segment of the endometrium. The indentation may best be appreciated in the transverse plane with subtle, focal, superior duplication of the endometrial echogenic complexes. No division of the uterine horns is noted (Homer et al 2000; Troiano and McCarthy 2004).

Hysterosalpingography shows a single uterine cavity with a saddle-shaped fundus (Fig. 1.8). MRI depicts normal fundal contour with small indentation at fundus. Subtle indentation of the peripheral subserosal arcuate vessels at the level of the fundus may be noted. The orientation mimics the pattern seen in the septate uterus and, hypothetically, may indicate a degree of vascular aberration (Clifford et al 1994; Raziel et al 1994; Maneschi et al 1995; Troiano and McCarthy 2004). Renal USG and IVP are usually recommended for patients with anomalies of the female genital tract (Fedele et al 1996b).

Preoperative evaluation: Data regarding the reproductive outcomes of patients with arcuate uterus are extremely limited and widely disparate. In small studies, both poor and good obstetric outcomes have been reported, although an arcuate configuration is generally thought to be compatible with normal-term gestation, with a quoted delivery rate of 85%. It has been proposed that when the ratio between the height of the fundal indentation and the distance between the lateral apices of the horns is less than 10% on the basis of HSG findings, an adverse reproductive outcome is not anticipated. Arcuate uterus is usually managed similar to septate uterus only in patients where there is recurrent pregnancy losses and no other cause can be established (Stampe 1983; Maneschi et al 1995; Troiano and McCarthy 2004).

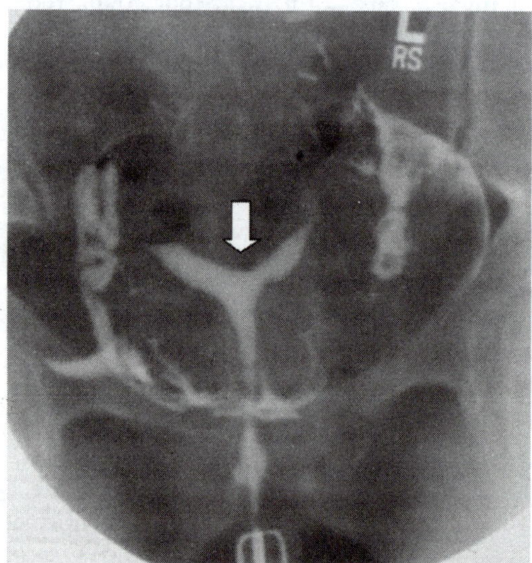

FIGURE 1.8: HYSTEROSALPINGOGRAPH SHOWING SEPTATE UTERUS WITH BILATERAL FREE SPILL. NOTE THE ANGLE BETWEEN THE TWO HORNS.

CLASS VII: DIETHYLSTILBESTROL (DES) RELATED ANOMALIES

A synthetic estrogen, diethylstilbestrol (DES), was prescribed for recurrent pregnancy loss and premature delivery. It has been shown to interfere with embryologic development of the mesenchyme of the genital tract.

An estimated 2–3 million women received DES, exposing 1.0–1.5 million offspring in utero. The adverse repercussions on reproductive potential are estimated to continue for the next 10–15 years (Rock and Jones 1977). Its use was banned in 1971 after its in utero exposure was shown to be associated with vaginal clear cell adenocarcinoma and other vaginal and cervical abnormalities (DeCherney et al 1981). Its exposure presented with T-shaped endometrial cavity, widened lower uterine segment, mid-fundal constriction, endometrial filling defects, irregular margins and a hypoplastic uterus. Cervical anomalies included hypoplasia, an anterior ridge, a collar and pseudopolyp formations. Vaginal adenosis and constrictions were also noted in some patients along with unusual vaginal clear cell carcinoma (DeCherney et al 1981; Winfield and Wentz 1992; Goldberg and Falcone 1999).

Diagnosis: Sixty-nine per cent of DES-exposed women had uterine abnormalities (detected on HSG). A T-shaped configuration of the endometrial cavity is the most commonly associated abnormality, seen in 31% of exposed women. Other uterine corpus anomalies include a small hypoplastic uterus, constriction bands, a widened lower uterine segment, a narrowed fundal segment of the endometrial canal, irregular endometrial margins, and intraluminal filling defects. Anomalies of the fallopian tube include foreshortening, sacculations and fimbrial deformities. On ultrasound, findings may be nonspecific, and definitive diagnosis may not be possible. On MR images, uterine hypoplasia, T configuration of the endometrial cavity and constriction bands can be demonstrated (DeCherney et al 1981; Kipersztok et al 1996; Goldberg and Falcone 1999).

Preoperative evaluation: It should be noted that not all women exposed to DES have reproductive problems. The amount of drug ingested, as well as when the drug was taken during gestation, have clinical implications. If the drug was taken very early in the first trimester or after 22 weeks gestation, structural abnormalities are not likely to occur. While there is no definitive evidence that women exposed to DES have decreased conception rates, they are known to be at a twofold increased risk for spontaneous abortion, and there is a ninefold increased risk for ectopic pregnancy. While some studies have failed to show associated adverse obstetric outcomes, the majority report an increased risk of premature labour and perinatal mortality. Prophylactic cervical cerclage has been advocated in selected women, especially those with a history of second-trimester losses and preterm births (DeCherney et al 1981; Ludmir et al 1987; Goldberg and Falcone 1999; Kaufman et al 2000).

OBSTRUCTED UTEROVAGINAL ANOMALIES—VAGINAL SEPTUM

In addition to obstruction associated with vaginal agenesis, obstruction from vaginal septa that arise from defects of vertical and lateral fusion are also seen in the spectrum of müllerian duct anomalies. Defects of vertical fusion include a transverse vaginal septum, which can occur anywhere along the vagina, although it occurs most frequently at the junction of the upper and middle third of the vagina. The septum is a membrane of fibrous connective tissue with vascular and muscular components. Resultant hematocolpos in patients with a uterus with functioning endometrium can cause marked distension of the vagina. Dilatation of the endometrium in hematometrocolpos is usually the presenting symptom.

A transverse vaginal septum may be present in any of the müllerian duct anomalies, or may occur independently. An imperforate hymen may mimic a low transverse septum with associated hematocolpos; however, an imperforate hymen is not a müllerian anomaly and should be distinguished from a transverse vaginal septum (Wenof et al 1979; Rock 1986; Raga et al 1996; Arnold et al 2001).

Diagnosis: Cyclic pain and primary amenorrhea are the usual presenting symptoms and the hematometra may be palpable on abdominal examination. Hysterosalpingography has little role in the evaluation of transverse septum and obstructed uterovaginal anomalies, given the fact that the cervix cannot be catheterised.

On ultrasound, hematometrocolpos manifests as a distended vagina and endometrium with a variable appearance, most often appearing as a cystic mass with diffuse low-level echoes. A solid appearance and a completely anechoic collection have also been described. It may not always be possible to visualise a discrete attenuated transverse septum.

MR imaging is an important modality in helping define the complexity of the anomaly. On MR, hematometrocolpos is characterised by a distended vagina with imperceptible walls: on T1-weighted images the blood is demonstrated as increased signal intensity, and on T2-weighted images the variable age of the retained blood causes variable signal intensity. Hematometros is well delineated given the preserved zonal anatomy of the uterus (Wenof et al 1979; Rock 1992; Raga et al 1996; Arnold et al 2001; Troiano and McCarthy 2004).

Preoperative evaluation: The treatment is excision of the septum and timely drainage of the hematocolpos and hematometra. The incidence of endometriosis is very high in these patients.

Conclusion: Congenital uterine anomalies are clinically important, especially in women who present with infertility and/ or recurrent pregnancy losses. Müllerian duct anomalies encompass a wide spectrum of clinical and imaging findings, and while many of the anomalies will be diagnosed initially at HSG or two-dimensional US, further imaging with MR and, potentially, three-dimensional US will often be required for a definitive diagnosis. Laparoscopy and hysteroscopy are then reserved for women, in whom interventional therapy is being undertaken, thus reducing healthcare expenditure and sparing women invasive diagnostic procedures. Precise imaging characterisation is essential, given the different clinical manifestations, treatment regimens and prognoses for fetal salvage.

References

Acien P. 1997. Shall we operate on müllerian defects? Incidence of müllerian defects in fertile and infertile women. *Hum Reprod* 12:1372–1376.

American Fertility Society. 1988. The American Fertility Society classifications of adnexal adhesions, distal tubal obstruction, tubal occlusion secondary to tubal ligation, tubal pregnancies, müllerian anomalies and intrauterine adhesions. *Fertil Steril* 49:944–955.

Andrews MC and HW Jones Jr. 1982. Impaired reproductive performances of the unicornuate uterus: IUGR, infertility, recurrent abortion. *Am J Obstet Gynecol* 144 (4):73–76.

Arnold BW, M Gilfeather, PJ Woodward. 2001. Müllerian duct anomalies complicated by obstruction: Evaluation with pelvic magnetic resonance imaging. *J Women's Imaging* 3:146–152.

Aughton DJ. 1993. Müllerian duct anomalies and galactosaemia heterozygosity: A family report. *Clin Dysmorphol* 2(1):56–61.

Baramki TA. 1984. Treatment of congenital anomalies in girls and women. *J Reprod Med* 29(6): 376–384.

Brody JM, SL Koelliker, GN Frishman. 1998. Unicornuate uterus: Imaging appearance, associated anomalies, and clinical applications. *Am J Roentgenol* 171:1341–1347.

Buss JG and RA Lee. 1989. McIndoe procedure for vaginal agenesis: Result and complications. *Mayo Clin Proc* 64(7):758–761.

Buttram VC and WE Gibbons. 1979. Müllerian anomalies: A proposed classification (an analysis of 144 cases). *Fertil Steril* 32:40–46.

Byrne J, A Nussbaum-Blask, WS Taylor et al. 2000. Prevalence of müllerian duct anomalies detected at ultrasound. *Am J Med Genet* 94:9–12.

Clifford K, R Rai, H Watson, L Regan. 1994. An informative protocol for the investigation of recurrent miscarriage: Preliminary experience of 500 consecutive cases. *Hum Reprod* 9:1328–1332.

Coney P. 1992. Effect of vaginal agenesis on adolescent: Prognosis for normal sexual and psychological adjustment. *Adol Pediatr Gynecol* 5:8.

Cramer DW, VA Ravnikar, M Craighill et al. 1988. Müllerian aplasia associated with maternal deficiency of galactose-1-phosphate uridyl transferase. *Fertil Steril* 47(6):930–934.

Daly DC, CA Witten, CE Soto-Albors, DH Riddick. 1983. Hysteroscopic metroplasty: Surgical technique and obstetric outcome. *Fertil Steril* 39:623–628.

David A, D Carmil, E Bar-David, DM Serr. 1975. Congenital absence of the vagina: Clinical and psychologic aspects. *Obstet Gynecol* 46(4):407–409.

DeCherney AH, I Cholst, F Naftolin. 1981. Structure and function of the fallopian tubes following exposure to diethylstilbestrol (DES) during gestation. *Fertil Steril* 36:741–745.

Donnez J and M Nisolle. 1997. Endoscopic laser treatment of uterine malformations. *Hum Reprod* 12(7):1381–1387.

Doyle MB. 1992. MRI in Müllerian fusion defects. *J Reprod Med* 37(1):33–38.

Fedele L and S Bianchi. 1995. Hysteroscopic metroplasty for septate uterus. *Obstet Gynecol Clin North Am* 2(3):473–489.

Fedele L, S Bianchi, B Agnoli, L Tozzi, M Vignali. 1996a. Urinary tract anomalies associated with unicornuate uterus. *J Urol* 155:847–848.

Fedele L, S Bianchi, M Marchini, R Mezzopane, G DiNola, L Tozzi. 1996b. Residual uterine septum of less than 1 cm after hysteroscopic metroplasty does not impair reproductive outcome. *Hum Reprod* 11:727–729.

Forstner R and H Hricak. 1994. Congenital malformations of uterus and vagina. *Radiology* 34(7): 397–404.

Goerzen JL, GP Gidwani, MM Bailez. 1994. Outcome of surgical reconstructive procedures for the treatment of vaginal anomalies. *Adol Pediatr Gynecol* 7:76.

Golan A, R Langer, I Bukovsky, E Caspi. 1989. Congenital anomalies of the müllerian system. *Fertil Steril* 51:747–755.

Golan A, R Langer, S Wexler, E Seceg, D Niv, PD Menachem. 1990. Cervical cerclage: Its role in the pregnant anomalous uterus. *Int J Fertil* 35:164–170.

Goldberg JM, T Falcone, M Attaran. 1997. Sonohysterographic evaluation of uterine anomalies noted on hysterosalpingography. *Hum Reprod* 12:2151–2153.

Goldberg JM and T Falcone. 1999. Effect of diethylstilbestrol on reproductive function. *Fertil Steril* 72:1–7.

Gray SE, DK Roberts, RR Franklin. 1984. Fertility after metroplasty of the uterus. *J Reprod Med* 29:185–188.

Green LK and RE Harris. 1976. Uterine anomalies: Frequency of diagnosis and obstetric complications. *Obstet Gynecol* 47:427–433.

Griffin JE, C Edwards, JD Madden et al. 1976. Congenital absence of the vagina. The Mayer-Rokitansky-Kuster-Hauser Syndrome. *Ann Intern Med* 85(2):224–236.

Harger JH, DF Archer, SG Marchese, M Muracca-Clemens, KL Garver. 1983. Etiology of recurrent pregnancy losses and outcome of subsequent pregnancies. *Obstet Gynecol* 62:574–581.

Heinonen PK. 1997. Unicornuate uterus and rudimentary horn. *Fertil Steril* 68:224–230.

Homer HA, TC Li, ID Cooke. 2000. The septate uterus: A review of management and reproductive outcome. *Fertil Steril* 73:1–14.

Jackson ND and PL Rosenblatt. 1994. Use of Interceed absorbable adhesion barrier for vaginoplasty. *Obstet Gynecol* 84(6):1048–1050.

Kaufman RH, E Adam, EE Hatch et al. 2000. Continued follow-up of pregnancy outcomes in diethylstilbestrol-exposed offspring. *Obstet Gynecol* 96:483–489.

Kipersztok S, M Javitt, MC Hill, RJ Stillman. 1996. Comparison of magnetic resonance imaging and transvaginal sonography with hysterosonography in the evaluation of women exposed to diethylstilbestrol. *J Reprod Med* 41:347–335.

Kupesic S and A Kurjak. 1998. Septate uterus: Detection and prediction of obstetrical complications by different forms of ultrasonography. *J Ultrasound Med* 17:631–636.

Kupesic S and A Kurjak. 2000. Ultrasound and Doppler assessment of uterine anomalies. In *Ultrasound and infertility*, eds S Kupesic and D de Ziegler. New York: Parthenon, 147–153.

Larsen WJ. 1993. Development of the urogenital system. In *Human Embryology*. New York: Churchill Livingstone, 235–279.

Lee DM, R Osathanondh, J Yeh. 1998. Localization of bcl-2 in the human fetal müllerian tract. *Fertil Steril* 70:135–140.

Lindenman E, MK Shepard, OH Pescovitz. 1997. Müllerian agenesis: An update. *Obstet Gynecol* 90:307–12.

Ludmir J, MB Landon, SG Gabbe et al. 1987. Management of DES exposed pregnant patient. *Am J Obstet Gynecol* 157(3): 665–669.

Lyons JK. 1997. MURCS association: Müllerian duct, renal and cervical vertebral defects. In *Smith's recognizable patterns of human malformation.* 5th ed. Philadelphia: WB Saunders, 666

Maneschi F, E Zupi, D Marconi et al. 1995. Hysteroscopically detected asymptomatic müllerian anomalies: Prevalence and reproductive implications. *J Reprod Med* 40(10):684–688.

Michalas SP. 1991. Outcome of pregnancy in women with uterine malformation: Evaluation of 62 cases. *Int J Gynecol Obstet* 35(3):215–219.

Mitchell DG. 1992. Benign disease of uterus and ovaries: Applications of MRI. *Radiol Clin North Am* 30(4):777–787.

Moore KL and TV Persaud. 1998. The urogenital system: The development of the genital system. In *The developing human: Clinically oriented embryology.* 6th ed. Philadelphia: WB Saunders, 303.

Ott DJ, JA Fayez, RJ Zagoria. 1998. Congenital anomalies. In *Hysterosalpingography: A text and atlas.* 2nd ed. Baltimore: Williams and Wilkins, 59–69.

Pellerito JS, SM McCarthy, MB Doyle. 1992. Diagnosis of uterine anomalies: Relative accuracy of MRI and HSG. *Radiology* 183(3):795–800.

Persaud TN. 1993. Embryology of female genital tract and gonads. In *Textbook of Gynecology,* eds IJ Copeland, J Jarrell, Y McGergor. Philadelphia: WB Saunders, 321.

Propst AM and JA Hill III. 2000. Anatomic factors associated with recurrent pregnancy loss. *Semin Reprod Med* 18(4):341–350.

Raga F, F Bonilla-Musoles, J Blanes, NG Osborne. 1996. Congenital Müllerian anomalies: Diagnostic accuracy of three-dimensional USG. *Fertil Steril* 65(3):523–528.

Raga F, C Bauset, J Remohi, F Bonilla-Musoles, C Simon, A Pellicer. 1997. Reproductive impact of congenital müllerian anomalies. *Hum Reprod* 12:2277–2281.

Raziel A, S Arieli, I Bukovsky, E Caspi, A Golan. 1994. Investigation of the uterine cavity in recurrent aborters. *Fertil Steril* 62:1080–1082.

Rock JA and HW Jones. 1977. The clinical management of the double uterus. *Fertil Steril* 28:798–806.

Rock JA. 1986. Anomalous development of the vagina. *Semin Reprod Endocrinol* 4:13–31.

Rock JA. 1992. Surgery for anomalies of müllerian ducts. In *Te Linde's Operative gynaecology*, eds JD Thompson, JA Rock. 7th ed. Philadelphia: JB Lippincott, 603.

Rolen AC, AJ Choquette, JP Semmens. 1966. Rudimentary uterine horn: Obstetric and gynecologic implications. *Obstet Gynecol* 27:806–813.

Sadove RC and CE Horton. 1988. Utilizing full thickness skin grafts for vaginal reconstruction. *Clin Plast Surg* 5(3):443–448.

Speroff L, RH Glass, NG Kase. 1998. Development of the Müllerian system. In *Clinical gynecologic endocrinology and infertility*, ed C Mitchell. 6th ed. Baltimore: Lippincott Williams and Wilkins, 124.

Stampe SS. 1983. Fundal contour of the uterine cavity in the new syndrome of minor müllerian duct anomalies and oligomenorrhea: A prospective controlled study. *Am J Obstet Gynecol* 145:659–667.

Stampe SS. 1988. Estimated prevalence of müllerian duct anomalies. *Acta Obstet Gynecol Scand* 67: 441–445.

Strassman EO. 1966. Fertility and unification of pregnant uterus *Fertil Steril* 17:165.

Troiano RN and SM McCarthy. 2004. Müllerian duct anomalies: Imaging and clinical issues. Radiology 233:19–34.

Tulandi T, GH Arronet, RA McInnes. 1980. Arcuate and bicornuate uterine anomalies and infertility. *Fertil Steril* 34:362–364.

Valle RF. 1996. Hysteroscopic treatment of partial and complete uterine septum. *Int J Fertil Menopausal Studies* 41:310–315.

Wenof M, JV Reyniak, J Novendstern, MJ Castadot. 1979. Transverse vaginal septum. *Obstet Gynecol* 54:60–64.

Winfield AC and AC Wentz. 1992. Diethylstilbestrol exposure in utero: Diagnostic imaging of infertility. 2nd ed. Baltimore: Williams and Wilkins, 85–95.

2

Adolescent and Pediatric Gynecological Problems

Jayita Chakrabarti | Kusagradhi Ghosh

Adolescence is a period of transition between childhood and adulthood. The WHO (1999) defines adolescents as those between 10–19 years. It is a period of rapid biological and psychological development.

Gynecological problems of adolescents need special attention. One in five people in the world is an adolescent and in India, 22.1% of the female population is in the age group of 10–19 years. The physical and emotional changes in this decade of life have important lifelong implications. Better nutrition and sedentary lifestyle pose problems like obesity and polycystic ovarian syndrome, which have long term consequences. Rapid urbanization, along with early puberty and late marriage, increase the risk of unprotected sex, teenage pregnancies and sexually transmitted infections. In the developing countries, these problems are compounded by the presence of illiteracy, superstition, gender inequality and inadequate health facilities. As a result, adolescent girls are exposed to early marriage, repeated childbirth, sexual abuse and poor nutrition. As a gynecologist, one must be aware of these diverse issues and strive to protect the health of female adolescents (Sheil and Turner 1996).

Pediatric gynecological problems are quite different from those in adolescents and are relatively uncommon. However, they may often be life-threatening, such as, in ambiguous genitalia due to congenital adrenal hyperplasia. Also, a disorder such as mucocolpos may be the precuror of an adolescent complaint of amenorrhea in cases of imperforate hymen. Physiological conditions like discharge from the breast, 'witch's milk' or vaginal bleeding in a neonate can cause anxiety in the parents. A gynecologist must be aware of these pediatric problems.

A neoplasm in pediatric and adolescent girls is a challenge to the gynecologist since a balance has to be maintained between preservation of reproductive function and long-term survival.

History Taking and Physical Examination

Gynecological problems in an adolescent are difficult to manage. Girls in this age group are often shy. The sudden change in physical contour may cause embarrassment. Lack of knowledge and awareness about these changes often makes them feel 'different' compared to friends and sisters. Fear of social stigma prevents the sexually abused teenager from seeking medical advice. Therefore, in order to elicit a proper history, the gynecologist must be understanding, friendly, empathetic and compassionate.

An adolescent girl, if taken into confidence, can herself provide adequate history. Essential information like history of childhood diseases or pubertal milestones in siblings can be obtained from the mother or the guardian. Particular attention should be paid to some associations in order to elicit the underlying cause.

1. History of heart disease—müllerian/chromosomal anomalies, for example, Turner syndrome.
2. History of urological complaints—müllerian anomalies
3. Delayed milestones in childhood—hypothyroidism, hypothalamic disorder
4. Anorexia, weight loss—hypothalamic disorder
5. History of steroid intake—precocious puberty
6. History of hernia repair—gonadal disorder

It should be remembered that incoherent history and expression of facts often points to an exposure of unprotected sex or sexual abuse. In such cases, the doctor must be tactful and compassionate.

The physical examination of an adolescent girl should ideally be done in a separate clinic, away from the rush of a general gynecological OPD. The doctor should gain the confidence of the girl and her parents. There is considerable overlap between normal and abnormal findings in this age group and as the developmental changes of puberty are very gradual, only regular follow-up can reveal any aberration.

The physical examination must include a record of height, weight, general examination with appraisal of secondary sexual development and congenital anomalies. A careful inspection of the vulva and vagina can reveal evidence of infection, imperforate hymen, foreign body, ambiguous genitalia or neoplasm. To check for abdominopelvic lumps, per abdomen examination must be performed. Speculum and bimanual examinations are reserved for sexually active teenagers.

Investigations

Ultrasonography: This is an important diagnostic tool, especially to evaluate genital tract abnormalities, pelvic masses and menstrual dysfunctions such as amenorrhea, puberty menorrhagia and precocious puberty (Rajan 1999), and also for identification of kidneys.

However, the ultrasound has its limitations. A pre-pubertal ovary or a high and laterally placed gonad in müllerian agenesis may be missed on ultrasound (Duncan 1997). Similarly, an uncanalised uterus may appear normal.

Despite these issues, ultrasonography is still preferred as the first diagnostic tool in patients with amenorrhea and well developed secondary sexual characteristics, so as to differentiate müllerian agenesis and testicular feminisation (uterus absent in both these cases) from outflow tract obstruction (uterus present).

Karyotyping: Karyotype helps in differentiating müllerian agenesis (46,XX) from androgen insensitivity syndrome (46,XY) in cases of primary amenorrhea. It is also an essential diagnostic tool in delayed puberty or amenorrhea associated with short stature. Karyotyping should be done in cases of ambiguous genitalia and heterosexual pubertal developments.

Hormone assays: Hormone assays are the mainstay in diagnosis of ambiguous genitalia where congenital adrenal hyperplasia is suspected, 21hydroxylase deficiency being the commonest type. An FSH assay can differentiate between hypo- and hypergonadotrophic hypogonadism. Measurement of FSH and LH levels is advised in polycystic ovaries; measurement of thyroxine and prolactin levels is useful in delayed puberty and amenorrhea. Blood testosterone levels should be measured where presence of testicular tissue in patients with amenorrhea is suspected, and also in heterosexual development of puberty.

X-ray: Bone age estimation provides useful biological evidence when chronological age is not known (as in cases of delayed or precocious puberty). Intravenous pyelography may be performed where associated renal anomalies are suspected. Cranial CT scan and MRI are used only to exclude a hypothalamic or pituitary cause for aberrant pubertal development.

PUBERTY

Physical development during puberty is a gradual process and occurs over several years (Table 2.1)—the sequence of events and time of appearance may vary. The mean age of menarche in white American girls is 10 years (Herman–Giddens et al 1997), whereas for Indian girls it is assumed to be 13.5 years (Hegde and Hazra 1990). Tanner described the five stages of development of breasts and pubic hair (Table 2.2).

Table 2.1: Physical Changes during Puberty

Physical feature	*Age (years)*
Breast growth	9–13
Pubic hair growth	9–13
Axillary hair growth	10–14
Growth in height	10–14
Menstruation	11–15

Table 2.2: Tanner staging of breast and pubic hair development

Stage	*Breast*	*Pubic hair*
1. Stage 1 (prepubertal)	Elevation of papilla only. Areola < 2 cm	No sexually stimulated hair
2. Stage 2	Elevation of breast and papilla as small mound, areola diameter enlarged Median age: 9.8 years	Sparse, long, pigmented hair, chiefly along labia majora Median age: 10.5 years
3. Stage 3	Further enlargement without separation of breast and areola. When viewed from side, nipple is at/above the midplane of breast tissue Median age: 11.2 years	Dark, coarse, curly hair spread over mons Median age: 11.4 years
4. Stage 4	Secondary mound of areola and papilla formed Median age: 12.1 years	Adult type, abundant hair, but limited to mons Median age: 12.0 years
5. Stage 5	Breast is mature in contour. Nipple more pigmented and when viewed from side, nipple is below midplane of breast tissue Median age: 14.6 years	Adult type hair extending on to inner aspect of thigh Median age: 13.7 years

ABERRATIONS OF PUBERTAL DEVELOPMENT

Delayed puberty: Since there is wide variation in the normal pubertal development, it is difficult to define delayed puberty. The only pubertal milestone, which can be 'dated', is menarche; the other changes are gradual. It is generally agreed that delayed puberty exists in girls who fail to develop any secondary sexual characteristics by 13 years, have not had menarche by 16 years or in whom 5 or more years have passed since the onset of pubertal development without attainment of menarche (Rebar 1988). The causes of delayed puberty are enlisted in Table 2.3.

The diagnosis of constitutional or physiological delay of puberty often poses a problem. Height and weight records and experience of older siblings must be taken into account. The diagnosis is substantiated if bone age is less than chronological age and is below the upper limit for menstruation, that is, 14.5 years (Edmonds 1989). Patients who have not developed signs of puberty by 17 years are very likely to have a specific problem. It cannot be attributed to physiological delay (Speroff et al 1999).

The approach to the diagnosis and management is provided in Table 2.4. Some of the salient points are given below:

1. History and detailed physical examination with special emphasis on development of secondary sexual characteristics often point to the diagnosis.

TABLE 2.3: CAUSES OF DELAYED PUBERTY

Cause	%
1. Hypertropic hypogonadism	***43%***
a. Ovarian failure, abnormal karyotype (for example, 45X0, 45X0/46XX mosaic)	
b. Ovarian failure, normal karyotype (46XX or 46XY)	
Pure gonadal dysgenesis	
Resistant ovary syndrome	
2. Hypogonadotropic hypogonadism	***31%***
a. Reversible causes	
Constitutional delay	
Anorexia, weight loss, exercise or stress induced	
Adrenal disease, for example, Cushing syndrome	
Primary hypothyroidism	
Prolactinomas	
Congenital adrenal hyperplasia	
b. Irreversible causes	
GnRH deficiency, for example, Kallmann's syndrome, Laurence-Moon-Bardet-Biedl syndrome, Prader–Labhardt–Willi syndrome	
Hypopituitarism	
Congenital CNS defects	
Infiltration, irradiation of CNS	
Neoplasms, for example, craniopharyngiomas, pituitary adenomas, malignant pituitary tumours	
3. Eugonadism (with definite evidence of gonadal function)	***26%***
a. Anatomical causes, for example, müllerian agenesis, transverse vaginal septum, imperforate hymen	
b. Androgen insensitivity syndrome	
c. Inappropriate feedback anovulation, for example, polycystic ovarian syndrome	

Adapted from Reindollar et al 1981.

2. Gonadal dysgenesis with abnormal karyotype (Turner 45,XO or mosaic 46,XX/45,XO) is the single most common cause of delayed puberty.
3. Primary amenorrhea with well developed secondary sexual characteristics usually points to outflow tract obstruction (the most common being imperforate hymen), müllerian agenesis, androgen insensitivity syndrome or polycystic ovarian syndrome. The work-up of such cases is mentioned in Table 2.4.

TABLE 2.4: INVESTIGATION AND MANAGEMENT OF DELAYED PUBERTY

Cause	*Investigation*	*Treatment*
1. Ovarian failure, abnormal karyotype	• FSH↑ LH↑ • Estrogen usually low. • Ultrasonography streak gonads, normal uterus, tubes, vagina. • Karyotype—45X0, 45X/46XX, 45X/46XY,deletion($46XX_q$-$46XX_p$) • Laparoscopy and ovarian biopsy indicated if karyotype shows presence of Y chrosome • Investigation of renal, cardiovascular, blood sugar and thyroid functions are indicated as they are often associated	• Hormone therapy (See table 2.5) • Gonadectomy if presence of Y chromosome • ART for future pregnancy • Psychological support
2. Ovarian failure, normal karyotype	• Unlike those with abnormal karyotype, they are usually of average height and phenotypically female FSH, LH↑, estradiol ↓ Ovarian biopsy i. afollicular ii. follicular (resistant ovary syndrome)	• Hormone replacement • Surgical removal, if streak gonads • In resistant ovarian syndrome—oocyte donation
3. Constitutional delay	• History is suggestive • Bone age estimation	• Reassurance and wait
4. Hypothalamic/ pituitary failure of gonadotrophin production	• FSH ↓ LH ↓ • Skull Xray • CT scan • LHRH stimulation test to differentiate between hypothalamic/pituitary cause	• Hormone replacement • ART for future pregnancies • Surgical excision or radiotherapy for hypothalamic—pituitary tumours
5. Thyroid dysfunction (hypothyroidism)	• T_3 T_4 TSH estimation (usually ↑ TSH ↓T_3, ↓T_4)	• Thyroxine replacement
6. Cushing syndrome	• Cortsiol assay • ACTH suppression test	• Medical management

7. Congenital adrenal hyperplasia	• Ultrasonography: uterus, fallopian tubes, vagina, ovaries present • Karyotype: 46XX • 17 α OH progesterone ↑ (beyond 8 ng/ml) • Urinary pregnanetriol and 17 ketosteroids are markedly elevated	• Hydrocortisone: 10–20 ng/m^2/d to suppress ACTH. Monitoring to be done by bone age and growth velocity. • Mineralocorticoid replacement • Reconstructive surgery → clitoral recession, vaginoplasty
8. Müllerian agenesis (Mayer–Rokitansky–Kuster–Hauser syndrome)	• Ultrasonography shows absent uterus (vagina may/may not be absent) • Laparoscopy—tubes may be present, normal ovaries • Karyotype—46XX • IVP—associated urinary tract abnormalities 15%—absent kidney 40%—double ureter Skeletal x-ray: 5–12% have skeletal system abnormalities involving vertebra, limbs, ribs	• Reconstructive surgery like vaginoplasty. • Psychological support. • Vaginoplasty and reconstructive surgery can restore the coital function. However, uterus being absent, ovum donation remains the only option for motherhood.
9. Imperforate hymen	• Clinical examination—presence of tense bulging bluish membrane at introitus due to hematocolpos • Ultrasonography: normal uterus, vagina, ovaries. In late case, hematometra, hematosalpinx may develop	Cruciate incision of hymen
10. Transverse vaginal septum	• Clinical examination—blind vagina, may be bulging, but pink (due to thickness of the septum) • Ultrasonography is very important to assess location of septum and any associated müllerian agenesis	• Resection of septum • May require abdomino–perineal approach
11. Androgen insentivity syndrome	• Ultrasonography—uterus absent (short blind vagina) • Laparoscopy—uterus and tubes absent • Labial or inguinal gonads • Serum testoterone ↑ • Karyotype: 46XY gonadal biopsy—testicular structure	• Gonadectomy • Hormone replacement • Vaginoplasty • Psychological support

4. Patients of delayed puberty often have associated disorders of CVS (for example, in gonadal dysgenesis), CNS (for example, in Kallmann syndrome), and renal and skeletal system (for example, in müllerian agenesis). Therefore, a detailed work-up along with consultation with specialist physicians is necessary for proper

Table 2.5: Hormone therapy for delayed puberty

- Exogenous estrogen should be initiated approximately at 12–13 years of age (Rebar 1996).
- Treatment should be started with low dose estrogen, such as conjugated estrogen 0.3 mg or estradiol 0.5 mg daily, orally.
- Progesterone (medroxyprogesterone 5–10 mg, orally) should be added for 12–14 days each month, after the patient first experiences vaginal bleeding or after 6 months to one year of unopposed estrogen, if the patient has not yet experienced bleeding.
- The dose of estrogen can be increased slowly over 1–2 years.
- Patients with gonadal dysgenesis must be monitored for development of hypertension, when on estrogen therapy.
- Growth hormone is recommended in those with isolated GH defiency and also in Turner syndrome (Rosenfeld et al 1992).
- Pulsatile GnRH treatment is both a logical and effective means of inducing puberty (Stanhope et al 1987). Expense and parenteral route of administration make this treatment impractical.

diagnosis and management.

v) Congenital adrenal hyperplasia is most commonly due to 21-hydroxylase deficiency. The classic form presents with genital ambiguity at birth; the late onset or nonclassical form presents at puberty with delayed puberty or heterosexual development. Again, untreated girls at childhood grow rapidly, bone age gets advanced and there is early closure of epiphysis resulting ultimately in short stature.

Precocious puberty: This is defined as onset of pubertal development at an age more than 2.5 SD below the mean. Though a substantial number of normal children are acquiring puberty at an earlier age nowadays, pubertal development below eight years is accepted as precocious. Precocious puberty is classified as:

1. GnRH dependent/true/complete/central precocious puberty: These terms signify an early activation of the hypothalamic–pituitary–gonadal axis. It is isosexual in nature, that is, puberty changes are common to the phenotypic sex of the individual.
2. GnRH independent/pseudo/incomplete/peripheral precocious puberty: These terms signify a sexual maturation independent of the hypothalamic–pituitary gonadotropin secretion. This may be isosexual or heterosexual (pubertal development of the opposite phenotypic sex).

Occasionally, patients may present with premature thelarche, premature menarche or premature adrenarche/pubarche. The causes of these and other subtypes of precocious puberty are listed in Table 2.6. The diagnosis of precocious puberty rests on detailed history, clinical examination including height and weight record, Tanner staging, examination of external genitalia, abdominopelvic examination and neurological examination. Though the most common cause of precocious puberty is idiopathic, this diagnosis should be made only after exclusion of other causes which might be life-threatening. Bone age estimation (x-ray of the wrist of the non-dominant hand) is often helpful. Prolonged follow-up is essential as many of the CNS abnormalities may become apparent only in adulthood.

Treatment: The treatment of precocious puberty should aim at the following:

1. Treatment of intracranial disease: surgery may be required.

Table 2.6: Causes of Precocious Puberty

1. GnRH Dependent/Central/True Precocious puberty
- a. Idiopathic/constitutional—most common, accounts for about 75% of cases
- b. CNS problems:
  - i. Hypothalamic neoplasms, for example, hamartomas (most common), craniopharyngiomas, astrocytomas
  - ii. Congenital malformations, for example, hydrocephalus, arachnoid cysts, craniostenosis
  - iii. Infections, for example, tuberculosis, encephalitis, meningitis
  - iv. Infiltrative processes, for example, Langerhans cell-type histiocytosis
  - v. Irradiation
  - vi. Trauma
- c. Primary hypothyroidism

2. GnRH Independent/Peripheral/Precocious Pseudopuberty
- a. Gonadrotrophin-secreting neoplasms
  - i. hCG secreting neoplasms, for example, pinealomas, hepatoblastomas, teratomas, choriocarcinomas
  - ii. LH secreting, for example, pituitary adenomas
- b. Gonadal neoplasms
  - i. Estrogen secreting, for example, granulosa-theca cell tumours, gonadal sex-cord tumours, functional ovarian cysts
  - ii. Androgen secreting, for example, arrhenoblastomas
- c. Adrenal causes
  - i. Congenital adrenal hyperplasia
  - ii. Cushing syndrome
  - iii. Adrenal neoplasms, for example, adenoma, carcinoma.
- d. Autonomous gonadal hypersecretion, for example, McCune-Albright syndrome
- e. Iatrogenic ingestion

2. Neoplasia of ovaries and adrenals should be managed surgically.
3. Precocious maturation should be arrested till the normal pubertal age, with special emphasis on prevention of premature epiphysial closure.
4. Psychosocial support, prevention of sexual abuse, contraceptive advice.

Features of hypothyroidism and those of McCune–Albright syndrome (cystic bony lesions, café au lait skin spots) must be sought for. Laboratory investigations include:

- Bone age estimation
- CT scan or MRI of head
- Ultrasound of abdomen and pelvis
- Thyroid function tests
- Hormone assays: FSH, LH, hCG, prolactin, steroids (for example, DHEAS, testosterone, estradiol, progesterone, 17α-OHP).

GnRH analogues are the drug of choice for the treatment of precocious puberty with the aim of suppression of the HPO axis (Pescowitz 1986). These agents may be administered subcutaneously, intranasally daily or as long-term depot preparations. Substantial regression of pubertal characteristics, amenorrhea and reduction in growth velocity are rapidly achieved and maintained within the first year of treatment (Wheeler and Styne 1991). Treatment is more effective if started before the bone age of 12 years (Kaull et al 1997).

Besides GnRH analogues, medroxy progesterone acetate, cyproterone acetate or danazol can also be used.

PREMATURE THELARCHE: It is usually a self-limiting condition seen in the first few years of life and does not require any therapy other than counselling. It may be unilateral or bilateral. Follow-up is essential to rule out precocious puberty.

PREMATURE MENARCHE: Isolated premature menarche without other features of pubertal development is very rare. Infection, foreign body, sexual abuse, trauma and local neoplasm should be excluded.

PREMATURE ADRENARCHE: Isolated appearance of pubic hair before the age of 8 years is termed premature adrenarche/premature pubarche. It is believed to be due to an increase in adrenal androgens—androstenedione, DHEA and DHEAS. Diagnosis is confirmed by increased 24-hour urinary 17-ketosteroids and increased serum DHEAS. No treatment is required, but surveillance should continue because this may be the first manifestation of precocious puberty. These patients have an increased chance of development of anovulation, hirsutism and hyperinsulinemia in later life (Ibanez et al 1997).

HETEROSEXUAL PUBERTY: Heterosexual puberty is the development of characteristics of the opposite sex occurring at the expected age of puberty.

The causes of heterosexual puberty are as follows:

1. Polycystic ovarian syndrome
2. Congenital adrenal hyperplasia—non-classic forms
3. Mixed gonadal dysgenesis
4. Male pseudohermaphroditism
5. Cushing syndrome
6. Androgen secreting tumours of adrenals or ovaries
7. Idiopathic hirsutism

While a detailed discussion of these is beyond the scope of this book, a few clinical points must be kept in mind when dealing with patients with heterosexual puberty.

- In polycystic ovarian syndrome, due to elevated levels of androgen and presence of circulating estrogen, girls are both feminised and masculinised. This is in contrast to those patients of CAH who present with only masculinising features at puberty.
- Distinguishing PCO from non-classic forms of CAH is problematic and controversial (Chrousos et al 1982), yet a basal level of 17α-OH progesterone higher than 800 mg/ml is virtually diagnostic of CAH.
- In mixed gonadal dysgenesis, there is asymmetric gonadal development with testis (or germ cell tumour) on one side and streak gonad on the other. In these patients, the karyotype is usually 45,XO/46,XY and they are reared as females (who later masculinise at puberty). Gonadectomy is indicated to eliminate the risk of neoplasia of the gonads and also to remove the masculinising effect.
- Male pseudohermaphrodites have male gonads but female external genitalia. The 5α-reductase deficiency (Reifenstein syndrome) presents at puberty with heterosexual development. The karyotype is XY, external genitalia are feminine whereas breast development is as in males. Hormone assays reveal increased ratio of dihydrotestone (as 5α-reductase is required to convert testosterone to dihydrotestosterone).
- Management of XY females involves gonadectomy, hormone replacement, external genitalia reconstruction and psychological support.

MENSTRUAL IRREGULARITIES

Disturbances of menstruation are the most common presenting symptoms of adolescents in a gynecological OPD. In a study by Balachandar et al (1993), 54.25% of 400 adolescent patients had menstrual disorders. They can be classified as follows:

i. Amenorrhea: a) primary; b) secondary
ii. Irregular periods: a) polymenorrhea b) oligomenorrhea
iii. Menorrhagia
iv. Dysmenorrhea
v. Premenstrual syndrome

Amenorrhea: Primary amenorrhea is defined as the absence of periods by age 16 years in the presence of normal secondary

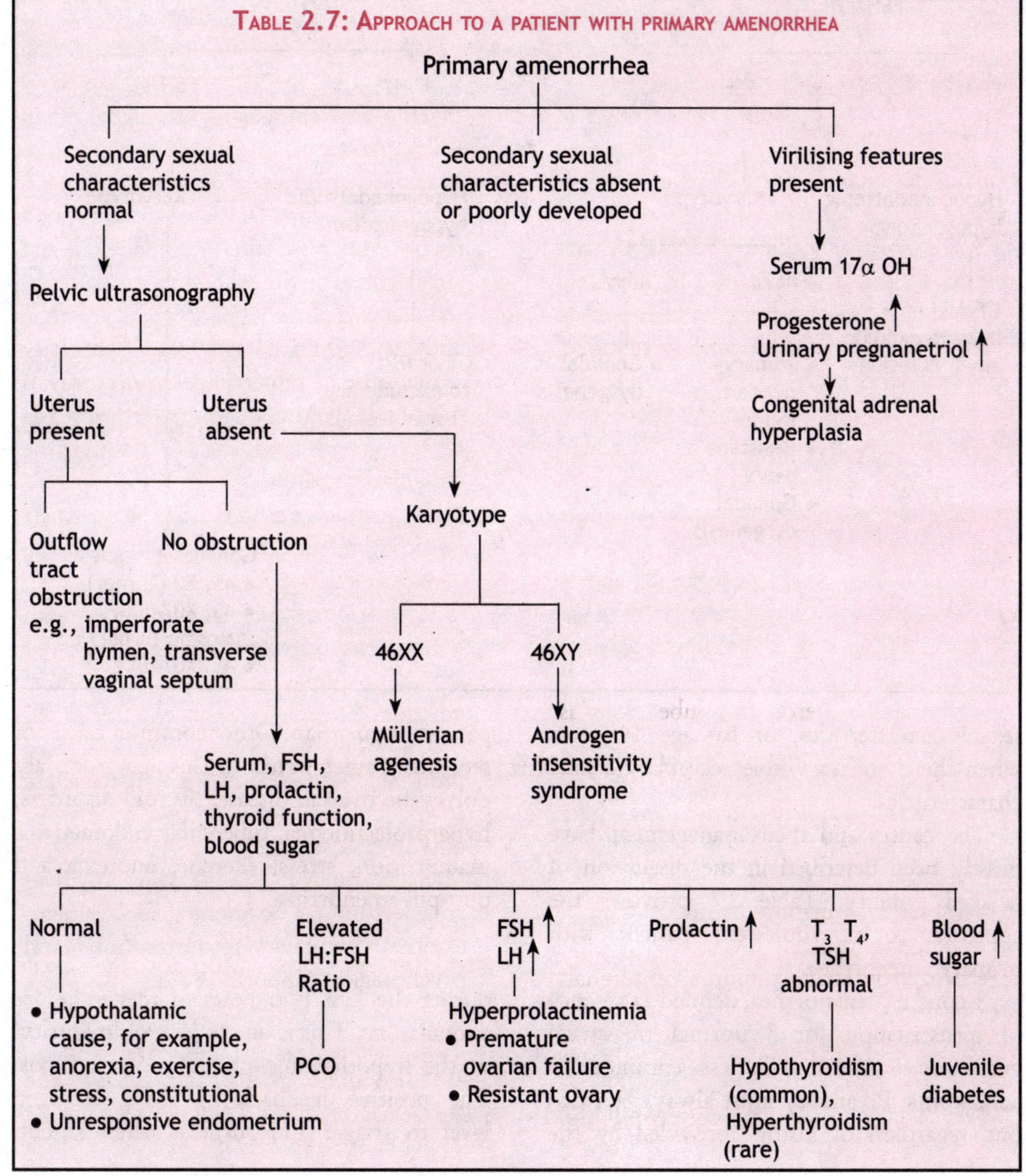

TABLE 2.7: APPROACH TO A PATIENT WITH PRIMARY AMENORRHEA

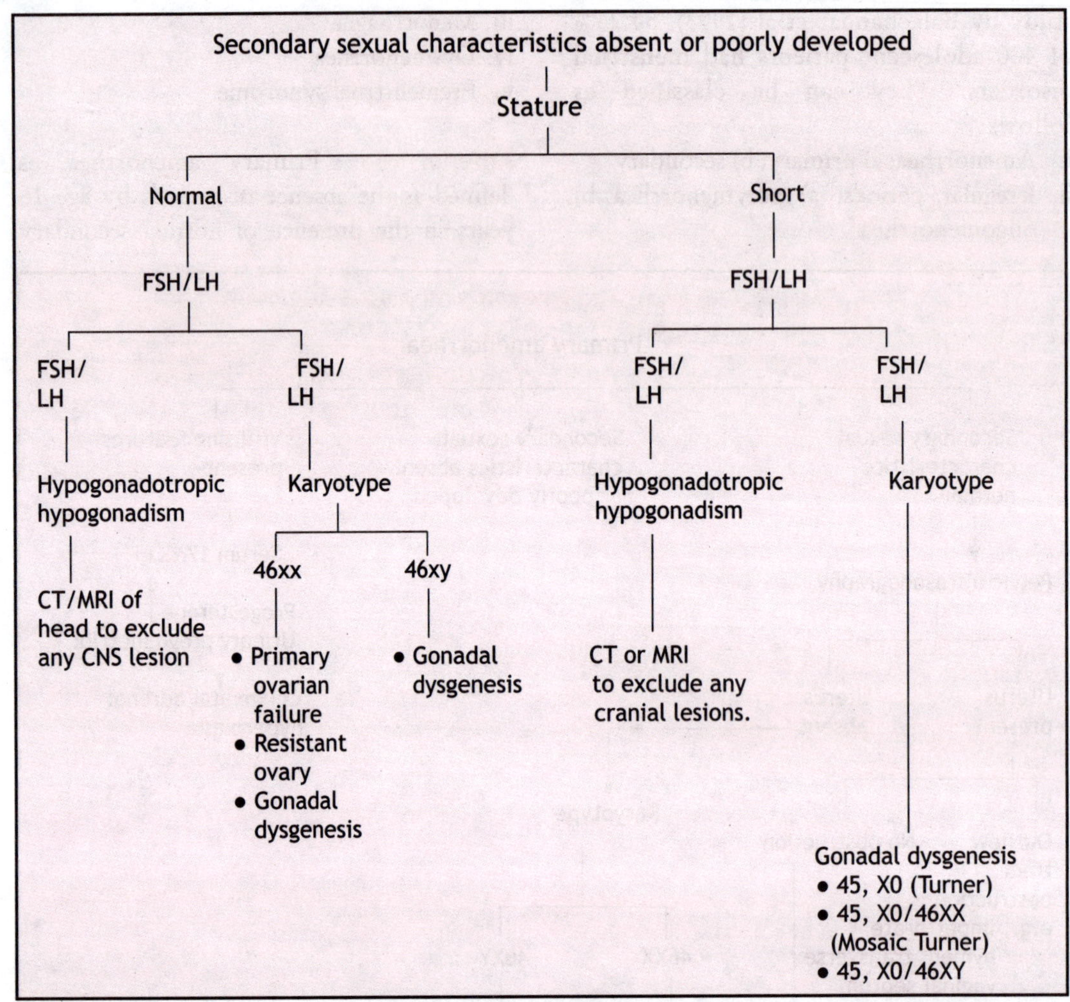

sexual characteristics, or by age 14 years when there are no visible secondary sexual characteristics.

The causes and their management have mostly been described in the discussion of delayed puberty. Table 2.7 provides the approach to an adolescent patient with primary amenorrhea.

Secondary amenorrhea, defined as absence of menstruation for 3 normal menstrual cycles or 6 months, is less common in adolescents. Pregnancy must always be ruled out, regardless of history provided by the patient or guardian. Other common causes of secondary amenorrhea in this age group are polycystic ovarian disease, thyroid disorders, hyperprolactinemia, tubercular endometritis, malnutrition, stress, exercise, anorexia and post-pill amenorrhea.

Irregular periods: Most of the cycles during the first two years of menarche are anovulatory. This is due to lack of 'maturity' of the hypothalamic–pituitary ovarian axis. The positive feedback of rising estrogen level to trigger LH surge is often absent.

As the regularity of cycles depends much on ovulation, it is not surprising that these anovular cycles during adolescence will be irregular. Yet, cycles longer than 42 days or shorter than 21 days and bleeding lasting more than 7 days should be considered as being out of the ordinary, particularly after the first two years from the onset of menarche (Hillard 1996). Oligomenorrhea (cycle length less than 40–42 days) is more common than polymenorrhea (cycle length more than 21 days).

When an adolescent patient presents with these menstrual irregularities, it is important for the clinician to determine if the patient knows how to calculate the duration of the cycle. Moreover, these menstrual irregularities cause anxiety in their mothers as they associate these disorders with future fertility. The gynecologist must counsel the mother regarding the ubiquity and normalcy of this disorder and at the same time, investigate and diagnose any underlying pathology which might be responsible for these symptoms (Table 2.8). One must always consider pregnancy and pregnancy-related bleeding per vaginum in an adolescent with irregular periods, although the history may not suggest it.

Diagnosis mainly depends on careful elicitation of history and physical examination to rule out any cause for abnormal bleeding. Investigations include measurement of serum LH/FSH ratio, serum androgens, thyroid function tests, serum prolactin. Ultrasonography of the pelvis is indicated. Rarely, a cranial CT/MRI is done to detect pituitary adenoma.

Treatment mainly consists of reassurance and correction of underlying cause if detected. Sometimes low dose combined OCPs may help restore the cyclicity of periods. If hirsutism is present, cyproterone acetate and ethinyl estradiol combined preparations are helpful, especially in those with polycystic ovaries. Polymenorrhea in adolescents is usually due to luteal phase defect and a progestogenic preparation in the luteal phase is helpful.

Menorrhagia: Puberty menorrhagia is a definite clinical entity that requires attention and proper management. The adolescent girl, who has just started menstruating, might find the normal flow and duration to be problematic and may complain of 'menorrhagia'. As mentioned before, the anovular cycles in the first few years may result in endometrial hyperplasia due to unopposed action of estrogen and result in prolonged shedding of the endometrium. These episodes

Table 2.8: Conditions associated with anovulation and abnormal bleeding

1. Eating disorders, for example, anorexia nervosa, bulimia nervosa
2. Emotional stress
3. Acute weight loss, excessive exercise
4. Androgen excess syndromes, for example, PCO, CAH, Cushing syndrome
5. Thyroid disorders, hypothyroidism, hyperthyroidism
6. Hyperprolactinemia
7. Chronic illness
8. Diabetes mellitus
9. Drugs and alcohol abuse
10. Exogenous hormones, for example, contraceptive pills causing breakthrough bleeding

of heavy flow might alarm the young girl as well as her parents. Untreated menorrhagia in this age group may lead to anemia and chronic ill health. Again, puberty menorrhagia might often be the first sign of underlying hemostatic disorders like von Willebrand disease and idiopathic thrombocytopenic purpura (ITP). Endocrine disorders, especially hypothyroidism, and genital tract infections like early stages of tuberculosis and chlamydia can also cause menorrhagia in this age group (Wolner-Hansen et al 1984). Rarely, puberty menorrhagia might also be due to hepatic disorders, hematological malignancies like leukemia or genital tract neoplasias.

A detailed history, with special emphasis on the exact duration of bleeding, number of pads required and passage of clots can reveal the true magnitude of the problem. History must also include information about easy bruising and any postoperative excess blood loss (indicating blood dyscrasias). Physical examination to detect anemia, purpuric spots, goitre, abdominopelvic lump should be performed. Inspection of vulva and vagina help rule out a local cause.

Investigations include a complete blood count, coagulation profile, thyroid function tests and ultrasonography. Any adolescent with abnormal bleeding should undergo a pregnancy test regardless of the history provided (Hillard 1996).

Norethisterone acetate progestogens are haemostatic progestogens. A higher dose of 10 mg three times a day for three to five days followed by reduction to 10mg twice a day will reduce or stop the bleeding drastically in most of the women.

The management of puberty menorrhagia is given in Table 2.9.

Dysmenorrhea: Adolescent girls often present with dysmenorrhea, especially after the first year of menarche, when their cycles become ovular. It can be classified as primary (more common) and secondary. Primary dysmenorrhea starts on the first day of menstruation, usually lasts for 24 hours and does not signify any underlying pathology. Secondary dysmenorrhea, the less common type, usually lasts for the duration of menstruation. In adolescents, secondary dysmenorrhea can be due to the presence of underlying endometriosis, uterine anomalies, genital tuberculosis and other pelvic inflammatory diseases and (in rare cases) benign or malignant neoplasias.

A detailed history and physical examination should help rule out a secondary cause. Reassurance and analgesics like the prostaglandin synthetase inhibitors (for example, mefenamic acid) are sufficient to relieve pain. Primary dysmenorrhea not responding to NSAIDs could be treated with low dose combined OCPs. Dysmenorrhea persisting after NSAIDs and OCP should be further investigated by ultrasonography to diagnose any underlying pathology.

Premenstrual syndrome (PMS): PMS, though not commonly recognised in the adolescent age group, is a difficult problem to manage. It is defined as cyclic appearance of one or more of a large number of symptoms in the luteal phase of each menstrual cycle, severe enough to disturb lifestyle or work, with an entirely symptom-free period for the rest of the cycle. It is not related to any underlying organic pathology. A number of psychological and physical symptoms have been recognised; the more common ones are shown in Table 2.10.

The exact pathophysiology is as yet unknown. However, various theories have been postulated:

1. Altered estrogen to progesterone ratio

Table 2.9: Management protocol of puberty menorrhagia

1. Mild bleeding:	i. Reassurance ii. Rest and nutritious diet iii. Iron supplementation iv. Deworming (to prevent further deterioration of anemia) v. Prostaglandin synthetase inhibitor (like mefanamic acid) can be given vi. Low dose OCP (21 days on, 7 days off) indicated if above measures fail. vii. Medroxy progesterone (5–10 mg/day) for 10–13 days every 1–2 months can prevent endometrial hyperplasia due to unopposed estrogen stimulation of endometrium
2. Moderate bleeding: (not requiring hospitalisation)	Other than rest, nutrition and hematinics, the following are required: i. OCP (combined monophasic type preferred) 1 tablet every 6 hrs x 4–7 days ↓ dose gradually tapered or stopped ↓ withdrawal flow occurs ii. Low dose OCP started when withdrawal flow occurs and continued for 3–6 cycles
3. Acute heavy bleeding: requiring emergency management	i. Hospitalisation ii. Blood transfusion, if patient is not hemodynamically stable or in compromised patients with pre-existing anemia. iii. Investigation to rule out non-pelvic causes is an essential step. iv. If DUB (dysfunctional uterine bleeding) is diagnosed, following are instituted:- a) Conjugated estrogen 25–40 mg i.v. every 6 hrs/2.5 mg orally every 6 hrs

- If responsive
  - Progesterone required to stabilise endometrium. OCP 50 μg estrogen started
  - Regimen tapered, then stopped
  - Withdrawal bleeding occurs
  - Combination low dose OCP x 3–6 cycles
- If unresponsive
  - Re-assessment of diagnosis
  - EUA and D/C biopsy may be required

TABLE 2.10: COMMON SYMPTOMS OF PMS

Psychological	*Physical*
1. Aggression, anger	1. Breast tenderness and breast swelling
2. Anxiety and tension	2. Headache
3. Sense of bloating	3. Edema
4. Sudden crying bouts	4. Joint or muscle pain
5. Depression	5. Bloatedness and true weight gain
6. Irritability	
7. Lack of concentration	
8. Loss of libido	
9. Decreased interest in usual activities	
10. Hypersomnia, insomnia	

2. Increased aldosterone activity
3. Increased renin–angiotensin activity
4. Decreased serotonin production
5. Withdrawal of endogenous endorphins
6. Vitamin deficiencies
7. Excess prolactin production

Treatment of PMS consists of reassurance, avoidance of salt, caffeine, alcohol and smoking, reduction in stress levels, regular exercise and adequate sleep. In severe and non-responsive cases, the following medication may be prescribed:

- Alprazolam may alleviate depression and anxiety.
- Fluoxetine may decrease psychic and behavioural symptoms
- Spironolactone may alleviate bloating and symptoms related to mood changes.
- Vitamin B_6, often proves helpful by correcting tryptopan metabolism, though results are inconclusive.
- Bromocriptine may decrease breast tenderness.
- GnRH analogues act by causing 'pseudomenopause'. However, the expense and risk of osteoporosis (must be supported by addback therapy) limit their use.

HIRSUTISM

Excessive growth of androgen-dependent sexual hair is termed hirsutism. It is actually the conversion of vellus hair to androgen-dependent sexual hair of male pattern in a female. Hirsutism in an adolescent girl not only disrupts the self-image but might also be a sign of underlying endocrine pathology or neoplasm. The causes of hirsutism are listed in Table 2.11.

A detailed history and physical examination may point to the underlying cause. History should include the age of onset, nature of progress, associated amenorrhea, family history, history of intake of drugs etc. General and abdominopelvic examination must be performed and the genitalia inspected.

Investigations include measurement of serum testosterone, 17α-OHP, DHEAS, thyroid profile and prolactin levels; and ultrasonography to check for the presence of an adrenal or ovarian mass. A CT scan and MR imaging may only be required in special circumstances.

Serum ACTH and ACTH stimulation test and dexamethasone suppression test may occasionally be necessary to differentiate

TABLE 2:11: CAUSES OF HIRSUITISM

1. Ovarian	i. Polycystic ovarian syndrome ii. Tumours like Sertoli–Leydig cell tumour, Hillus tumour, Lipoid cell tumour iii. Luteoma of pregnancy
2. Adrenal	i. Congenital adrenal hyperplasia (21-hydroxylase and II hydroxylase deficiency) ii. Neoplasms–adenoma, adenocarcinoma iii. Cushing syndrome
3. Pituitary	i. Cushing's disease (ACTH secreting) ii. Prolactin secreting tumours iii. Growth hormone secreting-acromegaly
4. Ectopic ACTH	Rare—from tumours of thymus, bronchus
5. Iatrogenic	Androgenic drugs like corticocteroids, danazol, phenytoin
6. Juvenile hypothyroidism	
7. Idiopathic	

between Cushing's disease, adrenal hyperplasia, adrenal neoplasia and ACTH-producing tumours.

The management depends on the underlying cause. Idiopathic or PCO-associated hirsutism is best managed with a combined preparation of ethinyl estradiol and cyproterone acetate, or cyproterone acetate alone. The response is relatively slow and at least 6 months of treatment is required to assess any improvement in the condition. Anti-androgens like spironolactone or finasteride should be added to the therapy in those who do not respond to initial therapy. GnRH analogues are used when anti-androgens fail to produce a response. For cosmetic improvement, epilation, waxing or electrolysis are beneficial.

TABLE 2.12: CAUSES OF ABDOMINOPELVIC MASS IN NEONATES, CHILDREN AND ADOLESCENTS

Age group	*Common causes*
1. Neonates	i. Functional ovarian cysts ii. Ovarian tumour, commonly germ cell tumour iii. Distended bladder due to mucocolpos caused by imperforate hymen
2. Prepubertal	i. Ovarian tumour ii. Hematocolpos, hematometra iii. Distended bladder
3. Adolescents	i. Functional ovarian cysts ii. Ovarian tumours—dermoid and other germ cell tumours, epithelial ovarian tumours iii. Hematometra, hematocolpos due to obstructing vaginal or uterine anomalies iv. Pregnancy v. Tubo-ovarian masses due to infection vi. Full bladder vii. Rarely, fibroid uterus

ABDOMINOPELVIC MASSES IN CHILDHOOD/ADOLESCENCE

An abdominopelvic mass in a neonate, child or adolescent can cause anxiety and concern in the parents. The mass may be gynecologic in origin or may even arise from the urinary tract (for example, Wilm's tumour), GI tract (for example, volvulus) or may be a tumour of the lymphatic system or musculoskeletal system. The common causes of such masses are given in Table 2.12.

Functional follicular cysts may occur in fetuses and newborns due to stimulation of ovaries by circulating maternal hormones. These usually regress within the first few months of life. Functional cysts persisting or developing in prepubertal children may lead to sexual precocity. The incidence of functional cysts again increases after menarche.

Ovarian malignancies are rare in children and adolescents. Of all ovarian masses confirmed surgically in childhood and adolescence, only 6% are malignant neoplasms (Diamond et al 1988). Germ cell tumours are the most common tumours in the first decade of life and decrease in frequency during adolescence (Hilard 1996). Mature cystic teratoma is the most frequent neoplastic tumour among children and adolescents, accounting for more than 50% of ovarian neoplasms in women below 20 years (Breen and Maxson 1977). Epithelial neoplasms are comparatively rare in this age group.

A transverse vaginal septum, or more commonly an imperforate hymen, may cause accumulation of cervical and vaginal secretions in the vagina leading to mucocolpos in neonates and children. This same entity can cause hematocolpos, hematometra and in late cases, hematosalpinx, when the menarchal blood collects in the vagina, uterus or tubes respectively. Hematocolpos may cause stretching of the urethra resulting in a distended bladder. Careful inspection of the vulval region and a gentle per rectum examination will reveal the entity.

Obstructing uterovaginal anomalies such as cervical or vaginal agenesis with a normally functioning endometrium may cause hematometra, leading to an abdominopelvic lump. A functioning non-communicating rudimentary uterine horn can also cause similar problems.

Abdominopelvic lumps in adolescents can often be due to pelvic infections, especially if associated with pain, temperature, mucopurulent vaginal discharge and abdominal and cervical tenderness. History of sexual abuse must be sought in these patients. In India, a tubo-ovarian mass may often be tubercular in origin.

In adolescents, pregnancy should always be ruled out as a cause of an abdominopelvic lump. A patient with an abdominopelvic mass may present with symptoms of vague dragging sensation in the lower abdomen and fullness, or acute pain due to torsion, intracystic hemorrhage or infection. Hematocolpos or hematometra may typically present with cystic pain and amenorrhea. Detailed history and an abdominopelvic examination, including a rectoabdominal examination, are important for the diagnosis. Investigations should include urine for pregnancy test, especially in adolescents, and ultrasonography. CT and MRI are required only if ultrasonography results are inconclusive. MRI, however, may often be more useful in evaluating rare uterovaginal malformations (Mitchell and Outwater 1995).

Management of abdominopelvic mass in children and adolescents should always be approached logically so as to balance conservation of uterus and ovaries for future pregnancy and eradication of disease process. Unilocular cystic masses are best managed conservatively as the risk of malignancy is low.

Ovarian dysgerminomas should be managed with unilateral oophorectomy followed by radiation (De Palo et al 1987) or preferably chemotherapy (Advani and Nair 1995). Other germ cell tumours such as endodermal sinus tumour, embryonal carcinoma, immature teratoma and choriocarcinoma are rare and mostly unilateral. Unilateral oophorectomy or salpingo-oophorectomy followed by chemotherapy may be effective and can preserve fertility as well. BEP (bleomycin, etoposide, cisplatin), VBP (vinblastine, bleomycin, cisplatin), and POMB-ACE (cisplatin, vincristine, methotrexate, bleomycin, actinomycin D, cyclophosphamide and etoposide) are common combination chemotherapies used for germ cell tumours of the ovary (Gershenson et al 1990; Williams et al 1991). For choriocarcinoma of the ovary, MAC (methotrexate, actinomycin D and

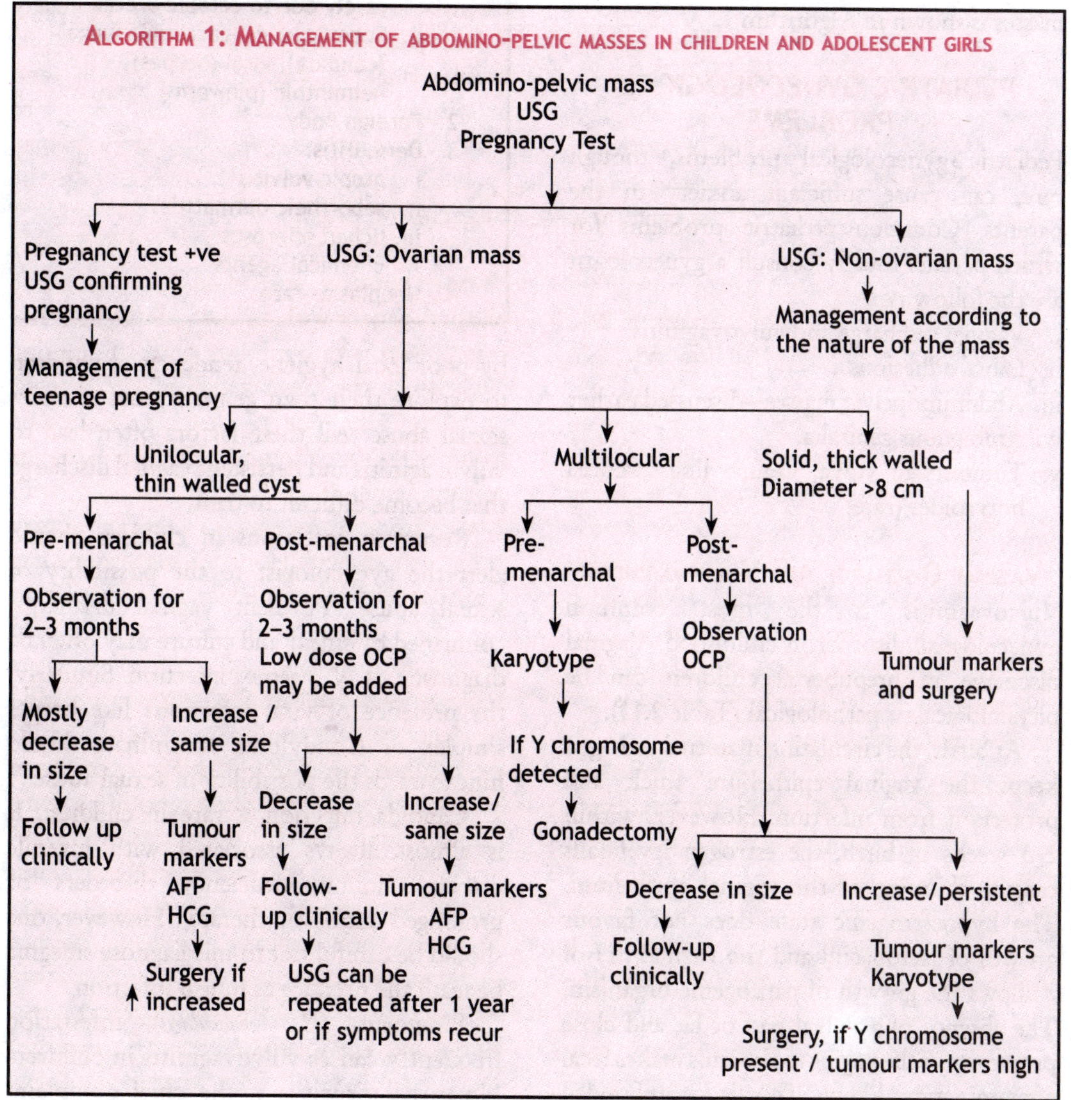

cyclophosphamide) regimen used in a manner described for gestational trophoblastic disease is effective (Berek et al 1996).

Tubo-ovarian masses, infective in origin are best managed by broadspectrum antibiotics and anti-tubercular drugs. Laparoscopic diagnosis and management, in the hands of a skilled surgeon can be curative and conservative as well, thereby maintaining the reproductive potential. A schematic approach to management of such pelvi-abdominal masses is shown in Algorithm 1.

PEDIATRIC GYNECOLOGICAL PROBLEMS

Pediatric gynecological problems, though rare, can cause sufficient anxiety in the parents. Common pediatric problems for which parents usually consult a gynecologist are the following:

i. Vaginal discharge and vulvovaginitis
ii. Labial adhesions
iii. Abdominopelvic masses—discussed earlier
iv. Ambiguous genitalia
v. Tumours of vulva, vagina, like sarcoma botyroides (rare)

Vaginal Discharge And Vulvovaginitis

Vulvovaginitis is the most common gynecological disorder in childhood. Vaginal discharge in prepubertal children can be physiological or pathological (Table 2.13).

Table 2.13: Causes of vaginal discharge in children

A. Physiological
   Neonatal—due to circulating maternal estrogen
   Preceding menarche—due to increasing estrogen levels
B. Pathological
   1. Infection
      i. Non-specific mixed infection, especially due to poor hygiene, enuresis, fecal contamination or rarely due to ectopic ureter
      ii. Specific, e.g., bacterial, fungal (candida), viral (herpes), helminthic (pinworm)
   2. Foreign body
   3. Dermatitis:
      i. atopic vulvitis
      ii. seborrheic dermatitis
      iii. lichen sclerosus
      iv. chemical agents
   4. Neoplasia—rare

At birth, the circulating maternal estrogen keeps the vaginal epithelium thick and protects it from infection. However, within 2–3 weeks of birth, the estrogen level falls causing thinning of the vaginal epithelium. The hypoestrogenic state does not favour growth of lactobacilli and the vaginal pH of 7 allows the growth of pathogenic organism. The absence of a vulval pad of fat and close proximity of the vagina to the anus makes fecal contamination likely. This is compounded by poor local hygiene, tendency of children to explore their own genitalia, and at times sexual abuse. All these factors often lead to vulvovaginitis and persistent vaginal discharge that become difficult to treat.

Recurrent infections in children should alert the gynecologist to the possibility of sexual abuse. Purulent vaginal discharge, confirmed by smear and culture may often be diagnostic of *N. gonorrhea* infection. Similarly, the presence of viral infections like herpes simplex or Condyloma accuminata should hint towards the possibility of sexual abuse.

Candida infection is rare in children. It is almost always associated with juvenile diabetes, immunodeficiency disorders or prolonged antibiotic therapy. However, one should be careful not to misdiagnose smegma beneath the prepuce as fungal infection.

Pinworm (*E. vermicularis*) infestation frequently causes vulvovaginitis in children. Nocturnal pruritus is the chief complaint because the pinworm lays eggs mainly at night around the anus causing itching in the perineal region.

Vulval skin disease is not uncommon in children. Lichen sclerosus has a characteristic 'cigarette paper' appearance in keyhole distribution around the vulva and anus (Hilard 1996). The skin becomes atrophic and fissures appear, making it very susceptible to secondary infection (Edmonds 1999).

It is mandatory to exclude the presence of any foreign body inside the vagina in children presenting with vaginal discharge (O'Brien 1995).

Diagnosis begins with proper inspection of the vulva and vagina under good illumination. Some clinicians prefer to use an otoscope or a nasal speculum for better vision to rule out the presence of a foreign body. Another aspect of the diagnosis is to collect specimens from inside the vagina without causing contamination or discomfort; a cotton wool swab may be used, though a pipette is preferable. Pokorny (Pokorny and Stormer 1987) has described a method using a catheter-within-a-catheter for this purpose. The narrow tubing of a scalp vein set is passed through a sterile urethral catheter, which in turn is passed through the introitus. Normal saline 1–2 ml is injected into the vagina, aspirated and sent for bacterial culture. This method can also be used to flush out small foreign bodies from the vagina.

Treatment mainly consists of reassurance and advice regarding maintenance of perineal hygiene. Parents must teach children to keep the vulva clean and dry. Washing after defecation, should be from front to back to avoid fecal contamination. Excessive washing should be discouraged as this might cause excessive exfoliation of the vulval skin. Scented soaps and tight synthetic undergarments are to be avoided.

Topical application of antibacterial or antifungal cream or ointment cures bacterial and fungal vulvovaginitis. Sometimes estrogen cream may be used for 2–3 weeks, but not exceeding one month. Mebendazole usually cures the helminthic infestation. Skin diseases are best managed by dermatologists.

Labial Adhesions/Adhesive Vulvitis/ Synechia Vulvae/Labial Agglutination

This is a minor disorder in which the labia minora fuse in the midline, usually from below upwards. Recurrent or chronic vulvovaginitis, due to any cause (listed in Table 2.13), causes denudation of the surface epithelium. The raw surface of the labia then adheres at the midline. Rarely, the ventral surface of the clitoris may bind to this adhesion.

This condition, although easy to treat, often causes anxiety in the parents who believe this to be absence of vagina or imperforate hymen. A translucent, dark, vertical line in the midline where the adhesions are thinnest can be seen in these conditions, which differentiate these from congenital absence of vagina (Edmonds 1999).

A hypoestrogenic state favours labial adhesions. Therefore, these are encountered usually in young children between six months and six years (Krishna and Salvi 2003). The condition is asymptomatic; however, in some cases there may be spraying of urine during micturition. Treatment consists of reassurance and cure of the chronic vulvovaginitis. Local estrogen cream may be applied for 2–3 weeks. Gentle digital separation followed by maintenance of local hygiene and application of a bland cream cures the condition. Rarely, separation with a probe under general anesthesia may be necessary.

Ambiguous Genitalia

The presence of ambiguous genitalia in a

newborn or prepubertal child is a medical and social challenge. The most common cause of ambiguous genitalia, congenital adrenal hyperplasia, must be diagnosed and managed early as the salt-losing type is often life-threatening. Moreover, the child's 'gender identity' needs to be established as early as possible, so as to provide it social and psychological assurance. It is best to assign sexual identity within 18 months of birth: reassignment of gender after the age of 2 years may cause psychological trauma to the child.

It should be understood that a correct diagnosis may not be possible by examination of the external genitalia alone. Ultrasonography, karyotype and hormone assays are required to establish the correct diagnosis. In these circumstances, counselling of the parents is vital. Instead of classifying the child as 'hermaphrodite' it is easier and comfortable to explain to the parents that the genitalia are 'unfinished' (Speroff et al 1999). Patients who present a few years after birth and have oriented to a specific gender role should not be advised to change the role, whatever the clinical diagnosis.

Finally, the clinical judgement to assign sex should not depend upon the karyotype alone. After all investigations, gender assignment should take into account the projected physical appearance at puberty, coital function and future chance of fertility.

The causes of ambiguous genitalia are as follows:

Though the appearance of the external genitalia in neonates and children may be similar, a detailed history and meticulous examination can point to the underlying cause. The following points should be remembered:

i. A gonad located in the labioscrotal or inguinal region is almost always a testis or contains testicular tissue.
ii. A testis is softer in consistency than ovary or a streak gonad.
iii. A gonad with variable consistency may be an ovotestis or a gonad with neoplastic transformation.
iv. The length of the phallus, measured from the pubic ramus to the tip of the glans of a stretched phallus, provides a clue for it to be clitoris or penis. Normal newborn clitoris measures less than 1 cm and a stretched penile length of less than 2.5 cm is 2.5 standard deviation below

TABLE 2.14: CAUSES OF AMBIGUOUS GENITALIA

Feature	*Cause*
Masculinisation of female fetus	Congenital adrenal hyperplasia - 21 hydroxylase deficiency being the most common Intrauterine exposure to increased androgens in maternal circulation: *Drugs*: e.g. Testosterone enanthate, Methylandrostenediol, Danazol *Disease*: e.g. Androgen secreting tumours, polycystic ovaries, Krukenburg tumours (Forrest et al 1978)
Incompletely masculinised males often associated with abnormal karyotypes	Androgen insensitivity syndrome—complete or partial 5α-reductase deficiency. Testosterone biosynthesis defect. Anti-müllerian hormone deficiency True hermaphrodites Gonadal dysgenesis

the mean for a newborn of 40 weeks (Myers–Seifer and Charest 1992).

v. A single midline frenulum on the ventral side of phallus indicates it to be a male one, whereas a "female phallus" usually has two frenula extending from lateral aspect to the labia minora.

vi. The degree of labioscrotal fusion has to be assessed. If the ratio of the distance from anus to edge of vagina and distance from anus to base of clitoris is 0.5 labioscrotal fusion is indicated (Speroff et al 1999).

vii. The position of the urethral meatus should be noted. Check for presence of a blind vagina or urogenital sinus.

viii. A gentle per rectum examination may reveal a midline structure that can be the uterus.

Investigations include measurement of serum 17α-OH progesterone to diagnose congenital adrenal hyperplasia (21-hydroxylase deficiency). Elevated levels of 11-deoxycorticosterone and 11-deoxycortisol are found in 11β-hydroxylase deficiency while 17 hydroxypregnenolone and dehydroepiandrosterone are high in 3β-hydroxysteroid dehydrogenase deficiency. Karyotyping should be done. Ultrasonography is indicated to check for presence of internal genitalia. Recent studies show MRI to be the most effective in determining the presence of any müllerian deviations (Hricak et al 1991).

TABLE 2.15: EMBRYOLOGY OF GONADAL DEVELOPMENT

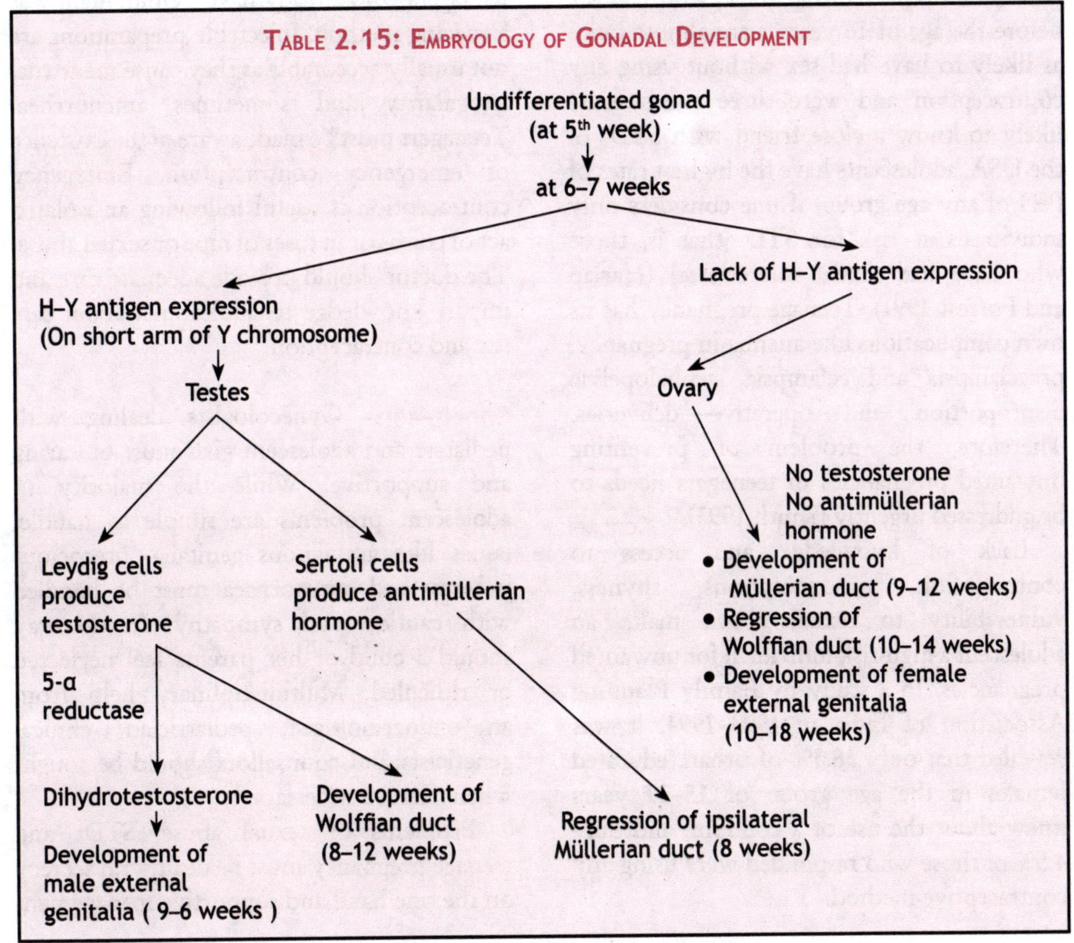

While Table 2.14 deals with the causes of ambiguous genitalia, the schematic representation in Table 2.15 will help us understand the embryology of gonadal development.

ADOLESCENT SEXUALITY, TEENAGE PREGNANCY AND CONTRACEPTION

Widespread use of media in different forms, nuclear families and unrestrained mixing has caused an increase in sexual activity among adolescents. Unprotected sexual activity increases the chance of sexually transmitted infections including AIDS, unwanted pregnancy and illegal abortion. Mellanby et al (1993) reported that those who had sex before the age of 16 years were almost twice as likely to have had sex without using any contraception and were three times more likely to know a close friend with STD. In the USA, adolescents have the highest rates of PID of any age group, if one considers only individuals at risk for STD (that is, those who have had sexual intercourse) (Harlap and Forrest 1991). Teenage pregnancy has its own complications like anemia in pregnancy, preeclampsia and eclampsia, cephalopelvic disproportion and operative deliveries. Therefore, the problem of preventing unwanted pregnancies in teenagers needs to be addressed urgently (Smith 1993).

Lack of knowledge and access to contraception, misconceptions, shyness, vulnerability to sexual abuse make an adolescent a high-risk individual for unwanted pregnancies. In a study by Family Planning Association of India in 1993–1994, it was revealed that only 36.3% of urban, educated females in the age group of 15–29 years knew about the use of a condom, and only 4.5% of those who responded were using any contraceptive method.

Barrier contraception, male or female condoms, is effective for teenagers. These should be recommended, especially to those with multiple sexual partners. However, as adolescents do not usually plan sexual encounters, barrier methods cannot be the only option for contraception.

Oral contraceptive pills may be an acceptable choice, provided there are no absolute contraindications. They are not recommended for those with multiple partners. They have benefits such as regularising menstrual cycles, decreasing dysmenorrhea, menorrhagia and PMS, and correcting anemia in this age group. Intrauterine contraceptive devices can only be prescribed to those teenagers who already have a child, mainly as a spacing method. Injectable preparations are not usually acceptable as they cause menstrual irregularity and sometimes amenorrhea. Teenagers must be made aware of the existence of emergency contraception. Emergency contraception is useful following an isolated act of coitus or in cases of rape or sexual abuse. The doctor should provide adequate care and impart knowledge to adolescents about safe sex and contraception.

Conclusion: Gynecologists dealing with pediatric and adolescent girls must be caring and supportive. While the majority of adolescent problems are simple to handle, issues like ambiguous genitalia, precocious puberty and amenorrhea must be handled with caution and sympathy. In no way should a child or her parents feel neglected or ridiculed. Multidisciplinary help from an endocrinologist, pediatrician, clinical geneticists and counsellors should be sought when deemed necessary.

Problems of sexual abuse, STDs and teenage pregnancy must be dealt with secrecy on the one hand and supportive management on the other.

Pediatric and adolescent gynecology deals with problems in those who will be, in coming years, the future generation of the nation. Protecting and promoting their health is the obligation of each individual especially the doctors. Establishment of specialised adolescent clinics, formulation of legal policies and cooperation of the media are positive steps towards such a goal.

References

Advani SM and R Nair. 1995. New frontiers in cancer chemotherapy in gynaecology In *Frontiers in Obstetrics and Gynaecology*, ed VS Patwardhan, D K Tank, D Dave, UB Saraiya. New Delhi: Jaypee Brothers,

Balachandar G, SS Raghavan, P Rajaram. 1993. Gynaecological problems in Adolescents. *J Obstet Gynaecol India* 43 (4): 599–604.

Berek JS, YS Fu, NF Hacker. 1996. Ovarian cancer In Novak's *Gynaecology* 12th edn, ed JS Berek, EY Adasni, PA Hillard, 1155–1230. Williams and Wilkins.

Breen JL and WS Maxson. 1977. Ovarian tumors in children and adolescents. *Clin Obstet Gynaecol* 20: 607–623.

Chrousos GP, DI Loriaux, DI Mann, GB Cutler. 1982. Late-onset 21-hydroxylase deficiency mimicking idiopathic hirsuitism or polycystic ovarian disease. *Ann. Intern Med* 96: 143–148.

De Palo G, A Lattuada, R Kenda et al. 1987. Germcell tumour of the ovary: The experience of the National Cancer Institute of Milan. *Dysgerminoma Inst T Radiat Oncol Biol Phy*; 13: 853–860.

Diamond MP, JW Baxter, GC Peerman Jr, Burnett LS 1988. Occurrence of ovarian malignancy in childhood and adolescence: A community-wide evaluation. *Obstet Gynaecol*; 71: 858–860.

Duncan SLB. 1997. Disorders of puberty In *Gynaecology* ed RW Shaw, WP Souther, SL Stanton, 185–199. Churchill Livingstone.

Edmonds DK 1989. Delayed Puberty In *Dewhurst's Practical Paediatric and Adolescent Gynaecology* 2nd edn, 71–85. London: Butterworth.

Edmonds DK. 1999. Gynaecological disorders of childhood and adolescence In *Dewhurst's Textbook of Obstetrics and Gynaecology for Postgraduates* 6th edn, ed DK Edmonds, 12–16. Blackwell Science Ltd.

Gershenson DM, M Morris, A Cangir, JJ Kavanaugh, CA Stringer, CL Edwards et al. 1990. Treatment of malignant germ cell tumors of the ovary with bleomycin, etoposide and cisplatin. *J Clin Oncol* 8: 715–720.

Harlap S and JD Kost Kaud Forrest. 1991. *Preventing Pregnancy Protecting Health: A New Look at Birth Control Choices in the United States*. New York: The Alan Gottmacher Institute.

Hegde K and M Desaipand Hazra. 1990. Adolescent menstrual patterns. *J Obstet Gynaecol India.* 40: 269–274.

Herman–Giddens MF, FJ Slora, RC Wasserman, CJ Bourdony, MV Bhapkar, GG Koch, CM Hasemeier. 1997. Secondary sexual characteristics and menses in young girls seen in office practice: A study from the Paediatric Research Office Settings Network. *Paediatrics* 99: 505.

Hilard PA. 1996. Benign Diseases of the Female Reproductive Tract: Symptoms and Signs. In *Novak's Gynaecology* 12th edn, ed JS Berek, EY Adashi, PA Hilard, 331–397. Williams and Wilkins.

Hricak H, YCF Chang, S Thurner. 1991. Vagina: evaluation with MR Imaging, Part I: Normal anatomy and congenital anomalies. *Radiology*: 179: 593.

Ibanez L, N Potau, M Zampolli, S Rique, P Saenger, A Carrascosa. 1997. Hyperinsulinemia and decreased insulin-like growth factor binding protein are common features in prepubertal and pubertal girls with a history of premature pubarche. *J Cin Endocrinol Metab.* 82: 2283.

Kaull R, A Galatzer, L Kornreich, L Lazar, A Pertzelan, Z Laron. 1997. Final height of girls with central precocious puberty, untreated vs. treated with cyproterone acetate or GnRH analogue: A comparative study with re-evaluation of predictions by the Bailey–Pinneau method. *Horm Res* 47: 54.

Mellanby A, F Phelps, JH Tripp. 1993. Teenagers, sex and risk taking. *BMJ* 307:25.

Mitchell DG and EK Outwater. 1995. Benign gynaecologic diseases: Applications of magnetic resonance imaging. *Top Magn Reson Imaging.* 7: 26–43.

Myers-Seifer CH and NJ Charest. 1992. Diagnosis and management of patients with ambiguous genitalia. *Semin Perinatol* 16: 332.

O' Brien TJ. 1995. Paediatric vulvovaginitis. *Aust J Derm* 56: 216–218.

Pescowitz OH, F Conite, K Hench et al. 1986. The NH experience with precocious puberty: Diagnostic subgroups and response to short-term leuthuising hormone releasing hormone analogue therapy. *J Pediatr* 108: 47–54.

Pokorny SF and LVN Stormer. 1987. Atraumatic removal of secretions from the prepubertal vagina. *Am J Obstet Gynaecol:* 156: 581–582.

Rajan R. 1999. Ultrasonography in the adolescent girl In *The Adolescent Girl*, ed U Krishna, S Parulekar, V Salvi, 216–224. Federation of Obstetric and Gynaecological Societies of India, Mumbai.

Rebar RW. 1996. Puberty In *Novak's Gynaecology* 12th edn, ed J S Berek, EY Adashi, PA Hilard. London: Williams and Wilkins. 771–807.

Reindollar RH, PG McDonough, JR Byrd. 1981. Delayed sexual development: A study of 252 patients. *Am Jr of Obs & Gyn* 140: 371–380.

Rosenfeld RG, J Frane, KM Attie, JA Brazel, S Burstein et al. 1992. Six-year results of a randomized prospective trial of human growth hormone and oxandrolone in Turner syndrome. *J Pedlatr* 121; 49–55.

Sheil O and M Turner. 1996. Adolescent gynaecology In Vol 12 of *Progress in Obstetrics & Gynaecology*, ed J Studd, 215–232. Churchill Livingstone.

Smith T. 1993. Influence of socio-economic factors on attaining targets for reducing teenage pregnancies. *Br. Med J* 306: 1232–1235.

Speroff L, RH Glass, NG Kase, 1999. Abnormal puberty and growth problems. In *Clinical Gynaecologic Endocrinology and Infertility* 6th edn. 381–419. Lippincott Williams & Wilkins.

Speroff L, RH Glass, NG Kase. 1999. Normal and abnormal sexual development. In *Clinical Gynaecologic Endocrinology and Infertility* 6th edn. 339–379. London: Lippincott Williams & Wilkins.

Stanhope R, PJ Pringle, CGD Brook, SJ Adam, HS Jacobs. 1987. Induction of puberty by pulsatile gonadotropin releasing hormone. *Lancet* ii: 552–557.

WHO. 1999. Programming for adolescent health and development. WHO Tech. Report Series 886, WHO, Geneva, 11.

Wheeler MD and DM Styne. 1991. The treatment of precocious puberty. *Endocrinol Metab Clin North Am* 20:183.

Williams SD, JA Blessing, K Hatch, HD Homesley. 1991. Chemotherapy of advanced ovarian dysgerminoma: trials of the Gynaecologic Oncology Group. *J Clin Oncol* 9: 1950–1955.

Wolner-Hanssen P, NB Kiviat, KK Holmes. 1984. A typical pelvic inflammatory disease: subacute, chronic or subclinical upper genital tract infection in women In *Sexually Transmitted Diseases.* 2nd edn, ed KK Holmes, PA Mardh, PF Sparling, PJ Wiesner, W Jr Cates, SM Lemon et al. 615–619. New York: McGraw-Hill.

3

Amenorrhea

Thankam Rama Varma

Introduction Amenorrhea is the absence of menstruation, either a lack of onset or the cessation of normal menstruation. Absence of menstruation may occur for a variety of reasons. It is very important for any woman who has stopped menstruating to consult a medical practitioner.

Pregnancy and menopause are two very natural reasons for menstruation to cease; amenorrhea due to these causes is known as **physiological amenorrhea.** The late onset of menstruation is often a cause of concern for young girls and their parents. If puberty has progressed normally, the girl is of normal weight and height and there are no other abnormal physical signs, there is usually no cause for concern in girls under 16 years of age. **Primary amenorrhea** is usually diagnosed if a girl has not started menstruation by 16 years of age. This type of amenorrhea is usually the result of a disorder of the pituitary and/or hypothalamus, chromosomal abnormality or abnormal development of the ovaries or uterus.

Secondary amenorrhea is a relatively more common problem. This condition is often the result of stress, vigorous athletic training or an extreme change in body weight (anorexia nervosa) or polycystic ovary syndrome. Other possible conditions are hyperprolactinemia, androgen producing tumours, intrauterine adhesions and thyroid dysfunction.

The intent of this chapter is to provide a simple mechanism for the differential diagnosis of amenorrhea of all types and chronology, using procedures available to all clinicians. One needs to pinpoint the organ system locus of disorder leading to the presenting symptom of amenorrhea. Once this is accomplished, the detailed evidence confirming the diagnosis can be sought and the assistance of appropriate specialists confidently chosen. In the end, the patient receives the most reliable diagnosis and therapy at minimum cost and optimum convenience.

BASIC PRINCIPLES OF MENSTRUAL FUNCTION

The clinical demonstration of menstrual function is on seeing menstrual discharge. This requires an intact outflow tract that connects the internal genital source of blood flow with the outside. Hence, the outflow tract requires patency and continuity of the vaginal orifice, the vaginal canal and the endocervix with the uterine cavity. Figure 3.1 indicates the basic principles of menstrual function.

At 6–8 weeks gestation, the first sign of ovarian differentiation is reflected in the rapid mitotic multiplication of germ cells, reaching 6–7 million oogonia by 16–20 weeks (Baker

Figure 3.1: Basic principles of menstrual function

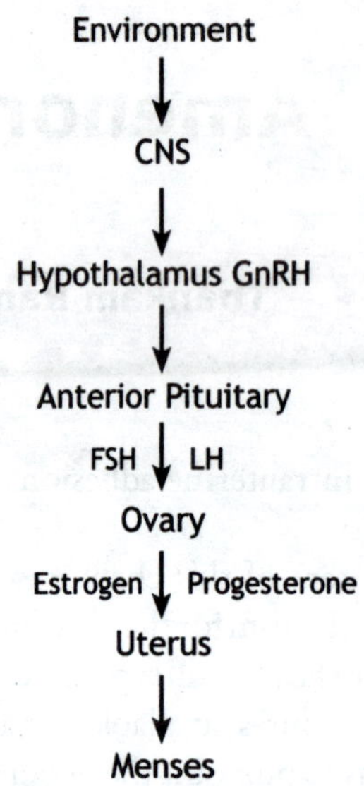

1963; Gondos et al 1971). Subsequently, the germ cell count decreases until some 50 years later, the store of oocytes will be finally exhausted. Chromosomal anomalies can accelerate germ cell loss. Rapid loss of oogonia leaves the gonad without a follicle at birth and it appears as a fibrous streak.

Failure to establish menstruation by the age of 16 years, in the presence of secondary sexual characteristics, or by the age of 14 years in their absence, constitutes primary amenorrhea. The arbitrary classification of amenorrhea into primary and secondary can lead to a degree of overlap in terms of etiology.

Diagnosis

It is useful to employ a diagnostic evaluation that segregates causes of amenorrhea into four sites which controls the reproductive function.

- Disorders of the outflow tract or uterine target organ
- Disorders of the ovary
- Disorders of the anterior pituitary
- Disorders of the central nervous system, hypothalamus factors

The age of onset of menstruation or menarche varies between 10 and 16 years and is influenced by geographical, racial and socio-economic factors. The average age of menarche is 13.2 years ± 0.04 years in North Indian girls (Sharma 1990).

Evaluation of amenorrhea

- A careful history and a thorough physical examination are mandatory
- One should look for psychological dysfunction or emotional stress, family history of genetic anomalies, signs of physical problem with a focus on nutritional status, abnormal growth and development, presence of a normal reproductive tract, and evidence of CNS disease
- Presence of galactorrhea, will channel the investigation to assess the condition
- Ultrasound of the abdomen and pelvis will give information of the presence or absence of uterus and ovaries.

Initial assessment (Figure 3.2)

- At the first assessment, exclude pregnancy
- Once pregnancy is excluded, a measurement of thyroid stimulating hormone (TSH), prolactin level and a progestational challenge test should be done
- If patients present with galactorrea, assessment of TSH and prolactin level should be considered. The longer the duration of hypothyroidism, the higher the incidence of galactorrhea and the higher the prolactin level (Contreras et al 1991). Patients with primary hypothyroidism and hyperprolactinemia may present with either primary or secondary amenorrhea (Poretsky et al 1986).

FIGURE 3.2: INITIAL ASSESSMENT TO MANAGE AMENORRHEA

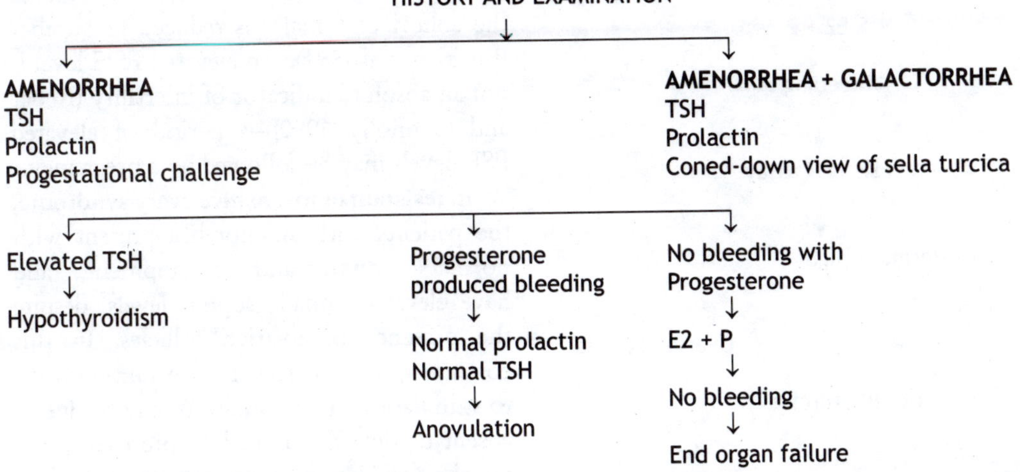

- The purpose of the progestational challenge is to assess the level of endogenous estrogen and the competence of the outflow tract. A progestational agent, totally devoid of estrogenic activity, is the choice.
- If the patient bleeds, it confirms the presence of a normal genital tract and a primed endometrium with estrogen. Some function of the ovary, pituitary and central nervous system (CNS) is established. Further evaluation is unnecessary.
- If the progestional medication does not produce withdrawal bleed (Fig. 3.3), it indicates that either the target organ outflow tract is inoperative or preliminary estrogen priming has not occurred.
- In that case, combined estrogen + progestin (E_2 + P) should be given for a period of 21 days to assess whether there is withdrawal bleed. If there is no withdrawal bleed, the diagnosis of a defect in the endometrium or outflow tract can be made
- If withdrawal bleed occurs with estrogen + progestin, the endometrium and the outflow tract is intact and estrogen priming will restore that function. From a practical point of view, in a patient with normal external and internal genitalia by pelvic examination, abnormality of the outflow tract is unlikely.
- Outflow tract problems include either destruction of the endometrium, generally the result of overzealous curettage, or the result of infection, for example, tuberculosis or primary amenorrhea resulting from the discontinuity or disruption of the müllerian duct. Abnormalities in the outflow tract are not very common.

SUBSEQUENT WORK-UP FOR ABSENCE OF ESTROGEN PRIMING

- This involves assessing steroid production by the ovaries. In order to produce estrogen, the ovaries should have normal follicular apparatus and sufficient pituitary gonadotrophins to stimulate the follicular apparatus.
- The assessment is made to check if there is a fault in the ovaries or in the release of gonadotrophins.

FIGURE 3.3: NO PROGESTERONE WITHDRAWAL BLEED, FURTHER ASSESSMENT

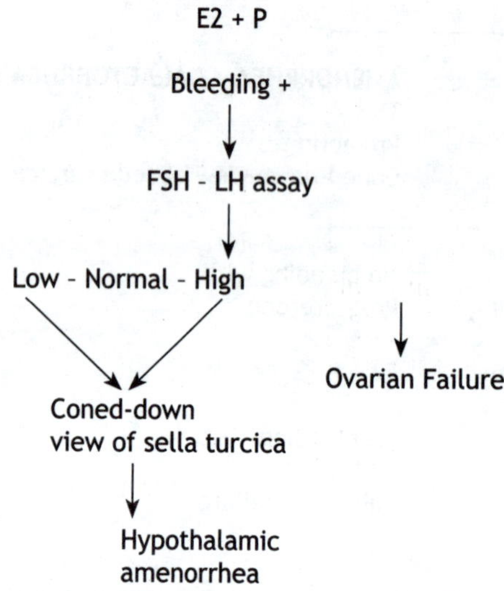

- The assessment involves measurement of gonadotrophins—**high level of gonadotrophins is interpreted as abnormal.**
- The lack of estrogen is due to a fault in the follicle or in the CNS–hypothalamic–pituitary axis.
- The gonadotrophin level in the amenorrheic woman who does not bleed following progestational agent will be abnormally **high,** abnormally **low** or in the **normal** range.

Elevated gonadotrophins can be due to a **gonadotrophin-secreting pituitary adenoma,** but they are not usually associated with hypogonadism or amenorrhea and it is difficult to diagnose this condition (Comtoise et al 1989; Katznelson et al 1992). These tumours may present with pressure symptoms such as headache and visual disturbances.

During the **peri-menopausal period,** it is normal for FSH levels to rise even before the cessation of the menstrual cycle. The rise in FSH prior to menopause is due to the declining inhibin production by either the less competent ovarian follicle or because the cohort of follicles is reduced in number (Buckler et al 1991). An elevated FSH level is not an absolute indicator of infertility (Rebar and Connolly 1990)—a period of elevated FSH levels may be followed by a pregnancy.

In **resistant or insensitive ovary syndrome,** the patients with amenorrhea present with normal growth and development, and have elevated gonadotrophin levels, despite the presence of ovarian follicles. In this condition, ovarian follicles are unresponsive to stimulation. This condition may be due to absent or defective gonadotrophin receptors on the follicles or a pre-receptor-signalling defect (Talbert et al 1984). Molecular biology studies have shown mutations in the gonadotrophin receptor genes that prevent ovarian response (Aittomaki et al 1995; 1996). Translocations between regions on X and Y chromosomes that share sequence homology have been reported in patients with secondary amenorrhea and ovarian failure (Delon et al 1997). It is important to remember that laparotomy for full-thickness biopsy is not recommended for every patient.

Secondary amenorrhea caused by premature ovarian failure may be associated with autoimmune disease (Alper and Garner 1985). The ovaries contain normal appearing primordial follicles, but developing follicles are surrounded by nests of lymphocytes and plasma cells with lymphatic infiltration of thecal layer of cells. However, antibodies blocking FSH and LH receptors have not been identified in immunoglobulin G from women with premature ovarian failure (Anasti et al 1995). Commonly, evidence of abnormal thyroid function is detected, hence complete thyroid function tests are recommended in all patients with premature ovarian failure.

Other rare conditions associated with premature ovarian failure include myasthenia gravis, idiopathic thrombocytopenic purpura, rheumatoid arthritis, vitiligo and autoimmune hemolytic anemia.

Because pregnancy is extremely unlikely, egg donation should be considered. However, an impressive pregnancy rate has been reported combining GnRH agonist, corticosteroids and induction of ovulation with high doses of exogenous gonadotrophins (Blumenfeld et al 1993).

Galactosemia is a rare inherited autosomal recessive disorder of galactose metabolism due to a deficiency of galactose-1-phosphate uridyl transferase. High gonadotrophin levels may be associated with **specific enzymatic deficiencies.**

Chromosome Evaluation

All patients under the age of 30 who have a diagnosis of premature ovarian failure on the basis of elevated gonadotrophins must have karyotyping done. The presence of mosaicism with a Y chromosome requires excision of the gonad because it increases the risk of developing malignant tumours. The secondary tumours arising from germ cells are highly malignant—gonadoblastomas, dysgerminomas, yolk sac tumours and choriocarcinoma. Most of the gonadal tumours appear before the age of 20 years, but a significant number are detected between 20 to 30 years (Manuel et al 1976; Troche and Hernandez 1986).

An individual with a mosaic karyotype (for example, XX/XO) may experience normal pubertal development, menses and even pregnancy before the onset of a premature menopause. It is therefore important to consider karyotyping, regardless of menstrual pattern, in an adolescent or young woman less than 60 inches tall. Spontaneous puberty has been reported in 10%–20% and spontaneous menstruation in 2%–5% of girls with Turner syndrome (Pasquino et al 1997).

Premature Ovarian Failure

Patients with repeatedly elevated gonadotrophins can be diagnosed as having ovarian failure and considered sterile. However, 10%–20% of patients presenting with secondary amenorrhea and elevated gonadotrophins with normal karyotype have resumed normal function after several months (Aiman and Smentek 1985; Rebar and Connolly 1990; Nelson et al 1994). However, periodic surveillance for adrenal function is recommended because ovarian failure usually precedes adrenal failure. Other than hypothyroidism, it is uncommon to encounter other disorders associated with premature ovarian failure.

Prior use of LHRH agonist to bring down levels of serum gonadotrophins is not associated with any benefit (Nelson et al 1992). Ovarian biopsy is not indicated; empirical treatment using gonadotrophins may show some benefit, though the response is often disappointing.

Gonadotrophins

Normal gonadotrophins: If normal gonadotrophins were present in the circulation, follicular growth should be present and estrogen levels would be adequate to provide a positive withdrawal bleed. Another rare possibility is an inherited disorder of gonadotrophin synthesis leading to the production of immunologically active but biologically inactive hormones (Axelrod et al 1979).

If the FSH and LH levels are in the normal range in a patient with a negative progestational withdrawal test, it is consistent with pituitary–CNS failure.

Low gonadotrophins: If the gonadotrophin assay is abnormally low, or in the normal range, localisation is required to distinguish between a pituitary or CNS hypothalamic cause for the amenorrhea.

The CT scan can be used to image the sella turcica, evaluate its contents as well as image the suprasellar area; however, total accuracy is not achieved (Teasdale et al 1986). Magnetic resonance imaging is more sensitive than the CT scan.

Microadenomas less than 10 mm in diameter do not require treatment unless associated with hyperprolactinemia. Spiroff et al (1999) recommend that the initial x-ray evaluation for amenorrheic patients, with or without galactorrhea, is the cone-down lateral view of the sella turcica. This will detect the presence of a large tumour. If the prolactin level is more than 100 ng/ml or if the cone-down view of the sella turcica is abnormal, further imaging with CT scan or MRI is recommended.

Large tumours are most frequently associated with prolactin levels greater than 100 ng/ml. Tumours which are large and associated with prolactin levels less than 100 ng/ml are more likely to be tumours other than prolactin-secreting adenomas, causing stalk compression and interruption of the normal dopamine regulation of prolactin secretion. Such tumours produce an abnormal coned-down view of the sella turcica.

No routine active management of microadenomas is necessary because microadenoma is very common, rarely grows during pregnancy, rarely progresses to macroadenomas, there is significant recurrence rates after surgery. There is no contraindication to HRT or oral contraceptives.

Hypogonadotrophic hypogonadism: A patient with amenorrhea and without galactorrhea who has normal imaging studies is classified as hypothalamic amenorrhea. Suppression of pulsatile GnRH secretion below its critical range can cause this problem.

Specific Disorders Related to Outflow Tract

Congenital abnormalities are limited to amenorrhea that presents in the pubertal period of life. Reindollar et al (1986) reported from a study they undertook in 262 patients with secondary amenorrhea, 7.0% presented with Asherman syndrome, abnormal chromosomes were seen in 0.5, prolactin tumours in 7.5% and anovulation in 28.0%, weight loss/anorexia in 10%, hypothalamic suppression in 10% and hypothyroidism in 1.0%.

Asherman syndrome: Secondary amenorrhea follows destruction of the endometrium (Asherman syndrome). This condition is produced by overzealous postpartum or post-abortal curettage resulting in intrauterine scarring or synechiae. Ideally, hysteroscopic examination should be done to assess the condition. The adhesions may partially or completely obliterate the endometrial cavity, the internal cervical os, the cervical canal, or a combination of these areas. Normally, hematometra does not occur. Asherman syndrome can occur following uterine surgery such as cesarean section, myomectomy or metroplasty.

Patients with Asherman syndrome may present with recurrent miscarriages, dysmenorrhea or hypomenorrhea or subfertility. Hysteroscopy will identify the problem. Tuberculosis can also destroy the endometrium and cause amenorrhea, more common in countries like India. Histopathological examination, culture of the menstrual discharge or endometrial biopsy

PCR should help to make the diagnosis. Schistosomiasis is another rare cause of end organ failure.

Hysteroscopy with direct lyses of adhesions by cutting cautery or laser yields better results than blind dilatation and curettage. To keep the uterine cavity from adhering, the use of pediatric Foley catheter for 7 days under antibiotic cover seems to be a better option than IUCD. The patient is given higher doses of estrogen, such as Premarin 2.5 mg, daily for three to four weeks with medroxy progesterone acetate, 10 mg daily, added during the last 7 days of the regimen.

Müllerian Anomalies

In primary amenorrhea, discontinuity by segmental disruptions of the müllerian tube should be ruled out. Direct observation should reveal imperforate hymen, obliteration of vaginal orifice, and lapses in continuity of the vaginal canals. The cervix or the entire uterus may be absent. Less commonly, the uterus is present but the cavity is absent or the endometrium will be lacking.

Imperforate hymen: Approximately 1 in 2000 girls are born with an imperforate hymen. Menstrual blood collects within the vagina and occasionally within the uterine cavity causing hematocolpos or even hematometra. It usually presents with cyclical abdominal pain, distension of lower abdomen and sometimes retention of urine. Abdominal mass may be palpable sometimes. Vulval inspection reveals a bluish, bulging membrane at the introitus. They can develop signs and symptoms of hemoperitoneum.

Ultrasonography confirms the hematocolpos and hematometra. All efforts are made to incise and drain from below at the points of closure of the müllerian tube, reestablishment of müllerian duct continuity usually can be achieved surgically. Prior to surgery, MRI may be used to identify the anatomical abnormality. A correct preoperative diagnosis will help in planning surgery.

Müllerian agenesis: Lack of müllerian development (Mayer-Rokitansky-Kuster-Hauser syndrome) is the diagnosis for the individual with primary amenorrhea and no apparent vagina. This is a relatively common cause (1 in 4000 female births) of primary amenorrhea, more frequent than congenital androgen insensitivity and second only to gonadal dysgenesis. These patients have an absence or hypoplasia of the vagina and usually an absence of the uterus and fallopian tubes. Rarely, the uterus may be present but there is no connection for outflow, or the outflow tracts may be rudimentary bicornuate cords. It is worthwhile to consider karyotyping to exclude male pseudohermaphroditism. Usually, ovarian function is normal. Growth and development are also normal. Affected girls possess a normal phenotype and usually have a normal karyotype (46,XX).

The exact cause is unknown—exposure to antimüllerian hormone (AMH) could be a cause. Other likely causes are mutations of the gene for antimüllerian hormone or the gene for the antimüllerian hormone receptor. A mutation has been identified in galactose-1-phosphate uridyl transferate in daughters with müllerian agenesis and their mothers (Cramer et al 1996).

Approximately a third of patients have urinary tract abnormalities, and 12% or more have skeletal anomalies, mostly involving the spine, although absent digits and syndactyly may occur.

Because of the difficulties and complications associated with surgical procedures, alternative methods such as the use of progressive dilatation of vagina should be tried (Frank 1938; Wabrek et al 1971). Operative treatment is reserved for women in whom the Frank method is not acceptable or has failed to achieve the desired outcome or a well-formed uterus is present and fertility might be preserved. If the cervix is atretic, it is better to remove the uterus (Bates and Wiser 1985). If the problem is of a minor nature such as an imperforate hymen or a transverse vaginal septum, surgery is indicated. It is usually not possible to preserve fertility in case of complete vaginal agenesis. Transverse vaginal septum is a failure of canalisation of the distal third of the vagina and presents with symptoms of obstruction and urinary frequency. It may be differentiated from an imperforate hymen by a lack of distension at the introitus with a valsalva's maneuver. Delay in surgical treatment for distal obstruction of the genital tract can lead to infertility and endometriosis. However, the oocytes collected from the mother and sperms from the genetic father can be fertilised and the embryos placed in a surrogate carrier (Batzer et al 1992).

Androgen insensitivity (testicular feminisation) syndrome: Complete androgen insensitivity is the likely diagnosis when a blind vaginal canal is diagnosed and the uterus is absent. This is the third most common cause of primary amenorrhea after gonadal dysgenesis and müllerian agenesis. The patient with testicular feminisation is a male pseudo-hermaphrodite, thus the individual has testes and XY karyotype—pseudo-hermaphrodite means that the genitalia are the opposite of the gonads. The individual is phenotypically female but with absent or meagre pubic and axillary hair. This is an X-linked disorder and occurs in 1 in 60,000 chromosomally male infants. Karyotype is 46,XY and testes are present, but androgenic effects are absent due to abnormalities of the androgen intracellular receptor.

The testes may be intra-abdominal or in the hernia. There is no spermatogenesis. The incidence of neoplasia in these gonads is high (22% to 52%) (Morris and Mahesh 1963); however, recent studies indicate a lower incidence of gonadal tumours (about 5%–10%) (Rutgers and Scully 1991; Griffin 1992). The gonads should be removed at age 16–18 years and the patient should receive hormone therapy. The only exception to the rule is that gonads with a Y chromosome should be removed as soon as a diagnosis is made.

Because antimüllerian hormone is present, development of antimüllerian duct is inhibited; hence the absence of uterus, tubes and upper vagina.

These women have normal female phenotype, normal male karyotype (46,XY) and abnormal or slightly elevated blood testosterone levels and high LH.

Incomplete androgen insensitivity: This condition is only a tenth as common as the complete androgen insensitivity syndrome and shows some androgen effect on examination. These individuals may have clitoral enlargement or may even have a phallus. Axillary and pubic hair develops along with breast growth. Gonadectomy should not be deferred in such cases; further virilisation needs to be prevented. A patient with a deficit in testicular 17β-hydroxy steroid dehydrogenase activity will have impaired testosterone production and will present clinically as having incomplete androgen insensitivity.

DISORDERS OF THE OVARIES

Gonadal dysgenesis: Problems in gonadal development can present with either primary or secondary amenorrhea. Streak gonads are present in 30%–40% of women presenting with primary amenorrhea, due to abnormal development (gonadal dysgenesis). They are categorised into three groups:

45,X (50%)
Mosaics (25%)
46,XY (25%)

Women with gonadal dysgenesis may also present with secondary amenorrhea; the karyotype varies and is given in the order of frequency:

46,XX (most common)
Mosaics (45,X/46,XX)
Deletion in short and long arms of X
47,XXX
45,X

Both X chromosomes must be present and active in oocytes to prevent the accelerated loss of follicles. Very often, a normal karyotype is found in patients with ovarian failure; this is perplexing. There may be unknown reasons for loss of activity; sometimes they may be due to specific gene alterations.

Turner syndrome: Among those with a female karyotype, 50% will have Turner syndrome, 25% will have mosaicism (45,X/46,XX) and the rest may possess a normal karyotype (25%). The typical characteristics of short stature, webbed neck, shield chest and increased carrying angle in the elbow, combined with hypergonadotrophic hypoestrogenic amenorrhea, make a diagnosis possible. Autoimmune disorders, cardiovascular abnormalities and various renal anomalies must be ruled out. All patients should undergo karyotyping. The presence of a pure syndrome 45,X chromosome single-cell line needs to be confirmed, 45% of individuals who appear to have Turner syndrome are mosaics or have structural aberrations in the X or Y chromosome.

Mosaicism: The presence of mosaicism should be ruled out because the presence of the Y chromosome would require removal of the gonad.

XY gonadal dysgenesis: A female patient with an XY karyotype who has a palpable müllerian system, normal female testosterone levels and lack of sexual development has Swyer syndrome.

Gonadal agenesis: Viral and metabolic influences in early gestation or undiscovered genetic mutations are suspected. The condition is not curable, results in hypergonadotrophic hypogonadism. In the absence of gonads, development is female. Surgical removal is mandatory to prevent the possibility of neoplasia.

The resistant ovary syndrome: Patient presents with amenorrhea, normal growth and development who has elevated gonadotrophins despite the presence of unstimulated ovarian follicle, and no evidence of autoimmune disease. There is follicle with no lymphocytes infiltration as seen with auto immune disease. FSH receptor mutations have been described in women with this diagnosis (Huhtanieni et al 1996).

Premature ovarian failure: In this common condition, early depletion of ovarian follicles occurs. Approximately 1% of women develop ovarian failure before the age of 40 years, and in women with amenorrhea, the prevalence ranges from 10% to 28% (Alper and Garner 1985; Coulam et al 1986). Etiology is not clear, it may be a genetic disorder with increased rate of follicle disappearance. Often, specific sex chromosome anomalies can be identified (Dewald and Spurbeck 1983).

History of hot flushes and other menopausal symptoms with raised gonadotrophins and a normal karyotype are diagnostic. Other genetic determinants of premature ovarian failure (POF) include FSH receptor mutations; fragile X permutation carrier status has also been linked with POF (Allingham-Hawkins et al 1999). Family history is an important predictor of this condition. Radio- and chemotherapy produces premature ovarian failure. A number of autoimmune diseases may co-exist in 10%–20% of women with POF (Conway et al 1996).

Using FISH, a higher percentage of cells containing a single X chromosome can be detected in women with premature ovarian failure (Devi et al 1998). The cause is most likely accelerated follicular atresia because even 45,X (Turner syndrome) patients begin with a full complement of germ cells.

Polycystic ovary syndrome (PCOS): This affects 5%–10% of women in the reproductive age group. This is the commonest cause for secondary amenorrhea. It is characterised by chronic anovulation and hyperandrogenism. Oligomenorrhea, hyperandrogenism in the absence of other endocrine disorders such as CAH, hyperprolactinemia, thyroid dysfunction and androgen secreting tumours are among the diagnostic criteria for PCOS (Dunaif and Thomas 2001). In recent years, insulin resistance has emerged as a key metabolic component of PCOS (Dunaif 1997).

Functioning ovarian tumours: Virilising tumours, such as arrhenoblastoma, may cause cessation of periods, hirsutism, male type baldness, acne and sometimes voice changes. Presence of clitoromegaly with secondary amenorrhea is suggestive of androgen-producing tumours.

DISORDERS OF THE ANTERIOR PITUITARY

Malignant tumours are almost never encountered but growth of a benign tumour can cause problems because it expands in a confined space. Elevated gonadotrophins in the presence of a pituitary microadenoma with amenorrhea are not a consequence of secretion by the tumour; another explanation must be sought (Algorithm 1).

Not all intrasellar masses are neoplastic. Cysts, tuberculosis, sarcoidosis and fat deposits have been reported as causes of pituitary compression leading to hypogonadrophic amenorrhea. Very rarely, lymphocytic hypophysitis can mimic a pituitary tumour, often occurring during pregnancy or in the first six months postpartum (Ezzat and Josse 1997).

Pituitary insufficiency may be secondary to ischemia and infarction and appear as a late sequelae to obstetric hemorrhage (Sheehan syndrome). Genetic disorders such as Laurence-Moon-Biedl and Prader-Willi syndromes are very rare and may need expert help in diagnosis. In a large series studied, 91% of sellar and parasellar masses were pituitary adenomas (Freda et al 1996).

Prolactin Secreting Pituitary Tumours

Hyperprolactinemia: Secretion of prolactin from the anterior pituitary is normally under the inhibitory control of hypothalamic dopamine—regulation of prolactin occurs via a short loop feedback in the hypophyseal portal system involving dopamine. Prolactin levels show a steep rise during pregnancy up to 4–20 times the normal value. In non-lactating women, these levels subside within 15–20 days following delivery. In lactating women, high circulating levels may be maintained for up to

ALGORITHM 1: MANAGEMENT OF PITUITARY ADENOMA

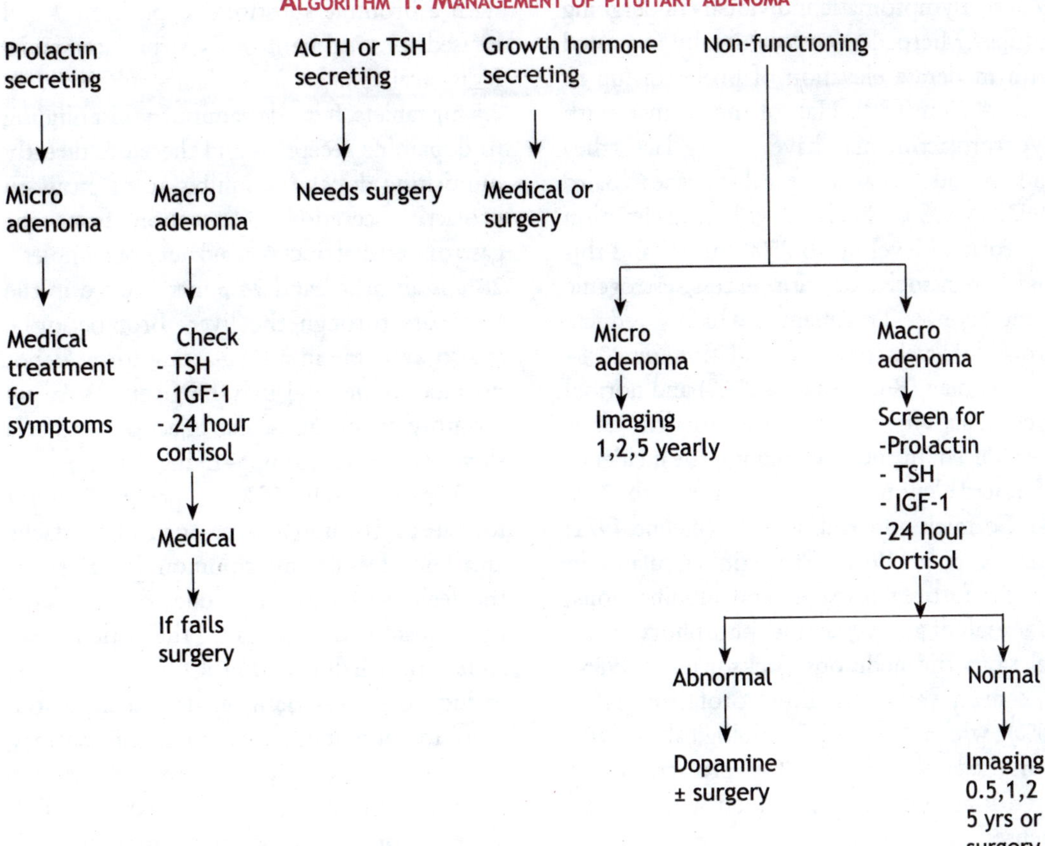

18–24 months. Hyperprolactinemia can cause ovarian inactivity and amenorrhea due to reduced or absent pulsatility of LH secretion, and a lack of a positive feedback response to estrogen.

Transient elevation in serum prolactin levels up to 700 min/l may occur during stressful situations and following breast examination. Hyperprolactinemia is also associated with drugs which inhibit the production or action of dopamine. These drugs include phenothiazines, butyrophenons (haloperidol), benzamides (metchlorpromide), cimetidine, reserpine and methyl dopa. Primary hypothyroidism can also cause hyperprolactinemia and is responsible for 3%–5% of cases.

The commonest causes of pathological hyperprolactinemia include pituitary adenomas accounting for 40%–50% and idiopathic hypersecretion. Most prolactin-secreting tumours are microadenomas (<1 cm), while a few may be larger in size (macroadenomas). Imaging of the pituitary fossa with MRI or CT scan will help identify a pituitary lesion from an extra pituitary one and a microadenoma from a macroadenoma. Macroadenomas carry a potential risk of optic nerve compression, pituitary adenomas are common and occur in

27% of asymptomatic individuals undergoing autopsy. Microadenomas are usually associated with moderate elevation of prolactin (up to 1500–4000 mIU/l). Half of the women with hyperprolactinemia have no galactorrhea and the other half have galactorrhea (Baird 1997). PCOS is associated with mild elevation of prolactin level up to 2500 mIU/l and this may be associated with excess estrogenic stimulation. Treatment which reduces prolactin levels restores ovulation in 80%–90% women (Randeva et al 2000) and normal cyclical activity returns once prolactin levels are reduced. In autopsy findings, the incidence of microadenoma varies from 9% to 27% (McCormick and Halmi 1971; Sheline 1971; Burrow et al 1981). Prolactin circulates in various forms with structural modifications, as a result of glycosylaction, phosphorylation, deletions and additions (Jackson et al 1985). The main variant is 'little' prolactin (80%–85%) which has more biological activity than the larger variants. 'Big' prolactin is the circulating prolactin in women with normal menses.

Very high prolactin levels (> 1000 ng/ml) are associated with invasive tumours—they can usually be effectively treated and controlled with a dopamine agonist.

Approximately a third of women with galactorrhea have normal menses (Speroff et al 1979). Trans-sphenoidal neurosurgery achieves immediate resolution of hyperprolactinemia with resumption of cyclic menses in approximately 30% of patients with macroadenomas and 70% of patients with microadenomas. Radiotherapy is less satisfactory than with surgery. The response is very slow.

DOPAMINE AGONIST TREATMENT

Bromocriptine is a lysergic acid derivative with a bromine substitute at position 2 and is used for treatment of hyperprolactinemia. It is available as a methane sulfonate, in 2.5 mg tablets. It is a dopamine agonist binding to dopamine receptors and therefore directly mimicking dopamine inhibition of pituitary prolactin secretion. Absorption from the gastrointestinal tract is rapid but not complete: 28% is absorbed and 94% metabolised in the first pass through the liver. Bromocriptine is also available in a long-acting form (depot bromocriptine) and may be given 50–75 mg monthly as intramuscular injection, and as a slow release oral form, 5–15 mg daily.

Approximately 10% of patients cannot tolerate oral bromocriptine—nausea, headache and faint feeling are common initial signs; the feeling of fainting is due to orthostatic hypotension. Occasionally, the patient may suffer from hallucination. Other side effects include dizziness, fatigue, nasal congestion, vomiting and abdominal cramps; these may be reduced if a small dose is given at bed time (starting with 1.25 mg and increased gradually). Vaginal administration of bromocriptine is an excellent method to avoid side effects, a 2.5 mg tablet is inserted high into the vagina at bedtime, absorption is nearly complete and avoids first pass effect. The responses of macroadenoma to bromocriptine is good and should be used when previous surgery or radiation has failed (Bevan et al 1992).

Other dopamine agonists: Pergolide is more potent, lasts longer and is sometimes better tolerated than bromocriptine. It is given as a single daily dose of 50–150 mg. Other agonists are lysuride, terguride, metergoline and cabergoline. Quinagolide is a non-ergot long-acting dopamine agonist given in a daily bedtime dose of 75–300 mg. Because quinagolide has a higher affinity for the dopamine receptor, tumours resistant to bromocriptine will respond to this drug and it tends to produce fewer side effects; it also has antidepressant properties (Brue et al 1992; Lappohn et al 1992).

Cabergoline: It is an ergot-derived dopamine agonist. Patients resistant to bromocriptine and quinagolide have been reported to respond to cabergoline. It is given orally at doses of 0.5 to 3.0 mg only once weekly—but may be given twice weekly; the side effects are minimal. The low rate of side effects and the once weekly dosage make cabergoline an attractive choice for initial treatment, replacing bromocriptine. The only reservation is the limited experience documenting fetal safety for patients being treated for infertility (Robert et al 1996). Cabergoline may also be given vaginally if needed.

Low dose contraceptives are given if the patient does not wish to become pregnant. Estrogen-induced tumour expansion or growth has not been a problem (Corenblum and Donovan 1993).

PREGNANCY AND PROLACTIN ADENOMAS

Approximately 80% of women with hyperprolactinemia achieve pregnancy with dopamine agonist treatment. Breastfeeding may be allowed without fear of stimulating tumour growth. There is no increase in pregnancy complications. However, 2% of women with hyperprolactinemia and microadenomas will develop signs and symptoms suggestive of tumour growth during pregnancy (Molitch 1985); none usually require surgical intervention. About 15% of women with macroadenoma may have tumour growth symptoms. They develop headache and visual disturbance; bilateral hemianopsia is a typical visual field finding. The latter symptoms respond to dopamine agonist treatment. Termination of pregnancy or neurosurgery is rarely necessary.

The empty sella syndrome: A patient may have an abnormal sella turcica rather than a tumour.

Sheehan syndrome: Acute infarction and necrosis of the pituitary gland due to postpartum hemorrhage and shock is known as Sheehan syndrome. The symptoms of hypopituitarism are seen in the early postpartum period, failure of lactation and loss of pubic and axillary hair. Deficiency in growth hormone and gonadotrophins are the most common, followed by ACTH and last by TSH (Veldhuis and Hammond 1980). Diabetes insipidus is not usually present (and is almost non-existent).

HETEROSEXUAL DEVELOPMENT

Congenital adrenal hyperplasia (CAH): This is an autosomal recessive disorder characterised by the deficiency of the enzymes involved in steroid pathways within the adrenal gland. While classic CAH usually presents in the neonate as a salt-losing crisis and ambiguous genitalia, other variants can lead to virilisation and primary amenorrhea. In rare cases, androgen secreting tumours from the ovary or adrenals may be the cause of virilisation and amenorrhea at puberty.

5α-reductase deficiency: This is an autosomal recessive condition characterised by incomplete male (46,XY) pseudohermaphroditism due to deficiency of the 5α-reductase enzyme. At birth, the external genitalia resemble those associated with androgen insensitivity syndrome.

CENTRAL NERVOUS SYSTEM DISORDERS

Hypothalamic amenorrhea: Higher centres within the cerebral cortex, control pulsatile hypothalamic secretion of GnRH. Ovarian follicular development is impaired if LH pulsatility falls to less than once every two hours.

Estrogen produced in adipose tissue by aromatisation of androgen, has a significant role in maintaining normal feedback control of the hypothalamic–pituitary–ovarian axis. Secretion of leptin from body fat can also regulate GnRH pulsatility; low levels of leptin are associated with amenorrhea (Groumenon et al 2003).

Experimental evidence suggests that corticotrophin-releasing hormone (CRH) inhibits gonadotrophin secretion, probably by augmenting endogenous opioid secretion—this could be the mechanism in stress-related problems (Olster and Ferin 1987) (Fig. 3.4). Women with hypothalamic amenorrhea have reduced FSH, LH and prolactin levels but increased cortisol levels (Olster and Ferin 1987; Berga et al 1989; Biller et al 1990).

Weight loss, anorexia, bulimia: For regular periods to occur, the adipose tissue should account for 22% of the body mass (Frisch 1984). Regular menses are unlikely to occur in those with BMI below 19 kg/m^2. Leptin, a protein hormone secreted exclusively from adipose tissue acts on the CNS pathways to regulate GnRH release from the hypothalamus (Yu et al 1997).

Anorexia nervosa occurs in women under 25. It is an eating disorder (when the person eats too little) and is often practised by the person to resolve a psychological problem, such as self-image. The incidence of this disorder is 1%.

Bulimia is a syndrome marked by episodic and secretive binge-eating followed by self-induced vomiting, fasting or the use of laxatives and diuretics. It appears to be a growing problem among young women (1%). Patients with bulimia have a high incidence of depressive symptoms. It is important to make an early diagnosis to allow psychologic intervention before the syndrome becomes entrenched and severe (Beaumont et al 1993).

Exercise and amenorrhea: Athletic activities, strenuous recreational exercise, ballet and modern dance produce menstrual irregularities and amenorrhea associated with hypothalamic suppression. As many as two-thirds of runners tend to have menstrual irregularities. If training starts before menarche, it may be delayed by three years or more.

There appear to be two major influences—a critical level of body fat and the effect of stress. Young women who weigh less than 115 pounds and lose more than 10 pounds while exercising are the most likely to develop the problem (Speroff and Redwine 1980), an association that supports the critical weight concept of Frisch (1985).

Studies indicate that ovarian activity may be affected by seasonal variation (Ronkainen et al 1985). Acute exercise decreases gonadotrophins and increases prolactin, growth hormone, testosterone, ACTH, the adrenal steroids and endorphin as a result of both enhanced secretion and reduced clearance (Cumming and Rebar 1985). Women athletes tend to have elevated daytime melatonin levels and amenorrheic athletes have an exaggerated nocturnal secretion of melatonin (Laughlin et al 1991) and appear to reflect suppression of GnRH pulsatile secretion. Athletes have relatively low T_4 levels, but amenorrheic athletes have an overall suppression of all circulating thyroid hormones, including reverse T_3 (Loucks et al 1992).

Amenorrheic athletes are in a state of negative energy balance—they have elevated levels of insulin-like growth factor binding protein-1 (IGFBP-1), increased insulin sensitivity/decreased insulin levels and decreased growth hormone levels (Laughlin and Yen 1996). The majority of women regain ovulation when stress and exercise diminish or cease (Stager et al 1984).

INHERITED GENETIC DEFECTS

Deficient secretion of GnRH is a consequence of Kallmann syndrome and the inherited disorder of adrenal hypoplasia. Amenorrhea and anosmia are a rare condition in women with congenital hypogonadotrophic hypogonadism syndrome due to deficient secretion of GnRH associated with anosmia or hyposmia (known as Kallmann syndrome) (Kallman et al 1944). This syndrome is characterised by primary amenorrhea, infantile sexual development, low gonadotrophins, a normal female karyotype, and the inability to perceive odours.

Hypogonadotrophic hypogonadism: This is characterised by reduced secretion of FSH and LH, which leads to failure of follicular development and estradiol production. When it occurs before puberty, those affected are likely to be short and devoid of secondary sexual characteristics. The common causes are congenital infections leading to hydrocephalus, cranial trauma and tumours (for example, craniopharyngioma). Turner syndrome is associated with short stature.

Most individuals with hypogonadotrophic amenorrhea respond to GnRH, this genetic defect is not common, and is worth pursuing only in patients who have family members with similar presentations.

Adrenal hypoplasia: Adrenal hypoplasia is an X-linked inherited disorder that results in adrenal deficiency, and in survivors, hypogonadotrophic hypogonadism. This is caused by mutations in the DAX-1 gene.

Post-pill amenorrhea: Amenorrhea following the use of steroids for contraception requires investigation. It was assumed that OCCP (combined OCP) and Depo-Provera produced secondary amenorrhea. Investigation is mandatory if the menstrual cycle is not established six months after the OCCP is discontinued or after 12 months following Depo-Provera stoppage. Post-pill amenorrhea affects about 1% of women and is more common among those who tend to experience significant weight loss during pill use. The cause is often not clear—it is possible that the withdrawal of the pill may unmask an underlying pathology such as PCO. Up to 30% of women on Depo-Provera may be amenorrheic, hence counselling the patient is mandatory.

SYSTEMIC DISEASE

Thyroid disease may cause anovulation and amenorrhea by compromising the normal activity of the HPO axis. Chronic renal

FIGURE 3.4: STRESS-RELATED AMENORRHEA

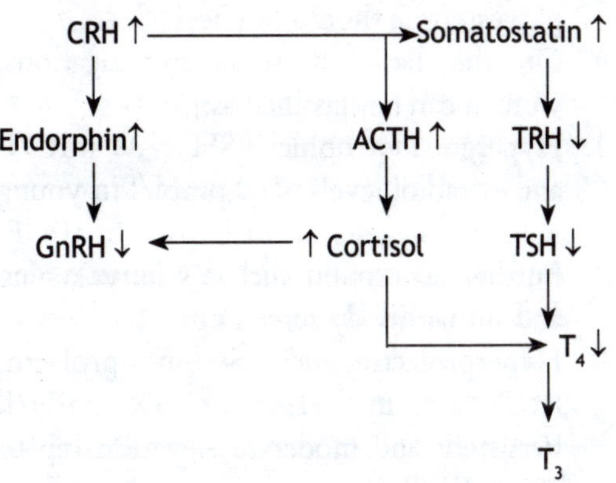

failure is an uncommon cause of secondary amenorrhea. Severe liver disease, particularly chronic active hepatitis can be associated with secondary amenorrhea. Tuberculosis involving the genital tract, especially destruction of the endometrium may cause amenorrhea.

EVALUATION AND MANAGEMENT

Secondary amenorrhea

- A detailed history should be taken to exclude pregnancy, menopause and concurrent medication
- Assessment for significant weight loss or gain, stress, vigorous exercise, anorexia nervosa, hirsutism, visual disturbances and galactorrhea
- A history of uterine curettage, chronic infective or metabolic illness needs to be excluded
- Family history of premature menopause examination should include body mass index (BMI) and signs of hyper-androgenic status, general and pelvic examination, followed by ultrasound assessment
- Endocrine investigations should include urinary or serum βhCG, serum FSH, LH, estradiol, prolactin, TSH, T_4 and T_3. When features of hirsutism or virilisation are present, levels of serum testosterone, androstenedione, DHEA, 17-OH progesterone should be checked.
- On the basis of these investigations, women can be classified as:

1. Hypergonadotrophic: FSH >30 mIU/L and estradiol levels <60 pmol/l in young women suggests a diagnosis of POF. Further assessment includes karyotyping and autoantibody screening
2. Hyperprolactinemic: Serum prolactin levels are in excess of 500 mIU/l. Persistent and moderate elevation (up to 700 mIU/l) is seen in hypothyroidism. A thyroid profile should be done before considering therapy. Women with PCOS may have raised prolactin levels and a full clinical assessment, ovarian scan and endocrine profile is needed prior to planning treatment. Progesterone challenge in these women should lead to uterine bleeding from the estrogen primed endometrium. When serum prolactin level is more than 1500 mIU/l, CT or MRI scan of the pituitary fossa is indicated. Serum prolactin level more than 5000 mIU/l is suggestive of macroprolactinoma.
3. Hypogonadotrophic: Amenorrhea is often triggered by stress, weight loss, with low BMI and low or undetectable levels of FSH, LH and estradiol.
4. Normogonadotrophic: These women account for up to a third of women with secondary amenorrhea. They have normal FSH levels. The LH/FSH ratio may be elevated in women with PCOS; on the other hand, women with uterine pathology have normal gonadotrophin levels. Progesterone challenge test using medroxy progesterone acetate, 10 mg orally, for five days may help to distinguish between the two. Withdrawal bleeding is indicative of an estrogen-primed endometrium and an intact outflow tract.

Therapeutic options

- Treatment depends on the specific cause.
- Hyperprolactinemia is treated medically with the help of dopaminergic agents. Bromocriptine is used extensively. Sometimes side effects are troublesome and include nausea, vomiting and hypotension. Cabergoline may be used as an alternative to bromocriptine; it is given twice weekly and has fewer side effects. Macroadenomas, unresponsive to drugs and producing pressure symptoms, need

trans-sphenoidal surgery. Women will require contraceptive advice; in case they do not wish to become pregnant, a barrier method can be offered. Women should be warned about the possibility of increase in size of the tumour during pregnancy. Regular visual field examination is mandatory during pregnancy.

- While planning treatment for women with PCOS it is mandatory to consider major problems such as infertility, hirsutism and irregular menstruation. Ovulation induction with clomiphene is the first line of treatment if pregnancy is desired. Failure with clomiphine may justify use of gonadotrophins or laparoscopic drilling. Anti-androgens such as cyproterone acetate with ethinyl estradiol (Dianette) or spironolactone may be tried for hirsutism. If fertility or hirsutism does not require treatment, the endometrium is protected using either OCCP or cyclical progestin. Overweight women are advised to lose weight—support and counselling should be offered. Insulin-sensitising agents such as metformin are used in women with PCOS.
- Women with POF need prophylactic treatment against osteoporosis as well as relief from symptoms, HRT or OCCP is used.
- Asherman syndrome could be treated with hysteroscopic adhesolysis
- Secondary amenorrhea may be physiological as in pregnancy or during lactation. Alternatively, it may be symptomatic of a number of serious disorders of the reproductive system—a systematic approach for evaluation and management is necessary. The treatment depends on the symptoms and the wishes of the patient.

Primary amenorrhea

- A detailed history should be elicited—delayed puberty/menarche in siblings or the mother is relevant in cases of constitutional delay.
- Enquiry into eating habits, exercise, weight change, periodic abdominal pains or acute retention of urine, headache and anosmia may be relevant
- Examination of the adolescent is best performed in the presence of the patient's mother and should include assessment of secondary sexual characteristics.
- Signs of hyperandrogenism and virilisation should be looked for
- An ultrasound examination to confirm the presence of uterus and ovaries should be performed
- MRI or CT scan may be necessary
- If the ultrasound suggests hematocolpos and hematometra, an examination under anesthesia should be done
- In case of an absent uterus, a karyotype should be done. MRKH syndrome may be diagnosed if the karyotype is 46,XX and the uterus is absent.
- A 46,XY karyotype suggests androgen insensitivity syndrome.
- When normal anatomy is confirmed, baseline gonadotrophins, prolactin and estradiol levels should be measured
- Further evaluation depends on the results of hormonal levels
- When serum FSH and LH levels are elevated, primary ovarian failure is the most likely diagnosis. The presence of 46,XY chromosome will identify cases of testicular dysgenesis. If the karyotype is XX, anti-ovarian antibodies may be the cause of ovarian failure. Related autoimmune disorders should be checked for.

- When FSH and LH levels are low, hypothalamic–pituitary imaging will confirm the presence of a tumour such as craniopharyngioma or a non-secreting pituitary adenoma.

It may be necessary to distinguish a hypothalamic cause from a pituitary one using a GnRH test (100 µg SC) after administering ethinyl estradiol orally at a dose of 5–10 µg a day for a week. This would assess the responsiveness of the pituitary and its capacity to secrete gonadotrophins. If the hypothalamus and pituitary are normal, the diagnosis is usually constitutional delay.

The normogonadotrophic group includes girls with PCOS, of whom 20%–30% may have normal ovaries on scanning. The elevation in LH, testosterone and occasionally prolactin levels, are helpful in confirming the diagnosis.

- A moderate elevation of serum prolactin is common in girls with hypothyroidism or PCOS. Serum concentrations above 1500 mIU/l warrant imaging of the pituitary fossa. MRI will detect the presence of pituitary macro- or microadenomas.
- The cause of amenorrhea and the clinical and social circumstances dictate the type and timing of treatment.
- Surgery is necessary in cases of imperforate hymen and transverse vaginal septum.
- Those with absent vagina and MRKH may be treated conservatively with vaginal dilators.
- When dilatation fails, surgery (vaginoplasty) is indicated.
- Gonadectomy is essential in an XY female between 16 and 18 years of age, once optimum height is achieved.
- Girls with estrogen deficiency may need replacement therapy to develop secondary sexual characteristics. It is important to prevent osteoporosis.
- For pubertal development, low dose ethinyl estradiol (2 µg daily) should be commenced and gradually increased according to breast response and age. Oral progesterone is added when breakthrough bleeding occurs or when ethinyl estradiol dose is 20 µg/day. She can be subsequently maintained on OCCP or conventional cyclic postmenopausal HRT.
- Primary amenorrhea is often a manifestation of an underlying disorder, identification of the precise cause is essential before treatment is contemplated. Interventions should be sensitive to the wishes of the patient, and tailored to her needs.

References

Aiman J and C Smentek. 1985. Premature ovarian failure. *Obstet Gynecol* 66:9.

Aittomaki K, JL Dieguez Lucena, P Pakarinen et al. 1995. Mutation in the follicle stimulating hormone receptor gene causes hereditary hypergonadotropic ovarian failure. *Cell* 82:959.

Aittomaki K, R Herva, VH Stenman et al. 1996. Clinical features of primary ovarian failure caused by a point mutation in the follicle stimulating hormone receptor gene. *J Clin Endocrinol Metab* 81:3722.

Allingham-Hawkins DJ, RR Babul-Hirji, D Chitayat et al. 1999. Fragile X permutation is a significant risk factor for premature ovarian failure. The international collaborative POF in fragile X study: Preliminary data. *Am J Med Gen* 83:322–325.

Alper MM and PR Garner. 1985. Premature ovarian failure: Its relationship to autoimmune disease. *Obstet Gynecol* 66:27.

Anasti JN, MR Flack, J Froehlich, LM Nelson. 1995. The use of human recombinant gonadotrophin receptors to search for immunoglobulin G-mediated premature ovarian failure. *J Clin Endocrinol Metab* 80:824.

Axelrod L, RM Neer, B Kilman. 1979. Hypogonadism in a male with immunologically active, biologically in active luteinizing hormone: An exception to a venerable rule. *J Clin Endocrinol Metab* 48:279.

Baird DT. 1997. Amenorrhoea. *Lancet* 35:275–279.

Baker TG. 1963. A quantitative and cytological study of germ cells in human ovaries. *Proc Roy Soc Lond* 158:417.

Bates GW and WL Wiser. 1985. A technique for uterine conservation in adolescents with vaginal agenesis and a functional uterus. *Obstet Gynecol* 66:290.

Batzer FR, ZL Corson, B Gocial, et al. 1992. Genetic offspring in patients with vaginal agenesis: Specific medical and legal issues. *Am J Obstet Gynecol* 167:1288.

Beaumont PJV, JD Russell, SW Touyz. 1993. Treatment of anorexia nervosa. *Lancet.* 341:1635.

Berga SL, JF Mortola, GB Suh et al. 1989. Neuroendocrine aberrations in women with functional hypothalamic amenorrhoea. *J Clin Endocrinol Metab* 68:301.

Bevan JS, Webster J, Burke CW, Scanion MF. 1992. Dopamine agonist and pituitary tumour shrinkage. *Endocr Rev* 13:220.

Biller BMK, HJ Federoff, JI Koering et al. 1990. Abnomral cortisol secretion and responses to corticotrophin releasing hormone in women with hypothalamic amenorrhoea. *J Clin Endocrinol Metab* 70:311.

Blumenfeld Z, S Halachmi, BA Peretz. 1993. Premature ovarian failure: The prognostic application of autoimmunity on conception after ovulation induction. *Fertil Steril* 59:750.

Brue T, I Pellegrini, G Gunz et al. 1992. Effects of the dopamine against CV 205-502 in human prolactinomas resistant to bromocriptine. *J Clin Endocrinol Metab* 74:577.

Buckler HM, A Evans, H Mamlora et al. 1991. Gonadotrophin, steroid and inhibin levels in women with incipient ovulation failure during anovulatory and ovulatory 'rebound' cycles. *J Clin Endocrinol Metab* 72:116.

Burrow GN, G Wortzman, NB Rewcastle et al. 1981. Microadenomas of the pituitary and abnormal sellar tomograms in an unselected auto series. *New Engl J Med* 304:156.

Comtoise R, J Bouchard, F Robert. 1989. Hypersecretion of gonadotrophins by a pituitary adenoma: Pituitary dynamic studies and treatment with bromocriptine in one patient. *Fertil Steril* 52:569.

Contreras P, G Genevini, H Michelson et al. 1981. Hyperprolactinemia and galactorrhea: Spontaneous versus iatrogenic hypothyroidism. *J Clin Endocrinol Metab* 53:1036.

Conway GS, G Kaltas, A Patel et al. 1996. Characteristics of idiopathic premature ovarian failure. *Fertil Steril* 65:339–341.

Corenblum B, I Donovan. 1993. The safety of physiological estrogen plus progestin replacement therapy and oral contraceptive therapy in women with pathological hyperprolactinemia. *Fertil Steril* 59:671.

Coulam CB, SB Adamsen, JF Annegers. 1986. Incidence of premature ovarian failure. *Obstet Gynecol* 67:604.

Cramer DW, DP Goldskin, C Fraer, JKV Reichardt. 1996. Vaginal agenesis. Mayer–Rokitansky–Kuster–Hauser syndrome associated with the N314D mutation of galactose-1-phosphate uridyl transferase. GALT. *Mol Hum Reprod* 2:145.

Cumming DC and RW Rebar. 1985. Hormonal changes with acute exercise and with training in women. *Semin Reprod Endocrinol* 3:55.

Delon B, H Lallaoui, C Abel-Lablanche et al. 1997. Fluorescent in situ hybridization and sequence-tagged sites for delineation of an XY translocation in a patient with secondary amenorrhoea. *Mol Hum Reprod* 3:439.

Devi AS, DA Metzzer, AA Luciano, PA Benn. 1998. 45 X/46 XX mosaicism in patients with idiopathic premature ovarian failure. *Fertil Steril* 70:89.

Dewald GW and Spurbeck JL. 1983. Sex chromosome anomalies associated with premature gonadal failure. *Semin Reprod Endocrinol* 1:79.

Dunaif A and A Thomas. 2001. Current concepts in the polycystic ovary syndrome. *Ann Rev Med* 52:401–419.

Dunaif A. 1997. Insulin resistance and the polycystic ovary syndrome mechanism and implications for pathogenesis. *Endocr Rev* 18:774–800.

Ezzat S and RG Josse. 1997. Autoimmune hypophysitis. *Trends Endocrinol Metab* 8:74.

Frank RT. 1938. Formation of artificial vagina without operation. *Am J Obstet Gynecol* 35:1053.

Freda PU, SL Wardlaw, KD Post. 1996. Unusual causes of sellar/para sellar masses in a large transphenoidal surgical series. *J Clin Endocrinol Metab* 81:3455.

Frisch RE. 1984. *Body fat puberty and fertility.* Biological reviews of the Cambridge Philosophical Society. 59:161–168.

Frisch RE. 1985. Body fat, menarche, and reproductive ability. *Semin Reprod Endocrinol* 3:45.

Gondos B, P Bhiraleus, C Hobel. 1971. Ultrastructural observations on germ cells in human fetal ovaries. *Am J Obstet Gynecol* 110:644.

Griffin JE. 1992. Androgen resistance: The clinical and molecular spectrum. *New Engl J Med* 326:611.

Groumenon AG, IM Mattaliotakis, GE Koumantakis et al. 2003. The role of leptin in fertility. *Eur J Obstet Gynecol Reprod Biol* 160(2):118–124.

Huhtanieni I, P Parkarinen, C Nilssen et al. 1996. Polymorphism and mutations of gonadotrophins and gonadotrophin genes. In *The ovary, regulation, dysfunction and treatment* eds M Filicori, C Flannigni. Amsterdam: Elsevier Science, 85–101.

Jackson RD, J Wortsman, WB Malarkey. 1985. Characteristic of a large molecular weight prolactin in women with idiopathic hyperprolactinemia and normal menses. *J Clin Endocrinol Metab* 61:258.

Kallmann FJ, WA Schoenfeld, SE Barrera. 1944. The genetic aspects of primary eunuchoidism. *Am J Ment Defic* 48:203.

Katznelson L, JM Alexander, HA Bikkal et al. 1992. Imbalanced follicle-stimulating hormone: Subunit hormone bio synthesis in human pituitary adenomas. *J Clin Endocrinol Metab* 74:1343.

Lappohn RÈ, HBM Van de Wiel, J Brownell. 1992. The effect of two dopaminergic drug on menstrual function and psychological state in hyperprolactinemia. *Fertil Steril* 58:321.

Laughlin GA, AB Loucks, SSC Yen. 1991. Marked augmentation of nocturnal melatonin secretion in amenorrheic athletes, but not in cycling athletes: Unaltered by opioidergic or dopaminergic blockade. *J Clin Endocrinol Metab* 73:1321.

Laughlin GA and SSC Yen. 1996. Nutritional and endocrine-metabolic aberrations in amenorrheic athletes. *J Clin Endocrinol Metab* 81:4301.

Loucks AB, GA Laughlin, JF Mortola et al. 1992. Hypothalamic–pituitary–thyroidal function in eumenorrheic and amenorrheic athletes. *J Clin Endocrinol Metab* 75:514.

Manuel M, KP Katayama, JR HW Jones. 1976. The age of occurrence of gonadal tumours in intersex patients with a Y chromosome. *Am J Obstet Gynecol* 124:293–300.

Mc Cormick WF, NS Halmi. 1971. Absence of chromophobe adenomas from a large series of pituitary tumours. *Arch Pathol* 92:231.

Molitch ME. 1985. Pregnancy and the hyperprolactinemic woman. *New Engl J Med* 312:1362.

Morris JM and VB Mahesh. 1963. Further observation on the syndrome "testicular feminization". *Am J Obstet Gynecol* 87:731.

Nelson LM, JN Anasti, LM Kimzay et al. 1994. Development of luteinized graafian follicles in patients with karyotypically normal spontaneous premature ovarian failure. *J Clin Endocrinol Metab* 79:1970.

Nelson LM, LM Kimzey, GR Merriam. 1992. Gonadotrophin suppression for the treatment of karyotypically normal spontaneous premature ovarian failure: A controlled trial. *Fertil Steril* 57:50.

Olster DH, Ferin M. 1987. Corticotrophin-releasing hormone inhibits gonadotrophin secretion in the ovariectomized rhesus monkey. *J Clin Endocrinol Metab* 65:262.

Pasquino AM, F Passeri, I Pucarelli et al. 1997. Spontaneous pubertal development in Turner's syndrome. *J Clin Endocrinol Metab* 82:1810.

Poretsky L, J Garber, J Kleefield. 1986. Primary amenorrhea and pseudoprolactinemia in a patient with primary hypothyroidism. *Am J Med* 81:180.

Randeva HS and M Davis. GM Prelevic. 2000. Prolactinoma and pregnancy. *Br J Obstet Gynaecol* 107:1064–1068.

Rebar RW and HV Connolly. 1990. Clinical feature of young women with hypergonadotropic amenorrhoea. *Fertil Steril* 53:804.

Reindollar RH, M Novak, SPT Tho, PG Mc Donough. 1986. Adult onset amenorrhea: A study of 262 patient. *Am J Obstet Gynecol* 155:531.

Robert E, L Musatti, G Piscitelli, CI Ferrari. 1996. Pregnancy outcome after treatment with ergot derivative, cabergoline. *Reprod Toxicol* 10:333.

Ronkainen H, A Pakarinen, P Kirkinen et al. 1985. Physical exercise induced changes and season associated differences in the pituitary–ovarian function of runners and joggers. *J Clin Endocrinol Metab* 60:416.

Rutgers JL and RE Scully. 1991. The androgen insensitivity syndrome, testicular feminization: A clinicopathologic study of 43 cases. *Int J Gynecol Path* 10:126.

Sharma K. 1990. Age at menarche in north west Indian females and review of Indian data. *Ann Human Biol* 17(2):159–162.

Sheline GE. 1971. Untreated and recurrent chromophobe adenomas of the pituitary. *Radiology* 112:768.

Speroff L, RH Glass, NG Kase. 1999. Amenorrhea *In Clinical gynecologic endocrinology and infertility*. 6th ed. Baltimore: Williams & Wilkins, 421.

Speroff L, RM Levin, RV Haning Jr, NG Kase. 1979. A practical approach for the evaluation of women with abnormal polytomography of elevated prolactin levels. *Am J Obstet Gynecol* 135:896.

Speroff I and DB Redwine. 1980. Exercise and menstrual function. *Physician Sport Med* 8:42.

Stager JM, RB Ritchie–Flanagan, D Robertshaw. 1984. Reversibility of amenorrhea in athletes. *New Engl J Med* 310:51.

Talbert LM, MHG Raj, MG Hammond et al. 1984. Endocrine and immunologic studies in a patient with resistant ovary syndrome. *Fertil Steril* 42:741.

Teasdale E, G Teasdale, F Mohsen, P Macpherson. 1986. High resolution computed tomography in pituitary micro adenoma. Is seeing believing? *Clin Radiol* 37:227.

Troche V and E Hernandez. 1986. Neoplasia arising in dysgenetic gonads. *Obstet Gynecol* 41:74.

Veldhuis JH and JM Hammond. 1980. Endocrine function after spontaneous infarction of the human pituitary, report, review and reappraisal. *Endocrinol Rev* 1:100.

Wabrek AJ, PR Millard, WB Wilson Jr, RJ Pion. 1971. Creation of neovagina by the Frank non-operative method. *Obstet Gynecol* 37:408.

Yu MH, M Kimura, A Walezewska et al. 1997. Role of leptin in hypothalamo-pituitary function. *Proc Natl Acad Sci* 94:1023–1028.

4

Sexual Ambiguity—Intersex Disorders

BN Chakravarty | NJ Gupta

Sexual ambiguity is defined as the existence of both male and female genital organs in the same individual. Ambiguity may involve external genital organs alone or both internal and external genital organs.

SEXUAL AMBIGUITY AND INTERSEX

Sexual ambiguity of the external genital organ is the most common, but not invariable, marker of all intersex problems. Three major intersex problems exist:

- Female intersex
- Male intersex
- True intersex

In Allen's classification (1985), 'mixed' gonadal dysgenesis with sexual ambiguity has also been included under the heading of intersex disorders.

For evaluation and treatment of sexual ambiguity, it is important to understand the normal embryology leading to the development of male and female genital organs.

Embryologic development of genital organs: Sexual differentiation, either to male or to female type, occurs in an embryo at weeks 7–8 of intrauterine life. There are two phases of sex organ differentiation.

The First Phase: This phase consists of formation of the gonads. This will depend on the chromosomal make-up of the embryo. When the chromosomal make-up is XX, an ovary will form; if it is XY, testis will develop. The chromosomal arrangement is completed at the time of fertilisation.

The molecular basis of gonadal development is complex. The gene sequence known as testis determining factor (TDF) on the Y chromosome appears to be responsible for testis development. In its absence, the ovary will form (Wiener and Gonzales 1996). In addition to TDF, other sex determining genes have been identified. These include SRY, DSS, DOX-9, DOX-3 etc. When either TDF or other sex determining gene(s) are absent or mutated, the testis cannot function properly even if the Y chromosome is present. This will lead to a clinical situation of intersex.

Immediately following development of the gonads, the external and internal genital organs start developing (Table 4.1). This brings about the second phase of sexual development. The external genital organs continue to develop till up to 20 weeks, whereas the development of the internal genital organs is completed within week 10 of intrauterine life.

Table 4.1: Normal sexual differentiation: first phase

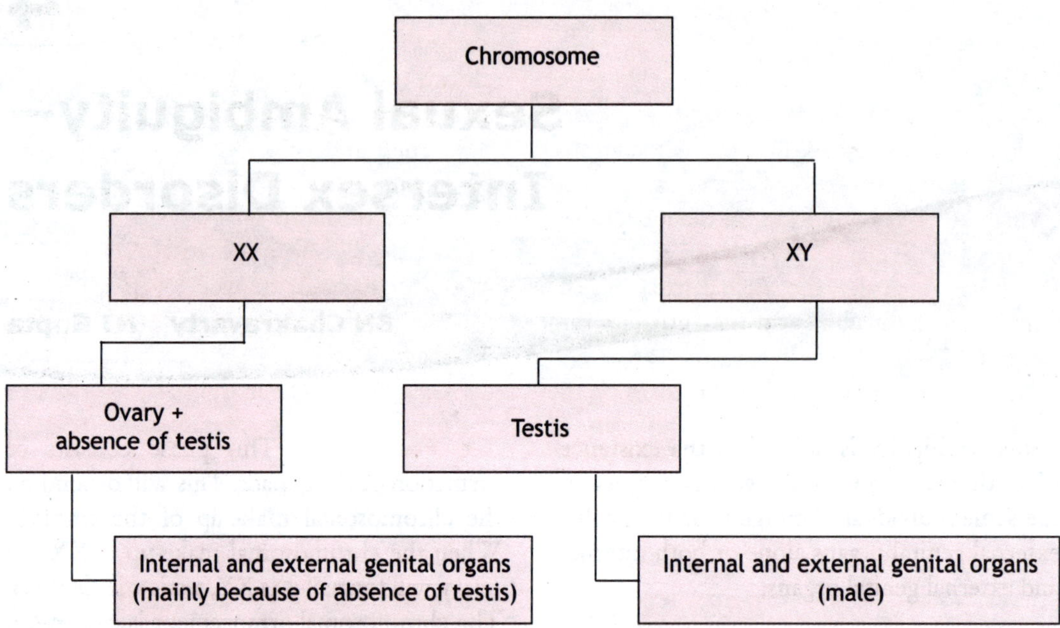

The Second Phase: With the formation of the gonads, external and internal genital organs begin developing—from two different sources:

a. From urogenital sinus derivatives (external genital organs)
b. From mesodermal derivatives (internal genital organs)

A communication is established between the external and internal genital organs, through the urogenital sinus. The external genital organs in association with the urinary bladder and the urethra (commonly known as urogenital organs), develop from primitive cloaca, which subdivides to form the ventral urogenital sinus and the dorsal cloaca.

The ventral urogenital sinus is further anatomically subdivided into two parts—cephalic and caudal. The cephalic end is the embryologic source of origin of the bladder and the ureteric diverticulum (metanephric duct) in both male and female (Fig. 4.1).

The caudal part of the urogenital sinus in the male will develop into the prostate, prostatic and membranous urethra into which the structure derived from the Wolffian duct (the vas deferens) will drain. The site of

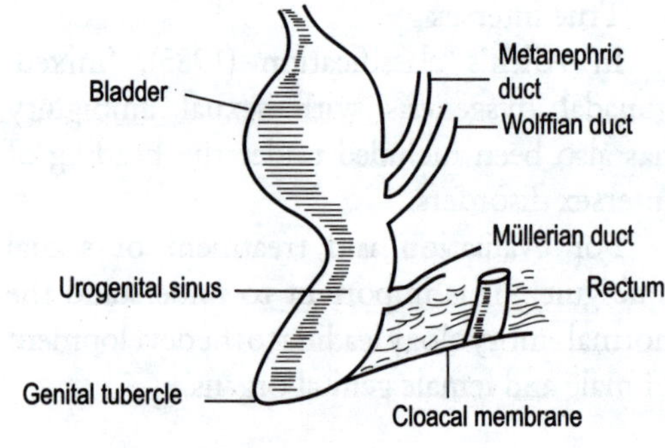

Figure 4.1: Embryologic source of development of external genital organs and the site of its communication with internal genital organs (*Adapted from "Intersexual Disorders" - Dewhurst and Gordon 1969*)

drainage into the urethra is known as the prostatic utricle (embryologic homologue of uterus).

In the male, the testis produces two types of hormones, testosterone and müllerian inhibitory substance (MIS). In the fetal testis, MIS will lead to regression of müllerian ducts, which otherwise will form the fallopian tubes, uterus and vagina.

In the female, the caudal part of the urogenital sinus will form the entire urethra and the vestibule into which the lower part of the müllerian duct will open forming the lower vagina. The site of contact between the lower part of the müllerian duct and dorsal wall of the caudal part of the urogenital sinus will form the sinovaginal bulb. Following canalisation, this area (sinovaginal bulb) will develop into the lower vagina, hymen and vestibule (Table 4.2).

Therefore, the caudal part of the urogenital sinus contributes mainly to the development of a communicating channel between the internal and external genital organs in both males and females. However, the more important components of the external genital organs originate from structures which lie in close proximity to the urogenital sinus (Table 4.3). These are:

a. Genital tubercle: This is the embryologic source of origin of the penis in the male and the clitoris in the female.
b. Genital fold: In the male, it forms the penile urethra and in the female it contributes to the formation of the labia minora.
c. Genital swelling: In the male, it leads to the formation of the scrotum; in the female, it contributes to the development of the labia majora.

Development of external genitalia in the male or female direction will primarily depend on the presence or absence of androgens (and androgen receptors) and not on chromosomes. Excess of androgen leads to the development of external genitalia tending towards male (for example, the virilising influence of CAH),

TABLE 4.2: NORMAL SEXUAL DIFFERENTIATION: SECOND PHASE

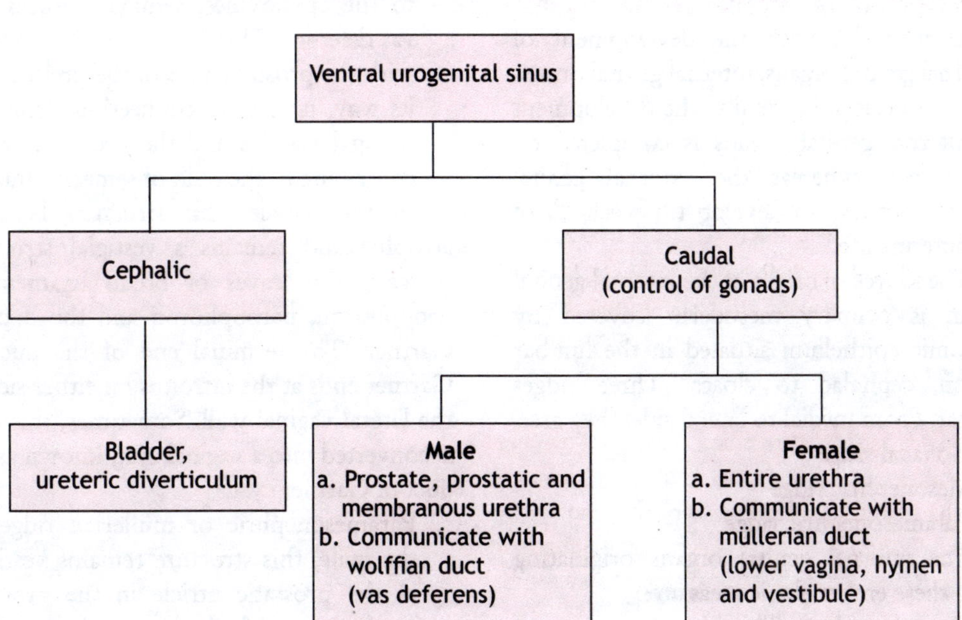

TABLE 4.3: EMBRYOLOGICAL ORIGIN OF EXTERNAL GENITAL ORGANS FROM AREAS IN THE PROXIMITY OF THE UROGENITAL SINUS (CHROMOSOMAL AND GONADAL INFLUENCE)

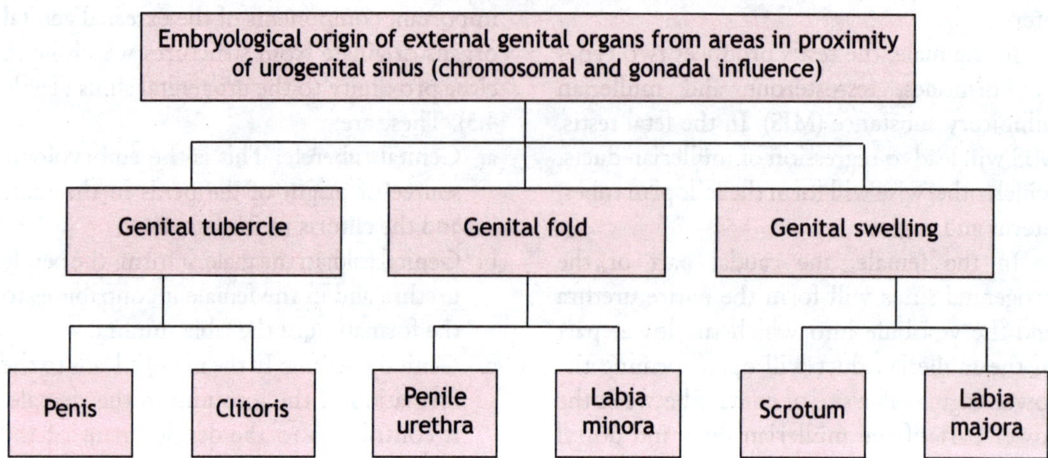

even when the chromosome pattern is 46,XX. On the other hand, if an adequate amount of androgens are present but no androgen receptors, the development of external genitalia will tend towards female (testicular feminising syndrome) in individuals with 46,XY chromosomes.

Development of internal genital organs:

Simultaneously, with the development of external genital organs, internal genital organs start to develop. Normally, the development of internal genital organs is completed by ten weeks, whereas the external genital organs continue to develop till week 20 of intrauterine life.

The source of origin of the internal genital organ is primary mesoderm covered by coelomic epithelium situated in the lumbar region, cephalad to cloaca. Three ridges appear. From medial to lateral side, they are:

- Gonadal ridge
- Mesonephric ridge
- Paramesonephric ridge

The internal genital organs originating from these embryologic areas are:

a. Genital ridge: This is the area of development of primitive gonads. In the male, the testis will develop and in females, the ovaries. Germ cells migrate to this area from the hindgut to form either male or female gametes (spermatocytes or oocytes) within the gonads.

b. Mesonephric ridge: In the male, this ridge forms the testicular duct which gives rise to the epididymes, seminal vesicles and vas deferens. This duct connects the testis with the prostatic part of the urethra. On its way, it receives connections from the seminal vesicles and the prostate, which contribute to the bulk of semen volume.

In the female, this structure becomes atrophic and remains a vestigial structure between the leaves of broad ligament as epoophoron, paroophoron and the duct of Gartner. The terminal end of the duct of Gartner ends at the introitus on either side of the lateral vaginal wall. Sometimes, this duct is converted into a vaginal cyst, known as the duct of Gartner cyst.

c. Paramesonephric or müllerian ridge: In the male, this structure remains vestigeal as the prostatic utricle in the prostatic urethra into which the ejaculatory duct, formed by the union of the seminal vesicle and vas deferens, will drain. In the female, this structure forms the fallopian tubes, uterus and upper two-thirds of the vagina.

To sum up, development of the external and internal sex organs will depend on chromosomal, gonadal, genetic and endocrinological factors. An abnormality in one or more of these factors will lead to sexual ambiguity. Clinical situations in which these factors may become relevant for the development of sexual ambiguity are briefly discussed below.

Chromosomal Anomalies: Chromosomal anomalies do not always lead to sexual ambiguity. For example, in Turner syndrome (45,XO) or in Klinefelter syndrome (47,XXY), there is no sexual ambiguity. In the classic variety of testicular feminising syndrome (male intersex), there is no ambiguity of external genitalia. However, in the incomplete variety of testicular feminising syndrome (another type of male intersex) and in true intersex, there may be ambiguity of external genitalia.

Gonadal Factors: The testis produces two types of hormones, testosterone and the antimüllerian hormone (AMH). The presence of testosterone combined with the absence of AMH will lead to the presence of the uterus and fallopian tube with male phenotype and male external genitalia. Such uterus, with fallopian tubes, is sometimes accidentally detected in the hernial sac in male intersex individuals. Similarly, deficient Leydig cell function will lead to subnormal testosterone production which may lead to a clinical situation of micropenis with cryptorchidism (a type of male intersex).

Genetic Factors: The presence of a Y chromosome is not enough for maleness. The presence of testis determining factor (TDF) is essential. A 46,XX phenotype boy (sex-reversed boy) can develop into a phenotypic male individual without sexual ambiguity. In this variety, translocation of male determining genetic material (TDF) would lead to male phenotype even in the absence of the Y chromosome (Donahoe 1987; Federman and Donahoe 1995; Blyth and Churchill 1996). Similarly, even in the presence of the Y chromosome, mutation or deletion of sex determining genes will lead to development of 46,XY female (classic testicular feminising syndrome—male intersex). Though these individuals have no ambiguity of external genitalia, there is an ambiguity between chromosomal, gonadal sex on the one hand and phenotypic sex on the other.

In addition, genetically determined enzymatic deficiency which is a receptor defect will lead to sexual ambiguity. Examples of sexual ambiguity due to enzymatic deficiency are 5-α reductase deficiency in male intersex and several enzymatic blocks in congenital adrenal hyperplasia (CAH), the commonest being 21-hydroxylase deficiency. An example of target organ androgen receptor block is the testicular feminising syndrome.

Endocrine Factors: Abnormal androgen production from a hyperactive adrenal cortex will virilise a female fetus with ambiguity of external genitalia. Similar ambiguity is also observed due to a virilising tumour in a female fetus or following administration of progestogens or androgens to the mother in the early months of pregnancy.

CLINICAL FINDINGS AND DIAGNOSIS OF DIFFERENT TYPES OF INTERSEX

Female Intersex

The most common cause of female intersex, after tumours and iatrogenic causes, is congenital adrenal hyperplasia (CAH). In clinical practice, it is also the most common cause of sexual ambiguity. The basic endocrinologic problem is a defect in the biosynthesis of cortisol.

If cortisol production is reduced or absent, the negative feedback control on the pituitary will be decreased, resulting in increased pituitary output of ACTH. The adrenal gland reacts to ACTH stimulation by increased production of androgens and estrogens from zona reticularis. In intrauterine life, androgen virilises the external genitalia of a female fetus. Depending on the time of onset, the amount of androgen secreted and the duration of exposure, there will be varying grades of labioscrotal fusion, clitoral enlargement and anatomical occlusion of the urethra and vagina (Figs 4.2–4.7).

The vagina and the urethra share a common urogenital sinus formed by the fusion of the labial folds. Complete vaginal suppression due to the virilising effect of congenital adrenal hyperplasia has rarely been reported. This is an important point of advantage during surgical correction. In the commonest type (in 21-hydroxylase deficiency), there is accumulation of dihydroepiandrosterone (DHEA) which is a weak androgen. Consequently, these affected girls are less masculinised. Therefore, in the majority, a separate vaginal and urethral opening can easily be identified.

Internal genital organs are not affected in CAH. This is because development of the internal genital organ is completed by weeks 10–12, whereas a significant amount of androgen secretion from the adrenal cortex starts thereafter. Moreover, there is no anomalous secretion of the antimüllerian hormone in females, affected with congenital adrenal hyperplasia.

In addition to ambiguity of external genitalia, excess androgens and estrogens have undesirable metabolic side effects. During infancy and childhood, bone growth

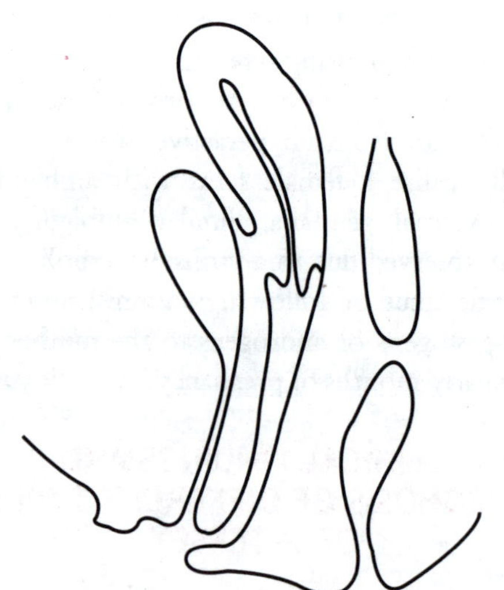

Figure 4.2: Slight enlargement of phallus; urethral and vaginal orifices are easily identified

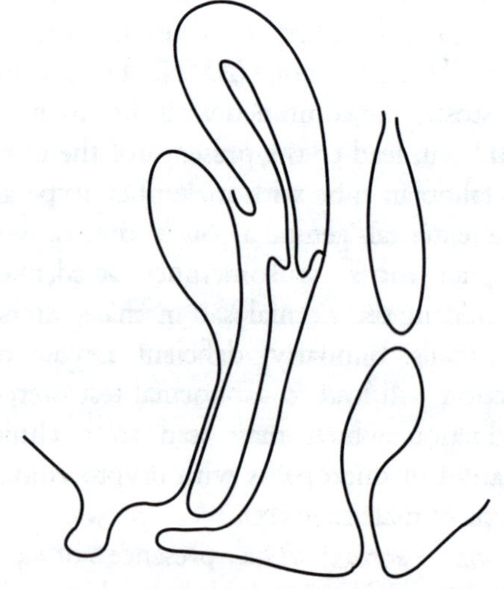

Figure 4.3: Moderate enlargement of phallus; urethral and vaginal orifices are difficult to locate

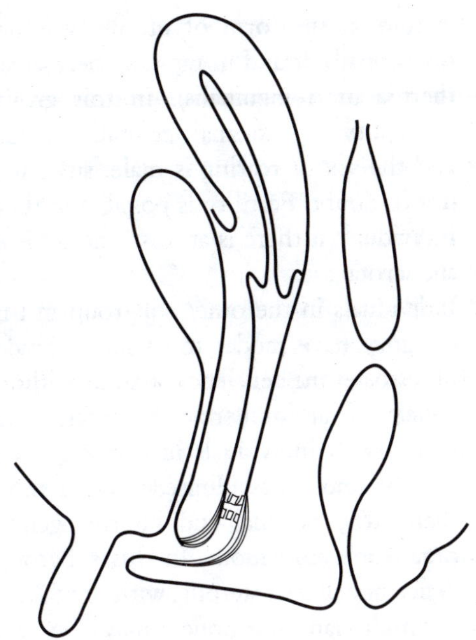

FIGURE 4.4: GROSS ENLARGEMENT OF PHALLUS, TOTAL CONCEALMENT OF URETHRAL AND VAGINAL OPENING, OCCASIONAL ABSENCE OF COMMUNICATION BETWEEN LOWER END OF MÜLLERIAN DUCT AND UPPER END OF UROGENITAL SINUS (EXTREMELY RARE)

is markedly stunted, and epiphyseal fusion occurs before attaining adult height. Static estrogen excess puts a negative feedback effect on the gonadotrophin function resulting in the absence of breast development and amenorrhea. Increased androgen levels may be responsible for increased hair on the face and body.

More than half of the patients with CAH will have a deficiency of the enzyme, 21-hydroxylase, which leads to elevated serum levels of 17-hydroxy progesterone (17-OHP) and increased urinary pregnanetriol (Allen 1985). Diagnosis of CAH is confirmed by estimation of serum 17-OHP. The normal level of serum 17-OHP in the morning should be less than 200 ng/dl.; levels higher than 800 ng/dl are diagnostic of CAH. Levels between 200 ng/dl and 800 ng/dl require an ACTH stimulation test for confirmation of diagnosis of CAH.

Immediately after birth, the 17-OHP level is elevated (1000–3000 ng/ml). This declines to a value of 100–200 ng/dl after 24 hours. In affected infants, the value of 17-OHP range between 3000 and 40,000 ng/dl. Many infants are at a risk of salt wasting, and therefore, to the risk of dehydration and hypotension. Deficiency of 11-hydroxylase (another variety of CAH) on the other hand, may be associated with salt retention and hypertension (Robertson and Walker 1975). 3-OL dehydrogenase deficiency is the rarest form of defects in CAH; these patients do not usually survive (because of severe salt wastage).

Prenatal Diagnosis of CAH: Amniocentesis and chorion villous biopsy may be helpful for prenatal diagnosis (Reindoller et al 1988). The objective is to institute treatment with dexamethasone before the female fetus is affected by genital ambiguity (Mulaikal et al 1987; Meyer-Bahlburg et al 1996.) However, as the prenatal diagnosis is not 100% accurate and there are potential hazards for such empirical therapy, this type of prenatal treatment has remained controversial and questionable (Pang et al 1992; Mercado et al 1995).

MALE INTERSEX

In this group, the chromosomal pattern is 46,XY and the gonads are invariably testes. About 80% of affected individuals have an altered phenotype caused by a genetically determined abnormal target organ response to testosterone (testicular feminising syndrome or feminised males), but usually with a normal response to antimüllerian hormone (absence of müllerian system). In such persons, the normal hypothalamic pituitary feedback loop is impaired resulting in elevated gonadotrophin and excess production of testosterone and androgens. However, in this type of male intersex, the presence of androgen does not make a difference because of deficient cellular response in the target organs. In the rest (the other type of male intersex), there is deficient testosterone and antimüllerian hormone production or both, in their testes (Rubenstein and Mandell 1993), resulting in a clinical state of under-masculinised males, with or without the existence of a müllerian system.

Etiological background of male intersex: There are two linked steps in the background of male intersex—deficiency of hormones and deletion or mutation of genes.

Direct Etiology: Deficiency of two hormones produced by the testes—testosterone and antimüllerian hormone (AMH)

Background Etiology: In the background of these defects, there is either deletion or mutation of the sex determining gene(s).

Clinical classification based on etiology: Based on the cause, these patients may be classified as follows:

A. Under-masculinised males

i. With deficiency of antimüllerian hormone and mild deficit of testosterone

ii. With moderate to severe grades of testosterone deficiency, with or without deficit of antimüllerian hormone

B. Feminised males or 46,XY females

i. Feminine external genitalia and usually absent müllerian system

ii. Typical ambiguous external genitalia with total absence of müllerian system

A. Under-masculinised males, usually reared as male

i. The first subgroup consists of individuals who have deficiency of the antimüllerian hormone and a mild deficit of testosterone. The external genitalia are therefore more masculine in appearance but occasionally with unilateral or bilateral undescended testes. They have persistence of müllerian system in the form of uterus and tube occasionally found in inguinal hernial sac (hernia uteri inguinalis). In this group, ambiguity of external genitalia is rare and the sex of rearing is male, since it is not in doubt. Fertility is possible in these individuals if there is at least one testis in the scrotal sac.

ii. Individuals in the other subgroup in this category have moderate to severe grades of testosterone deficiency with or without deficit of antimüllerian hormone. The majority of individuals in this group are grossly under-masculinised and in more than 50%, external and internal genital organs are ambiguous. In this subgroup, deficiency of testosterone, with or without antimüllerian hormone, may be due to several reasons. Some of the clinical evidence is given below:

a. Abnormal pituitary (counterfeit) gonadotrophin secretion (Siler-khodr et al 1974; Park et al 1975). These patients do not survive beyond the neonatal period; they may have ambiguous external genitalia.

b. Subnormal testicular testosterone biosynthesis due to enzymatic deficiency (Bongiovanni 1961; Dagenhart 1972; Cravioto et al 1986): These patients are under-masculinised without any evidence of müllerian system; some may have micropenis with cryptorchidism. Breast development is variable.

c. Defective biological expression (failure of testosterone being converted to dihydro testosterone[DHT]) at the target organ level due to deficiency of enzyme 5α-reductase (Imperato-Mcginley et al 1986)—DHT is more potent and more biologically active than testosterone. Wolffian duct derivatives namely epididymes, vas deferens and seminal vesicles are normally developed because these organs develop under the influence of testosterone. Urogenital sinus derivatives like prostate and membranous urethra are not well developed because they are under the influence of DHT. The urethra opens into the urogenital sinus giving it the appearance of hypospadias. Penile development is moderate because this is controlled by both testosterone and DHT. There is no facial hair indicating that facial hair is also under control of DHT. The majority will have sexual ambiguity of external genitalia.

d. Inadequacy of Leydig cell function (Jones 1992): External genitalia are feminised; ambiguity of external genitalia will depend on the degree of Leydig cell inadequacy. The müllerian system is inhibited, because the antimüllerian hormone (AMH) is normal.
e. Familial gonadal destruction leading to deficiency of both testosterone and antimüllerian hormone has been reported in literature (Park and Jones 1970; Rios et al 1974). These individuals had testes in embryonic life, but these were subsequently destroyed by genetic influence. When seen in adult life, there is hardly any evidence of identifiable testis. They are 46,XY individuals. The phenotype and appearance of external and internal genitalia will depend on the stage in embryonic life when testicular function was suppressed. Therefore, in these individuals, there may be müllerian remnants and ambiguity of external genitalia and the phenotype will be under-masculinised.

B. Feminised males or 46,XY females

Individuals in this group have a defect in the target organ cellular response to testosterone but normal response to antimüllerian hormone. The most common type of disorder in this group is testicular feminising syndrome (Fig. 4.8).

Morris (1953) collected several cases from literature and added two of his own and coined the term 'testicular feminising syndrome'. Keenan et al (1974) showed that the basic defect was an inability of the cytosol receptors to bind testosterone. Therefore, the target organs are unable to recognise testosterone and translate it into a biological reality. This is the reason why this syndrome is also known as androgen insensitivity syndrome. However, the current view is that there are a number of different mutations in sex determining genes that may result in androgen insensitivity (Brown and Migeon 1986).

There are two subgroups of this syndrome:

i. The majority in the first subgroup has external genitalia, typically feminine in appearances; the breasts are well developed. Pubic and axillary hair is absent and the gonads are externally palpable. Total absence of a müllerian system is the characteristic finding, but in a few cases, müllerian tissue is known to exist. In addition, the authors have also observed evidence of ovarian stromal cells and testicular seminiferous tubules or dysgenetic gonads (unpublished). In these cases, during laparoscopy, gonads are found within the abdominal cavity. This category has been designated '46,XY sex reversed females'.
ii. The other subgroup will have typical ambiguous external genitalia with total absence of a müllerian system. They have phallic enlargement with variable grades of urogenital sinus opening suppression. Pubic hair, though sparse, is present. Breasts are usually absent and if present are very poorly developed (incomplete testicular feminising syndrome).

Based on this information, the phenotype and external genitalia in male intersex can be broadly classified as follows:

- Tending towards typical male (10%)
- Mixed and gross ambiguity of external genitalia (10%)
- Typical female, sometimes with minor ambiguity of external genitalia (80%)

In this section, we are primarily concerned with individuals who are born with external genitalia, typical or tending towards female. This group has been further sub-classified as:

Complete variety of testicular feminising syndrome (also known as classic testicular feminising syndrome)

No müllerian system

Incomplete variety of testicular feminising syndrome

No müllerian system

Presence of sexual ambiguity

Sex reversed 46,XY female (special group)*

Presence of müllerian system

No sexual ambiguity

* This special group has been identified more in members of the same family and designated by us (in collaboration with Center for Cellular and Molecular Biology, Hyderabad) in the category of '46,XY sex reversed female'.

Tables 4.4 and 4.5 illustrate the differences between complete and incomplete varieties of testicular feminising syndrome and sex reversed 46,XY females.

In incomplete TFS, secondary sex characteristics are not well developed. Pubic and axillary hair may be present (totally absent in complete TFS). Moreover, in incomplete TFS, external genitalia are often ambiguous, sometimes with suppression of vaginal opening. However, a urogenital sinus opening always exists and vaginal reconstruction is possible.

In sex reversed 46,XY females (Fig. 4.9), rudimentary to normal size uterus and tubes have been found with occasional presence of ovarian stromal cells and seminiferous tubules or dysgenetic gonads. They were not cases of true intersex, because mosaicism, either in peripheral blood or in gonads, was not detected.

Background etiology: The basic defect leading to various clinical abnormalities in male intersex is due to either deletion or mutation of sex determining gene(s).

Sex Determining Genes: The known sex determining genes are SRY; SOX3, SOX9, DSS, ZFY, TDF. Literature survey

Table 4.4: Differences between complete (classic) and incomplete variety of testicular feminising syndrome

	Complete (classic)	*Incomplete (partial)*
Karyotype	46,XY	46,XY
Phenotype	Female	Female
Gonads	Ectopic (testes)	Ectopic (testes)
Müllerian system	Inhibited	Inhibited
Secondary sex characteristics	Well developed	May not be well developed
External genitalia	Typical female	Ambiguous
Vagina	Short, blind	Usually blind (remnant of UGS)
Pubic and axillary hair	Absent	May be present

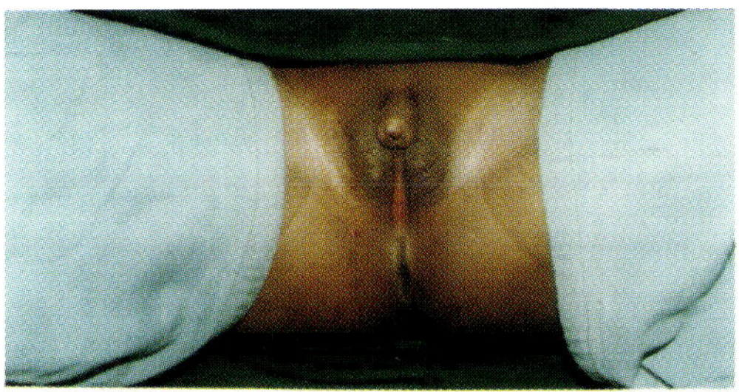

FIGURE 4.5: SEXUAL AMBIGUITY: CONGENITAL ADRENAL HYPERPLASIA IN A CHILD AGED 7 YEARS (COMMON OPENING OF URETHRA AND VAGINA THROUGH UROGENITAL SINUS WITH FUSION OF LABIOSCROTAL FOLDS, PHALLUS IS ENLARGED)

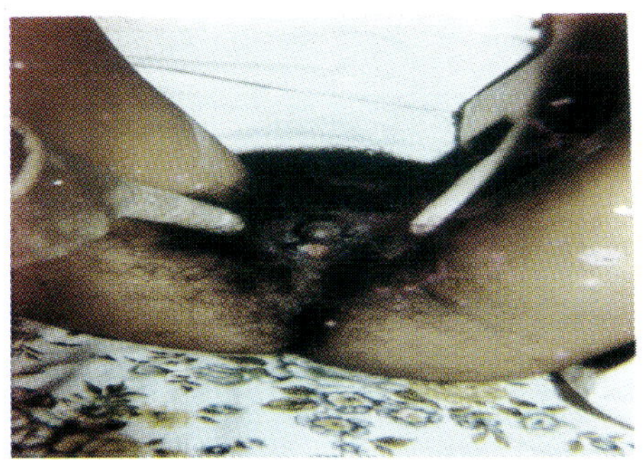

FIGURE 4.6: SEXUAL AMBIGUITY: CONGENITAL ADRENAL HYPERPLASIA IN AN ADOLESCENT. NOTE THE DEGREE OF VIRILISATION. COMMON OPENING OF VAGINA AND URETHRA THROUGH UROGENITAL SINUS WITH FUSION OF LABIOSCROTAL FOLD; PHALLUS IS ENLARGED

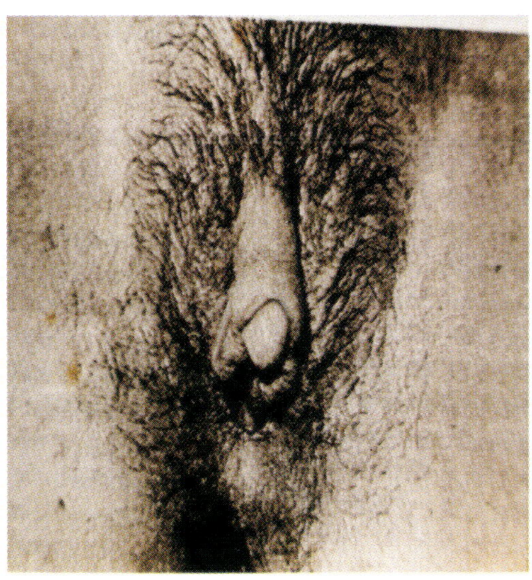

FIGURE 4.7: CONGENITAL ADRENAL HYPERPLASIA (LATE ONSET): GROSS ENLARGEMENT OF PHALLUS, MINIMUM LABIOSCROTAL FUSION; URETHRAL AND VAGINAL OPENING ARE VISIBLE (NOT IN THE PICTURE); OBVIOUSLY TIME OF ONSET OF SYNDROME IN THIS CASE WAS DELAYED. CLITORAL HYPERTROPHY DEPENDS ON AMOUNT OF ANDROGEN EXPOSURE AND NOT ON TIME OF ONSET OF THE SYNDROME

(Rubenstein and Mandell 1993) reveals that in 46,XY females, the müllerian system is totally inhibited and the sex determining gene is either deleted or mutated. However, the

TABLE 4.5: DIFFERENCES BETWEEN CLASSIC TESTICULAR FEMINISING SYNDROME AND 'SEX REVERSED' 46 XY FEMALE

	Typical TFS	*Sex-reversed XY females*
Karyotype	46,XY	46,XY
Phenotype	Female	Female
Secondary sex characteristics	Well developed	Well developed
External genitalia	Female	Female
Vagina	Short, blind	Normal
Gonads	Testes (ectopic)	Ovaries; sometimes ovaries and testes (normal situation for ovaries)
Müllerian tissues	Absent	Present: uterus and tubes usually rudimentary but sometimes normal in size

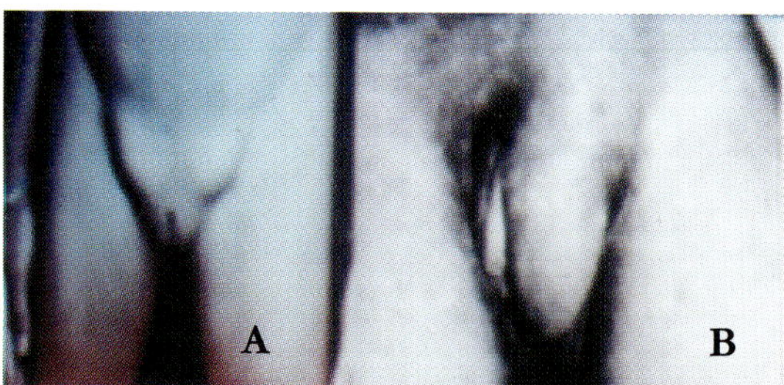

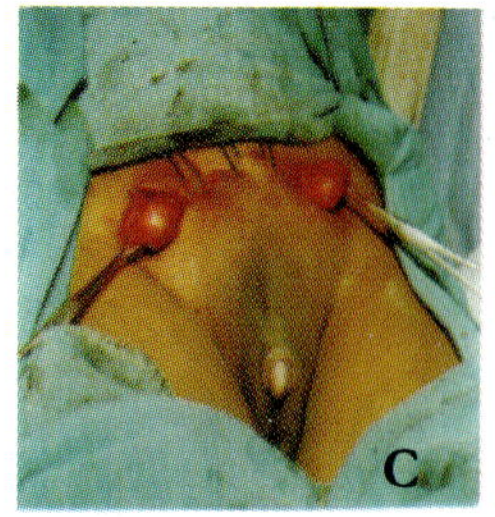

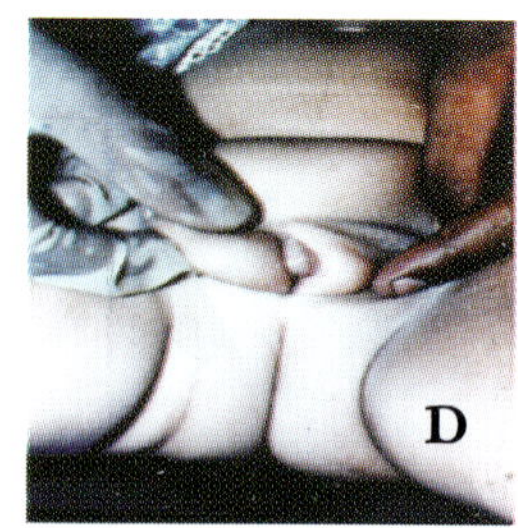

FIGURE 4.8 (A, B, C, D):
A. COMPLETE TESTICULAR FEMINISING SYNDROME, TYPICAL FEMININE EXTERNAL GENITALIA, NO PUBIC HAIR, BILATERAL INGUINAL GONADS
B. AND C. INCOMPLETE TESTICULAR FEMINISING SYNDROME IN TWO ADOLESCENT GIRLS. MILDLY ENLARGED PHALLUS, LABIAL GONAD IN B AND BILATERAL INGUINAL GONADS WITH MARKEDLY ENLARGED PHALLUS IN C
D. ANOTHER CASE OF INCOMPLETE TESTICULAR FEMINISING SYNDROME IN A CHILD—BILATERAL LABIAL, GONADS WITH PHALLIC ENLARGEMENT, LARGER THAN CLITORIS BUT SMALLER THAN PENIS; KARYOTYPE 46,XY

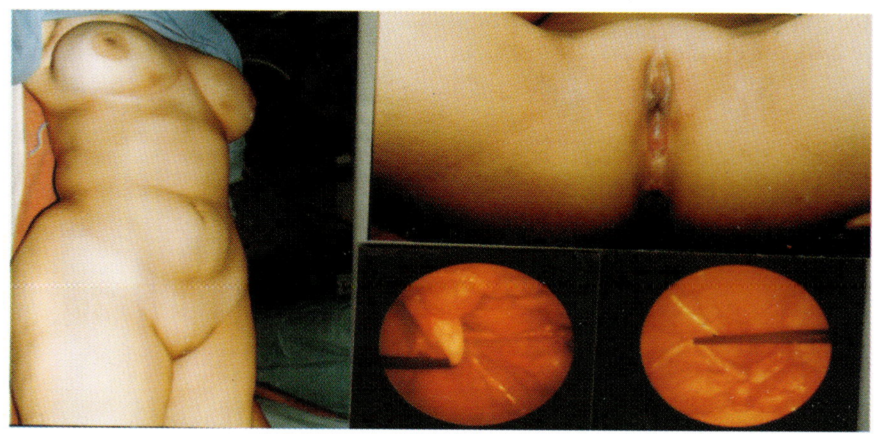

FIGURE 4.9A: PHENOTYPE OF SEX REVERSED 46 XY FEMALES SHOWS TYPICAL FEMININE EXTERNAL GENITALIA, ABSENCE OF PUBIC HAIR WITH WELL-DEVELOPED BREASTS. INSET SHOWS LAPAROSCOPIC VIEW OF INTERNAL GENITAL ORGANS. BIOPSY REVEALED OVARIAN STROMA ON ONE SIDE AND SEMINIFEROUS TUBULES CONTAINING SERTOLI CELLS ON THE OTHER SIDE. HYPOPLASTIC UTERUS IS SEEN IN THE INSET ON THE LEFT SIDE (MARKED BY ARROW)

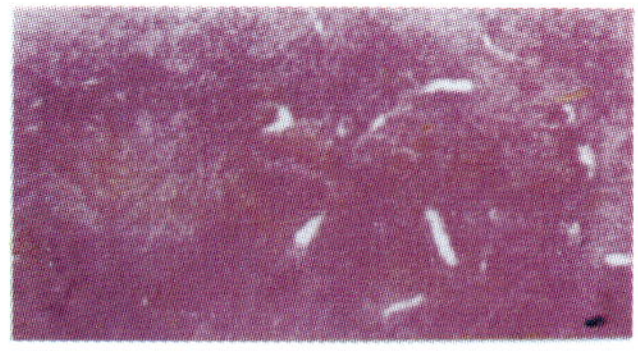

Sections of right gonadal tissue show histologic features compatible with ovarian stroma

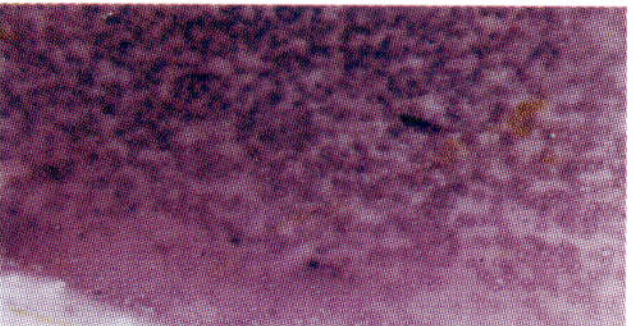

Left sided gonadal tissue revealed occasional seminiferous tubule containing sertoli cells only

FIGURE 4.9B: BIOPSY REVEALED OVARIAN STROMA ON ONE SIDE AND SEMINIFEROUS TUBULES CONTAINING SERTOLI CELLS ON THE OTHER SIDE. HYPOPLASTIC UTERUS IS SEEN IN THE INSET ON THE LEFT SIDE (MARKED BY ARROW)

authors' observation, based on evaluation of 52 cases of 46,XY females suggested that

a. Except in three patients, in all other cases of 46,XY females, these genes were intact
b. In 13 patients, there was evidences of a müllerian system and/or the presence of ovaries (sometimes streak/dysgenetic gonads)
c. They had no sexual ambiguity

Our observation of XY patients studied at the Institute Of Reproductive Medicine, Kolkata and CCMB Hyderabad, India is summed up below:

Total number of patients	52
Testicular feminisation	42
Sex reversed XY females	9
* XXY (Female Klinefelter)	1

* (Source: Thangaraj et al. 1998. A 47XXY female. Lancet)

In this group, there was one case of a 47,XXY female Klinefelter (Fig. 4.10) which has been reported for the first time in the world literature (Thangaraj et al 1998).

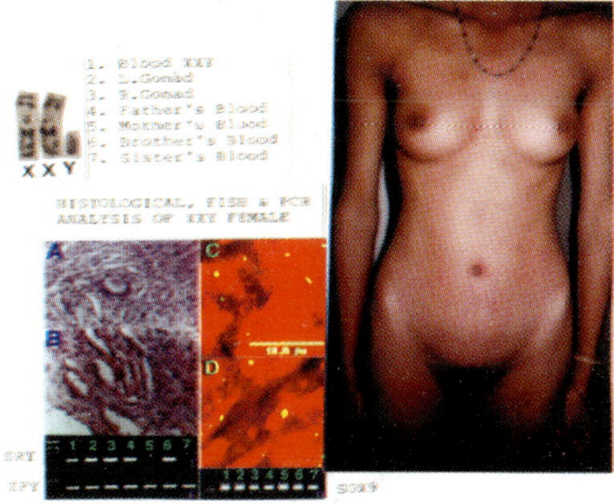

FIGURE 4.10: A CASE OF SEX REVERSAL (47,XXY FEMALE KLINEFELTER) SHOWING FEMALE SECONDARY SEX CHARACTERISTICS

SEX REVERSED 46,XY FEMALES

In the present study, we had 13 patients with so-called testicular feminising syndrome with a müllerian system and evidence of dysgenetic gonads or presence of seminiferons tubules and ovarian stromal cells in their gonads. This specific group of feminising male intersex does not fall in the category of 'typical' or 'classic' testicular feminising syndrome. In collaboration with the Center for Cellular and Molecular Biology, Hyderabad, the authors have therefore, placed them in a special category designated as '46,XY sex reversed female'. Successful pregnancies have been reported in this group following ovum donation and IVF (Kan et al 1997). Fig. 4.11 illustrates the family-tree pattern of three families of this subgroup; Fig 4.12 illustrates the proposed theory of inheritance of the 46,XY sex reversed female. The mother is the carrier of the affected gene. If the offspring is a female child, she becomes a carrier. If the offspring has 46,XY component, then the child is affected and becomes a sex-reversed XY female.

The findings of a recent study on genetic background of 46,XY female is as follows:

A marker locus has been observed by PCR technique in all cases, which is located on the X chromosome. The size of this locus is still not determined and this could involve many genes. Depending on the mutation/deletion in these genes, there may be phenotypic differentiation in 46,XY females, like typical testicular feminising syndrome, incomplete variety of testicular feminisation with ambiguous genitalia and total sex reversed XY females with presence of a müllerian system.

TRUE INTERSEX

These patients form the rarest group, accounting for less than 10% of all intersex disorders. Though the majority of individuals reported as true intersex have been reared as boys and men, the commonest chromosomal

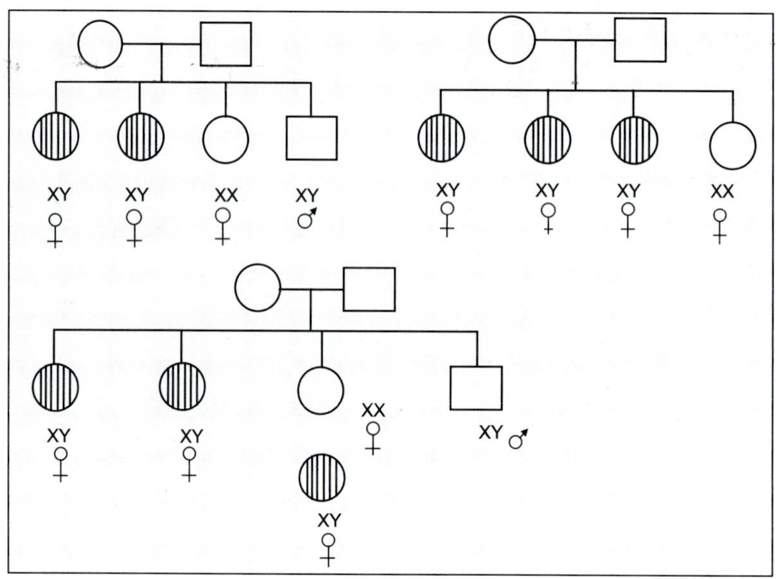

Figure 4.11: Three Families Of Sex Reversed XY Females

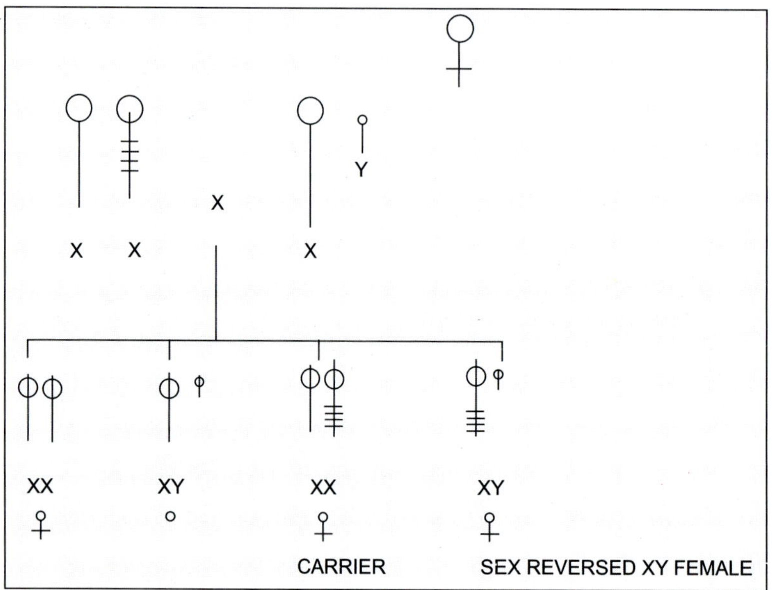

Figure 4.12: Proposed theory of inheritance of sex reversed XY female. The mother is the carrier of the affected gene. If the offspring is a female child she becomes a carrier. If the offspring has 46,XY component, then the child is an "Sex reversed XY female".

pattern is 46,XX. The common chromosomal finding in true intersex is of great interest, as it is very rare proof that a testis can develop without an apparent Y chromosome. Ten per cent have male genotype (46,XY) and the remaining are either mosaic (46,XX/46,XY) or chimeras with elements from two zygotes (Sivan et al 1995). These individuals may have either an ovary on one side and testes on the other or an ovary opposite to an ovotestis on the contralateral side. Bilateral ovotestis may exist in 20% of true intersex, while 10% of patients may have ovary and testis or ovotestes on the same side and no gonad on the other side. Though in the majority, the sex of rearing is male, breast development and menstruation occur in a substantial number of true intersex individuals. Patients who have external genitalia tending towards male are reared as male, while those with ambiguous external genitalia are usually reared as female. In all individuals with true intersex, the internal genital organs are of mixed type. Uterus and tubes are found on the side on which the ovary is present. The uterus may sometimes be malformed with evidence of hematometra. Vas deferens and seminiferous tubules are found on the side on which the testis is present. This may not always be true, especially in the presence of ovotestis. In these cases, remnants of müllerian and Wolffian duct structures may exist on the same side.

Mixed Gonadal Dysgenesis

These patients have a phenotypic appearance of classic Turner syndrome, but with ambiguous external genitalia. They have a chromosomal mosaicism (45,XO/46,XY). Internal findings consist of streak gonad associated with ipsilateral fallopian tube and uterus with a contralateral dysgenetic testis.

EVALUATION

Evaluation of ambiguous genitalia and sex assignment begins in the delivery room. It would be a mistake to assign the sex casually immediately after birth. If the physician assigns/hints at the gender immediately after birth and then there is a subsequent need to change the gender, the family will be deeply affected. Therefore, in the immediate neonatal period, gender-specific terms are to be avoided till the sex of rearing has been properly evaluated following the collection of as much information as possible.

Evaluation, for the assignment of appropriate sex of rearing, will depend on the following parameters:

- Physical examination
- Imaging—by ultrasonography, genitogram and MRI
- Chromosome analysis
- Biochemical assessment

Physical Examination

The presence or absence of an externally palpable gonad helps to establish a working diagnosis. Only an externally palpable gonad will exclude female intersex and will strongly suggest that the patient is either a male intersex or a true intersex.

Table 4.6 illustrates the provisional diagnosis in individuals with ambiguous external genitalia based on palpation of at least one gonad externally.

Apart from gonads, other features of external genitalia will be similar, whether the condition is due to masculinisation of a female fetus or under-masculinisation of male or due to true intersex. The phallus may be too large for female and too small for a male. In case of doubt, therapeutic trial with injection of depot testosterone may be

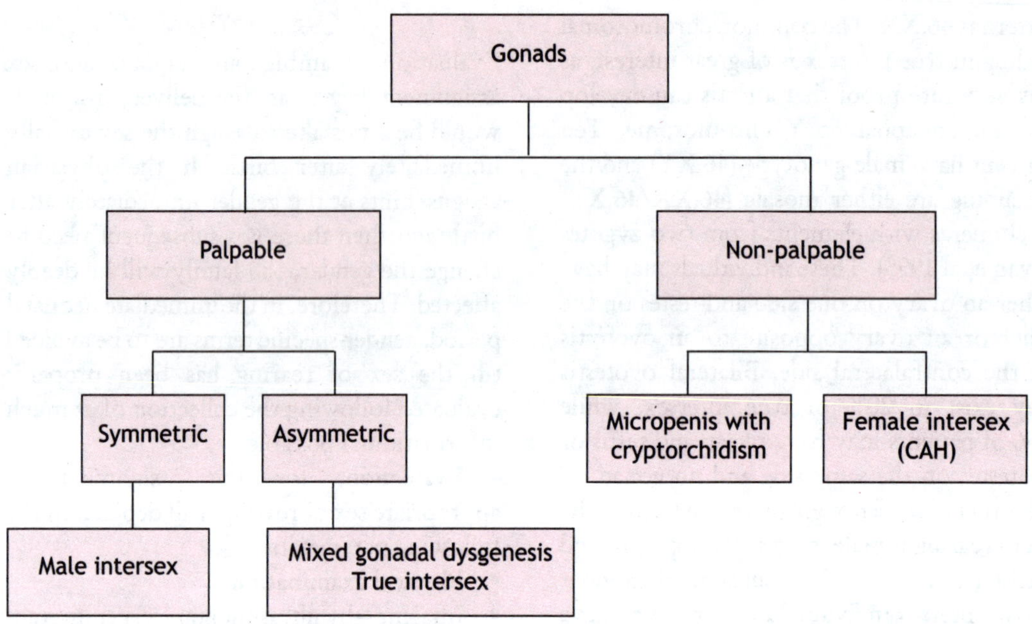

TABLE 4.6: PROVISIONAL DIAGNOSIS IN AMBIGUOUS GENITALIA

helpful. If the size of the phallus increases with depot testosterone, the sex of rearing will be male; otherwise sex assignment will be female with subsequent planned female genitoplasy. The scrotum will either look normal or like fused labia. The urethra will usually open on to the perineum but may be prolonged along the ventral surface of the phallus (Fig. 4.13).

However, the exact diagnosis of the cause of sexual ambiguity based on physical examination alone may not be possible. Hence, additional information by imaging, karyotype and biochemical assessments are essential.

IMAGING

Ultrasonography: Ultrasonographic imaging helps to identify internal genital organs like the uterus and ovaries (Kutteh et al 1995), and also enlarged adrenal glands in congenital adrenal hyperplasia (Wiener and Gonzales 1996).

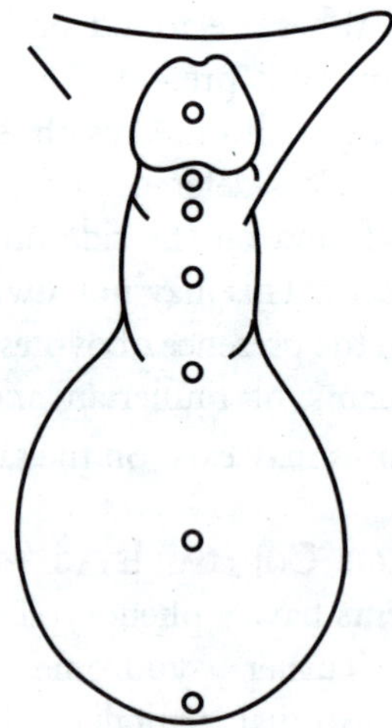

FIGURE 4.13: VARIOUS POTENTIAL LOCATIONS FOR THE URETHRAL MEATUS IN BOYS WITH HYPOSPADIAS

(Adapted from Abnormalities of The External Genitalia, Zaontz & Packer, 1997)

Genitogram: Sometimes there may be a single opening of the urogenital sinus into which both vagina and urethra will open. A genitogram can identify the urethra and bladder and the level of entry of vagina and the presence of other müllerian structures like the cervix, uterus and fallopian tubes. This may help in planning female genitoplasty, especially in congenital adrenal hyperplasia.

Magnetic resonance imaging (MRI): Though an expensive technology, the MRI is useful for morphologic evaluation of internal organs (Secaf et al 1994).

Chromosome Analysis

Karyotyping may help confirm diagnosis of intersex, but does not necessarily help to identify the sex of rearing. Nor does it help to decide the type of surgical reconstruction required. Chromosomal findings however, help in decision making regarding dysgenetic gonads and their risk of malignancies.

Appropriate Biochemical Assessment

This is essential, especially in a newborn with suspected congenital adrenal hyperplasia (CAH). Estimation of 17-OHP for confirmation of diagnosis and measurement of serum electrolytes is essential for immediate medical management. The salt-losing variety of adrenogenital syndrome will show hyperkalemia and hyponatremia.

In some cases of male intersex, when a decision has been taken in favour of feminising genitoplasty, measurement of serum testosterone before and after stimulation with hCG may be helpful in establishing the presence or absence of functional testicular tissue (Griffin and Wilson 1992). If present, this organ is to be removed.

Practical criteria for assignment of sex of rearing: The decision of sex of rearing at the neonatal age will depend upon availability of as much of the above information as possible. Of these, the following two criteria are of practical importance. The first criterion is whether the gonads are externally palpable or not. As a general rule, when the gonads are not palpable externally, the assigned sex of rearing should be female irrespective of other findings.

The second criterion is the size of the phallus. If it is more than 2.5 cm (except in CAH), the sex of rearing should be male. In case of doubt, therapeutic trial with depot testosterone will be helpful (see above).

SURGICAL CORRECTION

The following are the objectives of surgical correction:

- Acceptable gender assignment
- Better chance of coital function
- Additionally, improvement of reproductive potential, if possible

Types of Surgery Performed

a. Excision of unwanted genital organs and gonads
b. Construction of external genitalia in the desired line of sex of rearing.

Timing of Surgery: This will depend on the age of the person at the time of first visit. If the child is seen in the neonatal period and the decision regarding sex of rearing has been confirmed, external genitalia should be constructed in the desired line of sex of rearing, within 24 months of birth. This approach is likely to avoid psychological conflict and embarrassment for the child as well as for the family.

However, the following exceptions must be kept in mind:

a. Introitoplasty/vaginoplasty, especially in CAH or incomplete testicular feminising syndrome, should be performed when the child grows to the age of adolescence, for better exposure and handling
b. Gonadectomy: When the sex has been assigned as female like testicular feminising syndrome, the testis should be removed in adolescence after secondary sex characteristics have developed
c. Similarly, in true intersex, when sex has been assigned as male, mastectomy should be performed during adolescence. In the majority of true intersex persons reared as male (46,XX) the breasts are well developed by this time.

SURGICAL APPROACH: The majority of individuals with sexual ambiguity require feminising genitoplasty. Also, feminising genitoplasty is a relatively simpler procedure than masculinising genitoplasty.

SURGICAL ANATOMY: The nature of defect in the urogenital sinus derivatives is remarkably constant, regardless of the cause of the anomaly. It is essential to remember that without a virilising factor, either from normal embryonic testis or from an abnormal virilising source as in congenital adrenal hyperplasia, the urogenital sinus will develop in the female line. In the presence of a virilising source, there will be fusion of scrotolabial folds in such a manner that the vaginal opening is suppressed completely or concealed from the outside.

Vaginal communication is almost always in relation to caudal urogenital sinus derivatives (Fig. 4.14). This means that the vagina communicates with that part of the urogenital sinus which in the male will form the membranous part of urethra, and in the female the vestibule. The vagina (müllerian duct) never communicates with that part of the urogenital sinus which in the male forms the prostatic urethra and in the female forms the entire urethra (Bargy et al 1989). This is of considerable surgical importance because an anomalously persistent urogenital sinus may be boldly incised without apprehension of disturbing the urinary sphincteric continence.

Surgical correction of female intersex:

Surgical correction consists of:

- Phalloplasty
- Introitoplasty or vaginoplasty

In addition to surgical repair, all individuals with CAH will require dexamethasone or hydrocortisone throughout their life

PHALLOPLASTY: This can be performed in two ways:

i. Amputation of the phallus and reconstruction of the redundant part of the corpus to provide the shape for clitoris. Care should be taken not to injure the urethra, which lies just below the base of the enlarged phallus (Fig 4.15 a, b, c. See Page 89).
ii. Amputation of corpus with preservation of glans (for cosmetic reasons): The primary incision is the same. A broad clitoral flap is preserved to maintain the blood supply of the glans. The shaft of the phallus is

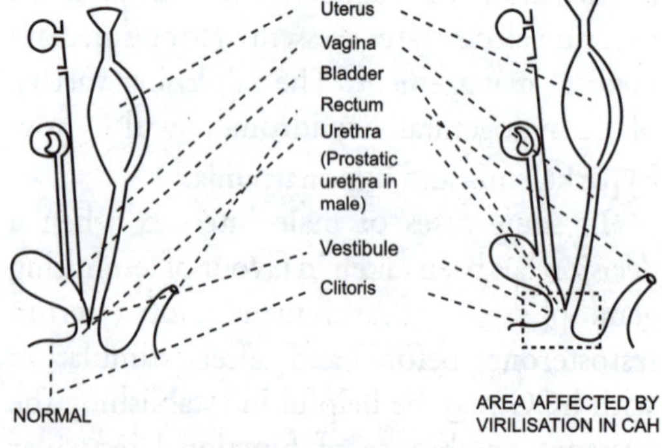

FIGURE 4.14: SURGICAL CORRECTION OF FEMALE INTERSEX—THE MOST COMMON IS CONGENITAL ADRENAL HYPERPLASIA (CAH)

removed; the space from which the corpus was removed is closed. This is followed by fixing the flap containing the preserved glans on the base of the shaft which has been left behind following removal of the corpus (Fig. 4.16).

VAGINOPLASTY: This will depend on the degree of virilisation. In the majority of persons affected by CAH there will be a single opening of the urogenital sinus, into which both urethra and vagina will open. Depending on the degree of virilisation, the sites of urethral and vaginal opening may be either easy or difficult to identify at the time of reconstructive surgery (see Figs 4.2, 4.3, 4.4).

Type I: In this group, through a narrow common urogenital sinus opening, vaginal and urethral orifices are easily identified. The steps are similar to those in Fenton's introitoplasty (Fig. 4.17A). In some cases, there may be labial fusion which may conceal urethral and vaginal openings. The fused area is usually very thin and can be vertically incised under the guidance of a probe or an artery forceps. The probe or artery forceps can be negotiated through the anterior opening of the fused labia (marked by an arrow below the enlarged phallus, Fig. 4.17B). The hidden urethral and vaginal orifices are then clearly visible. A few interrupted stitches may be necessary to cover the raw edges of the incised portion. Additional introitoplasty may not be necessary.

Type II: In this group, vaginal and urethral orifices are difficult to locate due to more aggressive scrotolabial fusion. An operative endoscope may be used to identify the urethral and vaginal openings (Fig. 4.18).

Even without using an endoscope, the urogenital sinus can be enlarged by midline perineal incision after putting a double-gloved finger in the rectum. The urethral and vaginal openings may then be seen separately. The vaginal mucous membrane will be dissected to a variable distance upwards. Again keeping the double-gloved finger in the rectum, perineal muscles are incised in the midline followed by apposition of the vaginal mucous membrane with skin.

Glans with intact clitoral flap

FIGURE 4.16: AMPUTATION OF CORPUS WITH PRESERVATION OF GLANS *(ADAPTED AND MODIFIED FROM "FEMALE REPRODUCTIVE SURGERY"; ED. ROCK, MURPHY AND JONES, 1992)*

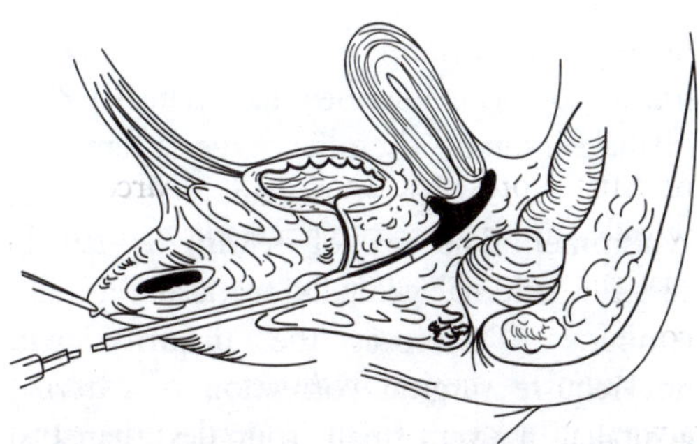

FIGURE 4.18: VAGINAL AND URETHRAL ORIFICIES ARE DIFFICULT TO IDENTIFY. THIS CAN BE IDENTIFIED WITH ENDOSCOPE OR THROUGH MIDLINE PERINEAL INCISION AFTER PLACING A DOUBLED GLOVED FINGER IN THE RECTUM *(ADAPTED AND MODIFIED FROM "FEMALE REPRODUCTIVE SURGERY"; ED. ROCK, MURPHY AND JONES, 1992)*

Type III: The vagina remains imperforate, that is, there is failure of communication between the lower end of the müllerian duct and the caudal end of the urogenital sinus. This is an extremely rare situation.

The abdomino-perineal approach has been recommended (Jones 1992). The abdominal route of approach is either through laparotomy or through laparoscope (the authors prefer open laparotomy). An ultrasound or guide is to be negotiated through the uterus or through the cervix (following bladder dissection). The tip of the sound or guide after passing through the cervix and upper vagina will push the perineal skin and can be palpated through the perineum. With the guide still in place, the skin and underlying urogenital sinus through the perineum can be palpated and incised (marked by arrow in the diagram). The edges of the vaginal epithelium, which can be identified, are brought down and sutured to the perineal skin (Fig. 4.19).

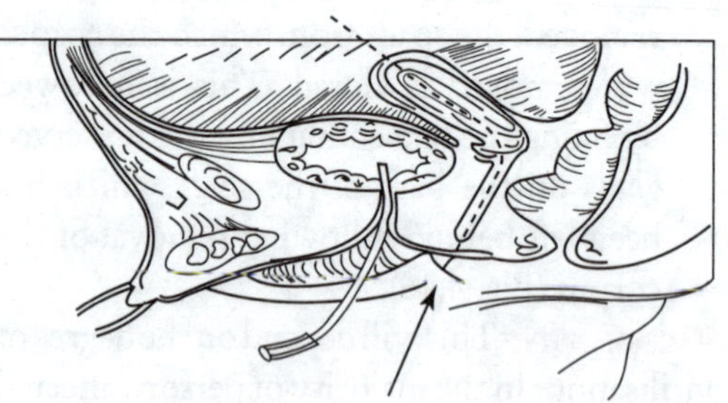

FIGURE 4.19: VAGINA IS IMPERFORATE (VERY RARE). A GUIDE IS NEGOTIATED THROUGH THE FUNDUS AFTER LAPAROTOMY OR LAPAROSCOPY. THE GUIDE PUSHES THE UROGENITAL SINUS AND PERINEAL SKIN (MARKED BY ARROW). THIS IS THE POINT OF INCISION OF PERINEAL SKIN. THROUGH THIS INCISION, THE VAGINAL MUCOUS MEMBRANE CAN BE BROUGHT DOWN AND SUTURED TO THE PERINEAL SKIN. *(ADAPTED AND MODIFIED FROM "FEMALE REPRODUCTIVE SURGERY"; ED. ROCK, MURPHY AND JONES, 1992)*

Obviously, such an operation can only be performed in adolescence, when the uterus and cervix have become reasonably big in size.

Surgical approach in male intersex: It has already been described that, in nearly 80% of male intersex, the phenotype is feminine (46,XY females—testicular feminising syndrome). The sex of rearing is female and the external genitalia are also typically feminine. Therefore, the majority will not require surgical correction of external genitalia. In a very small group (less than 1%) of patients with incomplete TFS (incomplete variety of testicular feminising syndrome) who have ambiguous external genitalia with phallic enlargement, surgical correction of the enlarged phallus (described under congenital adrenal hyperplasia) may be required. Vaginoplasty in these individuals may not be as easy as in congenital adrenal hyperplasia. They do not have a müllerian system, but certainly have a urogenital sinus below the orifice of the external urethral meatus. This may be widened surgically up to a depth of 2.5 to 4 cm and subsequently, the length may be increased by regular use of a plastic mould. However, in all these cases, the gonads are the testes and gonadectomy should be performed after the age of puberty (Fig 4.20). Estrogen substitution is essential for a few years.

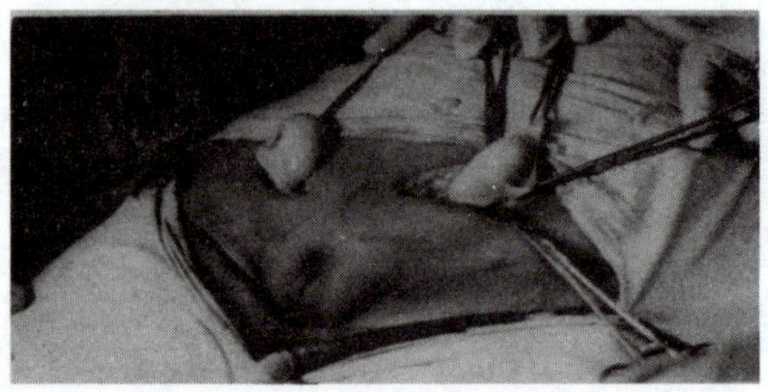

FIGURE 4.20: COMPLETE VARIETY OF TESTICULAR FEMINISING SYNDROME—FEMININE EXTERNAL GENITALIA—NO PUBIC HAIR, ECTOPIC GONADS ARE TESTES: GONADECTOMY IS BEING PERFORMED

In the 10% of individuals, who form the second group, who are reared as males, the external genitalia tend towards male (under-masculinised males). This group consists of those who may have Leydig cell insufficiency or deficiency of antimüllerian hormone. They may have remnants of müllerian tissue, either in the abdomen or in the inguinal region. These organs are to be removed.

The third group of male intersex (10%) may exhibit evidence of sexual ambiguity. Surgical correction will depend primarily on the length of the phallus, and secondarily on sex of rearing. Phallus size of more than 2.5 cm will indicate male genitoplasty, while a size less than that will indicate female genitoplasty. If the size cannot be measured, depot testosterone may be used as therapeutic trial. If the response is adequate, male genitoplasy is considered.

The entire plan of surgical approach for sexual ambiguity in male intersex can be outlined as follows (Algorithm 1).

Surgical approach to true intersex: Surgical approach in true intersex is more or less similar to that in male intersex. This includes removal of contradictory organs and reconstructing the external genitalia in keeping with the sex of rearing. The majority of these individuals are reared as males with average to normal penile development (possibly with minor grade of hypospadias), with unilateral testis located anywhere between the deep inguinal ring and scrotum (Fig. 4.21).

However, in this group a problem may

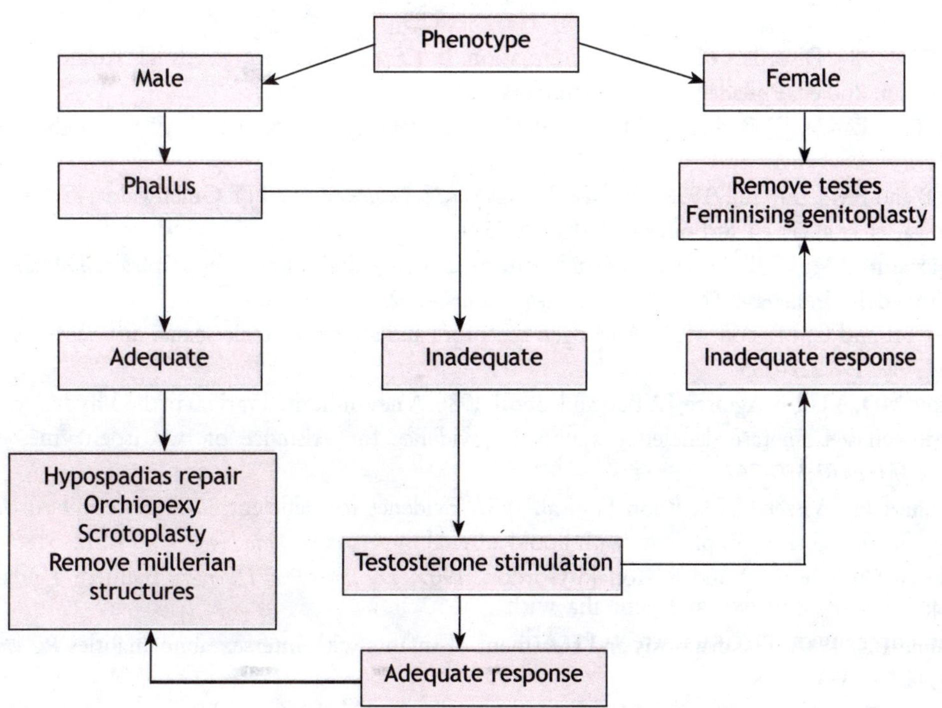

ALGORITHM 1: SURGICAL APPROACH TO MALE PSEUDOHERMAPHRODITISM (ADAPTED FROM ABNORMALITIES OF THE EXTERNAL GENITALIA, ZAONTZ & PACKER 1997)

arise during surgery, since the characteristic of the gonad (from the ovotestis) needs to be established. Since recognition by gross morphologic characteristics may not provide accurate identification, at the time of exploration, a biopsy should be taken and the gonad bisected and inspected so the contradictory gonad is not missed.

Surgical approach to mixed gonadal dysgenesis: These individuals have a Y chromosome with a streak gonad on one side and a dysgenetic testis on the other.

Conventional treatment is gonadectomy (to prevent the risk of malignancy) and sex organ reconstructed in the female line. In very rare cases, patients have undergone reconstruction as boys, with testes left in place, but these need very careful monitoring (Sivan et al 1995).

Conclusion: Sexual ambiguity, though rare, is a challenging clinical problem. Identification of the exact cause and appropriate management often becomes problematic and embarrassing. The commonest cause of sexual ambiguity encountered in clinical practice is due to congenital adrenal hyperplasia (female intersex) followed by testicular feminising syndrome (male intersex). True intersex and mixed gonadal dysgenesis are rare events. The objectives of surgical correction are primarily to assign the appropriate sex of rearing, and secondarily, to offer the scope of coital, and if possible, the reproductive function. In addition, unwanted organs and undesirable (which may be harmful) gonads are to be removed.

References

Allen TD. 1985. Disorders of sexual differentiation. In *Clinical pediatric urology,* eds KP Kelalis, LR King, BA Belman, 2nd ed. Philadelphia: WB Saunders, 904.

Bargy F, F Lande, JP Barbet, A Houtte. 1989. The anatomy of intersexuality. *Surg Radiol Anat* 11: 103–107.

Blyth B and BM Churchill. 1996. Intersex. In *Adult and pediatric urology*, ed JY Gillenwater, JT Grayhack, SS Howards, et al, 3rd ed. St Louis: CV Mosby, 2591.

Bongiovanni AM. 1961. Unusual steroid pattern in congenital adrenal hyperplasia: Deficiency of 3-hydroxydehydrogenase. *J Clin Endocrinol Metab* 21:860–862.

Brown TR and CJ Migeon. 1986. Androgen receptors and abnormal male sexual differentiation. *Adv Exp Med Biol* 196:227–255.

Cravioto MD, A Ulloa-Aguirre, JA Bermudez et al. 1986. A new inherited variant of the 3-hydroxysteroid de-hydrogenase-isomerase deficiency syndrome evidence for existence of two isoenzymes. *J Clin Endocrinol Metab* 63:360–367.

Dagenhart HJ, Visser HKA, Boon H et al. 1972. Evidence for deficient 20-cholesterol-hydroxylase activity in adrenal tissue of patients with lipoid adrenal hyperplasia. *Acta Endocrinol* 71:512–518.

Dewhurst Christopher J and R Ronald Gordon. 1969. *The Intersexual Disorders*. Bailliere Tindall and Cassell.

Donahoe PK. 1987. The diagnosis and treatment of infants with intersex abnormalities *Pediatric Clin North Am* 34:1333.

Federman DD and PK Donahoe. 1995. Ambiguous genitalia: Etiology, diagnosis and therapy. *Adv Endocrinol Metab* 6:91.

Griffin JE and JD Wilson. 1992. Disorder of sexual differentiation. In *Campbell's Urology* ed PC Walsh, AB Retik, TA Stamey et al, 6th ed. Philadelphia: WB Saunders, 1509.

Imperato-McGinley J, T Gautier, RE Peterson et al. 1986. The prevalence of 5α-reductase deficiency in children with ambiguous genitalia in the Dominican Republic. *J Urol* 136:867–873.

Kan AK, HI Abdalla, T Oskarsson. 1997. Two successful pregnancies in a 46,XY patient. *Hum Reprod* 12(7):1434–1435.

Keenan BS, WJ Meyer III, Hadian AJ et al. 1974. Syndrome of androgen insensivity in man: Absence of 5 alphadihydrotestosterone binding proteinin skin fibroblasts. *J Clin Endocrinol Metab* 38 (6): 1143–1146

Kutteh WH, R Santos-Ramos, LD Eramel. 1995. Accuracy of ultrasonic detection of the uterus in normal newborn infants: Implication for infants with ambiguous genitalia. *Ultrasound Obstet Gynecol* 5:109.

Mercado AB, RC Wilson, KC Cheng, J-Q Wei, MI New. 1995. Prenatal treatment and diagnosis of congenital adrenal hyperplasia owing to steroid 21-hydroxylase deficiency. *J Clin Endocrinol Metab* 80:2014.

Meyer-Bahlburg HF, RS Green, MI New, JJ Bell, A Morishima, M Shimshi et al. 1996. Gender change from female to male in classical congenital adrenal hyperplasia. *Horn Behav* 30:319.

Morris JM. 1953. Syndrome of testicular feminisation in male pseudohermaphrodites. *Am J Obstet Gynecol* 65:1192–1211.

Mulaikal RM, CJ Migeon, JA Rock. 1987. Fertility rates in female patients with congenital adrenal hyperplasia due to 21-hydroxylase deficiency. *New Engl J Med* 316:178.

Pang S, AT Clark, LC Freeman, LM Dolan, L Immken, OT Mueller et al. 1992. Maternal side effects of prenatal dexamethasone therapy for foetal congenital adrenal hyperplasia. *J Clin Endocrinol Metab* 75:249.

Park IJ, VE Aimakhu, HW Jones Jr. 1975. An etiologic and pathogenetic classification of male hermaphroditism. *Am J Obstet Gynecol* 123:505–518.

Park IJ, HW Jones Jr. 1970. Familial male hermaphrodite with ambiguous external genitalia. *Am J Obstet Gynecol* 108:1197–1205.

Reindoller RH, JB Lewis, PC White, PM Fernhoff, PG McDonough, JB Whitney III. 1988. Prenatal diagnosis of 21-hydroxylase deficiency by the complementary deoxyribonucleic acid probe for cytochrome p-450C-210 H. *Am J Obstet Gynecol* 158:545.

Rios EP, J Herrera, JA Bermudez. 1974. Endocrine and metabolic studies in an XY patient with gonadal agenesis. *J Clin Endocrinol Metab* 39:540–547.

Robertson M and D Walker. 1975. Psychological factors in hypospodias repair. *J Urol.* 113: 698–700

Rock JA, AA Murphy, HW Jones Jr. 1992. *Female reproductive surgery*. London: Williams and Wilkins, 311.

Rubenstein SC and J Mandell. 1993. Ambiguous genitalia in newborns. *Contemporary Pediatrics* 10:83.

Siler-Khodr TM, LL Morgenstern, FC Greenwood. 1974. Hormone synthesis and release from human fetal adrenohypophysis in vitro. *J Endocrine Metab* 39:891–905.

Sivan E, S Koch, EA Reece. 1995. Sonographic prenatal diagnosis of ambiguous genitalia. *Fet Diagn Ther* 10:311.

Secaf E, H Hricak, CA Gooding. 1994. Role of MRI in the evaluation of ambiguous genitalia. *Pediatr Radiol* 24:231.

Thangaraj K, NJ Gupta, BN Chakravarty, L Singh. 1998. A 47 XXY female. *Lancet* 352(3):1121.
Wiener JS and ET Gonzales. 1996. Intersex. *Curr Opin Urol* 6:320.
Zaontz MR and MG Packer. 1997. Abnormalities of the external genetalia. *Ped Clin North Am*, 44: 1267–1297.

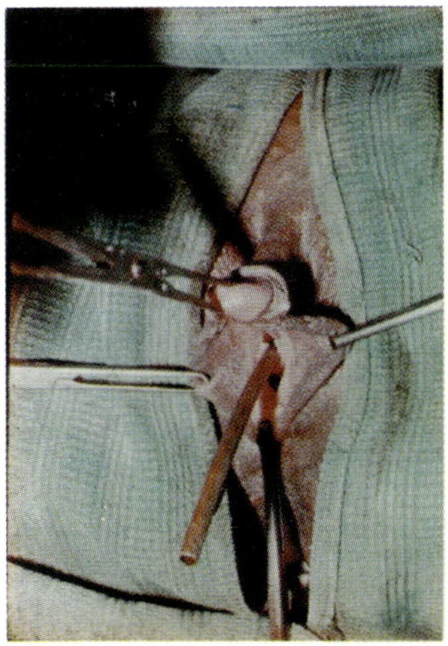

FIGURE 4.15A: ENLARGED PHALLUS, URETHRA AND VAGINAL OPENING ARE CLEARLY VISIBLE. METAL CATHETER INSIDE THE BLADDER

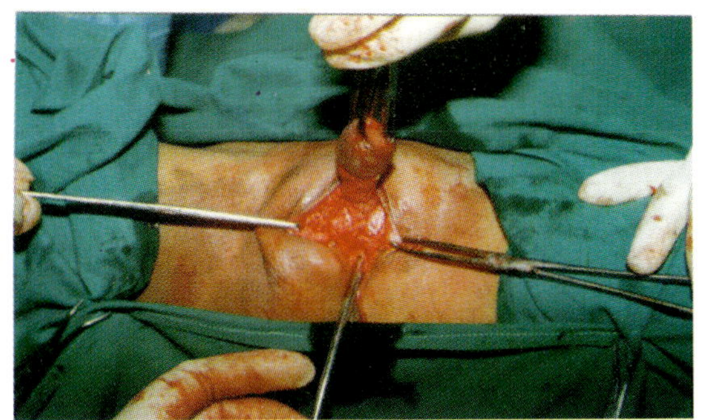

FIGURE 4.15B: ELLIPTICAL INCISION; DISSECTION OF CORPUS

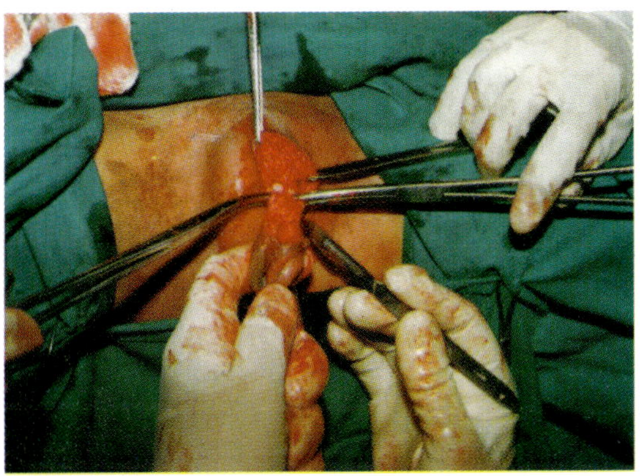

FIGURE 4.15C: CLAMPING AND EXCISION OF PHALLUS

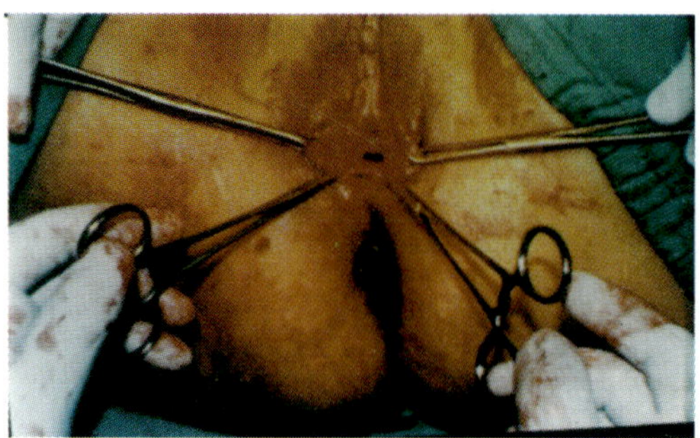

Figure 4.17a: Vaginoplasty in CAH in an adolescent girl (Vaginal and urethral orifices are easily identified)

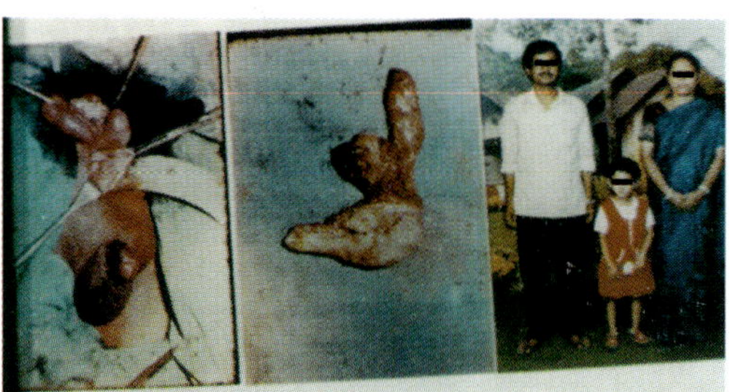

Figure 4.21: True intersex: Surgical removal of unwanted genital organs; uterus unilateral tube (hydrosalpinx) and ovary. The individual was reared up male with male external genitalia, unilateral testis, the other scrotal sac was empty. He presented at the age of 22 with periodic hematuria. He had a history of mastectomy at the age of 14, and reconstructive surgery of genital organs at the age of 23. Subsequently married and had a child by AIDS. A. Operative Step, B. Operative Specimen, C. Photograph of Patient with Wife and Child

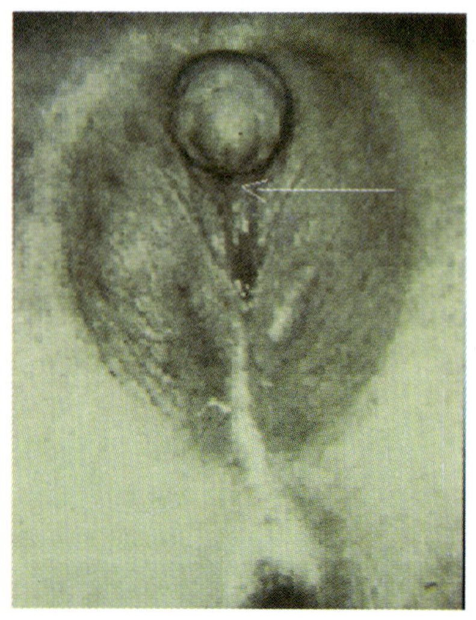

Figure 4.17b: Phalloplasty was performed at the age of 2 years in this girl

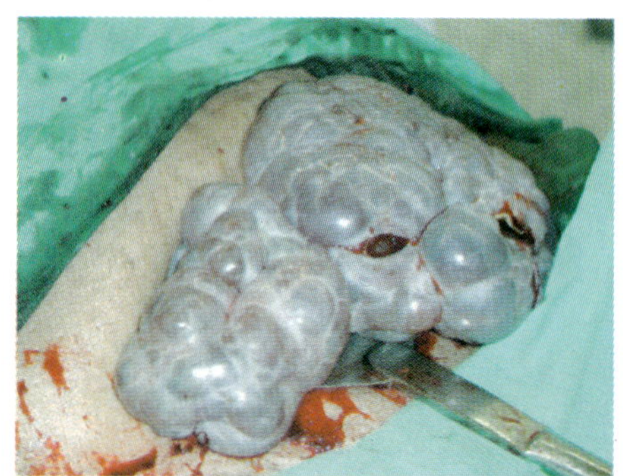

Figure 5.1: Massive polycystic ovaries seen at cesarean section in a patient who successfully conceived after in vitro fertilisation

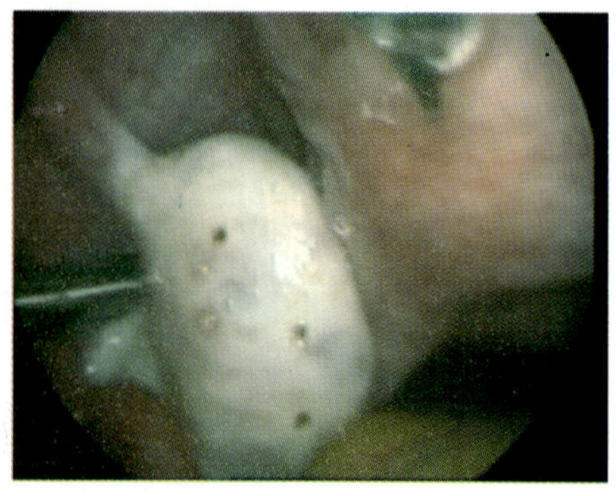

Figure 5.4: Laparoscopic ovarian drilling

5

Polycystic Ovary Syndrome

S Sevellaraja

Polycystic ovary syndrome (PCOS) was first described by Stein and Leventhal in 1935. It is probably the most common endocrine disorder in women, accounting for the majority of cases of hirsutism, menstrual disturbance and anovulatory infertility. It is also among the most poorly defined endocrinological conditions, with a complex pathophysiology that has produced considerable scientific debate. Currently, polycystic ovarian syndrome is believed to be a spectrum ranging from polycystic ovarian morphology with no overt abnormality at one end, to polycystic ovaries with severe clinical and biochemical disorders at the other end.

DIAGNOSIS

The diagnosis of a patient with PCOS will be based on three factors—clinical findings, biochemical findings and imaging (usually ultrasound).

Table 5.1: Clinical manifestations of polycystic ovary syndrome

1. Hyperandrogenism (acne, hirsutism, alopecia)
2. Infertility
3. Menstrual disturbances
4. Obesity
5. Sometimes asymptomatic

Clinical Features

The clinical features of PCOS are hyperandrogenism, menstrual irregularities and metabolic disorders such as obesity (Table 5.1).

Hyperandrogenism: This is characterised by hirsutism, alopecia and acne. Hirsutism is defined as the presence of excess terminal dark coarse hair in male pattern typically on the face, chest, lower abdomen or thighs. As many as 92% of women with this symptom have polycystic ovaries (PCO) on ultrasound (Adams et al 1986) (Fig. 5.1. See Page 90). Since hirsutism has a strong genetic basis, the family history for hirsutism should be elicited from the patient. The modified Ferriman–Gallwey scale of hirsutism or the Lorenzo scale of hirsutism may be used to assess hirsutism; however, these scores are subjective and few physicians in clinical practice actually use them (Diamanti-Kandarakis 1999; Rotterdam consensus 2004).

Approximately three-quarters of women who present with acne have PCO on ultrasound (Eden 1991) and more than 50% of adolescents who had PCOS were found to have moderate to severe acne (Dramusic et al 1997). Alopecia is less commonly reported in women with PCOS. Acanthosis nigricans is a skin eruption characterised by hyperkeratosis papillomatosis, an increased pigmentation seen most frequently at the back of the neck, the axilla, under the breasts and in the flexural areas. This skin condition is now recognised as a non-specific marker of moderate to severe insulin resistance (Dunaif 1992). In order to establish the diagnosis of PCOS, it is important to exclude other disorders with similar clinical presentations, such as congenital adrenal hyperplasia, Cushing syndrome, androgen secreting tumours of the adrenal or ovaries (Adams et al 1986) or the use of high-dose exogenous androgens (Pache et al 1991).

Menstrual disturbance: Menstrual disturbance, especially oligomenorrhea and amenorrhea, is one of the cardinal signs and symptoms of PCOS. In a large study (Balen et al 1991) using ultrasonically diagnosed polycystic ovaries as the marker, it was found that 29.7% had normal cycles, 47% oligomenorrhea, 19.2% amenorrhea, 2.7% polymenorrhea, and 1.4% menorrhagia. In another study, 87% of women with oligomenorrhea and 26% of those with amenorrhea presenting at a gynecological clinic were found to have polycystic ovaries on ultrasound examination (Adams et al 1986).

Obesity: There is a close association between obesity and PCOS. About 50% of women with PCOS have a body mass index (BMI) over 30 kg/m^2 and women with PCOS are on the average more obese than their non-PCOS counterparts (Norman et al 2002). It is possible that obesity drives polycystic ovaries to be more clinically manifest. The distribution of fat in women with polycystic ovaries results in an increased waist to hip ratio (Bringer et al 1993) and is frequently associated with greater insulin resistance than if fat is distributed predominantly in the lower body segment (Pasquali et al 1994). As a simple measure, waist circumference is thought to correlate more closely with obesity risk than BMI.

Polycystic ovary syndrome appears to be a heterogeneous condition with a wide variety of clinical presentations. The more severe the biochemical disturbance, the more likely the woman is to have a clinical presentation (Conway et al 1989; Balen et al 1991). It is unclear why some women present with anovulation with no hyperandrogenic manifestations, while others present with severe androgenic symptoms but remain ovulatory.

Ultrasound has been used extensively to diagnose PCOS. Presently, the transvaginal approach has greatly improved the accuracy of diagnosis of PCOS compared to transabdominal ultrasound (Fig. 5.2). The classic ultrasound features of PCOS are increased ovarian area or volume, increased roundness index (ovarian width/ovarian length ratio), decreased uterine width/ovarian length ratio (U/O), presence of microcysts <10 mm located peripherally near the surface of the ovary, increased echogenecity of ovarian stroma and increased surface of the ovarian stroma on cross-sectional cut (by computed measure) (Robert et al 2000). However, this finding on ultrasound does not confirm polycystic ovary syndrome.

Differential diagnosis: There are many differential diagnosis and the main one is multifollicular ovaries (MFO), which are encountered as normal findings in mid to late puberty, central precocious puberty, hyperprolactinemia, hypothalamic anovulation and most important, the early normal follicular phase in adult women before one follicle among the cohort becomes dominant (Adams et al 1985). Theoretically, polycystic ovaries differ from normal and multifollicular ovaries by being larger, more follicular and having a stromal hypertrophy. The follicle number is also higher in PCO, and in MFO, follicles seem to be randomly scattered throughout the ovaries. At an international consensus, the morphology of the polycystic ovary has been redefined as an ovary with 12 or more follicles measuring 2–9 mm in diameter and/or increased ovarian volume (10 cm^3) (Balen et al 2003).

Imaging

Besides ultrasound, magnetic resonance imaging (MRI) may be used to diagnose polycystic ovaries. It is only helpful in difficult situations such as severe hyperandrogenism, when ultrasonography is either not possible or is unhelpful (virgin or obese patients, respectively). Its main role is to exclude a virilising ovarian tumour; any ovary which appears larger in volume needs to be evaluated.

Three-dimensional ultrasound is being evaluated (Fig. 5.3). Doppler ultrasonography can be used to study the vasculature of ovaries—higher blood flow is seen in PCOS ovaries. However, its diagnostic usefulness is still questionable because of the overlap of the findings of increased blood flow with normal patients.

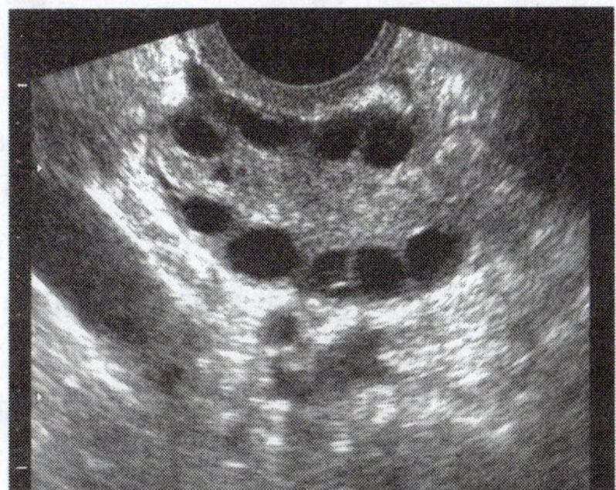

Figure 5.2: Transvaginal ultrasound scan of a polycystic ovary

Biochemical features: Biochemical feat-ures of PCOS can be confusing (Table 5.2). Both, the absolute level of circulating LH as well as its relation to FSH levels, are significantly elevated in women with PCOS as compared with controls (Taylor et al 1997). This is due to increased amplitude and frequency of LH pulses (Waldstreicher et al 1988). Elevated LH concentrations (above the 95th percentile of normal) may be observed in approximately 60% of women with PCOS (Laven et al 2002), whereas the LH/FSH ratio may be elevated in up to 95% of subjects (Taylor et al 1997), if women who have recently ovulated are excluded. LH levels may be influenced by the temporal relation to ovulation, which transiently normalises LH, by BMI (being higher in lean women with PCOS), as well as by the assay system used.

There is also elevation of one or more hormones, namely total testosterone, free testosterone, dehydroepiandrosterone sulphate (DHEAS), androstenedione or low levels of sex hormone binding globulin (SHBG). Hyperprolactinemia is also seen in PCOS.

Insulin resistance is a common feature of patients with PCOS. Anovulatory women who are hyperandrogenic should be assessed for insulin resistance and glucose tolerance with measurement of fasting glucose-insulin

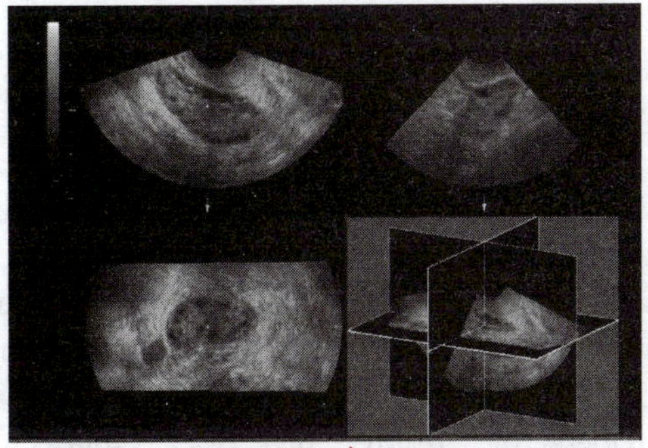

Figure 5.3: 3D ultrasound of a polycystic ovary

ratio followed by two-hour glucose tolerance test after a 75 g glucose load. A ratio of less than 4.5 is consistent with insulin resistance (Speroff et al 1999). However, testing for insulin resistance is being debated. Nestler et al (2002) in a review article stated that both lean and obese women with PCO can be assumed as having insulin resistance, and therefore testing for insulin resistance such as fasting insulin, glucose or glucose to insulin ratio are not very useful predictors of ovulatory response to insulin sensitising agents.

Since there are so many clinical and biochemical features in PCOS, the exact definition of PCOS can be confusing. At a recent joint consensus meeting of the European Society of Human Reproduction and the Embryology/American Society for Reproductive Medicine (ESHRE/ASRM), a refined definition of PCOS was agreed on:

The presence of two out of the following three criteria constitutes PCOS (Rotterdam consensus 2004):

1. Oligo- and/or anovulation
2. Hyperandrogenism (clinical and/or biochemical)
3. Polycystic ovaries, with the exclusion of other etiologies

MANAGEMENT

Since PCOS may affect a woman at any stage of life, the clinician will see a variety of clinical pictures. The adolescent, may present with menstrual irregularities, skin problems such as hirsutism, acne or alopecia, obesity or acanthosis nigicans. A woman in the reproductive age group may present with infertility. An older woman may present with problems related to long-term sequelae of PCOS such as gynecological cancer, diabetes or cardiovascular risk (Table 5.3). The management of a patient with PCOS will depend on her presenting problems.

Menstrual Irregularities

Many women with PCOS will report to their physician six menstrual periods per year—as long as these are not unduly heavy or painful, no particular medical therapy may be needed. Many others only have one or two periods a year—these women are at increased risk of endometrial carcinoma and anovulatory menorrhagia. In obese women, weight loss should be the first line of treatment. In patients who succeed in losing over 5% of their body weight, this alone may restore normal menstrual regularity (Kiddy et al 1992). A reduction in body weight of 5%–10% will cause a 30% reduction in visceral fat, which is often sufficient to restore ovulation and reduce markers of metabolic disease (Depres et al 2001). Others believe that weight loss of just 3 to 5 kg may be sufficient to restore the cycle. Weight loss is associated with a reduction of circulating insulin and androgen levels, which can also be achieved by using insulin-sensitising drugs (see next paragraph). However, there is still not enough evidence that insulin-sensitising agents can be recommended as a treatment when menstrual irregularity is the primary complaint (Balen et al 2005).

Often, oral contraceptives are prescribed to women with PCOS, since they have the benefit of contraception, protect against endometrial cancer and improve skin manifestations of polycystic ovaries such as hirsutism and acne. Diane 35® (Schering Healthcare Ltd) which contains 35 µg of ethinyl estradiol and 2 mg of cyprotenone acetate may be used in patients who also have hyperandrogenism (hirsutism and acne) associated with menstrual irregularity. As untreated PCOS may be regarded as a progressive syndrome, at least up to the age of 40, it is reasonable to assume that the treatment with this combination of ethinyl estradiol and

Table 5.2: Biochemical changes in polycystic ovary syndrome

1. Increase in LH/ usually normal FSH
2. Increase prolactin
3. Increase androgens (testosterone, androstenedione, dihydroepiandrosterone sulphate)
4. Increase fasting insulin
5. Abnormal glucose tolerance test
6. Increase in estradiol, estrone
7. Decrease SHBG

cyproterone acetate, which markedly reduces androgen concentrations and their untoward effects, will put the syndrome 'on hold', thus improving the prospects of success of fertility treatment when it is discontinued (Balen et al 2005).

Skin Manifestations

Skin manifestations of polycystic ovarian syndrome include acne, hirsutism, alopecia and acanthosis nigricans.

Acne: This is seen in approximately a third of PCOS patients (Conway et al 1989; Balen et al 1995; Franks 1998). Mild acne may be treated topically with keratolytics such as azaleic acid, retinoids, or with antibacterials such as benzoyl peroxide, clindamycin 1% lotion and erythromycin 2% gel (Cunliffe and Simpson 1998). More severe forms generally require oral antibiotics such as the tetracyclines, erythromycin and trimethoprim. For severe cases, isotretinoin is prescribed and produces long-term remission in more than 70% of patients.

In PCOS, anti-androgens are the most effective because acne occurs as a result of overstimulation of the pilosebaceous unit by androgens. Anti-androgens that can be used are cyroterone acetate, spironolactone, flutamide and finasteride. Cyproterone acetate can be given as a combined oral contraceptive pill (as mentioned above). This minimal dose has proven effective in almost 100% of cases (van Waygen and van den Ende 1995). In more severe cases, cyproterone acetate in a dose of 10–100 mg/day may be given on the first 10 days of the combined oral contraceptive pill. It will take three to five months for any improvement to become evident. Acne will be cleared in 60% of patients in six months, and after 12 months, 95% should be free of acne (Balen et al 2005).

Spironolactone, an aldosterone antagonist has anti-androgen action. A new combined contraceptive pill, Yasmin® (Schering Healthcare Ltd) contains drosperinone, a derivative of spironolactone, which has been found to be effective in the improvement of acne (Palel-Singh et al 2004). Flutamide, a non-steroidal anti-androgen, can be used for the treatment of hirsutism and acne. However, because of rare reports of hepatotoxicity, it is not commonly used. Finasteride acts by inhibiting 5α-reductase and can be taken orally in a dose of 1–5 mg/day. It does not have many side effects. When spironolactone, finasteride and flutamide is taken, contraception is advised to avoid the potential risk of feminisation of a male fetus. It is important to inform patients that clinical response takes time and patients have to be on long-term maintenance treatment to avoid relapse. The longer the duration of treatment (at least in the ethinyl estradiol/ cyproterone acetate oral contraceptive pills), the less the chance of relapse within a given period of time.

Hirsutism: Patients may present with excess hair as their main problem. Hirsutism can be treated with physical therapy such as bleaching, shaving, plucking, depilatory creams, electrolysis and laser. Bleaching with hydrogen peroxide disguises pigmented facial hair. Repeated plucking of hair may lead to permanent hair follicle matrix damage, resulting in finer, thinner hair (Hamilton and Potten 1974). Side effects include postinflammatory hyperpigmentation, folliculitis, pseudofolliculitis, and rarely, scarring (Olsen 1999).

Chemical depilators are usually thioglycates that disrupt the disulphide bonds of hair shaft. Electrolysis is a proven method of hair removal (Dawber 1998). Three forms exist, galvanic (direct current electrolysis), thermolysis (alternate current electrolysis) and the blend (galvanic electrolysis and thermolysis). The procedure is highly operator dependent. Laser such as ruby laser, alexandrite laser, semiconductor diode laser and YAG laser may be used to vapourise the target tissue. Side effects include erythema, hyperpigmentation and hypopigmentation, blistering and pain. Usually, several treatments in sittings or combination treatment improves efficacy.

A combined oral contraceptive pill will usually prevent growth of excess hair in newer areas but is rarely sufficient by itself to cause regression of excess hair. This usually necessitates the addition of anti-androgen therapy such as cyproterone acetate (CPA). Diane 35® (Schering Healthcare Ltd) is a very useful combined contraceptive pill for cases of mild to moderate hirsutism and/or acne. Severe cases usually require the use of 50 mg tablets of CPA. Typically, 1–2 tablets of CPA are taken with the first 10 active pills of Diane 35. Most women notice a regression of excess hair within four to six months, but typically, treatment needs to be continued for at least 1–2 years to substantially reduce hair growth and then maintenance therapy is required to keep the problem under control. Typically, this is a low-dose combined oral contraceptive pill. Another useful anti-androgenic treatment is spironolactone. This may be used alone or in combination with a contraceptive pill. Flutamide and finasteride are also drugs that help reduce hirsutism.

Table 5.3: Possible long-term problems of polycystic ovary syndrome

1. Diabetes mellitus
2. Endometrial cancer
3. Dyslipidemia
4. Hypertension, cardiovascular disease
5. Breast cancer (not proven)

Alopecia: Some patients may present with alopecia. Treatment includes psychological support, hairstyling and camouflage with wigs or sometimes hair transplantation.

Infertility

Infertility is a common presenting problem in patients with polycystic ovarian syndrome; approximately 80%–90% of women suffer from infertility due to anovulation (Adams et al 1986; Hull 1987). There are several methods of inducing ovulation, all of which use the basic principle of reducing insulin or LH concentrations, stimulating FSH stimulation or a combination of these principles (Balen et al 2005).

Weight Loss

The first step in ovulation induction is weight loss. Obese women (BMI > 30 kg/m^2) should be encouraged to lose weight. Even patients who are overweight (BMI > 27 kg/m^2) are associated with a reduced likelihood of ovulation. Weight loss improves the endocrine profile (Kiddy et al 1989, 1992), and thus the likelihood of ovulation and a healthy pregnancy. Achieving weight reduction is, however, extremely difficult, particularly as the metabolic status of the patient with

PCOS conspires against weight loss (Speroff et al 1999; Laven et al 2002). Different strategies may be used to lose weight. Dieting and exercise should be encouraged. Clarke et al used a realistic exercise programme with positive reinforcement of a suitable eating programme to achieve weight loss (Nestler et al 2002). Appetite suppressants should be reserved for the extremely obese (BMI >35 kg/m^2) because of the potential side effects (for example, pulmonary hypertension). Even with minimal weight reduction (4–5 kg), the patient may revert to ovulatory cycles and may be able to conceive spontaneously.

TREATMENT

Clomiphene Citrate

The simplest mode of ovulation induction is the use of clomiphene citrate. Patients may be given, to start with, 50 mg a day orally, for five days starting from day 2 to day 5 of a spontaneous or progesterone-induced bleed. At least the first cycle of treatment, if not all cycles, should be monitored. There are various ways to determine whether the patient is ovulating. The patient may be taught clinical signs and symptoms of ovulation, including changes in the cervical mucus, slight pelvic pain and breast tenderness. However, anovulatory patients usually find it difficult to identify these clinical signs and symptoms of ovulation. Serial transvaginal ultrasound may be used to examine the follicles. This may be done on day 10 of the cycle and depending on the presence and size of follicle, serial scans can help determine the patient's fertile period. Another method is the use of urinary LH test. Presence of a 'double line' indicates an LH surge and this can be used as a basis of determining when to have sexual intercourse.

The maximum dosage and the duration for treatment with clomiphene citrate are still under debate. If the patient does not ovulate with 50 mg of clomiphene citrate, then the dose may be increased to 100 mg. Some authors (Shepard et al 1979; Lobo et al 1982; Dickey et al 1997) believe that in overweight patients a higher dose of clomiphene citrate may be used (up to 250 mg of clomiphene citrate has been used). However, if the patient is ovulating with a low dose, there is no benefit in increasing the dose because high doses have other side effects, including thickening of the cervical mucus and antiestrogenic effect on the endometrium (Dickey et al 1993). A postcoital test should be considered when treatment is started.

As for the duration of use of clomiphene citrate, Balen and Jacobs suggested its use up to 12 months because of the expected increase in cumulative chance of pregnancy. They also suggested that the duration of therapy can also be increased from five days to ten days (Balen and Jacobs 2000). Adjuvant therapy with naltrexone has been tried in patients who are unresponsive to clomiphene citrate alone (Roozenberg et al 1997). FSH and LH can also be suppressed before ovulation induction by pretreatment with progesterone or even oral contraceptive pills. If there is evidence of unruptured follicle by ultrasound monitoring, hCG may be necessary (Polson et al 1989). Addition of dexamethasone at the follicular phase of the cycle has yielded better results (Parsanezhad et al 2002). Besides clomiphene citrate, tamoxifen (an antiestrogen) or letrozole (an oral aromatase inhibitor) may be used (Fisher et al 2002). Clomiphene citrate is currently licensed in the UK for only six months use.

Metformin

Metformin improves insulin sensitivity and 500 mg taken eight-hourly reduces hyperinsulinemia, basal and stimulated LH levels and free testosterone concentrations in overweight women with polycystic ovaries. However, it must only be used if there are no contraindications for metformin use. These include diminished renal function, cardiac diseases, severe pulmonary diseases, liver dysfunction, pancreatitis, concomitant use of diuretics and hypersensitivity to metformin. Patients must be informed about the adverse effects, which include gastrointestinal symptoms such as diarrhea, nausea, vomiting especially during the initial treatment period; these symptoms are usually transient and resolve spontaneously. Gastrointestinal symptoms may be avoided if metformin is taken with meals and if the dose is increased slowly. Probably because of the gastrointestinal side effects, some patients may lose weight. Patients may return to ovulatory cycles. However, there has been controversy, suggesting that the improvement in ovulation is a result of weight loss rather than the use of metformin (Speroff et al 1999). Insulin sensitising agent, troglitazone, appears to benefit PCOS patients but it has been withdrawn from the market because of reports of death from hepatotoxicity. The other thiazolidinedione that is being investigated is rosiglitazone.

In addition to difficulty in conceiving, women with PCOS are at increased risk of miscarriage following either spontaneous or assisted conception. Rates of early pregnancy loss defined as miscarriage during the first trimester, are reported to be 30%–50% in women with PCOS (Homburg et al 1988; Sagle et al 1988; Regan et al 1990; Balen et al 1993; Watson et al 1993), which is threefold higher than the rate of 10%–15% reported for normal women (Regan et al 1989; Gray and Wu 2000). Conversely, 36%–82% of women with recurrent early pregnancy loss are reported to have PCOS (Sagle et al 1988; Regan et al 1989; Clifford et al 1994; Liddell et al 1997). The intriguing question is will an insulin-sensitising drug prevent early pregnancy loss in PCOS? The result of a recent pilot study (Glucek et al 2001) and a preliminary report (Jakubowicz et al 2001), both of which reported a dramatic reduction of miscarriage in women with PCOS treated throughout pregnancy with metformin, suggest that it does. Glucek et al (2002) went further to report that metformin therapy throughout pregnancy reduces the development of gestational diabetes in women with PCOS.

In patients who do not ovulate while on metformin, clomiphene citrate may be added to induce ovulation. Nestler et al (1998) found that using metformin and clomiphene causes a higher incidence of ovulation and pregnancy compared with clomiphene alone.

If the above attempt fails, laparoscopic ovarian drilling or ovulation induction with parenteral gonadotrophic therapy may be attempted—which one should be done first is under debate.

Laparoscopic Ovarian Drilling

Gjonnaess reported the first series of patients who underwent ovarian diathermy; 90% of women ovulated, and 70% of the 62 women treated conceived (Gjonnaess 1994). Laparoscopic ovarian drilling is a simple procedure whereby several punctures are made in one or both the polycystic ovaries (Fig. 5.4. See Page 90) (This technique has superseded ovarian wedge resection). The controversy is how many diathermy points are to be drilled and what wattage is to be used during ovarian cautery. Gjonneass cauterised each ovary at five to eight points, for five to six seconds at each point with 300–400 W. Naether et al treated five to twenty points per ovary, with 400 W for one second (Naether et al 1991); Armer et al (1990) cauterised at four points; Balen and Jacobs (1994) only cauterised one ovary at four points using 40 W for four seconds and achieved ovarian activity. The risk of ovarian diathermy is periovarian adhesions and the possibility of ovarian failure. Abdominal lavage has helped reduce periovarian adhesions.

Besides diathermy, laser can be used for ovarian drilling. The laser provides controllable power density, sufficient depth of penetration and predictable thermodamage of surrounding tissues. It may also diminish the risk of adhesions (Huber et al 1988). Several types of laser have been used—carbon dioxide, argon, YAG. Almeida and Risk (1998) reported a case of ovarian drilling by microlaparoscopy under local anesthesia. Another technique that has been recently described is transvaginal hydrolaparoscopy and bipolar coagulation of the polycystic ovaries (Fernandez et al 2001).

Mio et al have shown in 18 patients with PCO that with transvaginal ultrasound-guided follicular aspiration they could obtain an 87%–100% ovulation rate per patient and 50% pregnancy (Mio et al 1991). Most of the persistent follicles were punctured and their contents aspirated during the midluteal phase. The same ovarian stimulation regimen as used in the previous cycles was administered in the cycles after the aspiration. A significant decrease of basal LH was observed. This method, simpler and less invasive than laparoscopy, could become very significant if further experiments confirm its efficacy.

The other issue is whether to wait after ovarian diathermy to await spontaneous ovulation or to immediately commence low-dose ovulation stimulation. Ostrzenski commenced all his patients on either clomiphene or FSH therapy immediately after laser wedge resection (1992). Farhi et al (1995) demonstrated an increased ovarian sensitivity to gonadotrophin therapy after laparoscopic ovarian diathermy.

Gonadotrophin Therapy

Gonadotrophin therapy is indicated in women with anovulatory PCOS who have been treated with antiestrogens, either if they have failed to ovulate or if they have a response to clomiphene that is likely to reduce their chance of conception (for example, persistent hypersecretion of LH, or negative postcoital tests due to the antiestogenic effect on cervical mucus). One of the greatest therapeutic challenges in all ovulation induction therapies is to predict the response to stimulation of women with polycystic ovaries. The polycystic ovary is characteristically quiescent (at least when viewed by ultrasound) before exhibiting an exuberant and explosive response to stimulation. The aim is for unifollicular development and this can be challenging. There are many protocols available but the most recent protocol is the sequential step-up–step-down protocol (Hugues 1996). Patients are started with very low-dose gonadotrophin (FSH) and the dose is gradually increased. When the leading follicle is 14 mm, the FSH threshold dose is reduced by half. This protocol appears to reduce the number of lead follicles when compared with a classic step-up protocol. The aim of this low dose step-up protocol is to reduce the risk of both multiple pregnancies and ovarian hyperstimulation syndrome, both of which are increased in women with polycystic ovaries. Treatment cycles may be up to 28–35 days. When the leading follicle reaches 17 mm in its largest diameter, hCG 10,000 units is given to trigger ovulation. Some believe that there may be benefit in waiting until the follicle becomes 20 mm (Silverberg et al 1991). Sometimes, there may be a sudden increase in the number of follicles. When this happens, the cycle may be cancelled or in vitro fertilisation may be attempted.

In clomiphene resistant PCOS, it is difficult to decide whether laparoscopic ovarian diathermy should be tried first or gonadotrophins. A recent meta-analysis of success rates of surgical treatment indicates that results for the former resemble those obtained by medical treatment (Farquhar et al 1999). Gonadotrophins are expensive even for unifollicular ovulation induction. The potential financial costs of a multiple pregnancy, particularly if neonatal intensive care facilities are required, are of course immense. Other costs have to be counted in terms of the successful outcome of treatment, a low rate of miscarriage and the birth of healthy, preferably singleton, babies, with no health risks to their mothers. It is here that laparoscopic ovarian surgery appears to provide a significant advantage—it is a single treatment that results in unifollicular ovulation, with correction of the endocrinopathy and an apparently low rate of miscarriage. Although there are risks associated with surgery and an anesthetic, women require a test of tubal patency prior to gonadotrophin therapy and therefore many would be subjected to a laparoscopy in any case. The main concerns are the formation of adhesions and the potential for significant reduction in viable ovarian tissue, with the possibility of inducing premature ovarian failure. The evidence to date, however, is reassuring.

In some patients, in vitro fertilisation (IVF), sometimes with intracytoplasmic sperm injection (ICSI), may be the only option for pregnancy. Patients with tubal blockage or whose partners have a low sperm count may have to undergo IVF or IVF–ICSI. Many protocols are available when performing IVF. The most commonly performed protocol for IVF is the long protocol using gonadotrophin agonist to downregulate, followed by gonadotrophin stimulation of the ovary. This protocol is ideal for patients with PCO. The reason is that PCO patients have high LH levels. This is detrimental to pregnancy rates and also causes high miscarriage rate (Dor et al 1990). As such, by pituitary downregulation, serum LH is reduced. It is also important to start these patients with low dose FSH. Balen and Jacobs (2000) recommend a dose of 75–150 IU of FSH or hMG for women under 35 years of age and 150 units for older women with PCO. These patients must also be monitored closely with daily ultrasound from day 8 of stimulation. Serial measurement of serum estradiol will also be helpful. The aim is to decrease the total number of follicles in the ovaries and thus reduce the incidence of OHSS. If there are too many follicles and serum estradiol levels are very high, then oocyte recovery and freezing of all the embryos and no fresh embryo transfer should be considered. Luteal phase support should not be given with hCG, and only progesterone support should be given.

Collection of immature oocytes from PCOS patients is being researched. The immature oocytes can be matured in vitro and ICSI could be performed (Trounson et al 1996); co-culture with Vero cells may be used to fertilise oocytes (Cha et al 1996). Although these techniques are still in the experimental stage, they may signify the future of patients with PCOS. The technique of freezing of mature and immature oocytes is being developed.

Long-term monitoring: There have been suggestions in the literature that women with PCOS are at increased risk of developing a number of chronic conditions and that consequently, their health should be monitored (Wild 1995; Bjorntorp 1996; Pettigrew and Hamilton-Fairley 1997; Hopkinson et al 1998).

Insulin resistance and the resulting hyperinsulinemia are known to be features of PCOS. It is now believed that insulin resistance is the underlying disorder of PCOS (Hopkinson et al 1998). Women with PCOS may be at increased risk of developing non-insulin dependent diabetes mellitus (NIDDM); however, there is inadequate evidence to support this. The extent to which NIDDM contributes to premature morbidity and mortality for women with PCOS remains unclear at present. It is also unclear whether PCOS itself, or the obesity that is a frequent attribute of the condition, or both, principally contribute to the observed excess of NIDDM among women with histologically proven PCOS (Venn and Shelly 2000).

Clinicians have been concerned about the possibility of an increase in cardiovascular disease in women with PCOS, due to the disturbance in insulin resistance and lipid profiles that often accompanies this diagnosis. Lipid studies showed that there are poorer lipid profiles among women with PCOS compared to the control group (Talbott et al 1998). However, Venn and Shelly concluded that the results of studies that have considered the relationship between PCOS and lipid level are inconsistent. HDL levels are a possible exception, with the majority of studies finding lower HDL levels among women with PCOS than among controls, regardless of the selection criteria for either cases or controls. The question of whether patients with PCOS have a greater tendency to develop high blood pressure also remains unanswered. There is very little evidence that women with PCOS are at increased risk of cardiovascular disease independent of NIDDM (Venn and Shelly 2000).

The association between exposure to unopposed estrogens and an increased risk of endometrial cancer has been well established. Obesity has been shown consistently to be an important risk factor for endometrial cancer (Parazzini et al 1997) and is therefore likely to contribute to cancer risk in overweight women with PCOS. Diabetes and hypertension have been associated with an increased risk of endometrial cancer in some studies but, overall, the findings have been inconsistent and the relationship is not well defined. So whether polycystic ovaries per se increase the risk of endometrial cancer is debatable, but with obesity and diabetes the risk is increased. There is also possibly no association between PCOS and breast cancer (Parazzini et al 1991; Anderson et al 1997; Modan et al 1998; Garland et al 1998). The risk of ovarian cancer in women with PCOS has not been studied adequately. In these patients, the recommendation of screening is similar to that in the general population. Women with polycystic ovaries may be monitored for endometrial hyperplasia.

Although it is not yet clear whether the predicted risks of health problems in women with PCOS actually translate into significant excess long-term morbidity and/or mortality, it has been suggested that women with PCOS could reduce their risk of NIDDM and cardiovascular disease through weight reduction and exercise—the use of medication that reduces insulin resistance might also be warranted (Guzick 1998; Hopkinson et al 1998). While weight loss and exercise may prove to be valuable interventions for overweight women with PCOS, the options for lean women are limited. Despite advice and efforts to lose weight, women with polycystic ovaries may find it very difficult to lose weight and maintain the recommended weight loss.

Conclusion: Polycystic ovarian syndrome is the most common endocrine disorder in women (prevalence 15%–20%), and is a heterogeneous condition. Diagnosis is made by ultrasound detection of polycystic ovaries and one or more of a combination of symptoms and signs (hyperandrogenism [acne, hirsutism, alopecia], obesity, menstrual cycle disturbance [oligo/amenorrhea] and biochemical abnormalities [hypersecretion of testosterone, luteinising hormone and insulin]). Management is symptom orientated. In obese patients, weight loss improves symptoms and endocrine profile.

Menstrual cycles may be regulated with cyclical oral contraceptives or progestogens. Hyperandrogenism may be managed with oral contraceptives containing ethinyl estradiol with cyproterone acetate. Insulin sensitising agents (such as metformin) are showing promise in the management of polycystic ovarian syndrome. Ovulation induction may be difficult since it requires various treatment strategies and patients must be monitored carefully. In patients with pure anovulatory infertility due to PCOS, whatever treatment options are used, there are a few who will be unable to conceive.

References

Adams JM, DW Polson, N Abulwadi et al.1985. Multifollicular ovaries: Clinical and endocrine features and response to pulsatile gonadotropin-releasing hormone. *Lancet* 2:1375–1378.

Adams J, DW Polson, S Franks. 1986. Prevalence of polycystic ovaries in women with anovulation and idiopathic hirsutism. *Br Med J* 293:355–359.

Almeida OD and B Risk. 1998 Microlaparoscopic ovarian drilling under local anesthesia. *Middle East Fertil Soc J* 3:189–191.

Anderson KE, TA Sellers, PL Chen et al. 1997. Association of Stein–Leventhal syndrome with the incidence of postmenopausal breast carcinoma in large prospective study of women in Iowa. *Cancer* 79:494–499.

Armar NA, HHG McGarrigle, JW Honour et al. 1990. Laparoscopic ovarian diathermy in the management of anovulatory infertility in women with polycystic ovaries: Endocrine changes and clinical outcome. *Fertil Steril* 53:45–49.

Balen AH and HS Jacobs. 1994. A prospective study comparing unilateral and bilateral laparoscopic ovarian diathermy in women with the polycystic ovary syndrome. *Fertil Steril* 62:921–925.

Balen A, G Conway, G Kaltsas, K Techatraisak, P Manning P. 1995. Polycystic ovary syndrome: The spectrum of the disorder in 1741 patients. *Hum Reprod* 10:2107–2111.

Balen AH, SL Tan, J MacDougall, HS Jacobs. 1993. Miscarriage rates following in vitro fertilisation are increased in women with polycystic ovaries and reduced by pituitary desensitisation with buserelin. *Hum Reprod* 8:959–964.

Balen AH, GS Conway, G Kaltsas et al. 1995. Polycystic ovary syndrome: The spectrum of the disorder in 1741 patients. *Hum Reprod* 10:2107–2111.

Balen AH, JSE Laven, SL Tan, D Dewailly. 2003. Ultrasound assessment of the polycystic ovary: International consensus definitions. *Hum Reprod Update* 9:505–514.

Balen AH, GS Conway, R Homburg, RS Legro. 2005. Polycystic ovary syndrome: *A guide to clinical management.* London: Taylor and Francis Group, 166.

Bjorntorp P. 1996. The android woman—a risky condition. *J Intl Med* 239:105–110.

Bringer J, P Lefebvre, F Boulet et al.1993. Body composition and regional fat distribution in polycystic ovarian syndrome. Relationship to hormonal and metabolic profiles. *Ann NY Acad Sci* 687:115–123, 853–861.

Cha KY, HM Chung, SY Han et al. 1996. Successful in vitro maturation, fertilisation and pregnancy by using immature follicular oocytes collected from unstimulated polycystic ovarian syndrome patients (Abstract 0–044) In Proceeding of the American Society of Reproductive Medicine, Boston, November 2–6, p. S23, Boston: American Society of Reproductive Medicine.

Clifford K, R Rai, H Watson, L Regan. 1994. An informative protocol for the investigation of recurrent miscarriage: Preliminary experience of 500 consecutive cases. *Hum Reprod* 9:1328–1332.

Conway G, J Honour, H Jacobs. 1989. Heterogeneity of the polycystic ovary syndrome: Clinical endocrine and ultrasound features in 556 patients. *Clin Endocrinol* 30:459–470.

Cunliffe W and N Simpson. 1998. Disorders of sebaceous glands. In *Rook Wilkinson Ebling Textbook of Dermatology*, ed R Champion, J Burton, D Burns and S Breathnach. Oxford: Blackwell Science, 1927–1984.

Dawber R. 1998. Facial and body hair. In *Cosmetic dermatology*, eds. R Baran and H Maibach. London: Martin Dunitz, 201–204.

Depres JP, I Lemieux, D Prud'homme. 2001. Treatment of obesity: Need to focus on high risk, abdominally obese patients. *Br Med J* 322:716–720.

Diamanti–Kandarakis E, CR Koulie, AT Bergiele, FA Filandra et al. 1999. A survey of the polycystic ovary syndrome in the Greek Island of Lesbos: A hormonal and metabolic profile. *J Clin Endocrinol Metab* 84:4006–4011.

Dickey RP, SN Taylor, DN Curole et al. 1997. Relationship of clomiphene dose and patient weight to successful treatment. *Hum Reprod* 12:449–453.

Dickey RP, TT Olar, Taylor SN et al. 1993. Relationship of biochemical pregnancy to preovulatory endometrial thickness and pattern in ovulation induction patients. *Hum Reprod* 8, 327–390.

Dor J, A Shulman, D Levran et al. 1990. The treatment of patients with polycystic ovary syndrome by in-vitro fertilisation: A comparison of results with those patients with tubal infertility. *Human Reproduction* 5, 816–818.

Dramusic V, U Rajan, YC Wong et al. 1997. Adolescent polycystic ovary syndrome. *Ann NY Acad Sci* 816:194–208.

Dunaif A. 1992. Insulin resistance and ovarian hyperandrogenism. *Endocrinologist* 2, 248–260.

Eden JA. 1991. The polycystic ovary syndrome presenting as resistant acne successfully treated with cyproterone acetate. *Med J Austr* 155:677–680.

Farhi J, S Soule, H Jacobs. 1995. Effect of laparoscopic ovarian electrocautery on ovarian response and outcome of treatment with gonadotrophins in clomiphene citrate resistant patients with PCOS. *Fertil Steril* 64:930–935.

Farquhar C, P Vanderkerckhove, M Arnot, R Lilford. 1999. *Laparoscopic 'drilling' by diathermy or laser for ovulation induction in anovulatory polycystic syndrome* (Cochrane Review). In The Cochrane Library, Issue 1. Oxford: Update Software.

Fernandez H, JD Alby, A Gervaise, R de Tayrac, R Frydman. 2001. Operative transvaginal hydrolaparoscopy for treatment of polycystic ovary syndrome: A new minimally invasive surgery. *Fertil Steril* 75(3):607–611.

Fisher SA, Reid RL, Van Vugt DA, Casper RF. 2002. A randomized double-blind comparison of the effects of clomiphene citrate and the aromatase inhibitor letrozole on ovulatory functiom in normal women. *Fertil Steril* 78(2):280–285.

Franks S. 1988. Polycystic ovary syndrome: A changing perspective. *Clin Endocrinol* 31:87–118.

Garland M, DJ Hunter, GA Colditz et al. 1998. Menstrual cycle characteristics and history of ovulatory infertility in relation to breast cancer risk in a large cohort of US women. *Am J Epidemiol* 147:636–643.

Gjonnaess H. 1984. Polycystic ovarian syndrome treated by ovarian electrocautery through the laparoscope. *Fertil Steril* 41:20–25.

Glucek CJ, Wang P, Kobayashi S, Philips H, Sieve-Smith L. 2002. Metformin therapy throughout pregnancy reduces the development of gestational diabetes in women with polycystic ovarian syndrome. *Fertil Steril* 77(3):520–525.

Glucek CJ, Phillips H, Cameron D, Sieve-Smith L, Wang P. 2001. Continuing metformin throughout pregnancy in women with polycystic ovary syndrome appears to safely reduce first-trimester spontaneous abortion: A pilot study. *Fertil Steril* 75:46–52.

Gray RH and Wu LY. 2000. Subfertility and the risk of spontaneous abortion. *Am J Public Health* 90:1452–1454.

Guzick D. 1998. Polycystic ovary syndrome: Symptomatology, pathophysiology and epidemiology. *Am J Obstet Gynecol* 179:S89–93

Hamilton E and C Potten. 1974. The effect of repeated plucking on mouse skincell kinetics. *J Invest Dermatol* 62:560–562.

Homburg R, NA Armar, A Eshel, J Adams, HS. Jacobs. 1988. Influence of serum luteinising hormone concentrations on ovulation, conception, and early pregnancy loss in polycystic ovary syndrome. *Br Med J* 297:1024–1026.

Hopkinson ZEC, Sattar N, Fleming R, Greer IA. 1998. Polycystic ovarian syndrome the metabolic syndrome comes to gynaecology. *Br Med J* 317:329–332.

Huber J, J Hosmann, J Spona. 1988. Polycystic ovarian syndrome treated by laser through the laparoscope. *Lancet* ii:215.

Hugues JN, I Cedrin-Durnerin I, C Avril C et al. 1996. Sequential step-up and step-down dose regimen: An alternative method for ovulation induction with FSH in polycystic ovary syndrome. *Hum Reprod* 11:2581–2584.

Hull MG. 1987. Epidemiology of infertility and polycystic ovarian disease: Endocrinological and demographic studies. *Gynaecol Endocrinol* 1:235–245.

Jakubowicz DJ, MJ Iuorno, S Jakubowicz, KA Roberts, JE Nestler. 2001. Metformin reduces early pregnancy loss in polycystic ovary syndrome abstractno. P2–147. In *Program and abstracts of the 83rd Annual Meeting of the Endocrine Society*, Denver, Colorado, 384.

Kiddy DS, D Hamilton-Fairley, M Seppala et al. 1989. Diet-induced changes in sex hormone binding globulin and free testosterone in women with normal or polycystic ovaries: correlation with serum insulin and insulin-like growth factor-1. *Clin Endocrinol (Oxford)* 31:757–763.

Kiddy DS, D Hamilton-Fairley, A Bush et al. 1992. Improvement in endocrine and ovarian function during dietary treatment of obese women with polycystic ovary syndrome. *Clin Endocrinol* 36: 105–111.

Laven JS, B Imani, MJ Eijkemans, BC Fauser. 2002. New approaches to PCOS and other forms of anovulation. *Obstet Gynecol Surv* 57:755–767.

Liddell HS, K Sowden, CM Farquhar. 1997. Recurrent miscarriage: Screening for polycystic ovaries and subsequent pregnancy outcome. *Aust NZ J Obstet Gynaecol* 37:402–406.

Lobo RA, M Gysler, CM March et al. 1982. Clinical and laboratory predictors of clomiphene response. *Fertil Steril* 37:168–174.

Michelmore K, AH Balen, D Dunger, M Vessey. 1999. Polycystic ovaries and associated clinical and biochemical features in young women in the normal population. *Clin Endocrinol* 51:779–786.

Mio Y, T Toda, M Tanikawa et al. 1991. Transvaginal ultrasound guided follicular aspiration in the management of anovulatory infertility associated with polycystic ovaries. *Fertil Steril* 56: 1060–1065.

Modan B, E Ron, L Lerner-Geva et al. 1998. Cancer incidence in cohort of infertile women. *Am J Epidemiol* 147:1038–1042.

Naether O, HC Weise, R Fischer. 1991. Treatment with electrocautery in sterility patients with polycystic ovarian disease. *Geburtsh Frauenheilk* 51:920–924.

Nestler JE, JN Clore, WG Blackard. 1989. The central role of obesity (hyperinsulinemia) in the pathogenesis of polycystic ovary syndrome. *Am J Obstet Gynecol* 5:1095–1097.

Nestler JE, DJ Jakubowicz, WS Evans, R Pasquali. 1998. Effects of metformin on spontaneous and clomiphene-induced ovulation in the polycystic ovary syndrome. *New Engl J Med* 338:1876–1880.

Nestler JE, D Stovall, N Akhter, MJ Iuorno, DJ Jakuboxicz. 2002. Strategies for the use of insulin sensitising drugs to treat infertility in women with polycystic ovarian syndrome. *Fertil Steril* 77 (2): 209–215.

Norman RJ, MJ Davies, J Lord, LJ Moran. 2002. The role of lifestyle modification in polycystic ovary syndrome. *Trends Endocrinol Metab* 13:251–257.

Olsen E. 1999. Methods of hair removal. *J Am Acad Dermatol* 40:143–157.

Ostrzenski A. 1992. Endoscopic carbon dioxide laser wedge resection in resistant PCO. *Intern J Fertil* 37:295–299.

Pache TD, S Chadha, LJ Gooren, WC Hop et al. 1991. Ovarian morphology in long term androgen treated female-to-male transsexuals. A human model for the study of PCOS? *Histopathol* 19: 445–452.

Palel-Singh M, JH Barth, K Mook, AH Balen. 2004. An observational study of Yasmin in the management of polycystic ovary syndrome. *Br J Fam Plann* 30:163–165.

Parazzini F, C la Vecchia, L Bocciolone, S Franceschi. 1991. The epidemiology of endometrial cancer. *Gynecol Oncol* 41:1–16.

Parazzini F, C La Vecchia, S Franceschi et al. 1997. Association of Stein–Leventhal syndrome with the incidence of postmenopausal breast carcinoma in a large prospective study of women in Iowa (letter). *Cancer* 80:1360–1362.

Parsanezhad ME, S Alborzi, S Motazedian, G Omrani. 2002. Use of dexamethasone and clomiphene citrate in the treatment of clomiphene citrate resistant patient with polycystic ovary syndrome and normal dehydroepiandrosterone sulfate levels: A prospective, double-blind placebo controlled trial. *Fertil Steril* 78(5):1001–1004.

Pasquali R, F Casmirri, D Venturoli. 1994. Body fat distribution has weight-independent effects on clinical, hormonal and metabolic features of women with polycystic ovary syndrome. *Metabolism* 6:706–713.

Pettigrew R and D Hamilton-Fairley. 1997. Obesity and female reproduction function. *Br Med Bull* 53:341–358.

Polson DW, DS Kiddy, HD Mason, S Franks. 1989. Induction of ovulation with clomiphene citrate in women with polycystic ovary syndrome: The difference between responders and nonresponders. *Fertil Steril* 51:30–34.

Regan L, PR Braude, PL Trembath. 1989. Influence of past reproductive performance on risk of spontaneous abortion. *Br Med J* 299:541–545.

Regan L, EJ Owen, HS Jacobs. 1990. Hypersecretion of luteinising hormone, infertility and miscarriage. *Lancet* 336:1141–1144.

Robert Y, Y Ardens, D Dewailly. 2000. Imaging polycystic ovaries. In *Polycystic ovary syndrome* ed GT Kovacs. Cambridge: Cambridge University Press.

Roozenberg BJ, HJHM van Dessel, JLH Evers, RSGM Bots. 1997. Successful induction of ovulation in normogonadotrophic clomiphene resistant anovulatory women by combined naltrexone and clomiphene citrate treatment. *Hum Reprod* 12:1720–1722.

Rotterdam ESHRE/ASRM–sponsored PCOS consensus workshop group: B Fauser, B Tarlazis, J Chang, R Azziz et al. 2004. Revised 2003 consensus on diagnostic criteria and long term health risks related to polycystic ovary syndrome (PCOS). *Hum Reprod* 19:41–47.

Sagle M, K Bishop, N Ridley, FM Alexander, M Michel, RC Bonney et al. 1988. Recurrent early miscarriage and polycystic ovaries. *Br Med J* 297:1027–1028.

Shepard MK, JP Balmaceda, CG Leija. 1979. Relationship of weight to successful induction of ovulation with clomiphene citrate. *Fertil Steril* 32:641–645.

Silverberg KM, DL Olive, WN Burns et al. 1991. Follicular size at the time of human chorionic gonadotrophin administration predicts ovulation outcome in human menopausal gonadotrophin-stimulated cycles. *Fertil Steril* 56:296–300.

Speroff L, RH Glass, NG Kase. 1999. *Clinical Gynaecologic Endocrinoology and Infertility*, 6th ed. Baltimore: Lippincott Williams & Wilkins, 171, 512.

Talbott E, A Clerici, SL Berga et al. 1998. Adverse lipid and coronary heart disease risk profiles in young women with polycystic ovary syndrome: Results of a case-control study. *J Clin Epidemiol* 51:415–422.

Taylor AE, B McCourt, K Martin, EJ Anderson, J Adams, D Schoebfeld et al. 1997. Determinants of abnormal gonadotropin secretion in clinically defined women with PCOS. *J Clin Endocrinol Metab* 82:2248–2256.

Trounson AO, A Bongso, A Szell et al. 1996. Maturation of human and bovine primary oocytes in vitro for fertilisation and embryo production. *Sing J Obstet Gynaecol* 27:78–84.

Van Waygen RG and A van den Ende. 1995. Experience in the long term treatment of hirsutism and/or acne with cyproterone acetate–containing preparations: Efficacy, metabolic and endocrine effects. *Expl Clin Endocrinol Diabetes* 103:241–251.

Venn A and J Shelly. 2000. Should there be long term monitoring of women with polycystic ovary syndrome? In *Polycystic ovary syndrome*, ed GT Kovacs. Cambridge: Cambridge University Press.

Waldstreicher J, NF Santoro, HJE Hall, M Filicori, WF Crowley. 1988. Hyperfunction of the hypothalamic-pituitary axis in women with polycystic ovarian disease: Indirect evidence of partial gonadotroph desensitisation. *J Clin Endocrinol Metab* 66:165–172

Watson H, DS Kiddy, D Hamilton-Fairley, MJ Scanlon, C Barnard, WP Collins et al. 1993. Hypersecretion of luteinizing hormone and ovarian steroids in women with recurrent early miscarriage. *Hum Reprod* 8:829–833.

Wild RA. 1995. Obesity, lipids, cardiovascular risk, androgen excess. *Am J Med* 98:27S–32S.

6

Management of Menorrhagia

Rajesh Bhakta

A normal menstrual cycle is 21–35 days in duration, bleeding lasts an average of seven days, and the flow is between 25 and 80 ml. Menorrhagia is menstruation at regular cycle intervals but with excessive flow and duration. Clinically, it is defined as total blood loss exceeding 80 ml per cycle or menses lasting longer than seven days in a patient with regular cycles.

Etiology: Menorrhagia may be due to systemic or pelvic pathology; however, no abnormality is found in 50% of cases—such patients are diagnosed as having dysfunctional uterine bleeding (DUB).

Causes of menorrhagia could belong to one of three categories:

Organic /or anatomic: Fibroid, adenomyosis, endometriosis, pelvic inflammatory disease (PID) endometrial polyp, (rarely) carcinoma of uterus

Endocrinological cause: Thyroid dysfunction, coagulation disorders

Iatrogenic cause: Intrauterine contraceptive device (IUCD), steroid hormones, medications like anticoagulants

Management: A detailed history should be elicited, including that of menstrual history of the last three cycles, its duration, rhythm and amount of bleeding—a pictorial blood assessment chart may be useful (Higham et al 1990). The presence of pelvic pain, either constant or premenstrual or with intercourse, may suggest pelvic pathology. Contraception usage or need, and the intention of having children in future should also be enquired into. A general as well as gynecological examination should be performed to include cervical cytology if necessary.

Investigations

The aim of investigations is to exclude any serious pathology and treat any underlying medical conditions.

Full blood count: A full blood count (including platelet count) provides extra information about the hematological indices and may reveal an iron deficiency state before anemia is reached. It should be remembered that coagulation disorders are found in almost 20% of adolescents with menorrhagia (Classens and Cowell 1981).

Thyroid function tests: There is no evidence linking menorrhagia with thyrotoxicosis (Ylikorkala and Viinikka 1983), but there have been several hypothyroid patients reporting an excess of menstrual irregularities, particularly menorrhagia (Nilsson and Rybo 1967). Routine screening for thyroid disease with thyroid function tests is not recommended for asymptomatic adults (Eldred and Thomas 1994).

Ultrasonography: Ultrasonography is the primary diagnostic tool in evaluating women with abnormal vaginal bleeding; it demonstrates anatomic findings not frequently detected during pelvic examination. These include leiomyoma, small ovarian cysts, as well as evaluation of the endometrium with respect to thickness, which would indirectly reflect the endometrial histology, and hormonal status of patients (Okaro et al 2003). Transvaginal ultrasound is the preferred modality to assess uterine shape, size and contour; endometrial thickness; and adnexal areas. Although MRI may be used, ultrasonography is more accurate, more economical, more convenient and probably better accepted than MRI.

Sonohysterography (SHG): This is also known by other names such as saline infusion hysterography or hysterosonography. In this procedure, saline is infused into the uterine cavity. This helps in separating and clarifying the relationships of anatomic lesions around the endometrial myometrial junction. It also helps visualise the mobility of an intracavitary lesion, such as polyps, within the liquid media. One study showed that SHG confirmed the presence of masses in 84% of consecutive cases of suspected intracavity lesions (De Kroon et al 2003).

Endometrial biopsy: Endometrial biopsy is a simple, quick, safe and convenient procedure, which can be performed on an ambulatory basis avoiding the need for anesthesia. The main purpose of an endometrial biopsy or aspirate is to exclude endometrial pathology like hyperplasia, endometrial disorders or malignancies. Routine endometrial biopsy should not be an initial investigation for menorrhagia, being indicated only if menorrhagia persists or when risk factors are present (RCOG 1998).

Hysteroscopy: This allows for examination of the whole endometrial cavity and cervical canal; it can detect small polyps or submucous fibroids that have been missed by ultrasonography, endometrial biopsy or blind curettage. The greatest advantage of hysteroscopy is its ability to allow directed biopsy in addition to direct visualisation of lesions.

In over 50% of women with menorrhagia no pathological cause is found. These women have been described as suffering from dysfunctional uterine bleeding (DUB).

Magnetic resonance imaging (MRI): is not a routine diagnostic tool. It allows for the differentiation of the fibroids from other pathological conditions such as adenomyosis, and delineates precisely the fibroid location within the uterus.

Others: Liver function and/or renal function tests, MRI

TREATMENT

Since improvement in quality of life is a key goal of therapy, it is important to assess the patient's preferences and take these into account when deciding on appropriate treatment. The patient's symptoms may be acute or chronic. Acute severe bleeding with unstable vital signs obviously requires aggressive management. Patients with a chronic problem can usually be treated in a stepwise manner incorporating NSAIDs and hormone-like progestogens to decrease bleeding. If menorrhagia is caused by defined pathology such as fibroid or hypothyroidism then appropriate treatment will result in cure.

When considering treatment options, the clinician, in collaboration with the woman, must make an assessment of the impact of the condition on the woman's quality of life and weigh this against the risks of treatment.

Treatment options can be divided into

a. Medical treatment
b. Surgical treatment

Medical treatment: Medical therapy must be tailored to the individual, taking into consideration the patient's age, no defined pelvic pathology like fibroid, adenomyosis, coexisting medical diseases, family history, and desire for fertility. Medication cost and adverse effects are also factored in because they may play a direct role in patient compliance.

The main classes of drugs employed for the medical treatment of menorrhagia are

A. Non-hormonal therapies:
   - Nonsteroidal anti-inflammatory drugs for example, mefanamic acid
   - Antifibrinolytics for example, tranexamic acid
   - Hemostatic agents
B. Hormonal therapies:
   - Oral contraceptive pill
   - Progestogens
   - Depot preparations
   - Intrauterine devices
   - Danazol
   - GnRH agents

Non-Steroidal antiinflammatory drugs (NSAIDs): These are widely used and are cost-effective. However, they have no effect on the rhythm of the menstrual cycle. They need to be taken regularly and should be commenced as soon as the bleeding starts, as they are less effective if commenced after the bleeding has become heavy. They are useful in women whose menorrhagia is secondary to an intrauterine coil, adenomyosis and coagulopathy. They can also be of benefit if dysmenorrhea is a significant symptom.

Mechanism of action: Research since the early 1980s indicated that prostaglandins are involved in the pathogenesis of heavy menstrual loss (Pickles et al 1965; Willman et al 1976; Cameron et al 1987). The endometrium is a rich source of prostaglandins (E_2 and $F_{2\alpha}$) and several studies have shown that prostaglandin concentrations are increased in the endometrium of women with menorrhagia. NSAIDs inhibit the cyclo-oxygenase enzyme system responsible for the conversion of arachidonic acid to prostaglandins and leukotrienes.

The most common NSAID used in the treatment of menorrhagia is mefanamic acid. Studies have shown a 25% reduction in menstrual blood loss associated with mefanamic acid (Dockeray et al 1989; Cameron et al 1990; Irvine and Cameron 1999). Other studies with other non-steroidals have shown reduction in menstrual loss from 20% to 80% in three-quarters of women with menorrhagia (Fraser and McCarron 1991; Milsom et al 1991). Mefanamic acid can be used for three cycles from the onset of menstruation, three times a day. Side effects are confined to gastric irritation, which may be minimised if taken with food. Serious side effects are very rare since they only need to be taken during menses.

Antifibrinolytics: Fibrinolysis is dependent on the production and release of activators and inhibitors of plasminogen. Significantly higher levels of plasminogen activator have been reported in extracts of late secretory endometrium from women with menorrhagia than in those with normal menstrual loss

(Shaw et al 1980). A strong correlation was evident between tissue plasminogen levels in the late secretory endometrium and menstrual blood loss (Sheppard et al 1990), indicating a key role for increased local release of fibrinolytic activators in the causation of excessive menstrual bleeding.

Tranexamic acid, an antifibrinolytic, is a synthetic derivative of the amino acid, lysine. Tranexamic acid has also been shown to reduce menstrual blood loss by 35%–51% in women whose objective menstrual loss is less than 80 ml, and is also effective when menorrhagia is caused by an intrauterine coil (Nilsson and Rybo 1967; Ylikorkala and Viinikka 1983).

Antifibrinolytic therapy causes a greater reduction in objective measurements of heavy menstrual blood loss compared to placebo or other medical therapies (Bonnar and Sheppard 1996; Lethaby et al 2003). Comparative studies have shown that tranexamic acid is better at lowering menstrual loss than NSAIDs, with reductions in loss of 56% and 44% following tranexamic acid and 21% and 24% after flurbiprofen and diclofenac, respectively (Ylikorkala and Viinikka 1983; Milsom et al 1991). The incidence of side effects is dose related and includes minor skin rashes, nausea and vomiting. As 90% of menstrual blood loss occurs in the first three days, treatment can be limited to these days, thus reducing the incidence of side effects.

The antifibrinolytics offer an effective first-line option for some women. They have a greater impact on reducing the degree of menstrual blood loss than NSAIDs. Both however, have the advantage of only being taken during menstruation itself, which aids compliance. The Royal College of Obstetricians and Gynaecologists recommends tranexamic acid and mefanamic acid as first-line drugs for women with menorrhagia who either do not require contraception or prefer non-hormonal treatment (RCOG 1998) for at least three months.

Hemostatics: Although endometrial hemostasis appears to be compromised in women with dysfunctional bleeding (Hourihan et al 1989; Sheppard et al 1990), ethamsylate, a medication that is believed to reduce capillary fragility and inhibit the prostaglandin pathway, has doubtful efficacy (Bonnar and Sheppard 1996). Therefore, ethamsylate is no longer considered to be an effective treatment of menorrhagia.

Hormone therapy: Hormones (estrogens and progestogens) should be taken on a cyclical or continuous basis. Hormones are not much of value, if taken only during the menstrual bleed. Their mechanism of action is to influence the hormonal environment either locally or systemically. As there is no hormonal defect in 80% of women with menorrhagia (Haynes et al 1977; Eldred and Thomas 1994), the use of hormone therapy does not correct an underlying disorder; it merely imposes an external control of the cycle. For many women, however, cycle control is as important an issue as the degree of menorrhagia.

Oral Contraceptive Pill: The continuous administration of estrogens and/or progestogens induces endometrial atrophy. The oral contraceptive pill (OCP) is effective treatment available for menorrhagia (Nilsson and Rybo 1971), as it reduces menstrual blood loss by about 50% (Irvine and Cameron 1999). The use of continuous administration of E and P is usually not acceptable as there is no menstruation; hence a cyclical OC pill is seen to be effective in reducing menstrual blood loss, and restoring regular rhythm to the cycle. Reduction in blood loss occurs in women with either menorrhagia or normal losses. The average blood loss in menstrual cycle is 30–50 ml. Patients receiving OC pills have menstrual blood loss less than 30 ml per cycle.

The OCP has the advantage of providing a regular rhythm to the cycle, reducing the incidence of dysmenorrhea and also provides contraception. It also reduces the long-term risk of endometrial and ovarian cancer. In women over the age of 40 years, who are low risk (that is, normal body mass index, non-smoker and normotensive), the combined pill may be used. In high-risk women, the progesterone-only pill can be used instead.

The side effects of OC pills can be classified as serious and less serious. Serious side effects are uncommon. The less serious side effects include nausea, vomiting, breast tenderness, headaches and mood changes, which may make it unacceptable to women. Other serious but uncommon side effects include thrombo-embolic disease, hypertension, impairment of liver function and hepatic tumours.

The Royal College of Obstetricians and Gynaecologists recommends the use of the combined oral contraceptive pill as a first-line drug for the management of menorrhagia in women requiring contraception (RCOG 1998).

Progestogens: Over the last 30 years, progestogens have been widely used often as a first-line treatment.

Oral: Norethisterone or medroxyprogesterone acetate is the most commonly prescribed preparation for menstrual problems. In anovulatory cycles, the progestogen induces secretory change in the endometrium. However, in ovulatory cycles, minimal change is produced and 80% of women with menorrhagia have ovulatory cycles. Despite this, cyclic progestogen is often used in the treatment of menorrhagia, particularly in primary care settings. Progestogens are also helpful in regulating menstruation and in preventing premenstrual spotting.

Progestogens can be used cyclically in two different treatment regimens—it can be taken at a low dose for 5–10 days in the luteal phase, or for 10–14 days; however, there is no significant decrease in menstrual blood loss (Coulter et al 1995). In patients with acute heavy bleeding, norethisterone acetate is preferred over medroxyprogesterone acetate due to its hemostatic benefit and can be given up to 30–40 mg in divided doses. Minor side effects such as abdominal bloating, weight gain, breast tenderness and increased appetite are common, and are often a reason why it may be unacceptable to some women. The prolonged use of high-dose progestogens is sometimes associated with irregular bleeding.

Depot preparations: These are available as medroxyprogesterone acetate and norethisterone. They are repeated at 8–12 week intervals, respectively. Injection medroxprogesterone acetate 150 mg IM is given once in three months and is to be repeated at three-month intervals for three doses.

Their mechanism of action is to induce endometrial atrophy. They induce amenorrhea in the majority of women after 3–6 months; however, irregular bleeding is a common side effect, particularly in the first three months. In addition, they also reduce dysmenorrhea and improve symptoms in women with pre-menstrual symptoms. Other side effects include bloatedness, breast tenderness, weight gain and depression and are the reasons why women discontinue this treatment. Up to 70% of users gain weight (up to 2 kg) in the first year (Bhathena 2001). A small reduction of bone density and changes in the lipid profile has been reported with use for more than five years (Cundy et al 1991; Guillebaud 1999). Also the duration of action can last up to 18 months on discontinuing treatment.

The Royal College of Obstetricians and Gynaecologists recommends the use of long acting progestogens as a first-line treatment for the management of menorrhagia in women requiring contraception (RCOG 1998).

Progestogen-releasing intrauterine system: The progestogen-only intrauterine device releases a steady amount of levonorgestrel (20 µg/ 24 h) from a steroid reservoir around the vertical stem of the device, which affects the endometrium locally, and only causes minimal systemic absorption. It can be left in situ for up to five years and is an excellent form of contraception. Studies from Scandinavia indicate that menstrual blood loss is decreased by as much as 90% in the majority of women (Berqvist and Rybo 1983; Milsom et al 1991; Andersson et al 1994) and 20% of women develop amenorrhea within a year of its insertion. Studies have shown that menstrual blood loss is decreased from a median of 176 ml before treatment to 24 ml at three months and 5 ml at 12 months (Andersson and Rybo 1990).

The efficacy of progestogen-only intrauterine device has also been compared to oral norethisterone—Irvine (1998) showed that there was no difference in adverse side effects between the two interventions, apart from intermenstrual spotting, which was seen in 53% with Mirena® IUS and 13% with oral progestogen. In another study, women with heavy menstrual loss were randomly allocated to Mirena® IUS or endometrial resection (Crosignani et al 1997). Blood loss was assessed semi-objectively and a general health questionnaire was completed after 12 months. Estimated blood loss was reduced by 79% and 89% in the Mirena® IUS and endometrial resection group, respectively. Satisfaction with treatment was 85% and 94%, respectively. Irregular bleeding is common, particularly in the early months and is the commonest reason why women discontinue its use. Due to its reduction in menstrual blood loss and minimal side effects, the Mirena® IUS is a good first-line treatment option for the management of menorrhagia, particularly in women who require contraception.

Danazol: This is an isoxazol derivative of 17-ethinyl testosterone, which has anti-estrogenic and anti-progestogenic activity. It suppresses the mid-cycle surge of follicle stimulating hormone and luteinising hormone, and inhibits ovulation without altering basal gonadotrophin levels. It also inhibits steriodogenesis in the corpus luteum. Menstrual blood loss reduction seems to be related to the dosage—taken in moderate to high dose (400 mg or more daily) it will induce amenorrhea in the majority of women. Studies have shown an overall reduction in menstrual blood loss of up to 50% (Dockeray et al 1989).

However, side effects are related to both its androgenic properties and hypo-estrogenic effect and tend to be dose related. High doses will frequently be accompanied by masculinising effects such as hirsutism, acne and irreversible voice change. Weight gain also occurs in 85% of women. Its use is contraindicated in liver disease, severe hypertension, congestive cardiac failure and impaired renal function. It is an effective treatment in the management of menorrhagia, but because of its side effects, it lacks acceptability; the need for continuing treatment limits its use (Dockeray et al 1989; Beaumount 2003; Roy and Bhattacharya 2004). It is therefore not a first-line treatment option in the management of menorrhagia.

Gonadotrophin-releasing hormone agonists (GNRH): GnRH analogues cause down-regulation of the pituitary and a subsequent decrease in gonadotrophins and ovarian steroids. This results in amenorrhoea in over 90% of women. Side effects tend to be related to the hypo-estrogenic state and are postmenopausal in type. Their use is also associated with osteoporosis with a decrease in bone mineral content of about 5% per year. These adverse effects can be minimised by concurrent hormone replacement therapy.

This is not a first-line option for most women, but may have a place in the short-term management of menorrhagia in women awaiting surgery or natural menopause.

Medical Versus Surgical Treatment

Medical treatment for menorrhagia is not as effective as surgery despite improvement in the control of bleeding. Oral medical therapy is associated with a higher incidence of side effects, and approximately 60% of women who had medical treatment would require surgery in two years. Surgery has been found to reduce menstrual bleeding more than medical treatment at one year, although the majority of women prefer medical treatment.

Surgical care: Surgical management has been the standard of treatment in menorrhagia due to organic causes (that is, fibroids) or when medical therapy fails to alleviate symptoms.

Surgical treatment ranges from a simple D & C to a full hysterectomy.

1. Dilatation and curettage
2. Endometrial destruction
   - First generation
     - Transcervical resection of the endometrium
     - Roller-ball endometrial ablation
     - Endometrial laser ablation
   - Second generation
     - Uterine balloon therapy
     - HydroTherm Ablator®
     - Microwave endometrial ablation alternative
3. Hysterectomy

Dilatation and curettage (D&C): Dilatation and curettage is used for diagnostic purposes. It is not used for treatment because it provides only short-term relief, typically for 1–2 months.

However, this procedure should not be the first line of treatment for menorrhagia, as the majority of cases of both acute and chronic menorrhagia can be managed with medical agents. The use of curettage for patients with an endocrinal etiology for their abnormal vaginal bleeding provides only a temporary cure.

Endometrial destruction/ablation: Endometrial ablation is used to treat menorrhagia in women with no intrauterine pathology. Endometrial destruction procedures are less invasive, more convenient and less expensive when no other gynecological condition is involved. It enables women to avoid major surgery and results in shorter hospital stay and convalescence. Complete removal of the endometrium may be accomplished by techniques, including resection with a diathermy wire loop or electrocoagulation using a diathermy roller ball under direct hysteroscopic guidance or by inserting a thermal coagulation probe into the uterine cavity, photocoagulation with Nd:YAG laser. There is little variation in the overall success rate between the different methods. Long-term follow-up studies have reported amenorrhea in 25%–50% of women and a significant decrease in menstrual loss in a further 45%–60%, giving a satisfactory rate of approximately 75%–80% (Derman et al 1991; Fraser and McCarron 1993; Garry et al 1995; Chullapram et al 1996; Baggish and Sze 1996; Thijssen 1997). The first-generation techniques involve lower costs than a hysterectomy, but the second-generation endometrial destruction techniques involve relatively high purchase and disposable supplies costs. However, these new techniques take less time to perform and have a lower incidence of intra-operative complications. The most significant complications after endometrial ablation are hemorrhage uterine perforation, fluid absorption leading to hyponatremia.

Hysterectomy: When medical or conservative surgery fails in adequately treating menorrhagia, hysterectomy becomes the treatment of choice. Hysterectomy is the most effective treatment yielding the highest level of satisfaction (Sculpher 1996). It is the only treatment that can guarantee a 100% cure rate. The route of hysterectomy should be decided in consultation with the patient, keeping in mind the uterine size, degree of uterine mobility, pubic arch angle, past surgical history, pelvic pathology, whether ovaries are to be removed, as well as the preference of the surgeon. The decision on whether the ovaries should be removed should rest with the patient after she has been counselled about the advantages and disadvantages of this procedure.

Conclusion: Menorrhagia is one of the most common presenting complaints for gynecological patients. Although this problem has many causes, it is generally possible to approach its diagnosis and management in an orderly fashion. When evaluating menorrhagic patients, it is important to work up towards a differential diagnosis that includes fibroid, adenomyosis, endometriosis, PID, IUCD and DUB. This differential approach can guide the types of historical data obtained from the patient, focus the physical examination and alert the gynecologist to the most appropriate investigation and suitable treatment for that patient.

References

Andersson JK and G Rybo. 1990. Levonorgestrel-releasing intrauterine device in the treatment of menorrhagia. *Br J Obstet Gynaecol* 97:690–694.

Andersson K, V Odlind and G Rybo. 1994. Levonorgestrel-releasing and copper-releasing (Nova-T) IUCDs during five years use: A randomised comparative trial. *Contraception* 49:56–72.

Baggish MS and EHM Sze. 1996. Endometrial ablation: A series of 568 patients treated over an 11 year period. *Am J Obstet Gynaecol* 174:908–913

Beaumount H, C Angood, K Duckitt, A Letnaby. 2002. Danazol for heavy menstrual bleeding. *Cochrane Database Systematic Review*, Issue 2, D001017, DOI 10. 1002/ 14651858. CD001017.

Berqvist A and G Rybo. 1983. Treatment of menorrhagia with intrauterine release of progesterone. *Br J Obstet Gynaecol* 90:255–258.

Bhathena RK. 2001. Long acting progestogen-only contraceptive injections: An update. *Br J Obstet Gynaecol* 108:3–8.

Bonnar J and BL Sheppard. 1996. Treatment of menorrhagia during menstruation: Randomized controlled trial of ethamsylate, mefanamic acid and tranexamic acid. *Br Med J* 313: 579–582.

Cameron IT, R Haining and MA Lumsden et al. 1990. The effects of mefanamic acid and norestesterone on measured menstrual blood loss. *Obstet Gynaecol* 76:85–88.

Cameron IT, Leask R and RW Kelly et al. 1987. Endometrial prostaglandins in women with abnormal uterine bleeding. *Prostaglandins Leukot Med* 29: 249–258.

Chullapram T, JY Song, IS Fraser. 1996. Medium-term follow up of women with menorrhagia treated by roller endometrial ablation. *Obstet Gynaecol* 88:71–76.

Classens EA and CA Cowell. 1981. Acute adolescent menorrhagia. *Am J Obstet Gynaecol* 139:277–280.

Coulter A, J Kelland, V Peto, MC Rees. 1995. Treating menorrhagia in primary care. An overview of drug trials and a survey of prescribing practice. *Int J Technol Assess Health Care* 11:456–471.

Crosignani PG, P Vercellini and P Mosconi et al. 1997. Levonorgestrel-releasing intrauterine device versus hysteroscopic endometrial resection in the treatment of dysfunctional uterine bleeding. *Obstet Gynaecol* 90:257–263.

Cundy T, M Evans, H. Roberts et al. 1991. Bone density in women receiving depot medroxy progesterone for contraception. *Br Med J* 303:13–16.

De Kroon CD, FW Jansen, LA Louwe et al. 2003. Technology assessment of saline contrast hysterosonography. *Am J Obstet Gynaecol* 188:945–949.

Derman SG, J Rehnstrom, RS Neuwirth. 1991. The long term effectiveness of hysteroscopic treatment of menorrhagia and leiomyomata. *Obstet and Gynaecol* 77:591–594.

Dockeray CJ, BL Sheppard and J Bonnar. 1989. Comparison between mefanamic acid and Danazol in the treatment of established menorrhagia. *Br J Obstet Gynaecol* 96:840–844.

Eldred JM and EJ Thomas. 1994. Pituitary and ovarian hormone levels in unexplained menorrhagia. *Obstet Gynaecol* 84:775–778.

Fraser IS. 1990. Treatment of ovulatory and anovulatory dysfunctional uterine bleeding with oral progestogens. *Aust NZ J Obstet Gynaecol* 30:353–356.

Fraser IS and G McCarron. 1991. Randomised trial of two hormonal and two prostaglandin-inhibiting agents in women with a complaint of menorrhagia, *Aust N Z J Obstet Gynaecol* 31:66–70.

Fraser IS, S Angsuwathana, F Mahmoud, S Yezerski, 1993. Short and medium-term outcomes after roller ball endometrial ablation for menorrhagia *Med J Aust* 158:454–457.

Garry R, D Shelley Jones, P Mooney, G Phillips. 1995. Six hundred endometrial laser ablations. *Obstet Gynaecol* 85:24–29

Guillebaud J. 1999. Oestrogen free hormonal contraception. In *Contraceptions: your questions answered*, ed J Guillebaud. Edinburgh: Churchill Livingstone, 311–316.

Haynes PJ, H Hodgson, ABM Anderson et al. 1977. Measurement of menstrual blood loss in patients complaining of menorrhagia, *Br J Obstet Gynaecol* 84:763–768.

Higham JM, PMS O Brien, RW Shaw. 1990. Assesment of menstrual blood loss using a pictorial chart *Br J Obstet Gynaecol* 97:734–739

Hourihan HM, BL Sheppard and J Bonnar. 1989. The morphologic characteristics of menstrual hemostasis in patients with unexplained menorrhagia *Inter J Gynaecol Pathol* 8: 221–229.

Irvine GA and IT Cameron. 1999. Medical management of dysfunctional uterine bleeding. *Baillieres Best Pract Res Clin Obstet Gynaecol* 13 (2):189–202.

Irvine GA, MB Campbell-Brown and MA Lumsden et al. 1998. Randomised comparative trial of the levonorgestrel intrauterine system and norethisterone for the treatment of idiopathic menorrhagia, *Br J Obstet Gynaecol* 105:592–598.

Lethaby A, G Irvine, I Cameron. 2003. Cyclical progestogens for heavy menstrual bleeding. *Cochrane Database Systematic Review* 15(3):215–218.

Milsom I, K Andersson, B Andersch et al. 1991. A comparison of flurbiprofen, tranexamic acid and levonorgestrel-releasing intrauterine contraceptive device in the treatment of idiopathic menorrhagia *Am J Obstet Gynaecol* 164: 879–883.

Nilsson L and G Rybo. 1967. Treatment of menorrhagia with an antifibrinolytic agent, tranexamic acid. *Acta Obstet Gynaecol Scand* 46:572–580.

Nilsson L and G Rybo. 1971. Treatment of menorrhagia. *Am J Obstet Gynaecol* 110: 713–720.

Okaro E, G Condous, T Bourne. 2003. The role of ultrasound in the management of menorrhagia. *Rev Gynaecol Prac* 3:16–25.

Roy SN and S Bhattacharya. 2004. Benefits and risks of pharmacological agents used for the treatment of menorrhagia *Drug Saf* 27 (2):75–90.

Royal College of Obstetricians and Gynaecologists. 1998. The initial management of menorrhagia in primary care. Evidence-based clinical guideline no. 1. London.

Sculpher MJ, N Dwyer, S Byford, GM Stirrat. 1996. Randomised controlled trial comparing hysterectomy and trans cervical endometrial resection: Effect on health related quality of life and costs two years after surgery. *Br J Obstet Gynaecol* 103:142–149.

Shaw ST, LK Macaulay, MS Tanaka et al. 1980. Plasminogen activator in human uterine tissue-relationship to location of sampling and time of ovarian cycle. *Biochem Med* 24:170–178.

Sheppard BL, M. Stack, M. Jordan et al. 1990. Plasminogen activator in the human uterus in normal menstruation and dysfunctional uterine bleeding. *Irish J Med Sci* 159:151.

Thijssen RFA. 1997. Radiofrequency induced endometrial ablation: An update. *Br J Obstet Gynaecol* 107:608–613.

Pickles VR, WJ Hall and FA Best et al. 1965. Prostaglandins in endometrium and menstrual fluid from normal and dysmenorrhoeic subjects. *J Obstet Gynaecol Br Commonw* 72:185–192.

Willman EA, WP Collins, SG Clayton.1976. Studies on the involvement of prostaglandins in uterine symptomatology and pathology. *Br J Obstet Gynaecol* 83:337.

Ylikorkala O and L Viinikka, 1983. Comparison between antifibrinolytic and antiprostaglandin treatment in the reduction of increased menstrual blood loss in women with intrauterine contraceptive devices. *Br J Obstet Gynaecol* 90:78–83.

7

Infertility

Pratap Kumar

Subfertility or infertility should be defined as failure to conceive after regular unprotected sexual intercourse for two years, in the absence of known reproductive pathology. The prevalence of infertility is about 10%. People who have not conceived after a year of regular unprotected sexual intercourse should be offered further clinical investigations. Where there is a history of predisposing factors (such as amenorrhea, oligomenorrhea, pelvic inflammatory disease or undescended testes), or where a woman is aged 35 years or over, earlier investigation should be offered if the couple seek advise for their inability to conceive.

History and clinical examination offer very few clues for infertility, unless there is evidence of polycystic ovarian disease (presence of oligomenorrhea, hirsutism and sometimes, obesity). Sexual history is important as a large number of couples may have some kind of problem which could be a factor for infertility. About 30% causes could be present in the female, 30% in the male, 20% combined; about 10% of causes are unexplained, and have not yet been understood.

WORK-UP OF A COUPLE WITH INFERTILITY

After a clinical examination, semen analysis and transvaginal sonography form the work-up of the couple

Semen analysis: The WHO reference values for semen analysis (Rowe 2000) are:

> Volume: 2.0 ml or more
> Liquefaction time: Within 60 minutes
> pH: 7.2 or more
> Sperm concentration: 20 million spermatozoa per millilitre or more
> Total sperm number: 40 million spermatozoa per ejaculate or more
> Motility: 50% or more motile (grades a* and b†) or
> 25% or more with progressive motility (grade a) within 60 minutes of ejaculation
> Morphology: 15% or 30%‡
> Vitality: 75% or more live
> White blood cells: fewer than one million per millilitre
>
> * Grade a: rapid progressive motility (sperm moving swiftly, usually in a straight line).
> † Grade b: slow or sluggish progressive motility (sperm may be less linear in their progression).
> ‡ Currently being reassessed by the WHO whether lower limit of 30% or 15% based on strict morphological criteria should be taken.

Terminology/definitions

Normozoospermia: Normal ejaculate as defined by the WHO reference values

Oligozoospermia: Sperm concentration less than the WHO reference values

Asthenozoospermia: Less than the WHO reference values for motility

Teratozoospermia: Less than the WHO reference values for morphology

Oligoasthenoteratozoospermia: Signifies disturbance of all three variables

Azoospermia: No spermatozoa in the ejaculate

Aspermia: No ejaculate

Cryptozoospermia: Few spermatozoa recovered after centrifugation

If the initial semen analysis is normal repeat analysis is not necessary. Ideally, three-day abstinence is required before semen is collected. To reduce false positives, it is suggested that a repeat semen analysis should be performed only if the result of the first analysis is abnormal (British Andrology Society 2002). Biologically, the optimal time for the second sample is at least three months after the initial sample because the spermatozoa take about three months to form (MacLeod 1964). However, if azoospermia or severe oligozoospermia is reported in the initial semen analysis, a repeat test could be undertaken within two to four weeks. If the repeat test is reported as normal, the semen may be regarded as normal and no further test is needed. However, these men may need further assessment of semen quality if assisted reproduction is being considered.

Sperm function tests: These tests vary in their ability to detect defects in the complex processes leading to fertilisation, and are of limited practical use (The ESHRE Capri Workshop 1996). The predictive value of subnormal semen variables is limited, except in the case of azoospermia. No functional test has yet been established that can unequivocally predict the fertilising capacity of spermatozoa.

Factors influencing semen collection:

- Incomplete samples should be tested again
- The sample should be protected from extremes of temperature (not <20°C and not >40°C) during transport
- The sample should be examined immediately after liquefaction, within an hour of ejaculation
- Low volume suggests abnormalities of accessory sex gland fluid
- Non-liquefaction suggests disturbances of the prostate
- Viscosity (semen through pipette >2 cm thread is abnormal)
- pH >8.0 suggests infection because of decreased secretion of prostatic fluid

Trial Wash: It is now believed that all semen samples should undergo a sperm wash to evaluate motile sperm counts; this is called trial wash.

- It is performed during semen analysis
- It evaluates semen for assisted conception procedures
- It helps select the appropriate sperm wash methods and helps to plan treatment.

In successful intrauterine insemination cases, the number of motile spermatozoa inseminated (NMSI) and their morphology has been studied. Their correlation is shown in Table 7.1 (Wainer et al 2004).

Hence, a post-wash sample with more than five million sperm count per ml of the total number of motile sperm inseminated (NMSI) leads to better pregnancy rates. However, in those who yield less NMSI, if a few cycles of intrauterine insemination (IUI) fail, assisted reproductive techniques (ART) should be considered.

MEDICAL MANAGEMENT FOR OLIGOSPERMIA

Several medications have been tried for

Table 7.1: Correlation between number of motile sperm inseminated and the pregnancy rate

Number of motile sperm inseminated (NMSI)	*Pregnancy rate/cycle*
<1 million	3.13
>2 million	12.91
<5 million, post-wash, N morphology <30%	5.43
>5 million, post-wash, N morphology >30%	18.42

oligospermia with varying rates of success. However, recently certain reviews have thrown some light in this direction.

Ten randomised controlled trials (RCTs) analysing the effect of clomiphene citrate (CC) and tamoxifen, it was shown that they did not have a beneficial effect on pregnancy rates when compared with placebo or no treatment for oligo/asthenozoospermia (Khan et al 1996). Gonadotrophin treatment for idiopathic male factor also with two RCTs showed no significant difference in pregnancy rates between gonadotrophin treatment vs placebo or no treatment (Matorras et al 1997). Medication, therefore, needs to be prescribed with care if the proposed benefit to the individual is unknown.

Varicocele and fertility: A varicocele is a collection of dilated veins in the spermatic cord and is a common physical anomaly. Varicoceles are found in 11.7% of men with normal semen and 25.4% of men with abnormal semen (WHO 1992). The mechanism by which varicoceles impair fertility and spermatogenesis is not clear. They may be associated with decreased ipsilateral testicular volume, elevated scrotal temperature and pain, as well as impaired semen quality (WHO 1992). Review of seven RCTs showed that varicocele repair did not improve pregnancy rates (Evers et al 2001).

Some studies on varicoceles are contrary. It was found that following varicocele surgery, a rise of sperm count was seen in 31% of patients when it was <5 million/ml prior to surgery (Cayan et al 2002). Hence, if an individual has fluctuating levels of sperm count and motility, then gross varicocele surgery may be attempted. If there is an improvement in the count and motility following varicocele surgery, some couples may benefit from IUI, rather than being limited to the options of in vitro fertilisation (IVF) or intracytoplasmic sperm injection (ICSI).

Management of Azoospermia

It is important to assess the size of the testis first and then check FSH levels—management would be directed by the results. There is no effective treatment to restore fertility in primary testicular failure.

Alternatively, surgical sperm retrieval with assisted reproduction or donor sperm may be considered. The diagnosis is based on normal testis size and normal serum FSH levels. This includes conditions such as congenital bilateral absence of vas deferens (CBAVD). CBAVD is commonly associated with cystic fibrosis mutations or renal tract abnormality (for example, an absent kidney). Serum FSH levels, three times the normal level, is the upper limit; above this, retrieval was not recommended (Ballessca et al 2000). Hence, if both testicles are small and FSH levels are high, biopsy of the testis is not recommended. The couple should be counselled for donor insemination or adoption.

Leucocytospermia has been associated

with adverse effects on semen parameters and function. Antibiotics have been considered in the treatment of leucocytospermia

- Spermatogenic cells and white cells are referred to as 'round cells'
- Peroxidase test reliably identifies granulocytes.

EVALUATION OF THE WOMAN

The first investigation in all women with suspected infertility is ultrasound of the pelvis.

Compared with bimanual pelvic examination, transvaginal ultrasound enables pelvic anatomy to be identified with more accuracy and reliability. Ultrasound can be used in the evaluation of pelvic pathology, such as endometrioma, cysts, endometrial polyp, leiomyoma, adnexal and ovarian abnormality, where such abnormalities are present (Frederick et al 1991). Diagnostic criteria for polycystic ovaries and PCOS, in which ultrasonic parameters play an important role, have been debated.

ANOVULATION AND PROBLEMS RELATED TO FERTILITY

Regular menstrual cycles are usually indicative of ovulation. Ovulation can be confirmed retrospectively by measurement of serum progesterone in the mid-luteal phase, approximately on day 21 of a 28-day cycle. Values range from 16 to 28 nmol/l as the lowest limit indicative of ovulation (ESHRE workshop 1996). Anovulation and oligo-ovulation are ovulatory disorders that are estimated to cause 21% of female infertility. The WHO classifies ovulation disorders into three groups (Rowe 1997).

Group 1—hypothalamic pituitary failure (hypothalamic amenorrhea or hypogonadotrophic hypogonadism): This group of disorders is characterised by low gonadotrophins, normal prolactin and low estrogen, and accounts for about 10% of ovulatory disorders. Failed ovarian follicular development results in hypo-estrogenic amenorrhea in this group of disorders.

Group 2—hypothalamic pituitary dysfunction: This group, which is characterised by gonadotrophin disorder and normal estrogen, accounts for about 85% of ovulatory disorders. This group of disorders results in anovulatory oligo/amenorrhea, predominately involving women with polycystic ovaries—present in about 80%–90% of women with oligomenorrhea and 30% of women with amenorrhea. About 30% of patients with PCOS are of normal weight.

The new definition for the diagnosis of PCOS requires the presence of at least two of the following three criteria (Rotterdam ESHRE/ASRM criteria 2004)

- Oligo- and/or anovulation
- Clinical and/or biochemical hyperandrogenism
- Polycystic ovaries, with the exclusion of other etiologies

Reduction in weight and increased pregnancy rates have been reported in obese infertile women who took up lifestyle improvement programmes involving increased exercise and weight loss as compared with conventional management (RCOG clinical guidelines 2004).

Group 3—ovarian failure: Ovarian failure, characterised by high gonadotrophins with hypogonadism and low estrogen, accounts for about 4%–5% of ovulatory disorders. Serum gonadotrophins (follicle-stimulating hormone and luteinising hormone) should be assessed on days 2 or 3 of the cycle to establish basal values.

Prolactin Measurement

Hyperprolactinemia is an endocrine disorder caused by an increased secretion of prolactin from the pituitary gland, resulting in galactorrhea, irregular menstruation and possible infertility. The incidence of raised prolactin in infertile but ovulatory women ranges from 3.8% to 11.5% (Vanrell et al 1983). Estimation of prolactin levels should be reserved for women with symptoms of an ovulatory disorder, galactorrhea or a pituitary tumour.

Assessing Ovarian Reserve

Female fecundability (ability to procreate) is related to the total number of primordial follicles remaining within the ovaries (referred to as ovarian reserve), which declines with age. It would be valuable if reliable estimates of ovarian reserve could be obtained before embarking on fertility therapy such as ovulation induction and IVF in women over the age of 35 years (Sharara et al 1998). Indirect measurements using endocrine markers, such as day 3 basal serum FSH, correlate well with the status of reserve of the ovary.

Elevated basal day 3 FSH is correlated with diminished ovarian reserve in women over 35 years and is associated with poor pregnancy rates after treatment with ovulation induction. Basal levels less than 10 mIU/ml is considered normal ovarian reserve. It has been reported that pregnancy rates decline significantly as day 3 FSH rises above 15 mIU/ml. Very few pregnancies were reported when FSH exceeded 25 mIU/ml (Scott er al 1989).

Direct measures of ovarian function such as inhibin B correlate inversely with age and FSH levels (Danforth et al 1998); also, inhibin B levels are reduced in women with diminished ovarian reserve.

Effect of body mass index/obesity on fertility

Effect of fat on hormones

- Excess fat affects not only gonadotrophin secretion but also 17β estradiol metabolism (which metabolises to a weaker estrogen—estriol)
- There is also conversion of androstenedione to estrone in peripheral adipose tissue

Body mass index (BMI): Women with BMI greater than 29 and who are not ovulating should be informed that losing weight is likely to increase their chance of conception (RCOG Clinical Guidelines 2004). *BMI of 30 is like having 30% excess fat, and is the point where problems of obesity begin.* Hence, bringing down the BMI for better response of ovulation induction will improve the chances of success in ovulation induction.

Thyroid function tests: Thyroid dysfunction can lead to menstrual and ovulatory disorders associated with infertility (Akande and Anderson 1975). Women with possible fertility problems are no more likely than the general population to have thyroid disease; therefore, routine measurement of thyroid function should not be offered. Estimation of thyroid function should be confined to women with symptoms of thyroid disease (RCOG Clinical Guidelines 2004).

Endometrial biopsy: Luteal-phase defect has been defined as either a defect of progesterone secretion by the corpus luteum or a defect in endometrial response to hormone stimulation, resulting in an endometrium unsuitable for blastocyst implantation and subsequent pregnancy. There is no consensus of opinion about the diagnosis or effective treatment of luteal-phase defect, and its role as a cause of infertility has been questioned. The benefit of treatment for luteal-phase defect on pregnancy rates has not been established (Karamardian and Grimes 1992). Women should not be offered an endometrial biopsy to evaluate the luteal phase as part of the investigation of fertility problems because there is no evidence that medical treatment of luteal-phase defect improves pregnancy rates. However, in a developing country when tuberculosis is suspected on seeing a thin endometrium by ultrasound, there is a role for endometrial curettage in selected cases.

Screening for chlamydia trachomatis: Chlamydia trachomatis is present in 11% of the sexually active population aged 19 years or less. It is a major cause of pelvic inflammatory disease, leading to chronic abdominal pain, ectopic pregnancy and tubal factor infertility (Westrom et al 1993). Asymptomatic chlamydial infection may go unrecognised and untreated. Both doxycycline and azithromycin are effective prophylaxis and treatment for chlamydia. There is evidence that screening for and treating cervical chlamydial infection can reduce the incidence of pelvic inflammatory disease in women at increased risk of chlamydia infection. Prophylactic antibiotics should be considered before uterine instrumentation if screening has not been carried out.

It has been found that women with positive Chlamydia testing often have distal tubal problems and hence it may be worthwhile considering a diagnostic laparoscopy in such women so that management could start without delay (den Hartog et al 2004). Elevated titres of chlamydial antibodies in women were significantly associated with tubal disease (Eggert-Kruse et al 1997).

Tubal patency tests: The tubal patency tests used most commonly are hysterosalpingography (HSG) and laparoscopy and dye (chromotubation). Both are invasive procedures, but HSG is less so. Although HSG is a not a reliable indicator of tubal occlusion, when HSG suggests that the tubes are patent, this will be confirmed at laparoscopy in 94% of women; it is therefore a reliable indicator of tubal patency. Results from another review suggest that HSG could be used as a screening test for couples with no history of pelvic infection, and if abnormal, confirmatory laparoscopy would follow (Opsahl et al 1993).

Women with possible co-morbidity such as pelvic and tubal diseases may need a laparoscopic assessment, based on positive symptoms, positive signs and positive ultrasound findings. Tubal pathology detected at laparoscopy has a greater effect on future fertility than that detected at HSG.

Women who have no known co-morbidities (such as pelvic inflammatory disease, previous ectopic pregnancy or endometriosis) can be offered HSG to screen for tubal occlusion because this is a reliable test for ruling out tubal occlusion, is less invasive and makes more efficient use of resources than laparoscopy.

Assessing Uterine Abnormalities

Uterine abnormalities such as adhesions, polyps, submucous leiomyomas and septae have been found in 10% to 15% of women seeking treatment for fertility problems (Wallach 1992). Compared with HSG, hysteroscopy is recognised as the gold standard test for identifying uterine abnormalities as it allows direct visualisation of the uterine cavity.

According to RCOG guidelines (2004), women should not be offered hysteroscopy as part of the initial investigation unless clinically indicated, because the effectiveness of surgical treatment of uterine abnormalities on improving pregnancy rates has not been established.

Postcoital testing of cervical mucus: The value of postcoital testing of cervical mucus for the presence of motile sperm is controversial and is a subject of continuing debate. The routine use of postcoital testing of cervical mucus in the investigation of fertility problems is not recommended because it has no predictive value on pregnancy rate.

STRATEGIES FOR MANAGEMENT OF FERTILITY PROBLEMS

If pathological conditions hampering fertility, such as endometriosis, fibroids, adhesions, are present, they have to be removed surgically. In the rest, active management such as ovulation induction, IUI, IVF or ICSI (depending on the sperm count and motility, trial wash as explained earlier) will need to be instituted.

WHO group I ovulation disorders: When the BMI is below the normal range, the BMI should be raised prior to attempting ovulation induction. Treatment for this group of women includes administering gonadotrophin releasing hormone (GnRH), a hypothalamic hormone which, if given in a pulsed fashion, induces the appropriate release of the pituitary gonadotrophin hormones FSH and LH. Alternatively, women can be treated with gonadotrophins which would be much more practical for clinical use. However, the dosage and the duration will vary according to the response of the patient to the drugs.

WHO group II ovulation disorders: Treatment strategies in women with WHO Group II ovulation disorders, such as PCOS, include three established options:

- Use of oral anti-estrogens
- Use of ovarian drilling
- Use of injectable gonadotrophins

Another option is the use of oral metformin. It is necessary to start metformin in women with BMI over 25. Clomiphene citrate may be introduced either along with metformin or after a few cycles since it improves pregnancy rates. Women prescribed metformin should be informed of the side effects associated with its use. Women with polycystic ovary syndrome who have not responded to clomifene citrate should be offered laparoscopic ovarian drilling because it is as effective as gonadotrophin treatment and is not associated with an increased risk of multiple pregnancy.

WHO group III ovulation disorders: These patients are diagnosed as having ovarian failure; oocyte donation is the management option.

Ovulation Induction

There are several approaches to ovulation induction therapy; the drugs used in ovulation induction therapy also form the basis of superovulation as used in IUI and IVF treatment.

Anti-estrogens: Two anti-estrogens are commonly used—clomiphene citrate (CC) and tamoxifen. They have a similar structure and properties. They induce gonadotrophin release by occupying the estrogen receptors in the hypothalamus, thereby interfering with the normal feedback mechanisms, increasing gonadotrophins and thus stimulating the ovary to have more follicles. The evidence relating to anti-estrogens predominantly involves clomiphene citrate. The adverse effects of antiestrogens such as CC include hot flushes, ovarian hyperstimulation, abdominal discomfort and multiple pregnancy. Ovulation occurs in about 70% of anovulatory women (Taymor 1990) at a dose of 50–100 mg of CC (Gysler et al 1982), the maximum dose being 250 mg. In clinical practice, however, we do not use more than 150 mg of CC per day for five days—anovulatory women who do not ovulate while receiving the 150 mg dose are considered to be resistant to the drug (Vandermolen et al 2001). In anovulatory women, there is a significant association between CC treatment failure and increased BMI (BMI greater than 27.2 kg/m^2 or greater than 30.6 kg/m^2)(Kousta et al 1997). A weight loss programme may improve ovulation and pregnancy outcomes in women who are obese and infertile for all forms of fertility treatment, including ovulation induction, IUI and IVF (Clark et al 1995).

Gonadotrophin use in ovulation induction therapy for ovulatory disorders: For women with WHO Group I ovulation disorders, treatment with human menopausal gonadotrophin (hMG), which includes FSH and LH, was reported to be more effective in improving ovulation than FSH alone (Shoham et al 1991). Women with WHO Group II ovulation disorders such as polycystic ovary syndrome who do not ovulate with clomiphene citrate (or tamoxifen) can be offered treatment with gonadotrophins. Human menopausal gonadotrophin, urinary follicle-stimulating hormone and recombinant follicle-stimulating hormone are equally effective in achieving pregnancy and cost-effectiveness should be kept in mind when prescribing these. Women with WHO Group II ovulation disorders (such as polycystic ovary syndrome) who ovulate with CC but have not become pregnant after six months of treatment should be offered CC-stimulated intrauterine insemination.

GnRH antagonists versus GnRH analogues: GnRH antagonists produce immediate and direct pituitary suppression. As part of in vitro fertilisation treatment, using GnRH agonist in addition to gonadotrophin stimulation facilitates cycle control and results in higher pregnancy rates than the use of gonadotrophins alone. The routine use of GnRH agonist in long protocols during in vitro fertilisation is therefore recommended.

Surgical Treatment in Female Infertility

Myomectomy: A good number of women with fibroids may not require surgery for the same; hence, patients for surgery must be selected with care. There are three types of fibroids—submucous, interstitial and subserous varieties. A systematic review of 11 cohort studies suggests that women with submucous myoma have lower pregnancy rates compared with women with other causes for their infertility. Myomectomy was not associated with an increase in live birth rate but was associated with a higher pregnancy rate (Pritts 2001). A case-control study found a lower pregnancy rate in women with myoma when compared with those without (11% versus 25%). The pregnancy rate in women following myomectomy was higher than that in women with untreated myoma (42% versus 25%) (Bulletti et al 1999).

Septa: The incidence of septae is not increased among women with infertility compared with other women (2%–3%) (Ashton et al 1988), it is more common in women who have had recurrent pregnancy loss or preterm birth.

Hysteroscopic metroplasty has not been shown to increase pregnancy rates in women with infertility, who have a septate uterus (Buttram Jr and Reiter 1981).

Intrauterine adhesions: Intrauterine adhesions are rare but may result from previous uterine evacuation or surgery. Women with amenorrhea who are found to have intrauterine adhesions should be offered hysteroscopic adhesiolysis because it is likely to restore menstruation and improve the chance of pregnancy.

Endometriosis: According to the RCOG guidelines (2004), women with minimal or mild endometriosis who undergo laparoscopy should be offered surgical ablation or resection of endometriosis plus laparoscopic adhesiolysis because this improves the chance of pregnancy. Women with ovarian endometriomas should be offered laparoscopic cystectomy, and women with moderate or severe endometriosis should be offered surgical treatment because it improves the chance of pregnancy. Post-operative medical treatment does not improve pregnancy rates in women with moderate to severe endometriosis and is not recommended. In the management of fertility problems associated with endometriosis, it is widely accepted that minimal and mild endometriosis may be considered equivalent to unexplained infertility and managed accordingly. Medical management, in the absence of pelvic pain, is no longer thought to be an appropriate strategy. Surgical management by the ablation of endometriotic lesions and the removal of endometriomas is an established approach.

Tubal disease: The management of tubal disease traditionally involved surgery, but IVF has become the preferred approach in recent years. However, microsurgery may be used in select cases.

The severity of tubal damage was linked closely to outcome—better results were seen in those with filmy adhesions and limited damage, compared to those with more extensive pathology. Success rates with tubal surgery are also thought to depend upon the severity of tubal damage as well as the age of the woman, duration of infertility and other associated infertility factors (Singhal et al 1991). Microsurgical tubocornual anastomosis has been regarded as the standard treatment for proximal tubal blockage. Since there are no RCTs or controlled observational studies comparing microsurgery with no treatment or with IVF, in the case of tubal problems, if surgery fails, IVF could be attempted. However, when multiple areas are blocked, IVF should be considered as the first line of treatment.

Uterine abnormalities: Uterine abnormalities such as adhesions, polyps, submucous leiomyomas and septae may be associated with infertility but their role in causing infertility is not clear. Laparoscopic ovarian drilling in PCOS is suggested only if there is no evidence for ovulation for several cycles after repeated trials (RCOG 2004).

Unexplained fertility problems: Unexplained (idiopathic) infertility is a diagnosis made by exclusion in couples who have not conceived and in whom standard investigations have not detected any abnormality. The spontaneous cumulative pregnancy rate has been estimated to lie between 33% and 60% at three years and 36% at seven years, although this is influenced by other known prognostic factors such as the age of the woman (Collins and Rowe 1989).

When the duration of infertility is longer, the prognosis falls by 25% per year and the prognosis is much poorer in women aged 35 years or over (Collins and Crosignani 1992). Many couples who have unexplained fertility problems are managed expectantly initially. Further management is essentially empirical—antiestrogens (usually clomiphene citrate) and IUI are usually used as intermediate options, with the final stage of management being IVF treatment.

Intrauterine Insemination

Intrauterine insemination (IUI) may involve timed insemination of sperm into the uterus in natural (unstimulated) cycles or insemination following stimulation of the ovaries using oral anti-estrogens or gonadotrophins. Couples with mild male factor fertility problems, unexplained fertility problems or minimal to mild endometriosis should be offered up to six cycles of IUI because this increases the chance of pregnancy (RCOG Guidelines 2004).

Where intrauterine insemination is used to manage unexplained fertility problems, both stimulated and unstimulated IUI are more effective than no treatment. Where it is undertaken, single rather than double insemination should be offered.

In Vitro Fertilisation (IVF) and Intracytoplasmic Sperm Injection (ICSI)

With the exception of ovulatory disorders, the final treatment option for most categories of fertility problems is IVF and its related technologies. The recognised indications for IVF treatment include:

- Male factor fertility problems where medical/surgical management and intrauterine insemination have not resulted in a live birth or are judged to be inappropriate
- Tubal disease where tubal surgery has not resulted in a live birth or is judged to be inappropriate
- Endometriosis where surgery and IUI have not resulted in a live birth or are judged to be inappropriate
- Unexplained fertility problems of three years duration where medical management and IUI have not resulted in a live birth or are judged to be inappropriate
- Failure of spermatogenesis caused by prior treatment for cancer where cryopreserved semen is unsuitable for IUI.

Intracytoplasmic sperm injection (ICSI) is a technique used within the IVF treatment process where it is necessary to use micromanipulation to achieve fertilisation. The standard approach in IVF is incubation of motile sperm with an egg; ICSI makes it possible for a single spermatozoon to fertilise the egg. It has therefore become the standard approach to treatment where the semen is of very poor quality or where spermatozoa have to be retrieved surgically because the man has azoospermia.

Use in couples with non-male subfertility: A systematic review of one RCT (n = 415) reported no difference in pregnancy rates between ICSI and IVF in couples with non-male subfertility. The RCT did not report live birth rates or miscarriage rates (Thonneau 1998)

The recognised indications for treatment by ICSI include:

- Severe deficits in semen quality
- Obstructive azoospermia
- Non-obstructive azoospermia

In addition, treatment by intracytoplasmic sperm injection should be considered for couples in whom a previous in vitro fertilisation treatment cycle has resulted in failed or very poor fertilisation.

There are no RCTs comparing ICSI with IVF (or other interventions) where semen quality is so poor that IVF would not achieve fertilisation. It is accepted that ICSI is the only treatment option in those circumstances.

A systematic review of ten RCTs compared ICSI versus IVF, ICSI versus additional IVF and ICSI versus subzonal sperm injection in couples with mild-moderate male factor infertility, unexplained infertility and tubal subfertility.

The recognised indications for treatment by ICSI include:

- Severe deficits in semen quality
- Obstructive azoospermia
- Non-obstructive azoospermia

In addition, treatment by intracytoplasmic sperm injection should be considered for couples in whom a previous in vitro fertilisation treatment cycle has resulted in failed or very poor fertilisation

Conclusion: In subfertility/infertility, choosing the appropriate evaluation techniques and management options is very important. Less invasive techniques are chosen for evaluation in a younger, short-term infertility couple; endoscopy could be reserved for those with positive gynecological symptoms and signs or positive ultrasound findings since at the time of endoscopy, an operative procedure for enhancing fertility could be conducted. However, when there is no pathology justifying surgical or medical intervention, the couple could be taken for enhancement of fertility by ovulation induction, intrauterine insemination, in vitro fertilisation or intracytoplasmic sperm injection. It is important to explain to all patients with infertility that there can be no assured success, since the physiology of implantation of the embryo has not yet been understood fully till date.

References

Akande EO and DC Anderson. 1975. Role of sex-hormone-binding globulin in hormonal changes and amenorrhea in thyrotoxic women. *Br J Obstet Gynaecol* 82:557–561.

Ashton D, HK Amin, RM Richart, RS Neuwirth. 1988. The incidence of asymptomatic uterine anomalies in women undergoing transcervical tubal sterilization. *Obstet Gynecol* 72:28–30.

Ballessca JL, J Balasch, JM Calafell, R Alvarez, F Fabreg, MJ de Osaba, C Ascaso. 2000. Serum Inhibin B determination is predictive of successful testicular sperm extraction in men with non-obstructive azoospermia. *Hum Reprod Aug* 15(8):1734–1738.

British Andrology Society. 2002. Education Sub-committee. *Seminal Fluid Analysis and Anti-sperm Antibody Testing. Standard Operating procedures—Laboratory Manual.* 1997. www.repromed.org.uk/bas/bas2000/Publications/labmanual.html

Bulletti C, D de Ziegler, V Polli, C Flamigni. 1999. The role of leiomyomas in infertility. *J Am Assoc Gynecol Laparosc* 6:441–445.

Buttram VC Jr and RC Reiter. 1981. Uterine leiomyomata: Etiology, symptomatology, and management. *Fertil Steril* 36:433–445.

Cayan S, Erdemir D, Ozbey I, Turek PJ, Kadioglu A, Tellaloglu S. 2002. Can varicocelectomy significantly change the way couples use assisted reproductive technologies? *J Urol* 167(4):1749–1752.

Clark AM, W Ledger, C Galletly, L Tomlinson, F Blaney, X Wang. 1995. Weight loss results in significant improvement in pregnancy and ovulation rates in anovulatory obese women. *Hum Reprod* 10:2705–2712.

Collins JA and PG Crosignani. 1992. Unexplained infertility: A review of diagnosis, prognosis, treatment efficacy and management. *Int J Gynaecol Obstet* 39:267–275.

Collins JA and TC Rowe. 1989. Age of the female partner is a prognostic factor in prolonged unexplained infertility: A multicenter study. *Fertil Steril* 52:15–20.

Danforth DR, LK Arbogast, J Mroueh, MH Kim, EA Kennard, DB Seifer. 1998. Dimeric inhibin: A direct marker of ovarian aging. *Fertil Steril* 70:119–123.

den Hartog JE, JA Land, FRM Stassen, MEP Van Drunnen Scobe, AGH Kessels, CA Bruggeman. 2004. The role of chlamydia genus-specific and species specific IgG antibody testing in predicting tubal disease in subfertile woman. *Hum Reprod* 19(6):1380–1384.

Eggert-Kruse W, G Rohr, T Demirakca, R Rusu, H Naher, D Petzoldt. 1997. Chlamydial serology in 1303 asymptomatic subfertile couples. *Hum Reprod* 12:1464–1475.

Evers JL et al. 2001. *Cochrane Database Systematic Review (1).* CD000479.

Frederick JL, RJ Paulson, MV Sauer. 1991. Routine use of vaginal ultrasonography in the preoperative evaluation of gynecologic patients. An adjunct to resident education. *J Reprod Med* 36:779–782.

Gysler M, CM March, DR Mishell Jr, EJ Bailey. 1982. A decade's experience with an individualized clomiphene treatment regimen including its effect on the postcoital test. *Fertil Steril* 37:161–167.

Karamardian LM and DA Grimes. 1992. Luteal phase deficiency: Effect of treatment on pregnancy rates. *Am J Obstet Gynecol* 167:1391–1398.

Khan KS, S Daya, A Jadad. 1996. The importance of quality of primary studies in producing unbiased systematic reviews. *Arch Intern Med* 156 (6):661–666.

Kousta E, DM White, S Franks. 1997 Modern use of clomiphene citrate in induction of ovulation. *Hum Reprod Update* 3:359–365.

RCOG Clinical Guidelines. 2004. Fertility assessment and treatment for people with fertility problems. http://www.rcog.org.uk/resources/Public/pdf/Fertility_full.pdf

MacLeod J. 1964. Human seminal cytology as a sensitive indicator of the germinal epithelium. *Int J Fertil* 9:281–295.

Matorras R, C Perez, B Corcostegui, JI Pijoan, O Ramon, P Delgado, FJ Rodrigues Escudero. 1997. Treatment of the male with follicle stimulating hormone in intrauterine insemination, with husband's spermatozoa: A randomized study. *Hum Reprod* 12(1):24–28.

Opsahl MS, B Miller, TA Klein. 1993. The predictive value of hysterosalpingography for tubal and peritoneal infertility factors. *Fertil Steril* 60:444–448.

Pritts EA. 2001. Fibroids and infertility: A systematic review of the evidence. *Obstet Gynecol Surv* 56: 483–491.

Rock JA . 1995. The revised American Fertility Society classification of endometriosis: Reproducibility of scoring. ZOLADEX Endometriosis Study Group. *Fertil Steril* 63:1108–1110.

Rowe PJ, FH Comhaire, TB Hargreave, AM Mahmoud. 2000. *WHO Manual for the Standardized Investigation, Diagnosis and Management of the Infertile Male.* Cambridge: Cambridge University Press.

Scott RT, JP Toner, SJ Muasher, S Oehninger, S Robinson, Z Rosenwaks. 1989. Follicle-stimulating hormone levels on cycle day 3 are predictive of in vitro fertilization outcome. *Fertil Steril* 51:651–654.

Sharara FI, RT Scott Jr, DB Seifer. 1998. The detection of diminished ovarian reserve in infertile women. *Am J Obstet Gynecol* 179:804–812.

Shoham Z, A Balen, A Patel, HS Jacobs. 1991. Results of ovulation induction using human menopausal gonadotropin or purified follicle stimulating hormone in hypogonadotropic hypogonadism patients. *Fertil Steril* 56:1048–1053.

Singhal V, TC Li, ID Cooke. 1991. An analysis of factors influencing the outcome of 232 consecutive tubal microsurgery cases. *Br J Obstet Gynaecol* 98:628–636.

Taymor ML. 1990. The use and misuse of ovulation-inducing drugs. *Infertil Reprod Med Clin North Am* 1:165–186.

The ESHRE Capri Workshop. 1996. Guidelines to the prevalence, diagnosis, treatment and management of infertility. *Hum Reprod* 11:1775–1807.

The Rotterdam ESHRE/ASRM-sponsored PCOS consensus workshop group. 2004. Revised 2003 consensus on diagnostic criteria and long-term health risks related to polycystic ovary syndrome (PCOS). *Hum Reprod* 1941–1947.

Thonneau P, L Bujan, L Multigner, R Mieusset. 1998. Occupational heat exposure and male fertility: A review. *Hum Reprod* 13:2122–2125.

Van Rumste MM, JL Evers, CM Farquhar, DA Blake. 2003. Intra-cytoplasmic sperm injection versus partial zona dissection, subzonal insemination and conventional techniques for oocyte insemination during in vitro fertilisation. *Cochrane Database Syst Rev* (2):CD001301.

Vandermolen DT, Ratts VS, Evans WS, Stovall DW, Kauma SW, Nestler JE. 2001. Metformin increases the ovulatory rate and pregnancy rate from clomiphene citrate in patients with polycystic ovary syndrome who are resistant to clomiphene citrate alone. *Fertil Steril* 75:310–5.

Vanrell JA and J Balasch. 1983. Prolactin in the evaluation of luteal phase in infertility. *Fertil Steril* 39:30–33.

Wainer R, M Albert, A Dorion, M Bailly, M Berger, R Combroso, M Gombault, J Selvea. 2004. Influence of the numbrt of motile spermatozoa inseminated and of their morphology on the success of intrauterine insemination. *Hum Reprod* 19(9):2060–2025.

Wallach EE. 1992. The uterine factor in infertility. *Fertil Steril* 23:138–158.

Westrom L and P Wolner-Hanssen. 1993. Pathogenesis of pelvic inflammatory disease. *Genitourin Med* 69:9–17.

World Health Organization. 1992. The influence of varicocele on parameters of fertility in a large group of men presenting to infertility clinics. *Fertil Steril* 57:1289–1293.

8

Endometriosis

C Soundaram | Kamal Ojha

Endometriosis is a benign disease defined by the presence of ectopic endometrial glands and stroma and associated with both pelvic pain and infertility. Endometriosis gives rise to a broad spectrum of clinical manifestations, is prone to progression and recurrence and often presents difficult clinical management problems for the patient and the clinician.

Epidemiology

True prevalence of endometriosis is not known because surgery is the gold standard for diagnosis and not all patients with symptoms of endometriosis undergo surgery to confirm the diagnosis. Diagnostic laparoscopy is usually not performed unless the symptoms are strongly suggestive of endometriosis. The prevalence of asymptomatic endometriosis is approximately 4% in women undergoing surgery for elective sterilisation (Mahmood and Templeton 1991).

Most estimates of prevalence of endometriosis have ranged between 5%–20% among women with pelvic pain and between 20%–40% among infertile women. The general prevalence ranges between 3%–10% in women in the reproductive age group (Speroff and Marc 2005).

Prevalence is known to vary according to geography and race, the highest being in the Japanese population, where the incidence of endometriosis is twice that of the Caucasian population (Miyazawa 1976).

Varied prevalence in the literature makes it difficult to interpret epidemiological data and counsel women; however, the epidemiology shows that if a woman has abdominal pain associated with menstruation and/or subfertility, then she should be referred for laparoscopy, as a significant proportion of women with these symptoms have endometriosis.

Etiology

Many theories have been propounded for the etiology of endometriosis, such as retrograde menstruation theory, coelomic metaplasia theory, vascular or lymphatic metastasis theory. However, no one single theory explains completely the occurrence of all cases of endometriosis.

Retrograde menstruation theory: Sampson's original theory (1927) is supported by the fact that retrograde menstruation is found in most normal women. Endometriosis is more common with obstructing müllerian anomalies, with early menarche, short cycles and menorrhagia. Endometriosis is commonly observed in the most dependent region of the pelvis, and can be experimentally induced in primates, which supports this theory.

Coelomic metaplasia theory: It explains the occurrence of endometriosis in prepubertal girls and endometriosis in sites distant from the pelvis.

Endometriosis disease theory: More recently, the 'endometriosis disease theory' (EDT) has been proposed (Koninckx et al 1999). According to this theory, superficial peritoneal lesions arise because of implantation and are regarded as physiological findings, which can regress spontaneously and there is no progression between minimal and severe disease. Severe, deeply infiltrating endometriosis and endometiotic cysts are pathological and arise from somatic mutations within cells, which then develop like a benign tumour, that is, changes occur in genetically predisposed individuals exposed to environmental risk factors such as dioxins and chlorinated biphenyl pollutants. These cells are embedded in the pelvic organs and escape regulation by the peritoneal fluid. The genetic concept underpinning this theory is supported by evidence of strong familial tendencies and at a molecular level, by the observation that cystic ovarian endometriosis is clonal in origin. Endometriosis is 6–7 times more common among first degree relatives of affected women compared to the general population (Moen and Magnus 1993).

Symptoms

The two most common presentations of endometriosis are pelvic pain and infertility.

Pathophysiology of pain in endometriosis: In the early stages of endometriosis, painful symptoms may be caused by the release of mediators, such as prostaglandins, bradykinins, interleukins and the inflammatory products of macrophages altering the receptive properties of the nociceptors in the pelvis. In the advanced stages, infiltrating endometriosis results in direct mechanical compression of the nociceptors, particularly around the uterosacral ligaments (Cornillie et al 1990; Perper et al 1995).

Pathophysiology of infertility in endometriosis: The pathogenesis of infertility in endometriosis is likely to be multifactorial (Table 8.1). In advanced endometriosis, there is obvious anatomical distortion of the pelvis which may interfere with the release or pickup of the oocytes. However, the cause–effect relationship of minimal endometriosis is more difficult to understand. Possible mechanisms include unruptured luteinised follicle syndrome, prostaglandin-induced luteolysis and oocyte maturation defects (Ingamells et al 1990; Brosens 1995). Currently there is no simple explanation for infertility in the presence of minimal and mild endometriosis.

Diagnosis

The traditional definition of endometriosis requires histological demonstration of ectopic endometrial glands and stroma; unfortunately there is no reliable non-invasive alternative to laparoscopy for the diagnosis of the disease. Laparoscopy with histological examination of excised lesions is the gold standard for the diagnosis of endometriosis.

Clinical diagnosis includes symptoms and physical examination. Symptoms suggestive of endometriosis are dysmenorrhea, intermenstrual pain, dyspareunia and subfertility. Dysmenorrhea often begins before the onset of menstrual flow and usually persists throughout menses. In adult women, dysmenorrhea may be especially suggestive of endometriosis if it begins after years of pain-free menses. The dyspareunia is usually new in onset, most intense with deep penetration and immediately prior to menstruation. The association between endometriosis and infertility is generally accepted in severe cases, but is controversial in minimal or mild endometriosis. However, endometriosis can be asymptomatic.

The often paradoxical relationship between the extent and severity of the pain and the stage and site of endometriosis is well recognised. Women with advanced disease may have little or no discomfort and those with minimal disease may have incapacitating pain (Vercellini et al 1996).

Physical examination may reveal a retroverted uterus, restricted mobility of the uterus, fixed adnexal mass, tenderness or nodularity. Compared with the laparoscopic (gold standard) diagnosis of endometriosis, physical examination has relatively poor sensitivity, specificity and predictive value (Spaczynski and Duleba 2003).

Transvaginal scan and magnetic resonance imaging have 90% sensitivity and almost 100% specificity in the detection and differentiation of endometriomas from other cystic ovarian masses but cannot image pelvic adhesions or superficial peritoneal foci of the disease (Arrive et al 1989; Patel et al 1999).

Classification

The American Society for Reproductive Medicine (ASRM) developed a classification system based on surgical findings that was modelled after those used for grading malignant disease. The current version of classification (ASRM 1997) is the most widely accepted tool for the classification but it still has serious limitations; chief among them is the poor correlation with pregnancy rates. Based on the scoring, endometriosis is classified into four stages.

Stage I (Minimal)
Stage II (Mild)
Stage III (Moderate)
Stage IV (Severe)

Table 8.1: Possible mechanisms of infertility in endometriosis

Hormonal dysfunction
Ovulatory dysfunction
Interference with implantation/ embryogenesis
Interference with sperm function
Interference with fertilisation
Interference with tubal function
Mechanical interference

Treatment

Treatment of endometriosis is symptom-based and the approach towards management differs depending on the presence of pain, infertility or both (Table 8.2). However, regardless of clinical profile, treatment of endometriosis is justified because endometriosis appears to progress in 30%–60% of patients within a year of diagnosis and it is not possible to predict which patients it will progress in (D'Hooge and Hill 2002). Treatment options are broadly classified into medical or surgical. The decision whether to treat endometriosis found incidentally on laparoscopy done for other reasons is debatable as endometriosis is a disease of progression, but not in all patients. When disease is less severe, medical treatment can effectively control pain in the large majority of women but has no effect on fertility. Surgery is at least as effective as medical treatment for relieving the pain and can also improve fertility (Prentice 2001).

Medical management: The basis of medical management is to reduce or eliminate cyclic menstruation, to suppress the growth and activity of the endometrium thereby anticipating that the same would occur in endometriotic implants (Table 8.3). Established medical treatments include danazol, progestins, cyclic or continuous oral contraceptives, gestrinone and GnRH agonists (Table 8.4). All available evidence indicates that they are equally effective and that no one treatment is to be preferred over others. Pain relief, subsequent pregnancy rates, recurrent rates are similar for all forms of medical treatment (Speroff and Marc 2005). Medical treatment is effective for pain associated with endometriosis, but there is no substantial evidence that medical treatment improves fertility (Prentice 2001). Medical treatment is not effective for all but the smallest of ovarian endometriomas (less than 1 cm). The choice between the combined oral contraceptive, progestogens, danazol and GnRH agonists depends principally upon their side-effect profiles because they relieve pain associated with endometriosis equally well.

Danazol: It is an isoxazol derivative of 17α-ethinyltestosterone which acts by inhibiting the midcycle LH surge and thereby inducing a chronic anovulatory state. It also inhibits other steroidogenic enzymes to yield a high-androgen, low-estrogen environment that inhibits endometriosis. The resulting amenorrhea decreases new seeding into the peritoneal cavity. Danazol at the recommended dose of 600–800 mg/day has significant androgenic and hypo-estrogenic side effects that limit the clinical utility of the drug. Most common of these effects are weight gain, fluid retention, fatigue, acne, oily skin, decreased breast size, atrophic vaginitis, hot flushes and mood disturbances. Less commonly, hirsutism and deepening of voice are noted.

Progestins: The progestins induce decidualisation leading to endometrial attenuation over time. The most extensively used progestin is medroxyprogesterone acetate both as oral (20–100 mg/day) and parentral therapy (150 mg per 3 months). Side effects include weight gain, fluid retention, breast tenderness, episodic breakthrough bleeding and depression. The incidence of side effects is similar for different types of progestins. Use of levonorgestrel intrauterine system (LNG-IUS) has recently been used in the treatment of rectovaginal endometriosis. Progestins can be used effectively to treat dysmenorrhea, dyspareunia and intermenstrual pain in women with endometriosis.

Oral contraceptives: Combined oral contraceptive pill, either in a continuous or cyclic fashion, has been used for a long time in the treatment of endometriosis. Continuous treatment has been dubbed as 'pseudopregnancy' as the amenorrhea with the high-estrogen and high-progesterone environment mimics pregnancy. The choice of pill is not significant, although a monophasic formulation seems more logical than a multiphasic pill for continuous therapy. The side effects of treatment are the same as those

Table 8.2: Diagnostic approach in endometriosis

History
Pelvic examination
Sonography
Computed tomography/MRI
Laparoscopy/Histology

Table 8.3: Phenotypic appearance of endometriotic implants

Nodular deep lesions
Superficial pigmented lesions
Superficial non-pigmented lesions
Peritoneal pockets
Endometrioma
Adhesions

associated with oral contraceptives.

GnRH (GONADOTROPHIN RELEASING HORMONE) AGONISTS: GnRH agonists induce a hypogonadal state that deprives the endometriotic tissue of estrogen support and amenorrhea which eliminates any possibility of new peritoneal seeding. GnRH agonists can be administered intramuscularly, subcutaneously or intranasally, the route varying with the specific drug. The side effects are those of hypogonadism and include hot flushes, vaginal dryness, decreased libido, depression, irritability, fatigue, headache, changes in skin texture and bone mineral depletion.

GESTRINONE: It is a 19-nortestosterone derivative steroid having androgenic, anti-progestogenic and anti-estrogenic actions. The advantage of the drug is less frequent administration (2.5–10 mg, two to three times a week). The side effects are similar to danazol but less pronounced.

Duration of therapy is limited for some drugs due to the side-effect profile. The combined pills and medroxyprogesterone acetate may be used long-term, but generally the use of gestagens, danazol and GnRH agonists is usually restricted to six months. GnRH agonist therapy is limited because up to 6% of bone mineral density may be lost in the first six months. However, the loss is restored almost completely two years after stopping GnRH treatment. 'Add-back' therapy (that is, progestogen with or without estrogen) can be used (with no loss of efficacy) to relieve menopausal side effects, to prevent bone loss and allow therapy to continue beyond six months. How long this regimen may safely be continued is unclear, but in a recent study using leuprolide acetate with hormonal add-back therapy, bone density was maintained at the same level over 12 months of treatment.

TABLE 8.4: AN APPROACH TO MEDICAL TREATMENT OF ENDOMETRIOSIS

Hypoestrogenism	GnRH analogues
Hyperandrogenism	Danazol
Hyperprogestational	Medroxyprogesterone Norethindrone Gestrinone

Surgical management: The objectives of surgical treatment of endometriosis are to restore anatomical relationships, to excise or destroy visible disease to the extent possible and to prevent or delay recurrence of the disease. Surgical treatment of endometriosis can be performed through laparoscopy or laparotomy. Laparoscopy offers the advantages of better visualisation, less tissue trauma and dessication, smaller incisions and a speedier postoperative recovery. Postoperative adhesions and complications may also be less than those that follow laparotomy. Most importantly, the results achieved with laparoscopy are equivalent or better than those observed with laparotomy (Sutton and Jones 2004).

Excision and ablation: Peritoneal implants can be ablated with unipolar or bipolar electrosurgical instruments or laser. Alternatively, they can excised by sharp dissection. There is no evidence to suggest that one is superior to the other. Because of the depth of the disease and anatomical distortion due to adhesions, excision is preferable to simple lysis.

Management of endometriomas: The optimal treatment of ovarian endometriomas is somewhat controversial. The modes of surgical treatment are stripping and drainage, with or without ablation of the cyst wall. The results of second-look laparoscopic studies suggest that residual deep ovarian disease is less likely after cystectomy or fenestration and ablation than drainage alone. Simply puncturing and draining the endometrioma has no beneficial role in the long term (Vercellini et al 1992).

Presacral neurectomy and laparoscopic uterosacral nerve ablation (LUNA): These procedures are used in the management of dysmenorrhea and central pelvic pain associated with endometriosis. Pre-sacral neurectomy involves interrupting the sympathetic innervation of the uterus at the level of the superior hypogastric plexus and LUNA involves the destruction of the middle portion of the uterosacral ligaments.

Management of rectovaginal disease: Deeply infiltrating endometriosis involving the rectovaginal septum requires extensive surgery. Surgery involves thorough dissection and exposure of the anterior rectum, the posterior vagina and nodular disease. Often a portion of the posterior vagina must be excised and sometimes a short segment of the rectum must be resected followed by anastomosis.

Radical surgery: In women with advanced symptomatic disease who have completed childbearing and those in whom medical and conservative surgical treatment fails, radical surgical treatment, hysterectomy with bilateral salpingo-oophorectomy, must be seriously considered.

SPECIAL CIRCUMSTANCES

HRT and endometriosis: Following bilateral oophorectomy, it has been suggested that women with endometriosis be given HRT with continuous estrogen and progesterone. In women with severe disease, especially involving bowel, bladder or ureters, a hormone-free period for up to six months may be advised before commencing combined therapy.

Extrapelvic endometriosis: Extrapelvic endometriosis is defined as the presence of endometriosis-like implants elsewhere in the peritoneal cavity or in other body cavities. Extrapelvic endometriosis has been reported in virtually every organ. The presence of cyclical symptoms related to the organ or system involved suggests the diagnosis of extrapelvic endometriosis. There may be involvement of the bladder, ureters, surgical scars, vagina, bowel and lung tissue. Hormonal therapy is of value as an interim measure, but recurrence is inevitable on cessation of medical treatment and surgical excision would be the eventual treatment of choice.

Recurrent endometriosis: It has been suggested that in only a third of cases the disease is progressive, while in the remainder the endometriosis remains in a steady state or eventually resolves spontaneously. After medical or surgical treatment, the endometriosis can regenerate in the same site or new disease can develop at new sites.

When choosing the therapeutic options there is no essential difference between primary and recurrent endometriosis. In many instances, repeat medical or repeat conservative surgical therapy is appropriate, but when symptoms are severe in recurrent endometriosis, a radical surgical approach may be an option for long-term pain relief.

Adenomyosis: This is endometrial tissue deep within the myometrium of the uterine wall. It affects women in the perimenopause age group and presents with symptoms similar to fibroid uterus. It shows a diffuse involvement of the uterus, which is usually enlarged, sometimes up to 14 weeks. It may respond to medical treatment but more commonly surgical management is undertaken in view of the patient's age and symptoms.

Carcinoma in endometriosis: The malignant potential of endometriosis is very low. Among all the endometrioid type of ovarian malignancy, up to 10% are seen in continuity with pre-existing endometriosis.

References

Arrive L, H Hricak, MC Martin. 1989. Pelvic endometriosis: MR imaging, *Radiology* 171:687.

Brosens I. 1990. Endometriosis related to infertility. *Curr Opin Obstet Gynecol* 3:205–210.

Cornillie FJ, D Ooterlynck, JM Lauweryns, PR Koninckx. 1990. Deeply infiltrating pelvic endometriosis: Histology and clinical significance. *Fertil Steril* 53: 978–983.

D'Hooge TM, JA Hill (ed.). 2002. Endometriosis. In *Novak's Gynecology*, 13th Edition. Philadelphia: Lippincott Williams & Wilkins. 931–970.

Ingamells S and EJ Thomas (ed). 1995. *Infertility and endometriosis. Endometriosis—Current understanding and management.* Oxford: Blackwell Science.

Koninckx PR, D Barlow, S Kennedy. 1999. Implantation versus infiltration: The Sampson versus endometriotic disease theory. *Gynaecol Obstett Inves* 47(suppl): 3–10.

Mahmood TA, A Templeton. 1991. Prevalence and genesis of endometriosis. *Hum Reprod* 6:544.

Miyazawa K. 1976. Incidence of endometriosis among Japanese women. *Obstet Gynecol* 48: 407–409.

Moen MH and P Magnus. 1993. The familial risk of endometriosis. *Acta Obstet Gynecol Scand* 72: 560.

Patel MD, VA Feldstein, DC Chen, SD Lipson, RA Filly. 1999. Endometriomas: Diagnostic performance of US. *Radiology* 210:739.

Perper MM, Nezhat F, H Goldstein, CH Nezhat, C Nezhat. 1995. Dysmenorrhea is related to the number of implants in endometriosis patients. *Fertil Steril* 63:500–503.

Prentice A (ed). 2001. Advances in the management of endometriosis related infertility. In *Recent advances in Obstetrics and Gynaecology* New York: Churchill Livingstone. 21:101–110.

Sampson JA. 1927. Peritoneal endometriosis due to menstrual dissemination of endometrial tissue into the peritoneal cavity. *Am J Obstet Gynaecol* 14:422–469.

Spaczynski RZ and AJ Duleba. 2003. Diagnosis of endometriosis. *Semin Reprod Med* 21:193.

Speroff L and AF Marc (ed). 2005. *Clinical gynaecological endocrinology and infertility*, 7th edition. Philadelphia: Lippincott Williams and Wilkins.

Sutton C, K Jones (ed). 2004. eds. *Endometriosis*. London: RCOG Press.

The American Society for Reproductive Medicine. 1997. Revised American Society for Reproductive Medicine classification for endometriosis. *Fertil Steril* 67:819.

Vercellini P, L Trespidi, O De Georgi, I Cortesi, F Parazzini, PG Crosignani. 1996. Endometriosis and pelvic pain: Relation to disease stage and localisation. *Fertil Steril* 65:299.

9

Current Trends in Early Diagnosis and Treatment of Tubal Pregnancy

Nutan Agarwal | Alka Kriplani

Ectopic pregnancy is implantation of the fertilised ovum outside the uterine cavity. The incidence of ectopic pregnancy has been rising steadily in the last four decades. In the USA, it has steadily increased from 4.5 per 1000 pregnancies in the 1970s to nearly 20 per 1000 pregnancies in the 1990s (Latchaw et al 1995). In the UK too, the incidence of ectopic pregnancy has been reported to rise 3.8-fold from 1966 to 1996. This is partly due to improved diagnosis (Rajkhowa et al 2000). Incidence in India was reported to be one in 300 by ICMR in 1989. Hospital admissions due to ectopic pregnancy also increased fourfold from the early 1970s to the late 1980s, but the late 1990s saw a decline in admissions due to changes in practice brought about by early diagnosis, and hence medical and conservative management, without admission (Cunningham et al 2001). Thus, despite increasing incidence, both hospital admissions and maternal deaths due to ectopic pregnancy are declining. Nevertheless, it still remains a leading cause of maternal death in the first trimester (Grimes 1995). The first successful surgical treatment of ectopic pregnancy was described by Tail in 1883. He performed salpingectomy in four cases and all survived. In 1940, blood bank facility developed and prognosis became better for these cases. Availability of the pregnancy test in 1960 and the ultrasound scan in 1970 were significant advances for early diagnosis of ectopic pregnancy.

Early and accurate diagnosis is possible using serum β hCG measurement as marker for ectopic pregnancy; this is key to medical management of ectopic pregnancy.

Risk Factors Of Tubal Pregnancy

Various factors that increase the risk of ectopic pregnancy include tubal factors, zygote abnormalities, ovarian factors, intrauterine devices (IUDs), etc. Among tubal factors, salpingitis increases the risk of ectopic pregnancy 2–4 times (WHO 1985), tubal ligation and recanalisation by 9–10 times (WHO 1985) and previous tubal surgery by 20-fold (Ankum et al 1996). In a woman who has already had one tubal pregnancy, the risk of having repeat ectopic pregnancy is seven to thirteen times greater than overall risk (Jeffcoate 2001).

Infertility increases the risk of ectopic pregnancy moderately, mainly because of tubal factors. This is particularly true for pregnancies that occur during infertility treatment. In multiparas with a history of infertility for 14 years there is a two to three times increased risk of ectopic pregnancy. The incidence of ectopic pregnancy following in vitro fertilisation (IVF) procedures is reported in up to 28% of cases, that is, a sixfold risk (Marcus and Brinsden 1995). Some studies have reported increased ectopic pregnancy rates with use of clomiphene citrate too (Cunningham et al 2001), probably due to altered tubal function as a result of hormone fluctuations (Karande et al 1991). Intrauterine devices prevent intrauterine pregnancy more effectively than tubal pregnancy and, therefore, if pregnancy occurs with an IUD in situ, it is more likely to be ectopic (Mol et al 1995). A higher proportion of ovarian ectopic pregnancies has been seen in IUD users (5.5% vs 0% in non-users) (Breen 1970; Raziel et al 1990).

Natural history of tubal pregnancy: Spontaneous resolution, either by regression or tubal abortion, is expected in up to 60% of cases (Ylostalo et al 1992). Tubal abortion is common when the ectopic pregnancy is situated at the ampullary or fimbrial region. Choriodecidual hemorrhage separates the ovum from the tube and thereafter one of four things may happen—it may resolve completely, present with hematosalpinx, or may keep trickling, resulting in persistent pain and the formation of a pelvic hematocele. Rarely, tubal abortion may result in secondary abdominal pregnancy. Acute tubal rupture is the classical course, which occurs more commonly at the isthmic site. The patient develops acute abdomen and hypovolemia. Sometimes tubal rupture may take a chronic course if bleeding at the site is not acute or severe.

Table 9.1: Symptoms and signs of ectopic pregnancy (Pisarska et al 1999)

Symptoms and signs	*Approximate percentage*
Abdominal pain	95%
Amenorrhea	85%
Vaginal bleeding	75%
Dizziness, fainting	25%
Passage of tissues	10%
Adnexal tenderness	80%
Adnexal mass	50%
Uterine enlargement	25%

Clinical features: There is a wide spectrum of symptoms and signs, ranging from the asymptomatic to the hemodynamically unstable (Table 9.1). Early ectopic pregnancy may be entirely asymptomatic. The most commonly reported symptoms are lower abdominal pain, amenorrhea and vaginal bleeding. The classical symptoms of ectopic pregnancy are found in 30% of cases and usually present at weeks 5 to 9 of amenorrhea (Tay et al 2000).

Abdominal pain has a wide spectrum ranging from mild to severe, lower to upper abdomen, unilateral or bilateral, localised or generalised, continuous or intermittent. Half the cases presenting with amenorrhea may experience spotting per vaginum at the time of the expected period. Vaginal bleeding occurs due to inadequate endocrine function. The failing trophoblast may lead to involution of the decidua and occasionally the entire decidua is sequestrated or expelled through the cervical canal (decidual cast), mimicking the passage of products of conception.

On examination, ipsilateral adnexal tenderness is frequently found. Cervical excitation, that is, tenderness on movement of the cervix, may be present in about two-thirds of cases. An adnexal mass may be palpable if it is over 3 cm in size (Graezykowski and Seifer 1999). Care must be taken while performing bimanual examination as vigorous manipulation may expedite rupture of the ectopic gestational mass. The patient may present with tachycardia, hypotension, abdominal distension, marked rebound tenderness and shoulder tip pain in cases of acute ruptured ectopic.

Early diagnosis: Nowadays, a larger number of pregnancies, especially those receiving infertility treatment, are monitored early and the diagnosis of ectopic pregnancy can be established before any symptoms manifest. Early diagnosis is essential to prevent maternal mortality and preserve future fertility—to achieve this, it is important to 'think' ectopic. The diagnosis of ectopic pregnancy should be suspected in any sexually active woman of reproductive age who presents with symptoms of lower abdominal pain and delayed menstruation, until proven otherwise. All women with a history of any of the predisposing factors such as infertility, pelvic inflammatory disease, previous ectopic pregnancy, tubal surgery, assisted reproductive techniques (ART) or IUD use must be screened for ectopic pregnancy. This is done by a urine pregnancy test, ultrasound and follow-up with serum β hCG, if required. Screening has been shown to reduce the risk of rupture from 2.1% to 0.6% (Mol et al 2002).

Diagnosis: The importance of symptoms and signs should not be underestimated despite the powerful diagnostic armamentarium. They not only help in diagnosing the condition, but also influence the choice of treatment. Thorough elicitation of history and physical examination can diagnose ectopic pregnancy with 60% accuracy (Barnhart et al 2002). However, various tests have become available over the last decade that have revolutionised the diagnosis of ectopic pregnancy. Of these, serum β hCG and ultrasound are the most important.

1. Serum β hCG
2. Transabdominal and transvaginal ultrasound
3. Uterine curettage
4. Serum progesterone
5. Doppler
6. Culdocentesis
7. Laparoscopy

Serum β hCG: This is the principal endocrine marker of pregnancy. It can be detected in maternal serum as early as 10 days after fertilisation. β hCG is positive in virtually all ectopic pregnancies. On very rare occasions, ectopic pregnancy may be found where β hCG cannot be detected in serum. It may be due to a very small volume of trophoblastic tissue which may be progressively degenerating. As the β hCG levels vary in pregnancy, a single measurement cannot distinguish between an ectopic and an intrauterine pregnancy, but repeating the measurement within 48–72 hours is useful. This is the normal doubling time of β hCG. In 85% of normal intrauterine pregnancies, the β hCG rises by 66% in 48 hours and 114% in 72 hours. In ectopic pregnancies on the other hand, 85% of ectopic pregnancies have no or $<66\%$ rise in 48 hours and their doubling time is usually $1 \geq 7$ days (Romero et al 1986).

Drawbacks of β hCG testing: Basing a diagnois on the results of β hCG alone, is unreliable for the following reasons:

1. In 15% of intrauterine pregnancies the rise is subnormal, whereas in 15% of ectopic pregnancies there is a normal rise of serum β hCG.
2. An abnormal pattern of serum β hCG levels in ectopic pregnancy cannot be distinguished from the one observed in a

failing intrauterine pregnancy.

3. Serum β hCG levels do not correlate with the size or site of the ectopic pregnancy.

ULTRASOUND: The introduction of ultrasonography has revolutionised the diagnosis and management of ectopic pregnancy. It can be used to evaluate the contents of the endometrial cavity, identify an adnexal mass as small as 10 mm and assess the amount of free peritoneal fluid.

Both transvaginal and transabdominal ultrasound are used to establish the diagnosis of ectopic pregnancy. The transvaginal ultrasound can be used to make the diagnosis a week earlier, with better visualisation and assessment of the fluid in the pouch of Douglas, whereas the transabdominal scan provides a broader view of the pelvis, detection of unusual sites and assessment of peritoneal fluid.

The ultrasound picture can be very variable in ectopic pregnancy—correlation with clinical findings and serum β hCG levels is required to establish the correct diagnosis.

1. Definite intrauterine pregnancy: If a definite intrauterine pregnancy is seen, the likelihood of a coexisting ectopic pregnancy is extremely low. The possibility of heterotopic pregnancy should be kept in mind in pregnancy after IVF. An intrauterine gestation sac is located eccentrically in the intrauterine cavity with a double decidual sac sign (DDSS) (Fig. 9.1). DDSS is an echogenic ring-like structure around the sac which has two thick consecutive lines due to the decidua capsularis–smooth chorion and the peripherally located decidua parietalis, and contains the fetal pole and yolk sac. It has to be differentiated from a pseudosac, which is seen in 10% of ectopic pregnancies (Maccato et al 1993). But pseudosacs are centrally located with no DDSS and no fetal pole (Fig. 9.2).
2. No definite intrauterine pregnancy: The level of β hCG at which an intrauterine pregnancy should be detectable on ultrasound is termed the discriminating zone (DZ) of serum β hCG. On transabdominal scanning, this is 6000 IU/l, whereas on transvaginal scan this is 2000 IU/l (Sadek and Schiotz 1995). If the uterus is empty at the DZ of serum β hCG, an ectopic pregnancy should be diagnosed, unless proven otherwise. In such a situation, there is a rare possibility of multiple pregnancy where higher serum β hCG levels can be expected in earlier gestation. If serum β hCG levels are low, the possibility of early pregnancy has to be kept in mind.
3. Abnormal intrauterine pregnancy: Various ultrasound features that can be seen at different stages of decay of the embryo include gestation sac with no fetal pole, no cardiac activity in the fetal pole, irregular crenated border of the gestation sac, larger sac with no DDSS or large, thin-walled yolk sac.

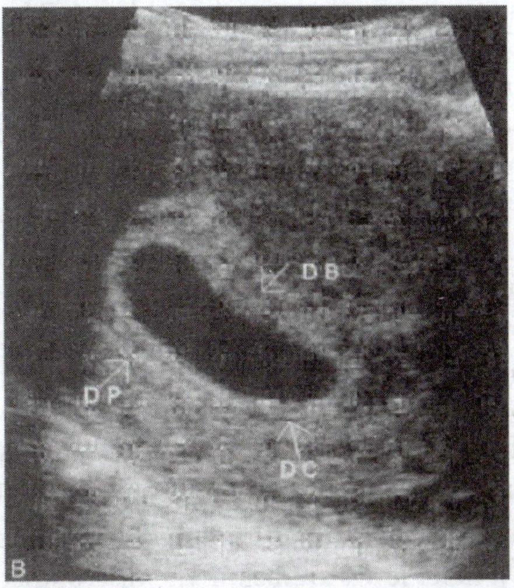

FIGURE 9.1: INTRAUTERINE GESTATIONAL SAC SHOWING DOUBLE DECIDUAL SAC SIGN (DDSS)

4. Probable ectopic: Presence of an adnexal mass, tenderness on probe palpation or fluid in the cul-de-sac suggest an ectopic pregnancy. Adnexal masses other than simple cysts of varying sizes are found. Adnexal masses due to ectopic pregnancy are complex masses with a solid and a cystic component formed by partially the collapsed gestational sac and hemorrhagic and thrombolic components. They are separate from the ovary. The gestation sac may be seen as a tubal ring (Bagel's ring) (Fig. 9.3), which is seen as a thick echogenic ring with a fluid sac (Kadar et al 1994).
5. Definite ectopic: Detection of an echogenic ring-like structure outside the uterine cavity with a fetal pole is diagnostic of definite ectopic pregnancy (Fig. 9.4).

Drawbacks of ultrasonography: Diagnosis by ultrasonography may be difficult in the following situations :

1. Differentiation between a pseudosac and a true intrauterine gestation sac may be difficult.
2. In the absence of an intrauterine pregnancy with low serum β hCG levels, the possibility of very early viable intrauterine pregnancy has to be kept in mind.
3. The absence of intrauterine pregnancy above DZ serum β hCG level does not rule out abortion.
4. There is a remote possibility of heterotopic pregnancy, especially after ART.
5. Other adnexal masses and corpus luteum can be misdiagnosed as ectopic.

Correlation of serum β hCG and ultrasonography: Proper evaluation, follow-up ultrasonography and serum β hCG levels may be required in certain situations to establish the diagnosis and plan the choice of treatment. If β hCG levels are below the discriminating zone and no intrauterine sac is seen, follow-up is required after 48 hours to assess the rise in β hCG as well as the appearance of a gestational sac once the DZ is reached. In high resolution scanners, the DZ it is reported to

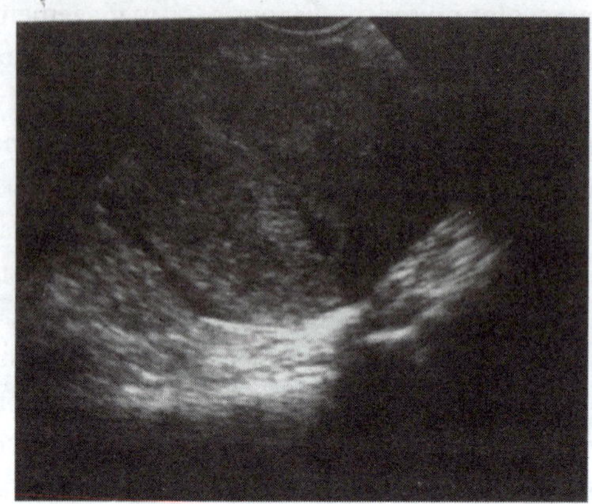

Figure 9.2: Pseudosac in case of ectopic gestation

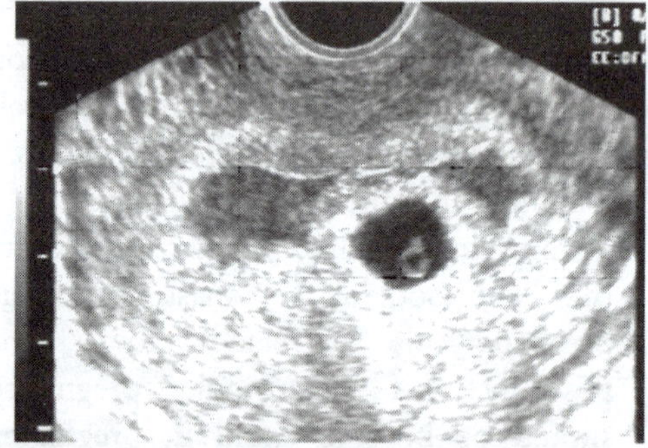

Figure 9.3: Gestational sac as a tubal ring in the fallopian tube

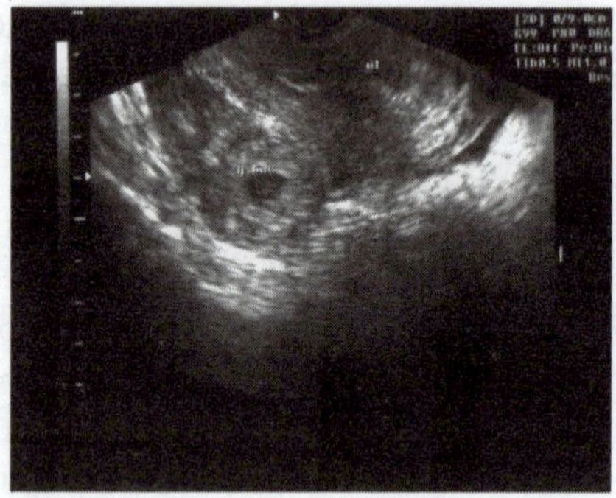

Figure 9.4: Live ectopic with fetal pole

be as low as 3000 IU/l for transabdominal and 1000 IU/l for transvaginal ultrasound (Cacciatore et al 1990), as an average gestational sac is detectable at 35 days at β hCG 1000 IU/l, the fetal pole at 40 days at β hCG 3000 IU/L and cardiac activity at 47 days at β hCG 3000 IU/l (Fossum et al 1988).

Other diagnostic modalities

Doppler ultrasound: It can help to differentiate between a true and pseudogestational sac. High velocity flow is seen in developing placentation, so it is seen at endometrium in normal or abnormal intrauterine pregnancy but not in ectopic pregnancy.

Dilatation and curettage (D&C): It can differentiate ectopic from non-viable intrauterine pregnancy. Villi can be checked immediately in normal saline after curettage—chorionic villi float, dediduas settle. Histological findings consistent with pregnancy confirm the clinical diagnosis. This can be further followed up with β hCG, a fall of ≥50% in 24 hours indicating abortion. Caution should be taken to avoid disruption of an early viable intrauterine pregnancy and D&C should be avoided as far as possible.

Serum progesterone: Serum progesterone testing takes only 2–3 hours and a single measurement may be helpful in identifying normal developing pregnancy. A level exceeding 25 ng/ml is associated with intrauterine viable pregnancy, whereas a value <5 ng/ml is highly suggestive of non-viable pregnancy. However, levels of 5–25 ng are inconclusive, so it has limited value (McCord et al 1996).

Culdocentesis: A significant amount of non-clotted blood is indicative of hemoperitoneum. In case of hemoperitoneum with positive pregnancy test, ectopic pregnancy is the most common cause. Presence of serous fluid or pus is a negative sign for ectopic pregnancy. Dry tap is inconclusive. In cases of ectopic pregnancy with little or no intraabdominal bleeding or organised pelvic hematocele, culdocentesis may be falsely negative. Because of the widespread availability of sonography, it is rarely indicated nowadays.

Differential Diagnosis Of Early Tubal Pregnancy

There are various conditions which may be confused with ectopic pregnancy:

1. Abortion: Abortion also presents with amenorrhea and uterine bleeding. Pain may be present but is not associated with fainting attacks. Adnexal tenderness is not a feature unless there is associated salpingitis.
2. Acute or subacute salpingitis: There may be irregular uterine bleeding and lower abdominal pain. Amenorrhea may not be present but patients had tenderness with or without adnexal mass; salpingitis is usually a bilateral condition.
3. Early pregnancy with corpus luteum: Sometimes a patient in early pregnancy may present with abdominal pain. If a corpus luteum is seen in the adnexa, tenderness is less likely to be present.
4. Torsion or rupture of ovarian cyst, sudden onset of pain with fainting attack of collapse along with findings of adnexal mass may confound the diagnosis.

Treatment

Treatment options for ectopic pregnancy are surgery, medical management or expectant management. Previously, surgery was regarded as mandatory because of the risk of rupture of ectopic pregnancy. Now, with early diagnosis, medical management or expectant management are viable alternatives. The choice of treatment depends on the characteristics of the patient, desire for future fertility, facilities and expertise available at the centre, compliance, socioeconomic status and preference of the patient.

Expectant management: The fact that some patients of ectopic pregnancy have spontaneous resolution, either through regression or through tubal abortion, is the basis of expectant management of ectopic pregnancy. Selection of patients for expectant management depends on the initial serum β hCG levels and size of the ectopic gestation. It is a reasonable option in very carefully selected patients. Stringent inclusion criteria include: ectopic mass <3 cm, β hCG <1000 IU/l and the absence of cardiac activity. Approximately 15%–20% cases of ectopic pregnancy may be appropriate for expectant management. The patient is closely monitored with clinical symptoms, hematocrit and weekly β hCG till undetectable. Transvaginal ultrasonography is performed if required. The overall success is approximately 70%. Complete resolution may take four weeks. Patients with persistent or increasing β hCG levels should be treated with medical or surgical therapy. The risk of tubal rupture on expectant management is reported to be about 2.5% (Kang et al 1998).

Medical management: If facilities for β hCG estimation and ultrasound exist, diagnosis of ectopic pregnancy can be made early and the need for surgical visualisation is eliminated in many cases. Medical treatment is effective and safe in carefully selected cases, provided a definite diagnosis of ectopic pregnancy can be made. The patient must be willing and eligible for medical management. All contraindications should be ruled out. Using the following criteria, about 40% of ectopic pregnancies are found to be appropriate for medical management (ACOG 1998):

Eligibility criteria for medical management

- Hemodynamically stable patient
- Unruptured ectopic
- Reliable and compliant patient, can return for follow-up
- Ectopic pregnancy <4 cm in size
- No contraindication for methotrexate
- Normal blood counts, liver and kidney function
- No suspected heterotopic pregnancy
- No history of prolonged pain (>24 hours)
- Desirous of future fertility

Presence of cardiac activity in the ectopic embryo and serum β hCG levels >10,000 mIU/ml are relative contraindications for medical management, although reports have shown successful outcome in such cases also (Lipscomb et al 1998). We have also used methotrexate successfully in two cases of live ectopic and two cases with high β hCG levels of 28,000 and 40,000 mIU/ml respectively. Close supervision in hospital is essential in these cases.

Treatment regimen Methotrexate is the drug of choice. Both single and multiple-dose regimens have been described. In the multidose regimen, methotrexate is given in a dose of 1 mg/kg IV or IM followed by leucovorin 0.1 mg/kg orally 24 hours later and the dose repeated every alternate day up to a maximum of four doses until β hCG level declines by 15%. Serum β hCG should be assessed at days 0, 3, 5 and 7 until hCG declines 15% from previous value (Barnhart et al 2000). Not all patients need four doses. The second, third or fourth dose is administered only if the β hCG value does not show response. After response is achieved, the patient is monitored with weekly β hCG levels until these are undetectable. If there is no response even after four doses, the patient is maintained drug-free for a week to decrease the risk of side effects (Stovall and Ling 1993).

The single dose regimen is more commonly used as it has fewer side effects. Methotrexate is given in a dose of 50 mg/m^2 IV or IM. β hCG is measured on days 0, 4 and 7. There should be a fall of 15% between day 4 and day 7. A rise in level is often seen on day 4 and does not indicate failure of response. In fact, an initial rise is sometimes caused by the release of trophoblastic tissues into circulation. If the β hCG levels are increased or plateau between day 4 and 7, a second weekly dose can be given (Timor-Tritsch et al 1988). Although most reports show administration of methotrexate by the intramuscular route, the authors prefer the intravenous route, because in two cases where the patient did not respond to IM injection they responded to IV injections. One patient received the first intramuscular injection at nearly 10,000 mIU/ml β hCG and did not respond (β hCG levels rose to 40,000 mIU/ml at DZ), she surprisingly responded to the second intravenous injection and did not require any surgery. Her β hCG became negative in 10 weeks.

Monitoring and follow-up: Most patients can be managed on an outpatient basis. While receiving methotrexate, the patient should be instructed not to take folic acid, salicylates or alcohol, should avoid exposure to the sun and maintain abstinence. She should be observed for heavy bleeding, pain, especially severe and persistent (> 12 hours) pain, any sign of rupture and hematocrit levels. The most difficult aspect is to distinguish between transient pain due to success of therapy from that of tubal rupture. Transient abdominal pain after three days for 4–12 hours is presumably due to tubal abortion (Cunningham et al 2001). About 80% of patients who have pain after medical management do not require surgery (Lipscomb et al 1999). The patient may be hospitalised, if required. Ultrasonography is not of much help (Buster and Pisarka 1999). The patient is followed with weekly β hCG monitoring till levels are undetectable. Resolution usually takes 5–7 weeks (Raziel et al 1990). Medical management is not considered successful until β hCG is no longer detectable in the serum. There are cases of treatment failure even with β hCG value as low as < 50 IU/l (Barnhart et al 1997).

Surgical Intervention

Surgical intervention may be necessary if there is orthostatic hypotension, decreasing hematocrit, persistent or severe pain, any sign of tubal rupture or impending tubal rupture. Surgery is indicated if the patient no longer wants to continue with medical therapy or if medical therapy fails.

Risk of tubal rupture: The risk of tubal rupture is greater with high levels of serum β hCG. The presence of cardiac activity is associated with a higher failure rate of 14% (vs 4.7% when cardiac activity is absent) (Lipscomb et al 1998). The tube is unlikely to rupture if the mass is < 2 cm and β hCG is < 2000 IU/l, although cases of rupture have been reported even with β hCG of < 5 IU/l (Sitka et al 1996).

Success rate: In a review of 26 studies, the overall success rate with the multiple-dose regimen is greater than with the single-dose regimen (95% vs 90%) (Saraj et al 1998). In the latter, 15% of cases need more than one dose. Multidose is less convenient and is associated with more side effects, 48% vs 29% in single dose. Comparison of medical management and conservative surgery has shown that success rate and patency is the same in both, whereas resolution is faster with salpingostomy (Cohen and Sauer 1999).

Surgically assisted medical management: Patients diagnosed before tubal rupture can be treated with alternative treatment options. Besides systemic medical management, local injections of tropholytic agents may be alternative options. These local injections may be injected either by ultrasound guidance or by laparoscopic guidance. Laparoscopically guided local injection does not seem to be a logical option as once the patient is exposed to laparoscopy, it is ideal to remove the ectopic gestation at the same sitting. However, ultrasound-guided salpingocentesis may be an option in certain cases of unruptured ectopic pregnancy to avoid the side effects of systemic drug. It is limited to those patients in whom ultrasound positively localises a tubal mass. Needle injection should be precisely and safely guided into the exact gestational target site. The most reliable ultrasound finding for ectopic pregnancy is the presence of a live embryo outside of the uterus. Tubal ring is another highly specific sonographic appearance; salpingocentesis can only be performed in patients with these specific findings.

Treatment agents including methotrexate 10 mg, hyperosmolar glucose and potassium chloride are used. There is lack of widespread acceptance of this technique. There are some distinct potential advantages:

- Avoidance of risk of laparoscopic surgery
- Lack of systemic toxicity of methotrexate, since it is delivered to a local point. However, its efficacy is considered to be the same as IM injection

However, it should be performed by an experienced practitioner. Other risks are infection, hemorrhage and tubal damage at the site of injection. The authors used potassium chloride (KCl) along with IV methotrexate in two cases with live ectopic pregnancy—both responded to the treatment.

Surgery: Surgery is the mainstay of treatment of all ectopic pregnancy. It is the preferred mode if the patient does not fulfil the criteria for medical management, or is not willing for the same or is not able to come for follow-up in early tubal pregnancy. Surgery may be conservative or radical. Conservative surgery, that is, salpingostomy or fimbrial expression is the logical option for women who wish to preserve their fertility. The subsequent intrauterine pregnancy rate is greater but there is also a higher recurrence risk of ectopic pregnancy (Fernandez et al 1994). Radical surgery, that is, salpingectomy, is indicated in cases of ruptured ectopic, uncontrolled bleeding, extensive tubal damage, large tubal pregnancy (>5 cm), recurrent ectopic on the same side or previous reconstructive surgery.

Laparoscopic surgery is minimally invasive and is therefore always preferable, unless the patient is hemodynamically unstable. Medical management can be offered in only 30%–40% of cases—it requires proper supervision with prolonged follow-up. Laparoscopic surgery is the ideal option, except in cases where the laparoscopic approach is expected to be difficult such as with previous surgery. Other relative contraindications include extensive pelvic adhesions, large blood clots, insufficient laparoscopic facilities or inexperience of the surgeon.

Linear salpingostomy: This is the standard conservative surgery for ectopic pregnancy. Ectopic pregnancy is identified and the tube is immobilised. A linear incision is made on the anti-mesosalpinx wall of the tube, at the point where it is maximally distended. Incision is made by unipolar electrocautery or laser. The products of conception are flushed out with irrigating solution at high pressure. A combination of blunt dissection and hydrodissection should be used. The specimen is grasped with claw forceps and removed—avoid removing the products piecemeal. Bleeding points can be coagulated. The tube is irrigated carefully and inspection should be done for hemostasis under water. The tubal incision is left open to heal.

Fimbrial expression by 'milking' the tube may be appropriate in cases of ampullary pregnancy if the pregnancy is aborting, trophoblastic tissues are expressed out by compressing the tube from proximal to distal side and further, the tube can be washed with irrigating solution. Thin suction cannula can be inserted from the fimbrial side and the solution can be flushed in under pressure. Tube should be thoroughly inspected for any retained products. Care should be taken to wash off all bits of trophoblastic tissue from the tube. Milking can lead to damage to the cilia. If there are large blood clots mini-laparotomy is often indicated in such cases.

The diagnosis of unruptured pregnancy is possible because of ultrasound. Conservative management, with or without surgery, has been explained in the chapter.

References

American College of Obstetricians and Gynecologists. 1998. *Medical management of tubal pregnancy*. Prac Bull No.3. Washington DC: ACOG.

Ankum WM, BWJ Bol, F Vander Veen, PMM Bossyut. 1996. Risk factors for ectopic pregnancy: A meta-analysis. *Fertil Steril* 65:1093–1099.

Barnhart KT, I Katz, A Hummel, CR Gracia. 2002. Presumed diagnosis of ectopic pregnancy. *Obstet Gynecol* 100(3):505–510.

Barnhart K, M Esposito, C Coutifaris. 2000. Update on the medical treatment of ectopic pregnancy. *Obstet Gynecol Clin N Am* 27(3):653–668.

Barnhart K, S Spandorfer, C Contifaris. 1997. Is the medical management of an interstitial pregnancy safe? A report of three failed cases. *J Reprod Med* 8:521–524.

Bhatla N ed. 2001. Jeffcoate's *Principles of Gynecology*, Sixth edition. New Delhi: Arnold Publishers.

Breen JL. 1970. A 21 year survey of 654 ectopic pregnancies. *Am J Obstet Gynecol* 106:1004.

Buster JE and MD Pisarka. 1999. Medical management of ectopic pregnancy. *Clin Obstet Gynecol* 42(1):23–30.

Cacciatore B, U Stenma, P Ylostalo. 1990. Diagnosis of ectopic pregnancy by vaginal ultrasonography in combination with discriminatory serum hCG level of 1000 IU/L (IRP). *Br J Obstet Gynaecol* 97:904–908.

Cohen MA and MV Sauer. 1999. Expectant management of ectopic pregnancy. *Clin Obstet Gynecol* 42(1):48–51.

Cunningham FG et al. 2001. Ectopic pregnancy In *Williams Obstetrics*, 21st ed. New York: McGraw-Hill, 883–910.

Fernandez H, P Bourget, Y Villi, C Lelaidier, R Frydman. 1994. Treatment of unruptured tubal pregnancy with methotrexate pharmacokinetic analysis of local versus intramuscular administration. *Fertil Steril* 62:943–947.

Fossum GT, V Davajan, OA Kletzky. 1988. Early detection of pregnancy with transvaginal ultrasound. *Fertil Steril* 49:789.

Graezykowski JW, DB Seifer. 1999. Diagnosis of acute and persistent ectopic. *Clin Obstet Gynecol* 42(1): 9–22.

Grimes DA. 1995. The morbidity and mortality of pregnancy: Still risky business. *Am J Obstet Gynecol.* 170:1489–1494.

Kadar N, M Bohrer, E Kemmann, R Shelden. 1994. The discriminatory human chorionic gonadotrophin zone for endovaginal sonography. A prospective, randomized study. *Fertil Steril* 61:1018.

Kang JY, EH Jeong, JS Roh, IU Ji, HS Kim. 1998. Expectant management of ectopic pregnancy. *Korean J Obstet Gynecol* 41(9):2377–2380.

Karande VC, JT Flood, N Heard, L Veeck, SJ Mousher. 1991. Analysis of ectopic pregnancies resulting from in vitro fertilisation and embryo transfer. *Hum Reprod* 6:446–449.

Latchaw G, P Takacs, L Gaitan, S Geren, J Burzawa. 1995. Ectopic pregnancy – United States: 1990–1992. *JAMA* 273:533.

Lipscomb GH, D Bran, ML McCord, JC Portera, Ling FW. 1998. Analysis of three hundred and fifteen ectopic pregnancies treated with single dose methotrexate. *Am J Obstet Gynecol* 178:1354–1358.

Lipscomb GH, KJ Puckett, D Bran, FW Lunk. 1999. Management of separation pain after single dose methotrexate therapy for ectopic pregnancy. *Obstet Gynaecol* 93(4):590–593.

Maccato ML, R Estrada, S Faro. 1993. Ectopic pregnancy with undetectable serum and urine β hCG levels and detection of β hCG in the ectopic trophoblast by immunocytochemical evaluation. *Obstet Gynecol* 81:878–880.

Marcus SF, PR Brinsden. 1995. Analysis of the incidence and risk factors associated with ectopic pregnancy following in vitro fertilisation and embryo transfer. *Hum Reprod* 10:199–203.

McCord M, D Muram, JE Buster, KL Arheart, TG Stoval, SA Carson. 1996. Single serum progesterone as a screen for ectopic pregnancy. Exchanging specificity and sensitivity to obtain optimal test performance. *Fertil Steril* 66:513–516.

Mol BW, WM Ankum, PMM Bossyut, F Vander Veen. 1995. Contraception and the risk of ectopic pregnancy. A meta-analysis. *Contraception* 52:337–341.

Mol BW, F Vander Veen, PMM Bossuyt. 2002. Symptom free women at increased risk of ectopic pregnancy. Should we screen? *Acta Obstet Gynecol Scand* 81(7):661–672.

Pisarska MD, SA Carson, JE Buster. 1999. Ectopic pregnancy. *Lancet* 351:115–120.

Rajkhowa M, MR Glass, AJ Rutherford, AH Balen, V Sharma, HS Cuckle. 2000. Trends in the incidence of ectopic pregnancy in England and Wales from 1966 to 1996. *Br J Obstet Gynaecol* 107: 369–374.

Raziel A, A Golan, M Pansky, EIR Ron, I Bukovsky, E Cospi. 1990. Ovarian pregnancy: A report of twenty cases in one institution. *Am J Obstet Gynecol* 163:1182–1185.

Romero R, H Kadar, D Castro. 1986. The value of serial human chorionic gonadotropin testing as a diagnostic tool in ectopic pregnancy. *Am J Obstet Gynecol* 155:392.

Sadek AL and HA Schiotz. 1995. Transvaginal sonography in the management of ectopic pregnancy. *Acta Obstet Gynecol Scand* 74:293–296.

Saraj AJ, Wilcox JG, Najmabadi S, Stein SM, Johnson MB, Paulsen RJ. 1998. Resolution of hormonal marker of ectopic gestation. A randomized trial comparing single dose intramuscular methotrexate with salpingectomy. *Obstet Gynaecol* 92:989–994.

Sitka CS, L Anderson, MD Frederiksen. 1996. Single dose methotrexate for the treatment of ectopic pregnancy. North Western memorial hospital three year experience. *Am J Obstet Gynecol* 174: 1840–1846.

Stovall TG, FW Ling, LA Gray, SA Larson, JE Buster. 1991. Methotrexate treatment of unruptured ectopic pregnancy. A report of 100 cases. *Obstet Gynecol* 77:749–753.

Stovall TG, FW Ling. Single dose methotrexate. An expanded clinical trial. 1993. *Am J Obstet Gynecol* 168:1759–1765.

Tay JI, J Moore, JJ Walker. 2000. Ectopic pregnancy. *Br Med J* 320:916–919.

Timor-Tritsch JE, MN Yeh, DB Peisner et al. 1988. The use of transvaginal ultrasound in the diagnosis of ectopic pregnancy. *Am J Obstet Gynecol* 161:157–161.

World Health Organization. 1985. Task force on intrauterine devices for fertility regulation. A multinational case control study of ectopic pregnancy. *Clin Reprod Fertil* 3:131–143.

Ylostalo P, B Cacciatore, J Sjoberg, M Kaariainen, A Tenhunen, UH Stenman. 1992. Expectant management of ectopic pregnancy. *Obstet Gynecol* 80:345–348.

10

Uterovaginal Prolapse

Pranathi Reddy

Genital prolapse refers to the protrusion or projection of the pelvic organs into the vagina or outside the vaginal opening. The prevalence of genital prolapse increases with age (Graves 1995). Because more women are living longer, genital prolapse will become even more common.

PELVIC SUPPORT SYSTEM: The pelvic support system maintains the pelvic organs in a physiologic position.

- The system consists of the levator ani muscles (fused posteriorly in the midline by the anococcygeal ligament to form the levator plate) and the endopelvic fascia (pubourethral, cardinal and uterosacral ligaments) (Delancey 1992).
- In a standing woman at rest, the levator plate lies nearly horizontal like a hammock. Three pairs of muscles form the levator ani—pubococcygeus, puborectalis and iliococygeus (Harris and Bent 1990; Delancey 1993). (Fig. 10.1).
- These muscles contain two types of fibres—slow twitch fibres form 70% (these are fatigue resistance fibres) and 30% are fast twitch fibres (responding to increases in intraabdominal pressure). The levator ani and sphincter muscles of the pelvic floor are innervated by the anterior sacral roots, S2 to S4 (Delancey 1992, 1993).
- The external anal sphincter and the striated urethral sphincter are innervated by branches of the pudendal nerve. This nerve arises from the same sacral roots (Delancey 1993; Handa et al 1993).
- The uterus, upper vagina and rectum lie parallel to and directly on the levator plate. Thus, increases in abdominal pressure push these organs against the plate. DeLancey described three levels or support that maintains genital organs in a physiologic position (Delancey 1992, 1993).

i. Level I suspension weakness is associated with uterine prolapse or vaginal cuff prolapse following a hysterectomy (Fig. 10.2).

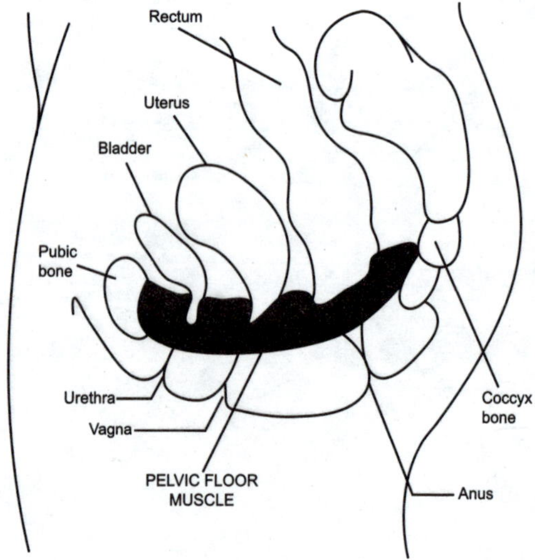

FIGURE 10.1: PELVIC FLOOR

ii. The paracolpium attaches to the vagina and the pelvic walls (level II). Level II weakness is associated with anterior and posterior vaginal prolapse (Harris and Bent 1990; Delancey 1992).
iii. The distal vagina does not have a paracolpium but attaches directly to the surrounding structures (level III) (Harris and Bent 1990; Delancey 1993) (Fig. 10.2).

Etiopathogenesis

Childbirth: This has constantly been put down as the main cause of pelvic floor damage. Frequent pregnancies, prolonged labour, difficult instrumental deliveries and poor repair of perineal damage may all contribute. The risk increases with each child but the rate of increase declines once a woman has had two children. An eleven-fold increase occurs in mothers of four or more children. A woman with two children has an eight times greater risk to prolapse than a nulliparous woman (Mant et al 1997). Prolonged strain and pressure on the levators and pressure on the pudendal nerve causes permanent muscle fibre damage, the quick acting fibres being more affected than the slow fibres. Long second stage of labour and heavier babies create more damage to the pelvic floor when seen on an electromyogram than factors like a forceps delivery or perineal tears There is need for an active management of labour to prevent this damage.

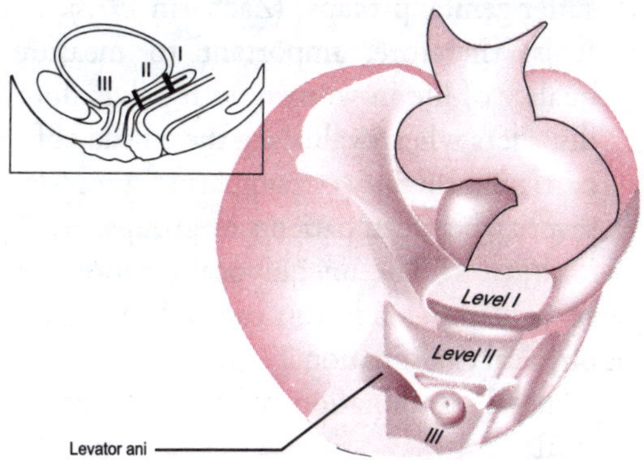

Figure 10.2: Levels of support

Congenital weakness: Congenital weakness of the supports is known to occur. The defect may be in the fascia where an abnormal distribution or structural defect of the collagen fibres would result in weakness. Prolapse in young nulliparous women is generally caused by this defect. Occult spina bifida has been correlated with development of this type of prolapse.

Table 10.1: Risk factors for development of incontinence and pelvic organ prolapse (Wein et al 2006)

Risk factor	Incontinence	Pelvic Organ Prolapse
Aging	+	+
Menopause	-	-
Pregnancy and parity	+	+
Episiotomy	?	?
Obesity	+	+
Surgery	+	+
Hysterectomy	?	+
Constipation	+	+
Chronic cough and respiratory disease	+	?
Exercise and heavy lifting	?+	?+
Genetic and neurologic conditions	+	+

Intraabdominal pressure: Increased intraabdominal pressure, if chronic, can cause stress on the pelvic support system. This coupled with a straightening of the uterovaginal axis would result in intraabdominal pressure driving the uterus down. Chronic cough or constipation, gross obesity, intraabdominal tumours and weight lifting increase the strain.

Role of estrogens: Due to the normal aging process there is a drop in the estrogen level leading to progressive deterioration in the collagen of the connective tissue and menopausal atrophy of the uterus and supporting structures causing prolapse of the uterus in postmenopausal women.

Evaluation of Genital Prolapse History

COMMON SYMPTOMS OF GENITAL PROLAPSE

- Traditionally, genital prolapse has been associated with lower urinary tract, bowel–rectum, sexual and other symptoms (Bump et al 1996).
- Common urinary symptoms include frequency, urgency, stress and urge incontinence, hesitancy, weak or prolonged urine stream, feelings of incomplete emptying, need for manual reduction of the prolapses of position changes to begin or complete voiding and urinary retention (Harris and Bent 1990; McGuire and Cespedes 1996).
- Common bowel symptoms include difficult defecation, incontinence of flatus, liquid or solid stools, staining of the underwear, urgency of defecation, discomfort with defecation, feeling of incomplete evacuation, and rectal protrusion during or after defecation (McGuire and Cespedes 1996).
- Common sexual symptoms of prolapse include loss of interest, lack of orgasm, inability to have vaginal intercourse, dyspareunia and incontinence during sexual activity (Harris and Bent 1990; Weber et al 1995; McGuire and Cespedes 1996).

QUALITY OF LIFE EVALUATION

- Disorders of the pelvic floor, such as urinary incontinence, fecal incontinence and pelvic organ prolapse, can have a significant impact on the woman's self-esteem and self-image (Harris and Bent 1990; Weber et al 1995).
- Especially in traditional societies, patients often so closely guard their symptoms that it was once reported that Chinese women were anatomically less predisposed to suffer genital prolapse (Zacharin 1977).
- It is, therefore, important to measure quality of life in women with pelvic floor disorders when evaluating the efficacy of a particular therapy or comparing symptom severity between patients or groups.

Examination: The unequivocal diagnosis of pelvic prolapse conditions can only be made on physical examination

- General examination with reference to BMI
- Hernial orifices

Local Examination:

- Lithotomy
- Sim's position: Most ideal position for examination
- Semi-upright
- Upright

Instruments:

- Sim's speculum
- Ruler/sponge forceps with markings

PRINCIPLES OF SYSTEMATIC EVALUATION OF PROLAPSE

- Anterior, apical and posterior prolapse
- Rectovaginal septum; perineal body and anal sphincter
- The levator ani muscles may also be assessed.

- It is important to have the patient strain while the examiner assesses each portion to avoid underestimating the degree of prolapse
- The hymenal ring, rather than the introitus, is defined as the fixed reference point for measuring the amount of prolapse

Anterior vaginal wall:

- The anterior vaginal wall and supports can be assessed by placing the speculum in the vagina to depress the posterior wall.
- The degree of anterior vaginal wall relaxation with and without straining is assessed.

Uterus and vagina or vaginal vault:

- With inadequate cardinal and uterosacral ligament support, the cervix may descend below the level of the ischial spines all the way below to the hymen (procidentia).
- After hysterectomy, the vaginal cuff will have dimples at the 3 and 9 o'clock areas, at the locations of the cardinal uterosacral ligament attachments
- The vaginal cuff may be well supported or may prolapse outside the hymen with other vaginal segments.

Enteroceles:

- Enteroceles are herniations of peritoneum-lined sacs containing abdominal contents such as small bowel or omentum
- Enteroceles can occur with or without concomitant vaginal vault prolapse or eversion.
- Vault eversions are accompanied by enteroceles in about 75%
- Although an enterocele may be obvious with severe degrees of prolapse, it may not be obvious with milder degrees.
- The cul-de-sac leading to the rectovaginal septum, where enteroceles most commonly appear, is normally at or above the level of the ischial spines
- Use two speculum blades to retract the anterior and posterior vaginal walls simultaneously.
- Distinction between an enterocele and a high rectocele is difficult.
- Palpation of the rectovaginal septum with the index finger in the rectal ampulla and thumb in the vagina may indicate a bulge between the rectum and the vagina.
- Having the patient stand and strain may make the enterocele more obvious.

Posterior vaginal wall:

- The speculum can be rotated to support the anterior wall while the posterior wall is examined.
- The posterior bulge can be demonstrated with the patient straining.
- Defects in the rectovaginal septum can be palpated with a finger in the rectum.
- The perineal body is examined along with the rectovaginal septum.
- In women with severe prolapse, the perineal body may be thinned or expanded.
- Anal sphincter tone can be evaluated by subjective digital testing of the strength of contraction.

Levator ani:

- Palpate the levator ani muscles with two gloved fingers in the posterior vagina, 2–4 cm above the hymen
- Ask the patient to squeeze the muscles she normally uses to hold urine and avoid passing gas

Grading and classification of genital prolapse

Pelvic organ prolapse quantification: Many estimates of the prevalence of pelvic organ prolapse (POP) define prolapse based on symptoms alone or on a nonvalidated genital examination. There are a number of classification systems (Porges 1963; Baden and

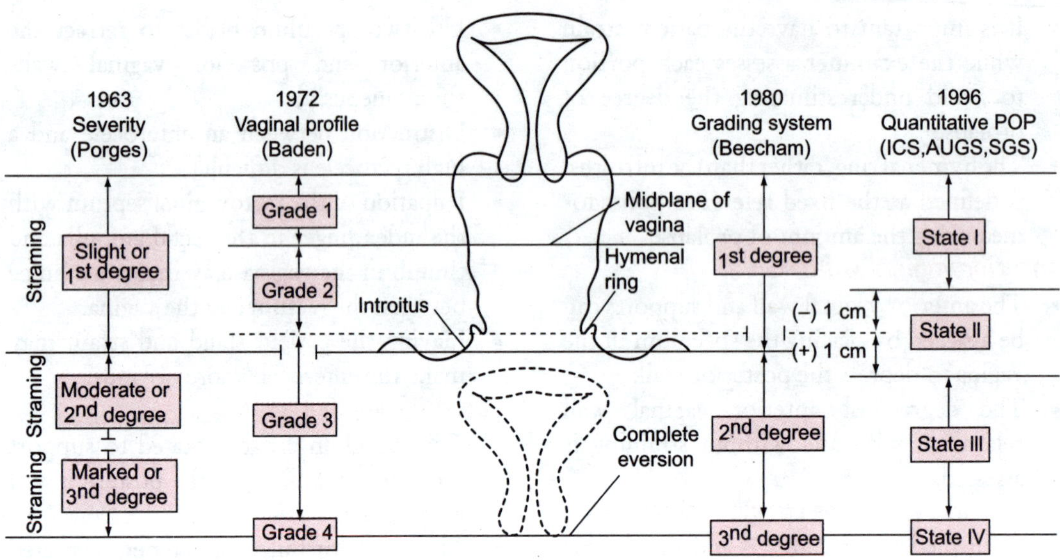

FIGURE 10.3: CLINICAL CLASSIFICATION OF PELVIC ORGAN PROLAPSE

Walker 1972; Beecham 1980). Until recently, none of the systems had been validated. The systems rely on a detailed pelvic examination and a presumptive diagnosis of the organ that has prolapsed (for example, cystocele, enterocele or rectocele) (Fig. 10.3).

Because there was a lack of an objective, universally accepted, and validated system for describing pelvic organ support, the International Continence Society (ICS) established an international, multidisciplinary terminology standardisation committee for prolapse in 1993 (Bump et al 1996).

The ICS recommends the use of the Pelvic Organ Prolapse Quantification (POPQ) scale. Based on this quantification system, new staging for POP was devised. The POPQ system uses the hymenal ring as the principal reference point (Figs 10.4, 10.5). The hymen was selected as the reference point (rather than the introitus used in the older classification systems), because it is more precisely identified. The POPQ system assigns negative numbers (in centimeters) to structures that have not prolapsed beyond the hymen and positive numbers to structures that protrude, with the plane of the hymen defined as zero (Fig. 10.6). The terminology avoids assigning a specific label, such as cystocele or rectocele, to the

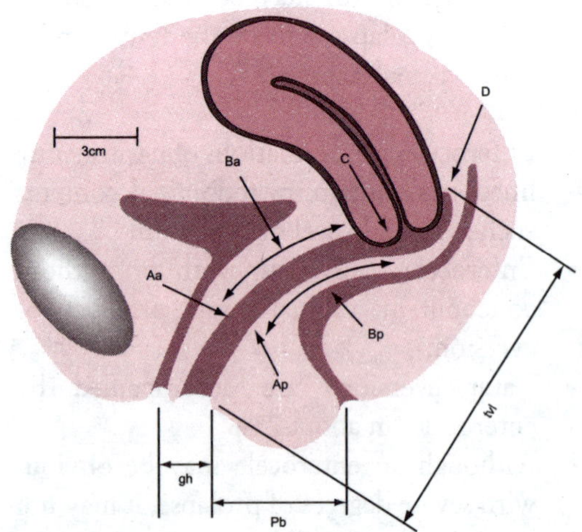

Three reference points anteriorly (Aa, Ba, and C)
Three reference points posteriorly (Ap, Bp, and D)

FIGURE 10.4: POP Q REFERENCE POINTS

Table 10.2: Stages of prolapse

Stage 0	No prolapse is demonstrated.
Stage I	The most distal portion of the prolapse is more than 1 cm above the level of the hymen.
Stage II	The most distal portion of the prolapse is 1 cm or less proximal or distal to the hymenal plane.
Stage III	The most distal portion of the prolapse protrudes more than 1 cm below the hymen but protrudes no farther than 2 cm less than the total vaginal length (that is, not all of the vagina has prolapsed).
Stage IV	Vaginal eversion is essentially complete.

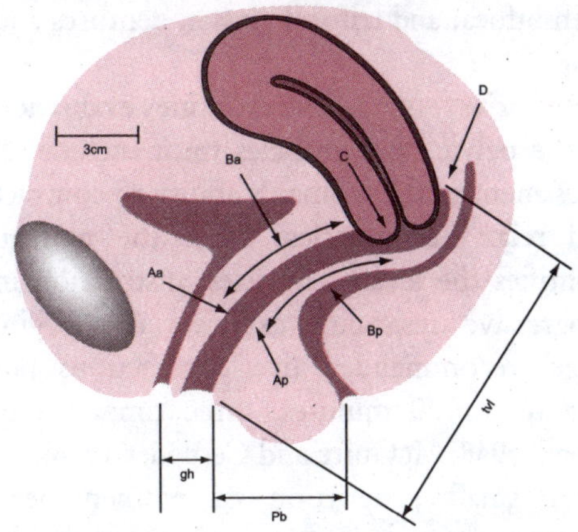

The vaginal length at rest, the genital hiatus (gh) from the middle of the urethral meatus to the posterior hymenal ring, the perineal body (Pb) from the posterior aspect of the genital hiatus to the midanal opening.
(Tvl) total vaginal length

Figure 10.5: POP Q Measurements

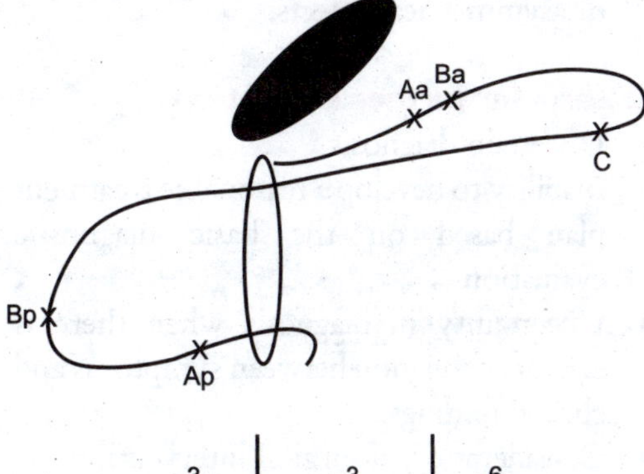

–3 Aa	–3 Ba	–6 C
4.5 gh	1 pb	8 tvl
Ap +2	Bp +5	–

Figure 10.6: POP Q Numbering

prolapsing part of the vagina, acknowledging that the actual organ(s) above the prolapse frequently cannot be determined on physical examination (Bump et al 1996; Theofrastous and Swift 1998).

Once the measurements are taken, the subjects are assigned to ordinal stages (Bump et al 1996) (Fig. 10.7) (Table 10.2).

Disadvantages of POP Q (Barber et al 2000; Auwad et al 2004):

- The system is more difficult to learn than the traditional staging, and overall

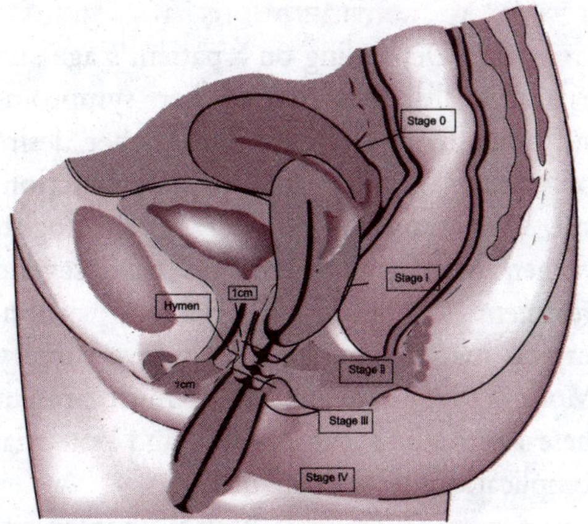

Figure 10.7: POP Q staging

adoption by specialists is about 40%.

- Patient position also affects reproducibility.
- The measurements are taken with the patient in the dorsal lithotomy position, and the degree of prolapse is assessed with patient straining.
- Prolapse may be more severe with the table raised at the head to a 45° angle.
- The system also does not identify unilateral or asymmetrical defects.

Criteria for further evaluation:

- Uncertain diagnosis
- Inability to develop a reasonable treatment plan based on the basic diagnostic evaluation
- Uncertainty in diagnosis when there is lack of correlation between symptoms and clinical findings
- Consideration of surgical intervention
- Hematuria without infection
- Abnormal postvoid residual urine
- A neurologic condition, such as multiple sclerosis and spinal cord lesions or injury.

Further evaluation may warrant urodynamics, cystoscopy, manometry and imaging.

Treatment considerations for genital prolapse: Depending on a patient's age and general health, severity of her symptoms and other medical complications, her desire for future fertility and coital function, and the training of her gynecologist, women with genital prolapse have several treatment options—observation, non-surgical management and corrective surgery (Morley 1996). The physician must present these alternatives, the benefits and potential complications to the patient.

Conservative management: Not all women are willing to have surgery; in some, a medical condition may prevent surgery, if only temporarily. In addition, genital prolapse only occasionally threatens life; an evisceration, for instance, requires prompt intervention. Moreover, pelvic organ prolapse in the majority of cases can be reduced. Thus, some women may defer surgery and may be more willing to accept a pessary. They may see the pessary as another accessory of older age, along with bifocal and trifocal glasses, dentures and canes.

Kegel Exercises: The routine evaluation of the pelvic floor muscles must include an assessment of the woman's ability to contract and relax her muscles. Once the woman identifies the levator muscles, instruction in progressive resistance exercises can begin. Kegel recommended five contractions per minute for 20 minutes, three times a day (Kegel 1948; McGuire and Cespedes 1996).

A small proportion of women need electrode stimulation and visual feedback. Others have improved by mechanical means, with the use of weighted vaginal cones.

Pessary: Genital prolapse and its therapy have been noted since the beginning of recorded history.

Hippocrates (400 BC) recommended several techniques, including a pessary consisting of half a pomegranate soaked in wine. Pessary materials have improved throughout the centuries, with most recent models manufactured from rubber, clear plastic, soft plastic with internal mouldable steel reinforcements, and silicone (Zeitlin and Lebherz 1992).

Currently most pessaries are made of silicone as it is considered non-allergenic, does not absorb odours or secretions, is resistant to repeat cleansing and autoclaving, and is soft and pliable. Latex pessaries have fallen out of favour because the general population has allergic reactions that can range from mild skin irritation to asthma and anaphylaxis (Slater 1994).

Pessary insertion: A pelvic examination determines the vaginal width. After measurement, reduce the prolapsed organs (a vaginal cream is often used). Then lubricate the vagina and pessary. Guide the pessary so that its wider diameter enters the vagina anteroposteriorly towards the vaginal vault. Sweep the index finger around the pessary and vaginal wall.

- The patient must feel comfortable when sitting, standing, squatting, bearing down and walking.
- When properly fitted, the patient does not feel the pessary and the pessary does not descend into the introitus during the Valsalva maneuver.
- A pessary may not be appropriate for women with genital anatomic anomalies, a space-occupying lesion or severe infection.

Pessary benefits: A pessary can facilitate preoperative healing of vaginal and cervical ulcers and improve mucosal hypertrophy, which commonly occurs in cases of genital prolapse (Clemons et al 2004).

Thus, a pessary can serve as a temporary measure while other conditions improve and the patient is ready for surgery. The Smith-Hodge vaginal pessary (size 2 and 3) can increase urethral functional length and urethral closure pressure. The pessary restored continence by stabilisation of the urethra and urethrovesical junction, allowing proper pressure transmission to the urethra. A trial of a pessary may assist in identifying women with genuine stress incontinence (Harris and Bent 1990; Morley 1996). The trial pessary may uncover stress incontinence, which will require evaluation before anatomic repair.

Complications associated with the pessary: A pessary that is too small will be expelled. Tight-fitting pessaries cause irritation, ulceration, bleeding and pain. Pessaries should be removed periodically for cleaning and evaluation of the genital mucosa (Morley 1996). As women with genital prolapse may also show estrogen deficiency, an estrogen vaginal cream is usually applied daily at the beginning. Later, and according to the condition of the genital mucosa, these applications are reduced to once or twice a week. Several complications have been associated with inadequate follow-up. Periodic care prevents such complications as leucorrhea, vaginitis, forgotten or incarcerated pessaries and vaginal cancer (Poma 1981). The literature describes vesico-vaginal fistula, bilateral hydronephrosis and sepsis, and even small bowel incarceration.

SURGICAL MANAGEMENT OF UTEROVAGINAL PROLAPSE

Surgical therapy has long been the mainstay of treatment. Surgical treatments in the treatment of POP can be best summarised through a compartmental approach to the pelvic floor. Pelvic floor prolapse may occur in the anterior, posterior and apical portions of the vagina. Cystoceles, urethroceles, predominate in the anterior aspect of the vagina.

Rectoceles predominate in the posterior portion of the vaginal vault. Uterine descensus and enteroceles predominate in the apical portion of the vaginal vault.

Aims of Surgery

- **Anatomic Objectives:** To restore normal anatomic positioning and structure.
- **Physiologic Objectives:** To restore normal function of pelvic floor (micturition, defecation, fecal and urinary continence and intercourse).

- **Patient Objectives:** To alleviate symptoms and prevent de novo problems.

Anterior compartment defects: Repair of anterior vaginal wall prolapse remains one of the most challenging components of pelvic floor reconstruction in terms of initial success and ultimate durability.

Anterior colporrhaphy/Kelly plication: Anterior colporrhaphy is recommended for midline defects and has been the traditional choice for the past century. The principle of the procedure is to plicate the layers of vaginal muscularis and adventitia that overlie the bladder (Nichols 1993b).

Method

1. A transverse incision is made in the vaginal mucosa near the apex. An additional clamp is placed below the external urethral meatus. If there is loss of the urethrovesical angle, the clamp is placed approximately 1 cm below the external urethral meatus, otherwise the angle is left undisturbed and the clamp placed below the urethrovesical angle.
2. Using Metzenbaum scissors and toothed pickups, the vaginal epithelium, including the muscularis, is separated in the midline to the level of the anterior clamp. The vagina is incised vertically in the midline.
3. Allis clamps (also known as Allis forceps) are then placed along the cut edge. The vaginal muscularis (pubocervical fascia) is carefully dissected from the vaginal epithelium (Fig. 10.8). The surgeon should ensure that the vaginal muscularis is not removed from the underlying detrusor muscle. It is important to be in the correct dissection plane for two reasons—first, bleeding tends to occur if the dissection is in the adventitial layer as described in the anatomical section and second, the aim is

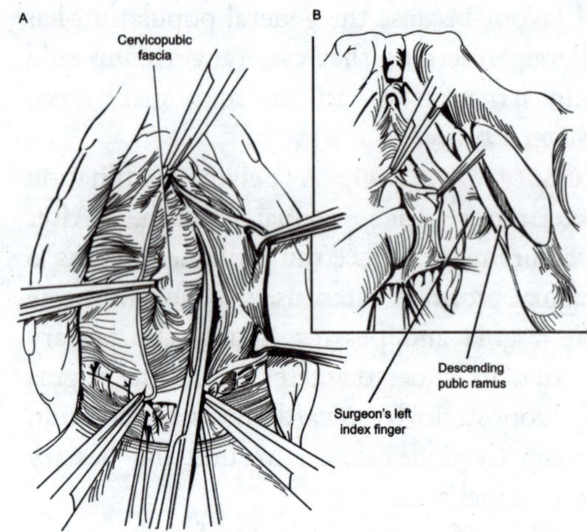

FIGURE 10.8: ANTERIOR REPAIR

to harvest as much vaginal muscularis as possible, as this forms the basis of the repair.

4. The vaginal muscularis is plicated using 2-0 absorbable suture material in an interrupted fashion. If there is loss of the urethrovesical angle, a plicating suture at the urethrovesical junction is placed to restore anatomy (the Kelly plication) (Fig. 10.9).
5. The redundant vaginal wall is then resected and the vaginal edges re-opposed using 2-0 absorbable suture in an interrupted

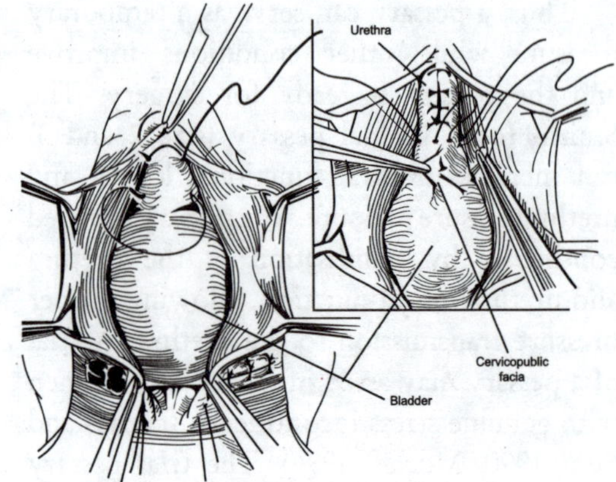

FIGURE 10.9: ANTERIOR REPAIR—FASCIAL BUTTRESSING

fashion, being careful to avoid the urethra and yet, at the same time, to pick up underlying vaginal muscularis to close the dead space (Fig. 10.10).

Key issues (Maher and Baessler 2006)

- Avoid separating vaginal muscularis from the bladder detrusor muscle. Leaving more tissue on the bladder and dissecting away only a thin layer of mucosa will help ensure that a strong support is left for the plication.
- Removing too much mucosa can lead to pain and development of paravaginal defects. Once the muscularis is plicated, trim off redundant mucosa so that the edges meet in the midline without tension.
- Closing the dead space between the mucosa and vaginal muscularis will help prevent development of a hematoma. When the mucosa is reapproximated, also incorporate a small amount of underlying tissue.

Paravaginal repair

Abdominal Approach

1. The retropubic space is entered and the bladder and vagina pulled medially to reveal the lateral defect due to avulsion of the vagina from the arcus tendineus fasciae pelvis.
2. The surgeon's non-dominant hand is placed in the vagina and elevates the antero-lateral vaginal sulcus and retracts the bladder medially.
3. A non-absorbable monofilament suture is placed through the full thickness of the vagina and then into the obturator internus fascia or arcus tendineus fasciae pelvis, 1–2 cm anterior to the ischial spine and 3–4 cm below the obturator canal. Subsequent sutures are placed 1 cm apart towards the pubic ramus. The obturator canal limits the distal aspect of the repair.

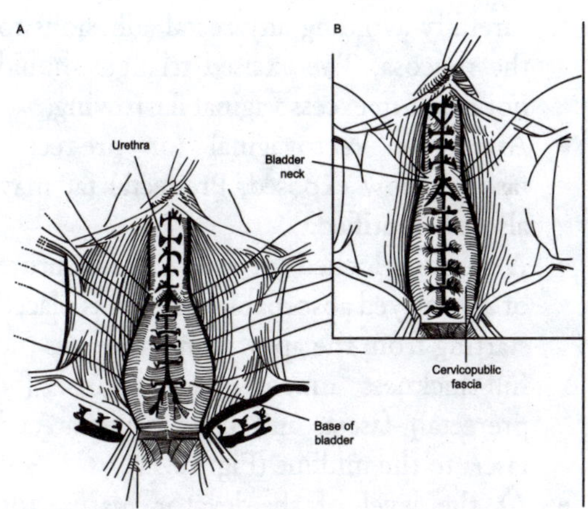

Figure 10.10: Anterior repair

Key issues (Richardson 1992)

- Dissection planes can be difficult in the presence of prior surgery in the retropubic space.
- The procedure can be combined with a modified Burch colposuspension in the presence of urodynamic stress incontinence.
- The disadvantages of the operation are related to the risks of complications and recovery linked to laparotomy.
- This is the most anatomical correction of the anterior vaginal wall defect.

The vaginal approach (Shull and Baden 1989)

1. The bladder neck and base are marked with sutures in the vaginal epithelium.
2. The vaginal epithelium is sharply dissected off the vaginal muscularis in a similar manner to anterior colporrhaphy. The dissection extends laterally to the pelvic side wall from behind the pubic ramus to the ischial spine.
3. If needed, a midline plication of the vaginal muscularis is performed.

4. Careful examination laterally confirms the paravaginal defect by revealing retropubic fat. Blunt finger dissection is used to gain complete access to the retropubic space.
5. A non-absorbable monofilament suture is placed in the white line, 1 cm proximal to the ischial spine, and a series of 4–6 sutures is placed along the arcus tendineus towards the inner aspect of the symphysis .
6. A three-point closure is then performed, incorporating the arcus tendineus, the lateral edge of the vaginal muscularis and the vaginal epithelium. The sutures are tied sequentially.
7. Vaginal tissue is not trimmed until all stitches are tied. After trimming, the anterior vagina is closed in a similar manner as for anterior colporrhaphy.

Key Issues (Mallipeddi et al 2001)

- The vaginal approach offers the benefit of avoiding laparotomy.
- The surgical challenge of identifying vaginal anatomy and reaching a level of support that may be beyond reach should be carefully weighed against the hurdles of laparotomy. This decision will vary, based on the surgeon and the woman's characteristics.
- Significant blood loss in the retropubic space is a real and serious complication. Cases of ureteral obstruction have been reported.

Posterior Compartment Defects: The aims of traditional posterior colporrhaphy for the repair of rectocele are to a) plicate the prerectal and pararectal fascia in the midline, b) narrow the posterior aspect of the levator hiatus with levator plication, and c) repair the perineal body (perineorrhaphy) (Raz et al 1998; Nichols 1993d). The repair effectively narrows the vaginal calibre.

Posterior Colporrhaphy and Perineorrhaphy

- With the patient in lithotomy position, a povidone iodine-soaked sponge is placed into the rectum which is isolated from the operative field.
- A Foley catheter is placed into the bladder, which is retracted upward with a Deaver retractor.
- Two Allis clamps are placed at a distance on each side of the introitus that, when brought together, form a new vaginal introitus that accommodates two to three fingers.
- A transverse incision is made to excise the skin between the two Allis clamps.
- The Allis clamps can be reapplied to the edge of the vaginal mucosa on the rectocele.
- The apex of the rectocele is marked.
- Saline solution is infiltrated bilaterally from the Allis clamps to the apex, and Metzenbaum scissors are inserted into a plane underneath the mucosa.
- The scissors are advanced and spread toward the apex while hugging the mucosa to avoid rectal injury
- The mucosa is incised with the scissors, and the triangular flap is excised while carefully avoiding any rectal adhesions to the mucosa. The excised triangle should not result in excess vaginal narrowing.
- Attenuated rectovaginal (or pre-rectal) fascia is now exposed. Pre-rectal fat may also be identified.
- A running locked (or interrupted) suture of 2-0 delayed absorbable material is placed starting from the apex. It incorporates the full-thickness mucosa, rectovaginal (or prerectal) fascia, and bites of pararectal fascia to the midline (Fig. 10.11).
- At the level of the levator hiatus, the

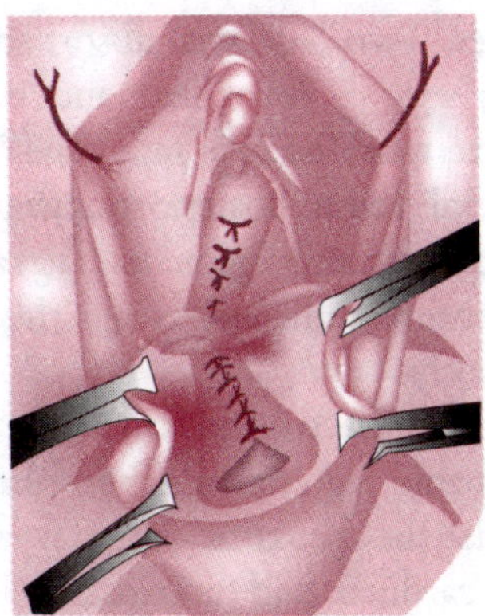

Figure 10.11: Posterior repair

running suture can include the levator fascia or muscles, or two or three interrupted sutures can be used to approximate the muscles. The running suture is continued to the distal end.

- The vaginal axis should be restored with a smooth posterior contour.
- The perineal body can be reconstructed (perineorrhaphy) when there is separation of the perineal muscles. The perineal body is reconstituted by placing interrupted U-shaped stitches to approximate the superficial and deep perineal muscles toward the midline (Fig. 10.12).
- The skin is approximated with subcuticular stitches. Care should be taken to avoid closing the introitus too tightly (Fig. 10.13).

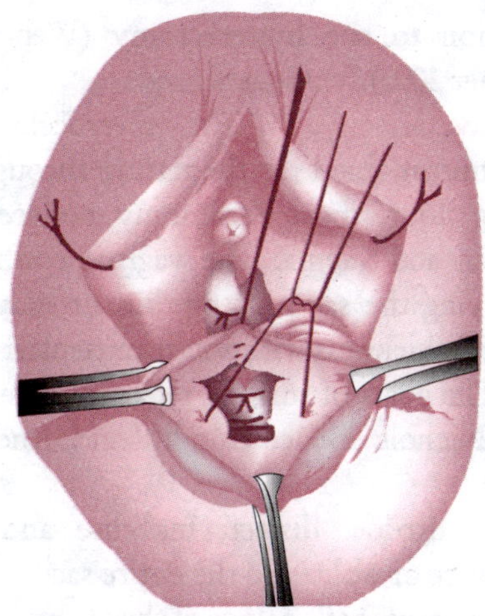

Figure 10.12: Posterior repair—fascial buttressing

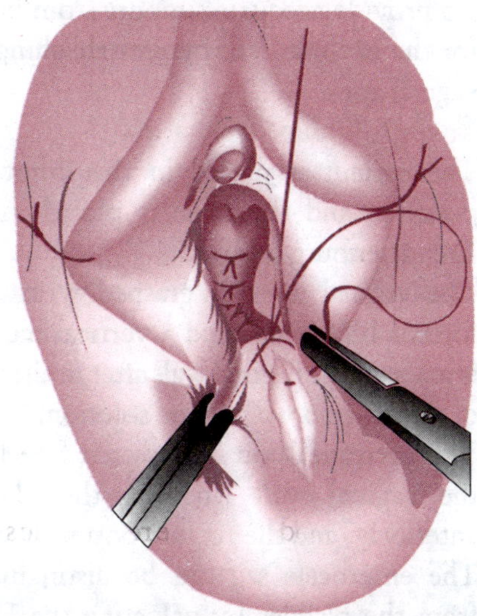

Figure 10.13: Perineoraphe

Middle compartment defects (Apical prolapse and enterocoele): Apical prolapse may include the uterus with or without enterocele and vaginal vault prolapse usually with enterocele. The standard treatment for symptomatic uterine prolapse is hysterectomy with procedure(s) to support the vaginal apex, address enterocele when indicated, repair coexisting anterior and posterior prolapse and perform anti-incontinence procedures as needed (Richardson 1995). However, there is a lack of evidence suggesting that hysterectomy improves the outcome of prolapse surgery. Descent of the uterus is thought to be a result, not a cause of prolapse (Brubaker et al 2005). When hysterectomy is performed for prolapse, hysterectomy alone, or with colporrhaphy, is insufficient; a specific vault suspension procedure must be performed in addition to the hysterectomy (Weber and Ritcher 2005).

Enterocele repairs: An enterocele is a peritoneum-lined sac herniating through the pelvic floor, most commonly between the rectum and vagina. The vaginal epithelium overlying the sac may be thin or may have normal thickness with intact muscularis

The goals of surgical repair of enterocele are (Nichols 1993c; Cundiff and Anderson 1998):

1. To expose, dissect, mobilise and then excise or obliterate the entire sac
2. To occlude the orifice of the sac by ligation as high as possible
3. To perform all indicated repairs
4. To provide adequate support from below for the occluded sac by reestablishing the vaginal apex

Surgical procedure:

- The patient is placed in the lithotomy position, and the table is placed in the Trendelenburg position.
- The vaginal apex is grasped with Allis forceps bilaterally, and a vertical incision is made in the vaginal wall after infiltration of the mucosa with saline solution.
- The peritoneal sac is dissected free from the vaginal wall laterally, the bladder anteriorly, and the rectum posteriorly.
- The enterocele sac can be distinguished from the bladder by palpating the Foley balloon or by a metal sound within the collapsed bladder, by the presence of preperitoneal fat, and by the appearance of peritoneal contents within the sac.
- The sac is opened in the midline, and the contents are packed into the peritoneal cavity. A small moist laparotomy sponge is inserted to protect the bowel.
- A Deaver retractor is used to expose the areas in which to put the culdoplasty stitches. Two 0 delayed absorbable purse-string sutures (proximal and distal) are placed that incorporate the anterior prerectal fascia posteriorly, the cardinal and uterosacral ligaments laterally, and the peritoneum overlying the bladder anteriorly.
- Two McCall sutures of No. 1 delayed absorbable material are then placed from outside the proximal vaginal wall into both cardinal and uterosacral ligaments through the peritoneal sac and back out of the vaginal wall
- The proximal and distal purse-string sutures are then tied to obliterate the cul-de-sac and elevate the peritoneum. The peritoneal sac is ligated at the base and may be excised.
- To facilitate repair of other defects, the McCall sutures are tied after the anterior wall and upper posterior wall are repaired.
- Excess vaginal wall is excised, and the incision is closed with continuous 2-0 delayed absorbable sutures.

Apical Suspension Procedures: See section on vaginal vault prolapse

Role of mesh: "Surgical results for cystocoele repair have been consistently poor for 80 years irrespective of operator skill or precise technique" (Freeman at the *IUGA Conference 2005, unpublished*).

Despite best practices, treatment failures for surgical repairs remain unacceptably high.

- 29% second surgery and 11% third surgery
- Overall failure 50% (Olson et al 1997)
- Objective failure rate of 60% within 2 years (Weber et al; AJOG 2001) (RCT at Cleveland Clinic)

In an attempt to improve the outcomes of incontinence and prolapse surgery, surgeons have used a large variety of synthetic or biologic materials. Using the hernia analogy, the focus shifted to the use of a synthetic mesh. This was an attempt deriving from the general surgeons' success in hernia repairs.

The mesh should be (Alexander et al 1967):

- Mechanically strong
- Chemically inert
- Non-carcinogenic
- Should not cause overwhelming inflammation
- Resistant to infection
- Available in convenient and affordable format for clinical use

The material should be inert, of good mechanical strength, knitted form, having higher bacterial adherence to multifilament material, of relevance when working in vagina as it is a potentially contaminated area. The filament diameter should be the smallest possible.

Pore size (Alexander et al 1967)

- Adequate to allow for migration and in-growth of fibroblasts, WBC, vascularised tissue
- Macrophages can be 50 microns, fibroblasts 15 microns
- Bacteria less than 1 micron

Rigidity

- Bend of material under its own weight
- Biomechanical calculation
- Mesh in vagina should be ideally less rigid

Total mesh content (Alexander et al 1967; Deffieux et al 2007)

- The lesser the foreign material, the better host acceptance and better tissue incorporation.
- Thinner mesh with less material gives a better result.

Ideal Mesh

The ideal mesh is of

- Small diameter, lightweight
- Polypropylene
- Filament type: monofilament
- Pore size : macroporous
- Total mesh content: thinner mesh with less material per given area

Significant complications have been associated with vaginal mesh, including (Alexander et al 1967; Flood et al 1998; Milani et al 2005):

- Infection and sinus tract formation: There is little in the literature on infection rates per se, but there is a four-fold increase in mesh erosion or infection when mesh is used vaginally compared with abdominally.
- Tape erosion: Rates of 20%–25% have been reported, with 1.4%–2% of all patients requiring mesh excision.
- Dyspareunia
- 'Hispareunia': A new term coined for the symptom of painful sexual intercourse experienced by the male partner, caused by the mesh fibres.

There is insufficient evidence, at present, to recommend the use of permanent meshes for genital prolapse. It may be wise to restrict the use of vaginally applied mesh to a tertiary referral setting until a larger evidence base is available.

Any surgeon deciding on the appropriate procedure should select the operation most appropriate to the needs of the woman and pay attention to their own success and failure rates.

VAGINAL VAULT PROLAPSE

Vaginal vault prolapse occurs when organs of the vagina descend from their normal position towards or through the vaginal introitus. This occurs by herniation through areas of weakness or breakage in the endopelvic fascia that covers the vagina.

The International Continence Society defines post-hysterectomy (apical) vaginal prolapse as descent of the vaginal cuff scar below a point that is 2 cm less than the total vaginal length above the plane of the hymen (Abrams et al 2002). The vaginal cuff scar corresponds to point C on the POPQ grid (Bump et al 1996).

Vaginal vault prolapse may occur on its own or together with a cystocele (when the bladder sags into the vagina), rectocele (when the front wall of the rectum bulges into the lower wall of the vagina) or enterocele (when the intestine bulges into the upper wall of the vagina).

Assessment: Assessment of the woman should be comprehensive and objective, addressing quality of life, looking for all pelvic floor defects and should be based on standard tools (Bump et al 1996).

All pelvic floor defects should be identified to enable surgical repair of significant and potential defects. Women with post-hysterectomy vaginal vault prolapse often have associated anterior or posterior vaginal wall prolapse. Failure to address such defects at the same time will lead to women presenting with recurrent prolapse from those defects left without support (indirect recurrence) (Harris and Bent 1990; Cundiff et al 1997).

Assessing occult stress incontinence of urine may be made with a full bladder after reducing the prolapse with a pessary or sponge holder (Harris and Bent 1990).

Conservative management: The role of conservative measures for post-hysterectomy vaginal vault prolapse is unclear (Hagen et al 2006). Conservative measures include pelvic-floor exercises (Kegel 1948) and different types of pessaries, of which ring and shelf are the most commonly used. These measures have been assessed for prolapse in general, rather than post-hysterectomy vaginal vault prolapse. They are therefore reserved for physically frail women, those considered unfit for surgery or when surgery is declined. Local estrogen can be used to improve atrophic changes, though there is no evidence to judge their value in relation to the frequency of pessary change (Cutner and Elneil 2004; Hagen et al 2006).

Surgical Procedures for Vaginal Vault Prolapse

Sacrospinous Ligament Fixation: (Nichols 1997)

- A surgical head lamp is strongly recommended for this procedure. A longitudinal incision is made in the vaginal mucosa extending to the posterior wall.
- The surgeon then palpates the ischial spine, with the index finger in the rectovaginal space, and traces the ligament that runs posteriorly to the hollow of the sacrum. (It is easier for a right-handed surgeon to use the right sacrospinous ligament.)
- The ligament must be exposed through a window in the soft tissue to allow suture placement.
- The rectal pillar, or lateral connective tissue between the rectum and the vagina, is penetrated either bluntly or with Mayo scissors to enter the pararectal space.
- The sacrospinous ligament/coccygeus muscle is palpated, and the window into the pararectal space is gently enlarged. Because the ligament is covered by the coccygeus muscle it is not visible.
- Flat long-blade retractors are placed

to retract the peritoneum and bladder upward and the rectum medially, and a shorter retractor may compress the distal portion of the pelvic diaphragm laterally.

- The sutures are placed 1.5 to 3 cm medial to the ischial spine, to avoid injury to the pudendal nerves and vessels, and through the substance of the ligament. The ligament can be grasped with a long Allis or Babcock clamp, and/or the sutures can be placed directly with a long needle driver or Deschamps ligature carrier and retrieved with a nerve hook (Fig. 10.14).
- Two No. 1 or No. 2 delayed absorbable sutures are placed. A gentle tug on the ligature carrier or on the suture should move the patient a little and confirm proper placement in the ligament.
- One end of each suture is then attached to the undersurface of the posterior vaginal wall at the apical area.
- If a posterior colporrhaphy is to be done, the suspension sutures are tied when the colporrhaphy closure reaches the midpoint of the vagina. The vaginal apex is then tied firmly to the ligament with no intervening bridge of suture material (Fig. 10.15).

Uterosacral ligament suspension: Suspension of the vaginal vault to the uterosacral ligaments is another approach and is based on McCall's original description that uses the uterosacrals as a support for the vaginal vault. It can be used prophylactically at hysterectomy or for treatment of vault prolapse. Its main advantages are a normal resultant vaginal axis and avoidance of suturing near neural or vascular structures.

Iliococcygeus suspension: The procedure involves an extraperitoneal exposure through a midline posterior incision. One or two suspension sutures are placed bilaterally into the fascia of the iliococcygeus muscle just anterior to the ischial spines and then attached to the vault. A potential benefit is the absence of critical structures in the area. Although the

FIGURE 10.14: IDENTIFYING THE SACROSPINOUS LIGAMENT

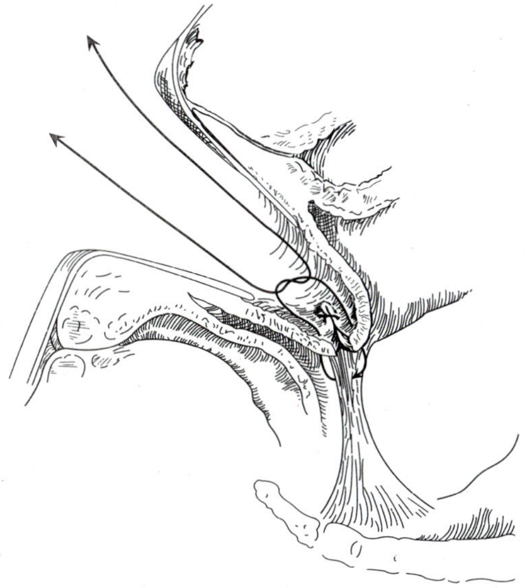

FIGURE 10.15: SACROSPINOUS LIGAMENT SUSPENSION

Table 10.3: Summary of principal risks and benefits of vaginal apical repairs (Weber and Richter 2005)		
Procedure	***Major Risks***	***Major Benefits***
Sacrospinous ligament fixation	Postoperative anterior prolapse; injury to pudendal and inferior gluteal arteries and pudendal and sciatic nerves; ligament may be atrophied in elderly; more difficult to teach and learn	No ureteral injury; rectal injury rare
Uterosacral ligament suspension	Entry into peritoneum; may be adhesions; possible bowel and ureteral injuries; ligaments may not be apparent or usable	Normal vaginal supports; resultant vaginal axis may be most physiologic
Iliococcygeus suspension	Possible shortened vagina; fewest reported cases	No vital structures nearby

suspension sutures maintain normal vaginal alignment, vaginal shortening may occur because the apex will lie anterior to the ischial spine.

Abdominal sacral colpopexy: The abdominal approach is indicated after failed vaginal repair, when concomitant abdominal surgery is required, or when the surgeon is unfamiliar with the vaginal approach.

The procedure involves attaching the vaginal vault to the sacrum using autologous, allograft or synthetic material to bridge the gap (Fig. 10.16). The suspension mesh is attached to the upper sacrum and promontory at the S1-S2 level, where blood vessels are more easily visualised and avoided

Abdominal sacrocolpopexy and sacrospinous fixation: Both these procedures have stood the test of time and are accepted as the standard of surgical practice for vaginal vault prolapse.

The following criteria should be considered when helping women choose between the two procedures. For a choice to be made, it is important that the surgeon is experienced in both procedures and is able to choose between them before surgery.

- Vaginal sacrospinous fixation requires adequate vaginal length and vault width to enable reaching the sacrospinous ligament (Brubaker et al 2005).
- Co-existent anterior and/or posterior vaginal wall prolapse can easily be managed by anterior and/or posterior repair while performing vaginal sacrospinous fixation. A separate vaginal procedure will be required for abdominal sacrocolpopexy.
- Vaginal sacrospinous fixation is more suitable for physically frail women,

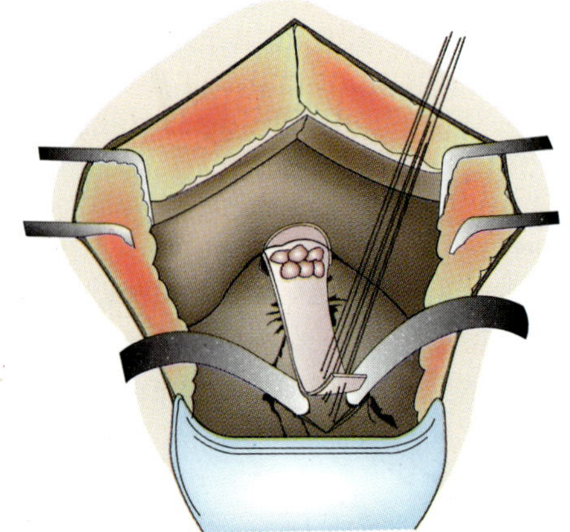

The graft has been attached to the vaginal apex. The proximal end of the graft will be attached to the sacral promontory.

Figure 10.16: Abdominal sacral colpopexy

because of the morbidity associated with abdominal surgery (Maher et al 2004; Brubaker et al 2005)

- Abdominal sacrocolpopexy can be carried out if women require laparotomy for other indication(s).
- Abdominal sacrocolpopexy is more suitable for sexually active women, as sacrospinous fixation is associated with exaggerated retroversion of the vagina, leading to a less physiological axis.
- Vaginal length is also well maintained after sacrocolpopexy, whereas sacrospinous fixation can cause vaginal narrowing and/ or shortening, especially when carried out alongside repair of anterior and/or posterior vaginal wall defects, leading to dyspareunia (Benson et al 1996; Brubaker et al 2005).
- **Complications** are rare but include (Benson et al 1996; Maher et al 2004; Brubaker et al 2005):

Sacrocolpopexy: hemorrhage requiring blood transfusion, bladder injury, incisional hernia, mesh rejection, wound infection

Sacrospinous fixation: hemorrhage requiring blood transfusion, bladder injury, rectovaginal hematoma, vaginal pain.

Abdominal sacrocolpopexy was associated with significantly longer operating time, slower return to normal activity and higher cost. There was no significant difference in terms of objective and subjective success, urinary, bowel or sexual dysfunction or quality of life. Given the available evidence, it is difficult to recommend one procedure over the other.

Vaginal wall repair: Anterior and posterior repair along with obliteration of the enterocele sac are inadequate for post-hysterectomy vaginal vault prolapse (Tooz-Hobson et al 1998).

The standard repair operation does not support the vaginal vault and risks vaginal narrowing and shortening, and thus dyspareunia, especially when posterior repair is carried out.

Colpocleisis: Colpocleisis entails closure of the vagina, which is suitable for frail women who do not want to retain sexual function. Different techniques have been described, including vaginectomy, pursestring closure of the vagina, colpocleisis after performing standard anterior and posterior vaginal wall repair (DeLancey and Morely 1997), purse-string closure of enterocele followed by approximation of pervesical and rectovaginal fascia and high levator plication (von Pechmann et al 2003) and LeFort colpocleisis, where a bridge of tissue is created between the anterior and posterior vaginal wall, to stop vault prolapse from protruding. It has a short operating time and low incidence of complications.

It is a safe and effective procedure that can be considered for those women who do not wish to retain sexual function (DeLancey and Morely 1997; von Pechmann et al 2003).

Laparoscopic procedures: These procedures involve a high level of expertise and longer operation times. Laparoscopic sacrocolpopexy appears to be as effective as open sacrocolpopexy. The ureters are particularly at risk during laparoscopic uterosacral ligament suspension. There is insufficient evidence to judge the value of other laparoscopic techniques.

Mesh reconstruction: A number of techniques are being introduced, whereby a sheet of synthetic mesh material is fixed at a number of points to act as a new pelvic floor. Complications, including mesh erosion and infection, as well as long-term effectiveness are specific areas of concern with these new techniques. There is insufficient evidence to judge the safety and effectiveness of total mesh reconstruction.

Prevention of post hysterectomy prolapse

1. McCall culdoplasty at the time of vaginal hysterectomy is a recommended measure to prevent enterocele formation. The technique involves approximating the uterosacral ligaments using continuous sutures, so as to obliterate the peritoneum of the posterior cul-de-sac as high as possible (McCall 1957). A similar approach has been described for abdominal hysterectomy.
2. Suturing the cardinal and uterosacral ligaments to the vaginal cuff at the time of hysterectomy is a recommended measure to avoid vault prolapse. Attaching the uterosacral and cardinal ligaments to the vaginal cuff and high circumferential obliteration of the pouch of Douglas has been suggested to prevent vault prolapse and enterocele formation.
3. Sacrospinous fixation at the time of vaginal hysterectomy is recommended when the vault descends to the introitus during closure. Prophylactic sacrospinous fixation has been suggested at the time of vaginal hysterectomy for marked uterovaginal prolapse, when the vault (point C on the POPQ system) could be pulled to the introitus at the end of anterior vaginal wall closure, which is a selected subgroup of those undergoing vaginal hysterectomy (Cruikshank and Cox 1990; Colombo and Milani 1998).

References

Abrams P, L Cardozo, M Fall, D Griffiths, P Rosier, U Ulmsten, et al. 2002. Standardisation Sub-Committee of the International Continence Society. The standardisation of terminology of lower urinary tract function: Report from the standardization sub-committee of the International Continence Society. *Neurourol Urodyn* 21:167–168.

Alexander JW, JZ Kaplan, WA Altemeier. 1967. Role of suture materials in the development of wound infection. *Ann Surg* 165:192–199. doi:10.1097/00000658-196702000-00005

Auwad W, RM Freeman, S Swift et al. 2004. Is the pelvic organ prolapse quantification system (POPQ) being used? A survey of members of the International Continence Society (ICS) and the American Urogynecologic Society (AUGS). *Int Urogynecol J Pelvic Floor Dysfunct* 15:324–327.

Baden WF and TA Walker. 1972. Genesis of the vaginal profile: A correlated classification of vaginal relaxation. *Clin Obstet Gynecol* 15:1048–1054.

Barber MD, A Lambers, AG Visco et al. 2000a. Effect of patient position on clinical evaluation of pelvic organ prolapse. *Obstet Gynecol* 96:18–22.

Beecham CT. 1980. Classification of vaginal relaxation. *Am J Obstet Gynecol* 136:957–958.

Benson JT, V Lucente, E McClellan. 1996. Vaginal versus abdominal reconstructive surgery for the treatment of pelvic support defects: A prospective randomized study with long-term outcome evaluation. *Am J Obstet Gynecol* 175:1418–1422.

Brubaker L, Bump R, Fynes MM et al. 2005. Surgery for pelvic organ prolapse. In Abrams P, Cardozo L, Khoury S, Wein A, ed. *Incontinence: 3rd International Consultation*, Plymouth, UK: Health Publications 1371–1401.

Bump RC, A Mattiasson, K Bo et al. 1996. The standardization of terminology of female pelvic organ prolapse and pelvic floor dysfunction. *Am J Obstet Gynecol* 175 ; 10–17

Clemons JL, VC Aguilar, TA Tillinghast et al., 2004. Patient satisfaction and changes in prolapse and urinary symptoms in women who were fitted successfully with a pessary for pelvic organ prolapse. *Am J Obstet Gynecol* 190:1025–1029.

Colombo M and R Milani. 1998. Sacrospinous ligament fixation and modified McCall culdoplasty during vaginal hysterectomy for advanced uterovaginal prolapse. *Am J Obstet Gynecol* 79: 13–20.

Cruikshank SH and DW Cox. 1990. Sacrospinous ligament fixation at the time of transvaginal hysterectomy. *Am J Obstet Gynecol* 162:1611–1619.

Cundiff GW and WA Addison, 1998. Cundiff, Addison: Management of pelvic organ prolapse. *Obstet Gynecol Clin North Am* 25:907–921.viii.

Cundiff GW, RL Harris, K Coates, VH Low, RC Bump, WA Addison. 1997. Abdominal sacral colpoperineopexy: A new approach for correction of posterior compartment descent associated with vaginal vault prolapse. *Am J Obstet Gynecol* 177:1345–1355.

Cutner AS and S Elneil. 2004. The vaginal vault. *Br J Obstet Gynaecol* 111(Suppl 1):79–83.

Deffieux Xde, R Tayrac, C Huel, J Bottero, A Gervaise, K Bonnet et al. 2007. Vaginal mesh erosion after transvaginal repair of cystocele using Gynemesh or Gynemesh-Soft in 138 women: A comparative study. *Int Urogynecol J Pelvic Floor Dysfunct* 18:73–79. doi:10.1007/s0192-005-0041-2

DeLancey JO and GW Morely. 1997. Total colpocleisis for vaginal eversion. *Am J Obstet Gynecol* 176:1228–1235.

Delancey JOL. 1992. Anatomic aspects of vaginal eversion after hysterectomy. *Am J Obstet Gynecol* 166: 1717–1728

DeLancey JOL. 1993. Anatomy and biomechanics of genital prolapse. *Chin Obstet Gynecol* 36: 897–909.

Flood CG, HP Drutz, L Waja. 1998. Anterior colporrhaphy reinforced with Marlex mesh for the treatment of cystoceles. *Int Urogynecol J Pelvic Floor Dysfunct* 9:200–4. doi:10.1007/BF01901604

Graves EJ. 1995. Detailed diagnosis and procedures: National Hospital Discharge survey, 1993: National Centre for Health Statistics. *Vital Health Stast* 13:50–128.

Hagen S, D Stark, C Maher, E Adams. 2006. Conservative management of pelvic organ prolapse in women. *Cochrane Database Syst Rev* 4:CD003882.

Handa VL and TA Harris, DR Ostergard. 1996. Protecting the pelvic floor: Obstetrical management to prevent incontinence and pelvic organ prolapse. *Obstet Gynecol* 88: 470–478.

Harris TA and AE Bent. 1990. Genital prolapse with and without urinary incontinence. *J Reprod Med* 35: 792–798.

Kegel AH. 1948. Progressive resistance exercise in the functional restoration of the perineal muscles. *Am J Obstet Gynecol* 58 : 238–248.

Maher C and K Baessler. 2006. Surgical management of anterior vaginal wall prolapse: An evidence based literature review. *Int Urogynecol J Pelvic Floor Dysfunct* 17:195–201. doi:10.1007/s00192-005-1296-3

Maher CF, AM Qatawneh, PL Dwyer, MP Carey, A Cornish, PJ Schluter. 2004. Abdominal sacral colpopexy or vaginal sacrospinous colpopexy for vaginal vault prolapse: A prospective randomized study. *Am J Obstet Gynecol* 190:20–26.

Mallipeddi PK, AC Steele, N Kohli, MM Karram. 2001. Anatomic and functional outcome of vaginal paravaginal repair in the correction of anterior vaginal wall prolapse. *Int Urogynecol J Pelvic Floor Dysfunct* 12:83–88.doi:10.1007/s001920170070

Mant J, R Painter, M Vessey. 1997. Epidemilology of genital prolapse: Observations from the Oxford Family Planning Association study. *Br J Obstet Gynecol* 104 : 579–585

McCall ML. 1957. Posterior culdoplasty: Surgical correction of enterocele during vaginal hysterectomy. A preliminary report. *Obstet Gynecol* 10:595–602.

McGuire EJ and RD Cespedes. 1996. Proper diagnosis: A must before surgery for stress incontinence. *J Endourol* 10 : 201–205.

Milani R, S Salvatore, M Soligo, P Pifarotti, M Meschia, M Cortese. 2005. Functional and anatomical outcome of anterior and posterior vaginal prolapse repair with prolene. *BJOG*;112:107–111. doi:10.1111/j.1471-0528.2004.00332.

Morley GW. 1996. Treatment of uterine and vaginal prolapse. *Clin Obstet Gynecol* 39: 959–696.

Nichols DH. 1993b. Cystocele In Nichols DH, ed. *Gynecologic and Obstetric Surgery*, St. Louis: CV Mosby; 334–362.

Nichols DH. 1993c. Enterocele In Nichols DH, ed. *Gynecologic and Obstetric Surgery*, St. Louis: CV Mosby; 1993:420–430.

Nichols DH. 1993d. Rectocele and perineal defect. In Nichols DH, ed. *Gynecologic and Obstetric Surgery*, St. Louis: CV Mosby 363–385.

Nichols DH. 1997. Nichols: Central compartment defects. In Rock JA, Thompson JD, ed. *Te Linde's Operative Gynecology*, Philadelphia: Lippincott-Raven; 1006–1030.

Poma PA. 1981. Management of incarcerated vaginal pessary. *J Am Geriatrics Soc* 29 : 325–327.

Porges RF. 1963. A practical system of diagnosis and classification of pelvic relaxations. *Surg Gynecol Obstet* 117:769–773.

Raz S, L Stothers, A Chopra et al. 1998. *Vaginal reconstructive surgery for incontinence and prolapse* In PC Walsh, A Retik, ED Vaughan Jr, AJ Wein ed. *Campbell's Urology*, 7th ed. Philadelphia: WB Saunders, 1059–1094.

Richardson AC. 1995. The anatomic defects in rectocele and enterocele. *J Pelvic Surg* 1:214–221.

Richardson AC. 1992. Cystocele. Paravaginal repair. In: *Female Pelvic Floor Disorders: Investigation and Management.* New York: WW Norton & Company;. p. 280–287.

Shull BL and WF Baden. 1989. A six-year experience with paravaginal defect repair for stress urinary incontinence. *Am J Obstet Gynecol* 1989;160:1432–1440.

Slater JE. 1994. Latex allergy. *J Allergy Clin Immunol* 94: 139–149.

Theofrastous JP and SE Swift. 1998. The clinical evaluation of pelvic floor dysfunction. *Obstet Gynecol Clin North Am* 25:783–804.

Toozs-Hobson P, K Boos, L Cardozo. 1998. Management of vaginal vault prolapse. *Br J Obstet Gynaecol* 105:13–17.

von Pechmann WS, M Mutone, J Fyffe, DS Hale. 2003. Total colpocleisis with high levator plication for the treatment of advanced pelvic organ prolapse. *Am J Obstet Gynecol*189:121–126

Weber AM, MD Walter, LR Schover, et al. 1995. Sexual function in women with uterovaginal prolapse and urinary incontinence. *Obstet Gynecol* 85: 483– 487.

Weber AM and HE Richter. 2005. Pelvic organ prolapse. *Obstet Gynecol* 106:615–634.

Wein AJ, LJ Kavoussi CA, Peters AC, Novick and AW Partin. 2006. Campbell-Walsh Urology, 9th edn. Elsevier Health Services

Zacharin RF. 1977. A Chinese anatomy: The pelvic supporting tissues of the Chinese and Occidental female compared and contrasted. *Aust NZ J Obstet Gynecol* 17: 1–11.

Zeitlin MP and TB Lebherz. 1992. Pessaries in the geriatric patient. *J Am Geriatr Soc* 40: 635–639.

11

Reproductive Tract Infections

Mahalakshmi Gorti | Edwin Chandraharan

Infections of the female reproductive tract are common and may be endogenous or due to sexually transmitted infections. Rarely, they may be iatrogenic following a variety of procedures. It is important to understand that the female reproductive tract may act as a pathway for infections to ascend from the vulva through the fallopian tubes, into the peritoneal cavity. Such an anatomical continuity may be potentially life threatening. Various 'protective mechanisms' are in place to prevent the ascension of infections. These include acidity of the vagina due to Doderlein's bacilli that causes competitive inhibition of the pathogens by the normal commensals and cervical mucus with its antimicrobial properties. Endometrial and tubal fluids and the movements of the cilia towards the uterine cavity also play a role. However, when these defense mechanisms are breached, the normally sterile upper genital tract (endometrium, tubes and the ovaries) is exposed to infection by a wide array of microorganisms.

Many women remain asymptomatic, whereas others may suffer from minor annoyances to a serious illness, which may even be fatal. The long-term consequences include chronic pelvic pain, infertility, ectopic pregnancy, dysmenorrhea and menstrual abnormalities. From the societal point of view, the economic and social costs of reproductive tract infections are enormous. During pregnancy, reproductive tract infections may cause miscarriages, congenital malformations, preterm births, intrauterine growth restriction (IUGR) and puerperal sepsis.

Epidemiology: Reproductive tract infections (RTI) contribute to a large proportion of the global burden of ill health. They are estimated to cause 750,000 deaths and 75 million illnesses among women each year. The World Health Organization (WHO) estimated that over 340 million new cases of four curable sexually transmitted infections (STI)—gonorrhea, chlamydia, syphilis and trichomoniasis—occurred in 1999 (WHO 2001). If viral STI such as the human papilloma virus (HPV), herpes simplex virus (HSV) and the human immunodeficiency virus (HIV) infections are included, the number of cases may be three times higher.

The consequences of RTI for reproductive health can be severe and life threatening. They include pelvic abscess, peritonitis, septicemia and complications of ectopic pregnancy, and can cause adverse pregnancy outcomes including miscarriage, stillbirth, preterm birth and congenital infections (Mullick et al 2005). They also increase the risk of HIV transmission (Sexton et al 2005). RTI are most commonly endogenous in origin but they may be iatrogenic or sexually transmitted.

ENDOGENOUS INFECTIONS

These result from the overgrowth of organisms normally found in the vagina and probably constitute the most common reproductive tract infections. Common endogenous infections are discussed below.

Bacterial Vaginosis

Bacterial vaginosis (BV) is a common cause of vaginal discharge. Though the actual pathogenesis is unclear, it is believed to be due to the replacement of the normal hydrogen peroxide-producing lactobacillus species in the vagina by a high concentration of anerobic bacteria like Gardenerella vaginalis, Mycoplasma hominis, Prevotella species and Mobilincus. Whether bacterial vaginosis is acquired sexually is still unclear. However, it has often been diagnosed in women being evaluated for sexually transmitted infections. Indeed, it has been reported that the growth of BV-related organisms mentioned above increases the risk of pelvic inflammatory disease (PID) (Ness et al 2005). Recently, it has also been shown that bacterial vaginosis was associated with practices that are associated with sexually transmitted infections in contrast to those observed with candidiasis (Bradshaw et al 2005).

Clinical features: Up to 50% of women may remain asymptomatic (BASHH 2002). It usually causes a profuse white discharge that coats the vagina smoothly, which may be offensive.

Diagnosis: In clinical practice, BV is diagnosed using the Amsel's criteria. At least three of the following four criteria should be present for the diagnosis to be confirmed:

- Thin, white, homogeneous discharge
- Clue cells on microscopy (vaginal epithelial cells 'coated' by Gram-variable coccobacilli)
- pH of vaginal fluid >4.5
- Release of a fishy odour on adding alkali (10% KOH).

Laboratory tests: Gram staining of the vaginal discharge demonstrates the 'altered' flora. An alternative is to use a Gram stained vaginal smear, with the Hay/Ison criteria (Ison and Hay, 2002):

- Grade 1 (Normal): Lactobacillus morphotypes predominate
- Grade 2 (Intermediate): Mixed flora with some lactobacilli present, but Gardenerella or Mobiliuncus morphotypes are also present
- Grade 3 (BV): predominantly Gardenerella and/or Mobiluncus morphotypes, few or absent lactobacilli.

Treatment: Patients should be advised to avoid vaginal douching, use of shower gel and use of antiseptic agents or shampoo in the bath. This is to avoid potential alteration in the normal flora of the vagina. Avoidance of tight nylon underwear may also help in this regard.

Specific treatment: All women who are symptomatic require treatment as are women who undergo surgical treatment and procedures. In selected cases, treatment may be instituted during pregnancy. However, the 'PREMET' study has very recently shown that the use of metronidazole in pregnancy may in fact increase the risk of preterm labour (Shennan et al 2006).

The recommended regimen is

metronidazole 400–500 mg orally twice a day for seven days or metronidazole gel (0.75%) one applicator full (5 g) intravaginally once a day for five days.

A single dose of metronidazole (2 g) is also recommended. Alternatively, Clindamycin cream (2%) one applicator full (5 g) intravaginally at bedtime for seven days may be used. All these treatments have been shown to achieve cure rates of 70%–80% after 4 weeks of treatment in various placebo controlled trials (BASHH 2002). Use of live yoghurt or lactobacillus acidophilus for recurrent bacterial vaginosis has not been shown to be of any benefit (Larsson 1992).

Common reproductive health morbidity associated with bacterial vaginosis include, post induced-abortion infection (leading to pelvic inflammatory disease), post-hysterectomy vaginal cuff cellulitis and infectious morbidity. A 15-fold increase in plasma cell endometritis has also been reported in patients with bacterial vaginosis (Korn et al 1995). During pregnancy it may be associated with amniotic fluid infection (Newton et al 1997), clinical chorioamnionitis, postpartum endometritis, prelabour rupture of the membranes, preterm delivery and low birth weight. The incidence of bacterial vaginosis is high in women with pelvic inflammatory disease (PID), but there is no evidence to support that treating symptomatic women for BV reduces their risk of developing PID subsequently.

Vulvovaginal Candidiasis

This is most commonly caused by *Candida albicans* (80%–92%), but occasionally it may be caused by other species like *Candida glabrata* and *Candida tropicalis* (BASHH 2002). Predisposing factors include diabetes mellitus, broadspectrum antibiotic use, immunosupression, corticosteroid use and sub-optimal perineal hygiene. There is an increased incidence of vulvovaginal candidiasis during pregnancy, possibly due to the altered immunology of pregnancy as well as an increase in the glycogen concentration in the vaginal epithelial cells. There is no evidence to suggest that the use of modern 'low dose' combined oral contraceptives increase the incidence of vulvovaginal candidiasis.

Clinical features: Patients present with vulval itching, soreness, discharge, superficial dyspareunia and dysuria. Speculum examination may demonstrate curdy white discharge, which may be associated with signs of inflammation or fissuring of the vaginal mucosa. In 10%–20% of women, candidiasis may be diagnosed incidentally during speculum examination performed as a part of their gynecological examination. Such women who harbour Candida species in the absence of symptoms do not require treatment (BASHH 2002).

Diagnosis: Gram stain of vaginal discharge demonstrates spores/pseudohyphae in 65%–68% of symptomatic cases, on microscopic examination (Emmerson et al 1994). Vaginal discharge treated with 10% potassium hydroxide (KOH) may demonstrate pseudohyphae with 70% sensitivity (Sobel 1997). Culture (Sabouraud's dextrose media) could be considered in symptomatic women where microscopy is inconclusive or when identification of the species is important (for example, the resistant cases).

Treatment: Candida species respond well to imidazole group of anti-fungals, with up to 80%–95% cure rates (Reef et al 1995). Clotrimazole pessary 500 mg as a single dose or clotrimazole pessary 200 mg every night for three nights, or clotrimazole 100 mg every night for six nights are the accepted regimens of treatment. Clotrimazole cream 10% (5 g daily) can be applied locally. Sometimes it may be prudent to eradicate the 'bowel reservoir' by the use of oral nystatin treatment. Other oral treatment regimens include fluconazole capsule 150 mg as a single dose or itraconazole capsule 200 mg two doses 12 hours apart.

Recurrent candidiasis: This refers to the occurrence of four or more episodes of symptomatic candidiasis annually and may affect 5% of women. The exact pathogenesis is unclear but is associated with diabetes mellitus, immunodeficiency, steroid use and frequent antibiotic use. Rarely, issues relating to personal hygiene may play a role. Patients are often distressed and may have received multiple treatments, sometimes 'self-prescribing' over-the-counter antifungal agents.

Treatment: Initial induction therapy should be followed by maintenance therapy for six months to suppress the organisms. However, it is important to exclude the possible contributory factors mentioned above. Women should be counselled that there is at least a 50% chance that cessation of therapy may result in a relapse. The following medications have been recommended (Spinollo et al 1997):

Fluconazole 100 mg weekly for six months

Clotrimazole pessary 500 mg weekly for six months.

Itraconazole 400 mg monthly for six months

Ketoconazole 100 mg daily for six months

Liver function tests (LFT) need to be monitored monthly in view of the possibility of drug induced hepatitis following long term treatment with imidazoles.

Non-Albicans Vulvovaginal Candidiasis: *Candida glabarata* and *Candida tropicalis* may rarely cause an infection. Candida glabrata does not form pseudohyphae or hyphae and is not easily recognised on microscopy. They are found in 10% of the patients with recurrent vulvovaginal candidiasis. There is no consensus regarding the optimal treatment regimen for these non-albicans species. Longer duration of treatment with clotrimazole for 7-14 days is recommended as first-line therapy. A recent worldwide study comparing the susceptibilities of candida species to fluconazole indicated that in 2001, 0.6% of *C. albicans* isolates were resistant as compared to 30.7% of *C. glabarata* isolates (Hazen et al 2003).

SEXUALLY TRANSMITTED INFECTIONS

Lymphogranuloma Venereum (LGV)

This is usually caused by L1, L2, L3 strains of *Chlamydia trachomatis* and contributes to about 5% of the cases presenting with genital ulcers. The primary lesion is a painless papule or pustule followed by inguinal and/or femoral lymphadenopathy. Vulval edema may be associated with the ulcer. This is followed by bubo formation. In the vast majority of patients, the infection clears without further sequelae. Complications include proctocolitis and chronic fissures around the anus. Diagnosis is by exclusion of other causes of genital ulcer and lymphadenopathy. Complement fixation titres higher than 1:64 is diagnostic of lymphogranuloma venereum (Frei's test).

The recommended treatment regimen is 100 mg of doxycycline twice daily for 21 days or erythromycin 500 mg four times daily for 21 days (CDC 2002).Women affected with LGV during pregnancy and lactation should be treated with erythromycin. Doxycycline is contraindicated in pregnancy and the safety of azithromycin in pregnancy has not yet been fully evaluated.

Granuloma Inguinale

This is a sexually transmitted infection caused by *Klebsiella granulomatis*. It manifests as genital ulceration which is usually painless, followed by spread to the inguinal lymph nodes. The overlying tissues can give rise to pseudo buboes. Diagnosis is by demonstration of Donovan bodies. The condition responds well to azithromycin 1 g weekly or 500 mg daily till the ulcer heals or for a three-week period. Pregnant women affected by granuloma inguinale should be treated with erythromycin 500 mg four times a day for three weeks.

Chancroid

This is caused by *Hemophilus ducreyi* and the incidence of chancroid caused by this organism is steadily decreasing. A co-infection with treponema and herpes simplex virus (HSV) is seen in 10% of the population: it is also an important cofactor in the transmission of the human immunodeficiency virus (CDC 2002).

Clinical features: The incubation period is 3–10 days, and is usually followed by a single painful, soft sore with necrotic base and ragged undermined edges. There is associated inguinal adenitis in 50% of the cases.

Diagnosis: Microscopy of a Gram-stained smear of scrapings from ulcer base or culture of the scrapings from the ulcer base would demonstrate Gram-negative coccobacilli with occasional chaining. The most sensitive test is the detection of the nucleic acid (DNA) by polymerase chain reaction (PCR) using nested technique.

Treatment: Chancroid responds well to azithromycin 1 g orally as a single dose. Alternatively, ceftriaxone 250 mg can be given intramuscularly (IM) or erythromycin 500 mg orally can be administered as a single dose. No adverse effects of chancroid have been reported on the pregnancy outcome. Erythromycin is the drug of choice during pregnancy.

Herpes Simplex (Type 1 and Type 2)

Herpes simplex causes a recurrent lifelong disease with no definitive cure. Patients may be symptomatic or asymptomatic and may harbour and shed the virus. Prior infection with herpes simplex type 1 (HSV-1) often modifies the clinical manifestation of first infection by herpes simplex type 2 (HSV-2). As a general rule HSV-1 causes lesions above the waist (oro-pharyngeal) whereas, HSV-2 causes lesions below the waist (genital tract). Increasingly, due to changing sexual practices (oro-genital contact), the former is being isolated from the genital lesions and HSV-1 may also cause lesions below the waist.

Following primary infection the virus becomes latent in local sensory ganglia, periodically reactivating to cause herpetic lesions. These lesions are infectious and are associated with viral shedding, irrespective of the presence or absence of symptoms. Recurrence rates decline over time in most individuals. The majority of individuals who initially have asymptomatic HSV-2 infection subsequently develop symptomatic lesions.

Clinical features: The patient may be asymptomatic and the lesions may be detected during routine examination of the lower genital tract. Patients who are symptomatic present with painful ulceration of the external genitalia with inguinal lymphadenopathy, vaginal discharge and painful sexual intercourse. There may be associated dysuria and systemic manifestations like fever and myalgia. Complications include autonomic neuropathy resulting in urinary retention and aseptic meningitis.

Diagnosis: This is based on the isolation of HSV from the genital lesions. Type-specific enzyme immunoassay (EIA) based on glycoprotein G or Western blot assays are being used. Most of the commercial tests for HSV antibodies are not type-specific and are not of much value.

Treatment: A sympathetic approach and measures like saline bathing, analgesics and judicious use of topical anesthetic agents may help alleviate pain and discomfort. Antiviral drugs are indicated within five days of the start of the episode and while new lesions are still forming. Aciclovir, valaciclovir and famciclovir are commonly used. They reduce the severity and duration of the episode and hence, the amount of viral shedding and infectivity. However, they do not alter the natural history of the disease. Topical agents are less effective than oral agents.

Commonly used regimens include aciclovir 200 mg five times daily for five days, famciclovir 250 mg three times daily for five days or valaciclovir 500 mg twice daily for five days. Compliance is better with famciclovir and valaciclovir (fewer doses), although they are more expensive. Hospitalisation may be required for urinary retention, meningism, and severe constitutional symptoms. Broad-spectrum antibiotics may be necessary to prevent or treat secondary bacterial infections.

Recurrent Genital Herpes

Patient may experience up to four recurrences per year after the first episode. Recurrences are self-limiting and generally cause minor symptoms. HSV-2 recurs six times more frequently than HSV-1 (Beauman 2005). The patient should be fully involved in the management, which includes supportive measures, episodic antiviral treatment and suppressive antiviral therapy. A recent survey in the UK indicated that 96% of clinics provided drug treatment for recurrent herpes (Hamill and Goldmeier 2005).

Episodic antiviral treatment involves initiation of specific treatment early in an episode as this has been shown to be effective. Aciclovir 200 mg five times daily for five days is commonly used. Alternatively, valaciclovir 500 mg twice daily or famciclovir 125 mg twice daily may be used for five days. Use of high dose of famciclovir (1000 mg, two doses) at the onset of lesions has been shown to reduce the time required for healing (Langley 2005).

The decision to start suppressive antiviral treatment is subjective. It is important to balance the frequency of recurrence of infection with the cost and inconvenience of treatment. Aciclovir 400 mg twice daily or 200 mg four times daily, or famciclovir 250 mg twice daily has been recommended for up to one year. The International Herpes Management Forum (IHMF) now recommends suppressive treatment to all immunocompetent individuals with valaciclovir (500 mg daily). This has been shown to reduce the transmission of HSV-2 by 48% and lower the risk of clinical disease in susceptible partners by 75% (Corey et al 2004).

Human Papilloma Virus (HPV)

The prevalence of this infection has been reported to be 14%–90%, with the highest prevalence among women with possible sexually transmitted disease (Revzina and Di Clemente 2005). At least 50% of sexually active men and women acquire genital HPV infection at some point in their lives. It is estimated that at least 80% of women will have acquired genital HPV infection by the age of 50. More than thirty types of HPV can infect the genital tract. Most HPV infections are asymptomatic, unrecognised or subclinical. Visible genital warts are caused by HPV types 6 or 11 and these serotypes are only very rarely associated with invasive squamous cell cancer. HPV types 16, 18, 31, 33 and 35 have been shown to be strongly associated with cervical neoplasia. Genital warts can affect the external genitalia, vagina, cervix, uterus, anus, urethra, whereas mouth may be involved due to oro-genital contact.

Treatment: Treatment of genital warts should be guided by the patient's preference, available resources and experience of the clinician in the management of genital warts in particular and sexually transmitted infections in general. It is difficult to predict the natural history as some warts may regress while others may grow in size and number. Patients may be distressed by their unsightly appearance. Recommended treatment options include podophyllotoxin (0.5% solution or gel) applied twice a day for three days, followed by four days of no treatment. This cycle may be repeated if necessary for up to four cycles. This has been recommended as the first line therapy as it is very cost-effective (Fox and Tung 2005). Alternatively, imiquimod (5% cream) may be applied once daily at bedtime, thrice weekly, for up to 16 weeks. Podophyllin resin 10%–25%, cryotherapy, surgical removal, laser and electrosurgery are other alternatives.

Gonorrhea

This is a sexually transmitted infection caused by the Gram-negative diplococcus, *Neisseria gonorrhoeae*. This organism commonly affects the mucous membranes of the urethra, endocervix, rectum, pharynx and conjunctiva. The primary site of urogenital gonococcal infection in females is the endocervix. Patients may be asymptomatic (50%) or may present with vaginal discharge (50%), lower abdominal pain (25%), dysuria and/or frequency of micturition (12%). Complications include pelvic inflammatory disease (PID), hematogenous dissemination resulting in skin lesions, arthralgia, arthritis and tenosynovitis. Rectal and pharyngeal infections are often asymptomatic. Gonorrheal infections are usually associated with trichomonas vaginalis, candidiasis and chlamydial infections.

Diagnosis: Gram stain of the secretions often demonstrate Gram-negative 'kidney-shaped' intracellular diplococci. Culture is more sensitive and specific. It is important to transport the specimen in special transport media like modified Stuart's medium or charcoal free Amie's medium. This is because the organism is extremely sensitive to environmental conditions like heat and drying. Isolation rate in the laboratory is approximately 100% in 12 hours and 90% in 24 hours, which indicates a decline in the number of colonies with time. Nucleic acid amplification tests (NAATS) and nucleic acid hybridisation test may help in the diagnosis.

Treatment: Third generation cephalosporins like ceftriaxone 250 mg IM as a single dose or cefixime 400 mg oral as a single dose are recommended as first line agents (Tyson, 2005). Alternatively, spectinomycin 2 g IM as a single dose may be used; however, ciprofloxacin is no longer recommended due to increasing drug resistance (Ison et al, 2004). Sexual partners should be treated for gonorrhea after evaluation of the other sexually acquired infection. Genital infection with chlamydia commonly coexists in up to 40% of the women. Adults with gonorrhea must routinely be screened for presence of *C. trachomatis*.

Trichomoniasis

This infection is caused by the protozoal parasite, *Trichomonas vaginalis,* and is usually sexually transmitted. Many of the infected women (10%–50%) are asymptomatic. The commonest symptom is offensive vaginal discharge, which is often associated with vulval itching, swelling and dysuria. The vaginal discharge, if present, varies in consistency from thin and scanty to profuse and thick in 70% of women. The classical 'frothy yellow-green discharge' occurs only in about 10%–30% of women. Approximately 2% of patients will have a 'strawberry cervix', a term used to describe the intensely inflamed cervix seen with trichomoniasis. This is sometimes described as the 'red, angry-looking cervix'. It is prudent to remember that approximately 5%–15% of women who harbour the organism will have no abnormality on speculum examination.

Diagnosis: Direct observation by a wet smear or acridine orange stained slide from the swab taken from the posterior fornix of the vagina demonstrates the organism in 40%–80% of cases. Vaginal secretions in saline when examined under a microscope may show the 'moving' trophozoites, which are of the same size as the red cells but have three flagella. Although 'spun urine' may also be used to screen for trichomonas, the pick-up rate is lower compared to that in vaginal secretions. Of late, polymerase chain reaction (PCR) is being used as a diagnostic tool in some centres as the sensitivity and specificity of this method has been reported to be higher than that of culture (Caliendo 2005).

Treatment: Sexual partners should be treated simultaneously and sexual abstinence advised until treatment is completed. Screening for other coexistent sexually transmitted infection should be undertaken. Metronidazole 2 g orally as a single dose or metronidazole 400–500 mg twice daily for seven days is recommended. The approximate cure rate is 95%. Topical metronidazole gel is not recommended as it is not absorbed well enough to produce sufficient blood levels to eradicate the organisms from the paraurethral glands of Skene and the urethra. Rarely, in metronidazole-resistant cases mebendazole and furazolidone may be tried.

Chlamydia Trachomatis

Genital infection with chlamydia is common and it is estimated that 3%–5% of sexually active women in the UK may have a chlamydial infection. The exact prevalence in the general population is unknown. The cost of treating chlamydial infection and its complications is estimated to be at least 50 million pounds annually in the UK. Up to 73% of infections occur in the younger age group (16–24 years). Fig 11.1 shows a steady increase in chlamydial infection in the UK over the last 10 years in this age group. Risk factors include age (<25 years), new sexual partner or more than one sexual partners, lack of barrier contraception and women undergoing termination of pregnancy. Complications of chlamydial infection include pelvic inflammatory disease (PID) and sequelae (tubal damage leading to infertility, ectopic pregnancy, chronic pelvic pain, dyspareunia), Fitz-Hugh Curtis syndrome (perihepatitis that may cause upper abdominal pain), vertical transmission to neonate (conjunctivitis, pneumonia) and sexually acquired reactive arthritis/

Reiter syndrome (more common in men). Approximately 40% of non-gonococcal urethritis is caused by *C. trachomatis*.

Clinical features: Many women (80%) may be asymptomatic and as a result, the disease is often not diagnosed until complications develop (called 'silent STD'). If symptoms occur, they usually do so within 1–3 weeks after exposure and may include intermittent vaginal bleeding or discharge, pain on urination, or ill-defined abdominal discomfort. Others may present with postcoital bleeding, intermenstrual bleeding and lower abdominal pain. On speculum examination, there may be profuse vaginal discharge and cervix may appear inflamed and sometimes be mistaken for 'cervical erosion'.

Diagnosis: It is recommended that the overlying cervical mucous should be removed and the swab inserted up to 1–2 cm inside the cervical canal. This should be then rotated for about 10–30 seconds and directly inoculated into the culture medium or in a transport medium. Cervical swabs consistently have sensitivities >80%, whereas urine has sensitivity of 44%–94%. Various antigen detection techniques like enzyme immunoassay (EIA) and direct immunofluorescence (DIF) are being used. It has been reported that EIA has a sensitivity and specificity of 88% and 99%, respectively (Clark et al 1992). Compared to culture methods which have a sensitivity of up to 60%–65%, recent DNA amplification techniques like polymerase chain reaction (PCR) and ligase chain reaction (LCR) have sensitivities of up to 90%. Hence, these are being increasingly used.

Treatment: Azithromycin 1 g orally as a single dose or doxycycline 100 mg orally twice a day for seven days may be used as first line agents. Alternate regimens include erythromycin 500 mg orally four times a day for seven days, ofloxacin 300 mg orally twice a day for seven days and levofloxacin 500 mg once daily orally for seven days.

Follow-up: Re-testing for chlamydia after completing treatment with doxycycline or azithromycin is not required unless symptoms persist or re-infection is suspected. A test of cure may be considered three weeks after completion of treatment with erythromycin. Patients should be advised to refer their sexual contacts for investigation and treatment ('contact tracing'), especially if they had sexual contact during the 60 days preceding onset of symptoms or diagnosis of chlamydia. It is a good practice to evaluate and treat, even if the time of the last sexual contact was >60 days before symptom onset or diagnosis. Patients should be advised to abstain from sexual intercourse until they and their sex partners have completed treatment. Abstinence should be continued until seven days after a single-dose regimen or after completion of a 7-day regimen. Such measures would help reduce the incidence of re-infection.

Drugs in pregnancy: Doxycycline and ofloxacin are contraindicated during pregnancy. Clinical experience and preliminary data suggest that azithromycin (1 g orally as a single dose) is safe and effective. However, currently there is no scientific evidence on its safety in pregnancy. Erythromycin base 500 mg orally four times a day for seven days is recommended during pregnancy. Repeat testing three weeks after completion of therapy is recommended for all pregnant women, because these regimens may not be highly efficacious and the frequent side effects of erythromycin might discourage patient compliance with this regimen.

Syphilis

Syphilis is a sexually transmitted disease with diverse clinical manifestations. It is caused by a spirochete, *Treponema pallidum* and is a systemic illness early from the outset. The primary pathology is vasculitis (endarteritis obliterans), involving many organs. Acquired syphilis can be divided into primary, secondary, latent and tertiary stages. The infection can be transmitted vertically resulting in congenital syphilis and occasionally by blood transfusion and non-sexual contact. Syphilis increases the risk of transmission of HIV infection. Conversely, HIV may cause more severe manifestations of early syphilis or more rapid progression to late syphilis, due to immunodeficiency. Syphilis is usually the second or third commonest cause of genital ulcer (chancroid or genital herpes being more common).

Clinical manifestation: The primary lesion is called 'chancre' and it commonly occurs in the anogenital region. The incubation period is 9–90 days. The ulcer is usually indurated and painless and they are often described as 'punched out ulcers'. Sometimes it may be atypical (painful and soft) due to a co-infection with chancroid and herpes. Spread to the regional lymph nodes results in enlarged rubbery lymph nodes. Other sites that the chancre can develop are lip, tongue and tonsils from oral sex and kissing. Nipple may be involved from kissing or nursing of infected babies, and finger with minor abrasion, from touching lesions.

Secondary syphilis presents with generalised rash affecting the palms and soles, generalised lymphadenopathy and orogenital mucosal lesions including snail tract ulcers and condylomata lata. Other manifestations include alopecia, anterior uveitis, retinitis, cranial nerve involvement, laryngitis, gastritis, hepatosplenomegaly and glomerulonephritis. This is followed by a latent phase and if untreated, about 40% of patients may proceed to tertiary stage. Tertiary syphilis is characterised by gumma, cardiovascular and neurological manifestations including tabes dorsalis and meningovascular syphilis.

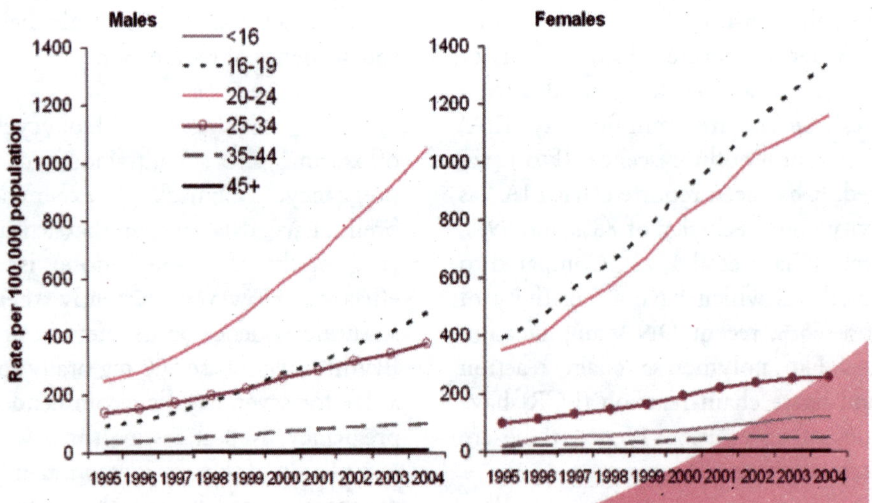

Figure 11.1: Rates of diagnosis of uncomplicated genital chlamydial infection by sex and age group in the UK, 1995-2004. Reproduced with permission from Health Protection Agency (HPA, U.K.)

Diagnosis: Treponemes may be identified using dark field microscopy, which shows organisms with 'cork-screw' movements. Direct fluorescent antibody staining of treponemes may also be useful. Serological tests that are commonly used are treponemal enzyme immunoassay (EIA), *T. pallidum* particle agglutination (TPPA) or hemagglutination (TPHA) and fluorescent antibody absorption tests (FTA-abs). The non-treponemal tests are Veneral Disease Research Laboratory (VDRL) or rapid plasma regain (RPR) test.

Primary syphilis is diagnosed by dark field microscopy or direct fluorescent antibody stain of serum from the ulcer. The diagnosis of secondary syphilis is by dark field microscopy of the specimen obtained from condyloma lata, genital lesions or lymph node aspirate and/or by serological tests. Latent and tertiary syphilis are diagnosed by the serological tests, whereas, neurosyphilis is diagnosed clinically and by abnormal cerebrospinal fluid. Presence of positive VDRL/RPR and a raised TPHA index in the CSF would help make a diagnosis of neurological syphilis.

Treatment: Benzathine penicillin 2.4 megaunits administered intramuscularly either as a single dose or weekly in two or three doses is the mainstay of management of early syphilis. In patients allergic to penicillin, doxycycline 100 mg twice daily for two weeks or tetracycline 500 mg four times daily for two weeks or azithromycin 500 mg daily for one week may be administered. Patients should be warned of the Jarisch–Herxheimer reaction that causes a flu-like illness within 24 hours of starting treatment. This is more of concern in patients with neuro/ocular/cardiovascular syphilis and is usually treated by prednisolone 10–20 mg three times a day for three days starting 24 hours before anti-treponemal treatment.

Pelvic Inflammatory Disease

Pelvic inflammatory disease (PID) is a result of ascending infection from the endocervix causing infection of the upper genital tract. This includes endometritis, salpingitis, parametritis, oophoritis, tubo-ovarian abscess and/or pelvic peritonitis, which may lead to septicemia. *Neisseria gonorrhoeae* and Chlamydia are probably the most common 'primary-pathogenic' organisms. *Gardenerella vaginalis*, anerobes and other organisms commonly found in the vagina may also be implicated.

Clinical features: Women may present with lower abdominal pain, dyspareunia, abnormal vaginal bleeding or vaginal discharge. Acute PID may be characterised by fever with chills, nausea, vomiting and profuse vaginal discharge. On examination, there may be bilateral tenderness in the lower abdomen. Adnexal tenderness and cervical excitation may also be noted and an 'adnexal mass' may be felt if there is a tubo-ovarian mass or abscess. About 15% of women with PID will require hospital admission and more than 20% will become infertile because of tubal disease; 3% may have an ectopic pregnancy.

Diagnosis: Women with PID may be asymptomatic. Clinical symptoms and signs lack sensitivity and specificity, whereas laparoscopy has the best specificity (Gaitan et al 2002). Screening for gonorrhea and chlamydia in the lower genital tract is recommended because a positive result may support the diagnosis of PID. However, the absence of infection at this site does not exclude PID. An elevated ESR or C-reactive protein (CRP) may help support the diagnosis of PID. Laparoscopy is useful in diagnosing PID but is not justified routinely as it may not be possible to identify mild intra-tubal inflammation or endometritis. There may be intra- and interobserver variation in diagnosing PID. There may be procedure-related complications including bowel and great vessel injury. Laparoscopy is invaluable in acute PID which does not respond to standard antibiotic therapy. In this situation, it may help in excluding other intraperitoneal pathology as well as in the drainage of pelvic abscess.

Management: Prompt and appropriate treatment is essential to reduce the incidence of long-term sequelae such as ectopic pregnancy, infertility and chronic pelvic pain. Lack of definitive diagnostic criteria coupled with risk of complications would require a low threshold for empiric treatment for PID. Broad spectrum antibiotic therapy is recommended to cover *N.gonorrheae*, Chlamydia, aerobic and anaerobic bacteria. Patients with mild PID may be managed as outpatients with a combination of oral ofloxacin 400 mg twice a day and oral metronidazole 400 mg twice a day, for 14 days. Alternatively, IM ceftriaxone 250 mg or IM cefoxitin 2 g may be administered immediately with oral probenecid (1 g) followed by oral doxycycline 100 mg twice a day plus metronidazole 400 mg twice a day for 14 days (RCOG 2003).

The following clinical situations may warrant hospitalisation—severe pelvic inflammatory disease, tubo-ovarian abscess, PID in pregnancy, lack of response to oral treatment and intolerance to oral therapy. Recommended regimens are intravenous cefoxitin 2 g three times a day and intravenous doxycycline 100 mg twice a day (oral doxycycline may be used if tolerated), followed by oral doxycycline 100 mg twice a day and oral metronidazole 400 mg twice, a day for a total of 14 days. Alternatively, intravenous clindamycin 900 mg three times a day and intravenous gentamicin (2 mg/kg loading dose followed by 1.5 mg/kg) three times a day (a single daily dose of 7 mg/kg may be substituted), followed by either oral clindamycin 450 mg four times a day to complete 14 days or oral doxycycline 100 mg twice a day and oral metronidazole 400 mg twice a day to complete 14 days may be used. Intravenous ofloxacin 400 mg twice a day plus IV metronidazole 500 mg three times a day for 14 days may be another option. Treatment with IV antibiotics should continue until 24 hours after clinical improvement. Laparoscopy/laparotomy should be considered for severe cases or when pelvic abscess is suspected. Adhesiolysis and drainage of the abscess may help in early resolution of the disease.

Conclusion: The incidence of reproductive tract infections has been increasing worldwide and should be considered a serious global health problem. The economic, reproductive and social consequences are enormous. Public health education, effective use of barrier contraception coupled with early diagnosis and prompt and appropriate treatment may help prevent complications and optimise reproductive health of women.

References

Barrett S, and C Taylor. 2005. A review on pelvic inflammatory disease. *Int J STD AIDS* 16(1): 715–720.

BASHH. 2002. 2001 National Guidelines for the Management of Bacterial Vaginosis. *British Association for Sexual Health and HIV*.

BASHH. 2002. 2001 National Guidelines for the Management of Vulvovaginal Candidiasis. *British Association for Sexual Health and HIV*.

Beauman JG. 2005. Genital herpes: A review. *Am Fam Physician* 72(8):1527–1534.

Borcklehurst P, M Hannah, H McDonald. 2005. Interventions for treating bacterial vaginosis in pregnancy. *Cochrane Database Syst Rev* CD000262.

Bradshaw CS, AN Morton, SM Garland et al. 2005. Higher–risk behavioural practices associated with bacterial vaginosis compared to vaginal candidiasis. *Obstet Gynecol* 106:105–114.

Caliendo AM, JA Jordan, AM Green et al. 2005. Real-time PCR improves detection of trichomonas vaginalis infection compared with culture using self-collected vaginal swabs. *Infect Dis Obstet Gynecol* 13(3):145–150.

Carey JC, MA Klebanoff, JC Hauth et al. 2000. Metronidazole to prevent preterm delivery in pregnant women with asymptomatic bacterial vaginosis. *N Engl J Med* 342(8):543–540.

Centers for Disease Control and Prevention. 2002. Sexually transmitted disease treatment guidelines. *Morbidity Mortality Weekly Report* 55:1–84.

Corey L, R Ashley. Valaciclovir HSV Transmission Study Group. 2004. Prevention of herpes simplex virus type 2 transmission with antiviral therapy. *Herpes* 11(S3):170A–174A.

Emmerson J, A Gunputrao, J Hawkswel et al. 1994. Sampling for vaginal candidiasis: How good is it? *Int J STD AIDS* 5:356–358.

Fox PA and MY Tung. 2005. Human papilloma virus: Burden of illness and treatment cost considerations. *Am J Clin Dermatol* 6(6):365–381.

Hamill M and D Goldmeier. 2005. Management of recurrent genital herpes: A survey of UK genitourinary medicine clinics in 2003. *Int J STD AIDS* 16(11):760–762.

Hazen KC, EJ Baron, AL Combo et al. 2003. Comparison of susceptibilities of the candida species to fluconozole and voriconazole in a 4-year global evaluation using disk diffusion. *J Clin Microbiol* 41(12):5623–5632.

Health Protection Agency UK. 2005. Epidemiological Data - Chlamydia http://www.hpa.org.uk/infections/topics_az/hiv_and_sti/sti-chlamydia/epidemiology/epidemiology.

Ison CA and PE Hay. 2002. Validation of a simplified grading of Gram-stained vaginal smear for use in GUM Clinics. *Sex Transm Infec* 78:413–415.

Ison CA, JW Mouton, K Jones et al. 2004. Which cephalosporin for gonorrhoea? *Sex Transm Infect* 80(5):386–388.

Korn AP, G Bolan, N Padian et al. 1995. Plasma cell endometritis in women with symptomatic bacterial vaginosis. *Obstet Gynecol* 85:387–390.

Langley RG. 2005. Famciclovir for the treatment of recurrent genital herpes lesions. *Skin Therapy Lett* 10(10): 5–7.

Larsson PG. 1992. Treatment of bacterial vaginosis. *Int J STD AIDS* 3:239–247.

McDonald HM, JA O'Laughlin, R Vigneswaran et al. 1997. Impact of metronidazole therapy on preterm birth in women with bacterial vaginosis flora: A randomised placebo controlled trial. *Br J Obstet Gynaecol* 104: 1391–1397.

Mullick S, D Watson-Jones, M Belinska, D Mabez. 2005. Sexually transmitted infections in pregnancy: Prevalence, impact on pregnancy outcomes and approach to treatment in development countries. *Sex Transm Infect* 81:294–302.

Ness RB, KE Kip, SL Hillier, et al. 2005. A cluster analysis of bacterial vaginosis associated microflora and pelvic inflammatory disease. *Am J Epidemiol* 162(6):585–590.

Newton ER, J Piper, W Peairs. 1997. Bacterial vaginosis and intra-amniotic infection. *Am J Obstet Gynecol* 176:672–677.

RCOG. 2003. *Management of Acute Pelvic Inflammatory disease.* Guideline No 32 of the RCOG. London: RCOG Press.

Reef SE, WC Levina, MM McNeil et al. 1995. Treatment options for vulvovaginal candidiasis. *Clin Infect Dis* 20(S1):580–590.

Revzina NV and RJ Diclemente. 2005. Prevalence and incidence of human papilloma virus infection in women in the USA: A systemic review. *Int J STD AIDS* 16(8):528–537.

Sexton J, G Carrett, JA Rottingen. 2005. Meta-analysis and meta-regression in interpreting study variability in the impact of sexually transmitted diseases on susceptibility to HIV infections. *Sex Transm Dis* 32(6):351–357.

Shennan A, S Crawshaw, A Briley. 2006. A randomised controlled trial of metronidazole for the prevention of preterm birth in women positive for cervicovaginal fibronectin: The PREMET Study. *Br J Obstet Gynaecol* 113(1):65–74.

Sobel JD. 1997. Vaginitis. *N Engl J Med* 337:1896–1903.

Spinollo A, C Colonna, G Piazzi et al. 1997. Managing recurrent vulvovaginal candidiasis: Intermittent prevention with itraconozole. *J Reprod Med* 42:83–87.

Tyson M. 2005. Guidance for first-line treatment of anogenital gonorrhoea infection. *Br J Nurs* 14(12):646–648.

Ugwumadu A, I Manyonda, F Reid, P Hay. 2003. Effect of early oral clindamycin on late miscarriage and preterm delivery in asymptomatic women with abnormal vaginal flora and bacterial vaginosis: A randomised controlled trial. *Lancet* 361(362):983–988.

World Health Organization. 2001. *Global prevalence and incidence of selected curable sexually transmitted infections: Overview and estimates.* Geneva: World Health Organization.

12

Epidemiology of Malignancies in the Reproductive Age Group

Neelanjana Mukhopadhaya | Sabaratnam Arulkumaran

One in three individuals develops cancer in their life time. Cancer is predominantly a disease of the elderly, but both men and women in their reproductive age are now being diagnosed with cancer more frequently. Setting aside the dermatological malignancies, the four most common cancers are lung, colorectal, breast and prostate (Fig. 12.1). In the year 2005, there were 153,491 deaths from cancer in the United Kingdom (Cancer Research UK 2007) which accounted for 26% of all deaths in the UK in 2005. Epidemiological studies have identified incidence and mortality trends and its association with factors such as environmental and lifestyle patterns which are the basis for many preventive strategies.

History of cancer reporting: National statutory death registration in England and Wales was initiated on 1 July 1837. The Registrar General has collected mortality data since then. Site and age specific data were gradually developed over the years. It has since become clear that specific occupational exposures, geographical distribution and lifestyle patterns have a major impact on the occurrence of cancer. Medical statisticians and epidemiologists had foreseen the importance of cancer data collection and in 1944, Harold Dorn (1944) in the United States highlighted the importance of cancer reporting in Public Health. Johannes Clemmensen (1955) in Denmark and Mitsuo Segi (1960) in Japan had by then pioneered cancer incidence data collection. In 1966, Doll et al published the first volume of 'Cancer Incidence in Five Continents'.

Cancer reporting in the UK: A national system was developed in 1945 (Stocks 1936), and from the year 1947 all data collected by the Registrar General was collated and incorporated into the Office of Population Censuses and Surveys (OPCS) and subsequently in the Office for National Statistics (ONS). Full national geographical coverage was attained in 1962 and held on computers since 1959. The ONS is the main reporting body in the UK. Cancer Research UK is the world's largest independent cancer research organisation dedicated to various types and aspects of cancer. It was formed by the merging of the Imperial Cancer Research Fund (ICRF) and the Cancer Research Campaign (CRC).

Problems with cancer reporting: Cancer Registries vary in their ways of registering deaths all over the world. These inconsistencies may account for discrepancies in the data and their interpretation. The degree of precision in reporting the cause of death affects the incidence and mortality data. Since 1911, mortality data in England and Wales has been coded according to the International Classification of Diseases (ICD). Reporting has been affected due to changes in the coding system. The advancement of technology in medicine, both diagnostic and therapeutic, has affected mortality all over the world. Screening programmes have led to an increase in the incidence rates as more prevalent cases are detected. However, this should be followed by a decrease in the incidence, with an effective screening programme. Reluctance in mentioning cancers in death certificates has been a problem in some countries. In cases where the death may be due to a secondary from a primary cancer site, there may be no mention of the primary site, thus leading to misinterpretation of the data. An improvement in death certification quality can help immensely by being more informative and identifying genuine temporal trends in cancer epidemiology (Percy and Muir 1989).

Causative factors

Genetic factors: Majority of the recognised carcinogens cause genetic mutations—the basis for carcinogenesis. The change in the gene expression by somatic cells is caused by an interaction between the individual's own genetic susceptibility and environmental carcinogens. One or more of these highly penetrating, dominantly inherited genetic susceptibilities could potentially exist in each individual; 2%–5% of all cancers can be attributed to genetic susceptibilities. Environmental factors can modify these individual susceptibilities by causing genetic polymorphism. For example, nutritional factors mediated by the carcinogens in food, ingestion of hormones and exposure to certain infection or lowering of immune resistance can exacerbate the genetic risk (Uauy and Solomons 2005).

Environmental factors: Environment constitutes a major etiological factor in many cancers, especially in those of the lung, bladder and breast. Specific exposures can lead to different cancers. Air pollutants like black smoke, sulphur dioxide, carbon monoxide and other volatile organic compounds have been implicated in the pathology of lung cancer. Inhalation of metal air pollutants like copper, chromium and zinc play a role in lung carcinogenesis (Coyle et al 2006). Exposures to ionising radiations, both natural (for example, cosmic, gamma and domestic radon) and artificial (for example, medical, occupational, fallout radiation, discharges) are known to cause thyroid cancers.

Solar ultraviolet radiation is the main causative factor in Non Melanoma Skin Cancers (NMSC). It not only plays a major role in the induction of NMSC but also serves as a complete carcinogen and a cancer promoter (Molho-Pessach and Lotem 2007).

Cancers with gender preponderance: Some cancers are more predominant in women than men and vice- versa. Possible reasons are smoking and alcohol habits, food and nutrient consumption, anthropometric characteristics, nature of occupation and physical exercise. Perhaps more importantly, many cancers are regulated and modulated by estrogen and progesterone receptor status and therefore can have gender preponderance.

Gall bladder and thyroid cancers are more common in women, while bladder, lung and liver cancer are preponderant in men. A high female to male ratio is seen in colon cancer in premenopausal women (McMichael and Potter 1980; Jensen 1984).

GEOGRAPHICAL AREAS: Colorectal cancer is Australia's most commonly occurring internal cancer (Towler et al 1998). Various lines of research suggest that there may be a great inter-individual variation in the susceptibility to external carcinogens based on the geographical area, lifestyle measures and metabolic phenotypes related to race and ethnic origin. In parts of India and South East Asia, tobacco and betel chewing predispose individuals to oral and pharyngeal cancers. Increasing alcohol and tobacco consumption in different geographical areas may account for esophageal cancer trends. Occupation, physical activity and environment vary geographically and account for epidemiological trends of cancer.

LIFESTYLE PATTERNS: This contributes significantly to the etiopathogenesis of cancers in general. Epidemiological studies have identified several factors that may be closely related to the development of cancers in certain areas of the world or ethnic groups. A study from Montreal showed that married individuals had a lower risk of developing colon cancer compared to their single counterparts. The authors attributed this to the food habits of the single individual. Constipation and use of laxatives increases the risk of colon cancer (Ghadirian et al 1998). It is evident from studies that lifestyle changes can be a significant factor in altering an individual's risk to developing cancer. Dietary deficiencies are associated with increased risk of esophageal cancer. Carotene, tocopherol and selenium reduce the mortality rates of gastric cancer. About 33%–50% cases of nasopharyngeal carcinoma are related to consumption of salt fish. Estrogens are associated with breast cancer, mainly as promoters rather than as a causal agent. Lifestyle factors have a major impact on disease development and progression (Wiseman 2004). Smoking and alcohol consumption are independent risk factors and have been implicated in the pathogenesis of many cancers. Smoking alone is the single largest avoidable cause of premature death and carcinogenesis. Cancers of the lung, larynx, oral cavity, pharynx, esophagus, pancreas, kidney and bladder are associated with tobacco smoking. Alcohol together with tobacco smoking accounts for oral cavity, pharynx, larynx and esophageal cancers. Alcohol alone contributes to the pathogenesis of liver and cancers of the breast and colon.

Cancer incidence and mortality: Cancer incidence and mortality data are obtained from cancer registries from all over the world. There has been a gradual increase in the mortality from cancer, for both men and women, over the years (Fig. 12.2). The possible reasons are improved standards of coding, documentation in death certificates and reporting. This is also reflective of better diagnosis and effective cancer screening programmes. The most recent cancer mortality statistics from the Cancer Research UK, England and Wales 2005 suggest that lung cancer is responsible for the highest cancer mortality (Fig. 12.1). The percentages are shown in Table 12.1.

Epidemiological risk factors and trends in individual cancers

LUNG CANCER: Once rare, this is a major killer today. Industrialisation and modernisation saw an epidemic of lung cancer. This was first noted among males in the USA and in several European countries in the 1940s. By the early 1950s there was sufficient epidemiological evidence to show that cigarette smoking was strongly related to lung cancer (Doll and Hill 1950).

Lung cancer has accounted for 1.35 million cases worldwide and 1.18 million deaths in 2005. It has a high case fatality ratio (ratio of mortality to incidence is 0.87). Cigarette smoking is associated with 88% of cases (WHO revised Global Burden of disease 2002). Most non-smoking related cases of lung cancers are adenocarcinomas. Factors that determine risk are number, type and duration of smoking (Wu-Williams and Samet 1994; Lubin and Caporaso 2006). Current hypothesis include individual susceptibilities like genetic factors, intake of anti-oxidant micronutrients like beta-carotene and synergism with other environmental factors. Certain genetic variations in the nucleotide excision repair present in some individuals may provide a protective effect from the carcinogens present in tobacco smoke (Garcia-Closas et al 2006). Environmental carcinogens like polycyclic aromatic hydrocarbons, heavy metal exposure (arsenic, asbestos, chromium and nickel), domestic radons and industrial fumes that contaminate air can also modify one's risk to developing lung cancer.

Histologically, most common malignant tumours are squamous cell carcinoma, adenocarcinoma, large cell and small cell carcinoma. Men are 10 times more likely to be affected than women (Fig.12.3). The disease affects men and women between 40 and 70 years.

It is imperative that research continues into the prevalence of smoking practices and lung cancer trends.

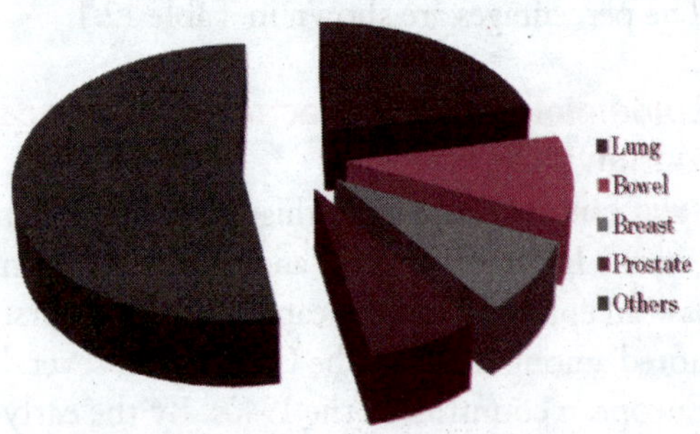

FIGURE 12.1: UK CANCER MORTALITY STATISTICS (DATA FROM CANCER RESEARCH UK)

TABLE 12.1: COMMON TYPES OF CANCER IN THE UK

Types of Cancer	*Percentage mortality*
Lung	22%
Bowel	10%
Breast	8%
Prostate	7%
Others	53%

Source: Courtesy of National Mortality Statistics 2005; *Cancer Research UK.*

BREAST CANCER: It is the second most prevalent cancer in the world (1.15 million new cases per year). It ranks fifth in mortality worldwide (it has a relatively favourable prognosis with a mortality to incidence ratio of 0.35).The incidence of non-hormone dependent cancer increases with age but the rate of increase slows after menopause. The age-frequency distribution for females is bimodal with peaks at 52 and 71 years of age, whereas it is unimodal in men with a peak at 71 years

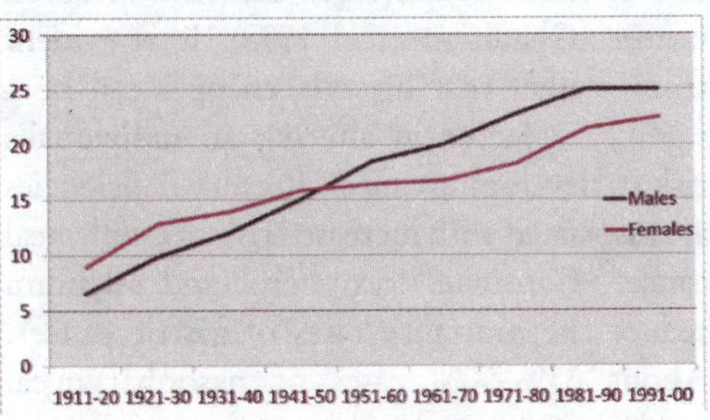

FIGURE 12.2: PERCENTAGE OF ALL DEATHS DUE TO NEOPLASMS ENGLAND AND WALES (CANCER RESEARCH UK)

Table 12.2: Million Women Study (Beral 2003)

Breast cancer incidence	*Relative Risk (95% CI)*
Never users	1.00
All past users	1.01
Current users:	
Oestrogen	1.30
Oestrogen/progestogen	2.00
Tibolone	1.45
Others/unknown types	1.44

(Anderson et al 2004). The lifetime odds of developing breast cancer are 1:8 women in North America and 1:12 in Western Europe (Benshushan and Brzenzinski 2002).

Various factors have been studied to understand their role in pathogenesis. Hormonal manipulations like hormone replacement therapy (HRT), oral contraceptives (OC) and anti-estrogens increase the risk of breast cancer. A decrease of one year at the age of menarche increases the risk by 10% and an increase in the age at menopause by one year increases risk by nearly 10%. Parity can influence breast cancer risk. For white women, the reduction in the risk of breast carcinoma per full term pregnancy was 13% among women between the ages of 35 and 49 and 10% between the ages of 50 and 64. The risk falls significantly with each full term pregnancy, irrespective of age and ethnicity. Duration of lactation is inversely related to breast cancer risk. Because women now have fewer children than in the past and fewer of them are breastfeeding, this may account for the possibility of a rise in breast cancer. Dietary factors, especially fat, are associated with the etiology of breast cancer as shown by intervention and ecological

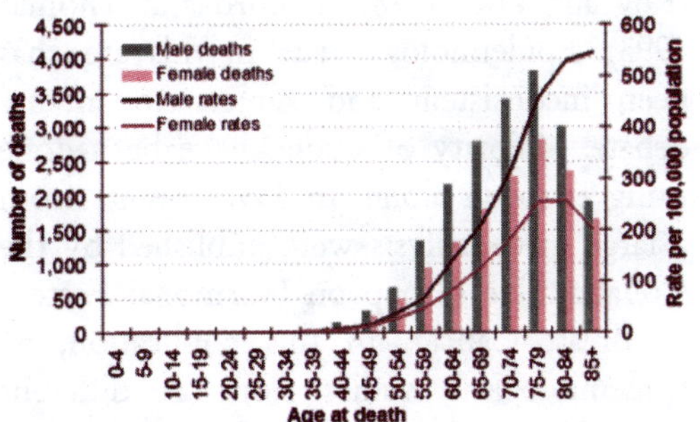

Figure 12.3: Lung cancer by sex in the UK, 2005 cancer research UK

correlation studies, but the evidence from case-control and cohort studies is inconsistent and contradictory (Wiseman 2000).

There is evidence that use of OC increases the risk to breast cancer. OC use and its relation to breast carcinoma has been a much debated topic for many years. Spicer and Pike (1994), in their review of literature, stratified women by their menopausal status at the time of diagnosis of breast carcinoma. They identified five population-based case controlled studies and three cohort studies in women less than 45 years of age. An increased risk of breast carcinoma was observed in this group of OC users in all the eight studies. Risk was estimated at 3.1% per year of use (Spicer and Pike1994). However, in the review of the three population-based case controlled studies and three cohort studies in women over 45 years of age, there was no increase in the incidence of breast cancer with OC. Brinton (1997) found an interesting link between the duration of OC use and age in African American women. A strong risk was observed in African American women between 40–54 years, but the risk was lower in those between the ages of 20 and 39.

Research suggests that combined HRT may increase breast cancer risk significantly compared with estrogen-only preparations

(Key and Pike 1988; Stanford and Thomas 1993). Epidemiologic data in this area has been inconsistent and subject to intense debate. Majority of studies have been done using estrogen alone. In 1997, results from a large meta-analysis were published by the Collaborative Group on Hormonal Factors in Breast Cancer. In this publication, 51 epidemiological studies from 21 different countries were analysed using more than 50,000 cases and 100,000 controls. A 2.3% increase in breast cancer for each year of HRT used in postmenopausal women was observed. Relative Risk (RR) for women who were current users of HRT for 5 years or longer was 1.35 (Collaborative Group on Hormonal Factors in Breast Cancer 1997).

More recently, the Million Women Study by Beral (2003) sparked a major interest both among clinicians and the public (Table 12.2). A total of 1,084,110 women aged 50–64 years were recruited into the study between the years 1996 and 2000. Current users of HRT were more likely to develop breast cancer with preparations containing estrogen only (RR 1.30 {95% CI 1.21–1.40} p=< 0.0001), estrogen-progestogen (2.00{1.88–2.12}, p<0.0001) and tibolone (1.45{1.25–1.68}, p<0.0001).

Testicular cancer: This is a rare disease accounting for <2% of all malignant neoplasms in males. It is relatively common in young and middle aged males (15–44 yrs). Majority of the tumours in young men are germ cell tumours. Testicular germ cell tumours can be subdivided into pure seminoma and teratoma (this includes embryonal carcinoma, choriocarcinoma, yolk-sac tumour and mixed tumours). The median age at diagnosis is about 10 years less for teratomas compared with seminomas. The teratomas usually occur in the age range of 25-29 years. The peak age for testicular tumours is 25–34 years. A gradual decline in incidence is observed with very few cases after 55 years of age. Swerdlow and Skeet (1988) showed an association between affluence and particular professions with testicular cancers. Occupation related rise in risk has been studied by many researchers. Risk of seminomas increased with the exposure to pesticides, organic solvents and textile dusts (Guo et al 2005). A significant risk factor is undescended testis (odds ratio 3.82; 95% 2.24–6.52) and inguinal hernia {1.91; 1.12-3.23} (United Kingdom Testicular Cancer Study Group 1994). Early orchidopexy was seen to reduce risks. Sedentary lifestyle, early puberty and infertility are also associated with an increase in the risk of testicular cancer. There was no association found with vasectomy.

Although incidence of testicular cancer has gone up, possibly due to better diagnostic aids and histological confirmation, mortality rates have improved due to appropriate and effective chemotherapy.

Thyroid cancer: It is a rare disease (0.5–10 per 100,000). Epidemiological studies have provided an insight into its etiopathogenesis. Possible causes are benign thyroid diseases (benign nodules and goitre), acromegaly (Barzilay et al 1991), reproductive factors (miscarriages, late pregnancies) and dietary habits such as lack or excess of iodine and protective effect of vegetables (Glattre et al 1993). Radiation, either following radioactive fallout as in the Chernobyl accident or cancer treatment in childhood, has been shown to increase one's risk to thyroid cancer. A study by Kazakov et al in 1992 conducted on subjects in the regions of Belarus and Russia showed an increase in thyroid cancer cases (four cases per year from 1986–89, to 55 cases per year in 1991). A study in the United States that explored etiology for rising rates of thyroid cancer identified radiation exposure in childhood as a strong risk factor in children treated for primary cancers (Ronckers et al 2005).

There are practical difficulties in most epidemiological studies with thyroid cancer. The risk factors apart from ionising radiation, are generally poorly defined. Histological differentiation is complicated. The thyroid gland contains follicular, parafollicular, connective tissue-fibroblast, vascular endothelium and lymphoid cells (each could give rise to histologically different tumours). Due to diagnostic problems, a 'pool'of individuals with occult cancer may be present even at a young age. In addition, diagnostic intensity and classification criteria vary from place to place.

Generally, there has been an upward temporal trend in incidence rates but mortality rates have remained stable.

Hodgkin's lymphoma (HD): MacMahon (1957) offered the first model that a viral infection with low infectivity causes the early age peak (MacMahon 1957). Epstein–Barr Virus (EBV), causing infectious mononucleosis remains the leading candidate in the pathogenesis of HD. Other risk factors include occupational risks like exposure to solvents, wood dust and agricultural chemicals. The incidence of HD varies from 0.5/100,000 in parts of Asia to 3/100,000 in parts of North America. The incidence is higher in younger adults and falls in older ages. There has been a sharp decline in mortality over the years.

Non-Hodgkin's lymphoma (NHL): NHL is a heterogenous group of T and B cell lymphomas arising in the lymph nodes (Ulcickas et al 2007). Although the rapid rise in the number of cases in recent years could be due to an increase in HIV infection, other risk factors have also been implicated. NHL accounts for 3.4% of cancer deaths in the United States (Alexander et al 2007). Cumulative incidence in the HIV population is 5%–10%. The risk factors for NHL are viral infection, immunosuppressive states, family history and occupational reasons in farmers exposed to pesticides and herbicides. Hepatitis B infection is also a risk factor as evident from a recent study. Rare genetic syndromes characterised by immunosuppression such as Wiskott-Aldrich syndrome, ataxia telengectasia and X-linked lymphoproliferative syndrome may predispose an individual to NHL. Immunosuppressive therapy with medication, as in transplant patients and viral infections, can also increase the risk of developing NHL (Filipovich et al 1992). Epidemiological trends suggest an increase in both incidence and mortality, steadily and almost universally during the past decades. Epidemiological research is needed to clarify the etiological factors and identify preventive approaches.

Cervical cancer: It is the second most common cancer in women worldwide. Age Standardised Incidence Rates of Cervical Cancer per 100,000 varies from 33.4–87.3 in some areas of the developing world to <9.4 in most developed countries. Eighty per cent of cervical cancers occur in developing countries. In the study of cervical cancer deaths in Europe for the year 2004, Arbyn et al 2007 estimated 14,000 deaths from cancer cervix of the approximately 31,000 affected women. The age-standardised incidence rates for 15 old and 10 new EU (European Union) member states was 9.5 versus 16.7; standardised mortality rates of 4.9 versus 10.7. The burden was lowest in Finland (cumulative incidence and mortality rates of 0.38% and 0.12%, respectively) and highest in Lithuania (cumulative incidence and mortality of 1.64% and 0.94%, respectively). In many Asian and African countries, screening for cervical cancer is still in its early days and may take many years to become universal. In addition, the prevalence of the Human Papilloma Virus (HPV) is high in these countries. In a study from China, HPV prevalence was found to be 16.8% overall and 13.6% among women without cervical abnormalities (age-standardised to world standard population is 16.6% and 12.4% respectively). The prevalence of HPV16 was the highest (3.4%), then HPV52 (2.5%), HPV58 (1.9%) and multiple infections in 31.3% of all infected women (Li et al 2006). Thomas et al (2004) studied the prevalence of HPV in an inner city of Nigeria and reported much higher rates. Thirty-two different HPV strains were found with an overall prevalence of 26.3% and 24.8% in women without cervical lesions. HPV 16, 31, 35 and 58 were most prevalent. 33.5% women had mixed HPV infection.

Possible causes include poverty-associated factors like early and frequent child bearing, nutritional deficiencies and high prevalence of sexually transmitted diseases. The dominant trend in cervical cancer is a decline in the incidence and mortality from the disease all over the world but this is more marked in the developed countries. Apart from better screening, other contributing factors are improvement in nutrition and genital hygiene, decline in early and frequent childbearing, increasing use of barrier contraception and decrease in the prevalence of sexually transmitted diseases.

There are factors which affect trends in cervical cancer epidemiology. Cancer registrations and death certificates for uterine cancers do not always specify precisely where the cancer is located, and many are reported as 'uterus unspecified'. The diagnostic and coding boundaries between cervical malignancy and cervical intraepithelial neoplasia have altered over the years, particularly as screening reveals many of the early disease stages. Hysterectomy rates influence the number of cervices that may have been affected by early disease. The changes in sexual behaviour with trends of younger age at first intercourse and multiple partners have affected the prevalence of HPV and the disease.

National Screening Programme in the UK started in 1964 and with the re-organisation in the programme in the mid 1980s, cancer mortality showed a decline. The decline has been rapid in the last 30 years in England, Wales and Scotland; however, it is slow in Northern Ireland. Unlike UK, mortality figures have increased in the Irish Republic where cancer screening is yet to become comprehensive (Comber and Gavin 2004).

Ovarian cancer: Ovarian cancer usually produces minimal symptoms and can present in late stages. Epithelial tumours account for 80%–90% of ovarian carcinomas (Baylis et al 1986).

Trends in ovarian cancer mortality over the period 1955–1989 were analysed for 25 European countries (excluding the Soviet Union and a few small countries) on the basis of the official death certification data from the World Health Organization database (La Vecchia et al 1992). The authors observed that overall variation in age-standardised ovarian cancer mortality at all ages had declined appreciably, from over 17-fold during the period 1955–1959 (that is, between 10.5/100,000 in Denmark and 0.6/100,000 in Spain, world standard) to 3.4-fold (that is, between 9.9/100,000 in Denmark and 2.9/100,000 in Spain) in the late 1980s. In another population-based study for germ cell tumours, the 30-year, age-adjusted incidence rate per 100,000 women-years was 0.338, decreasing by 29.4% for dysgerminomas ($p = 0.18$) and by 31.5% for mixed germ cell tumours ($p = 0.22$) (Smith et al 2006).

International trends in mortality and incidence varies between countries and age groups. Trends in most countries show a decline in mortality in women less than 55 years but a rise above 55 years. The incidence however, in younger women has shown little decline. Several risk factors have been identified such as family history of ovarian cancer, reproductive factors such as infertility, early age at menarche and late age at menopause, use of HRT, OC and parity.

Epidemiological trends have been affected by the advancement in both diagnostic and therapeutic technology. Major advances have taken place in the treatment of germ cell tumours that particularly affects younger women. However, most ovarian cancer is of epithelial origin and presents at a late stage in 80% of cases. Some difference in the incidence and mortality may be due to greater detection of less aggressive tumours through better and increased use of ultrasound.

Prostate cancer: This is a cancer of older males. Prostate cancer is rare between the ages of 35 and 45 years. Incidence and mortality from prostate cancer at age 50 years and above has risen. Asymptomatic prostate cancer is common in older men (12% of latent carcinoma) (Breslow et al 1977). A study by Vercelli et al (2000) evaluated the incidence and mortality trends from prostate cancer in EU countries. Incidence rates rose across the period considered, in almost all countries for elderly, middle aged and for younger adults, increasing more rapidly in younger men. Incidence trends showed a less clear geographic pattern than for mortality. The falling trends in mortality from prostate cancer in the US suggest that the trends in Europe should also show a downward trend in the near future.

Histological curettings from Trans-Urethral Resection of Prostate (TURP) leads to incidental diagnosis in a substantial proportion of cases. With rising rates of TURP for benign prostatic hypertrophy more cases are being diagnosed. The introduction of prostate specific antigen screening in 1990 accelerated diagnosis two-fold (Corder et al 1994).

Less is understood about risk factors associated with prostate cancer. Dietary fat consumption and dairy products have been implicated as risk factors but overall evidence is still inconsistent.

Pancreatic cancer: Pancreatic cancer is a cancer of late diagnosis and has a high case-fatality ratio. Smoking is the main risk factor but has a much lower attributable risk than for lung cancer. A study on smoking-related pancreatic cancers in men and women showed both groups to be equally affected (Muscat et al 1997). Compared to never-smokers, the odds ratio (OR) for current cigarette smokers was 1.6 [95% CI, 1.1–2.4] for men and 2.3 (95% CI, 1.4–3.5) for women. Decrease in incidence and mortality from pancreatic cancer is likely to be due to reduction in smoking practices. Difficulty in diagnosis with pancreatic cancer lies in late manifestation of symptoms and the need for histopathological confirmation of diagnosis. With the advance in imaging and cytological techniques like Computed Tomography (CT) and endoscopic retrograde cholagiopancreatography (ERCP) and magnetic resonance imaging (MRI), accurate diagnosis and resectabilty of the tumour can be achieved (Hochwald et al 1999).

Bladder cancer: Incidence and mortality from bladder cancer has shown a downward trend in most parts of the world. Tobacco smoking, exposure to aromatic amines and phenacetin containing analgesics are important factors in its causation. Urolithiasis and repeated urinary infections may cause bladder irritation and predispose one to bladder cancer (Pelucchi et al 2006).

LIVER CANCER: Variable trends in incidence and mortality has been observed in different parts of the world. There has been an increasing trend of primary live cancer in Japan, stabilising and a decreasing trend in Sweden and a definite drop in the incidence in Singapore. A study conducted between 1982–1994 showed the age-standardised incidence was highest in southern Europe (12/100,000 in men and 3/100,000 in women in 1992–94) and lowest in northern Europe, where incidence was similar to that of the United States (3/100,000 in men, <1/100,000 in women) (Capocaccia et al 2007). Increasing incidence in southern Europe is probably related to hepatitis B and C infection and increasing alcohol intake, while improving survival may be due to better surveillance for cirrhosis.

Hepatocellular carcinoma is by far the most common liver cancer. Rates are highest in South East Asia and lowest in the UK. It generally affects more men than women in all registries. Hepatitis B virus (HBV) (Beasley et al 1981) and Hepatitis C Virus (HCV) (Zavitsanos et al 1992) are known predisposing factors. Aflatoxin (International Agency for Research on Cancer 1987), tobacco smoking and alcohol are etiopathogens.

Apparent changes in incidence and mortality are due to revisions in classification, coding, diagnosis and certification and newer modalities of treatment.

COLORECTAL CANCERS: It is a cancer affecting the older age group. It is the second most common cause of cancer death in developed countries. Australia has one of the highest incidence rates in the world. Risk factors include diet (lack of fibre), high body mass index (Sedio et al 2007) and alcohol consumption.

In 1971, Denis Burkitt put forward his hypothesis that a low fibre diet predisposed an individual to colorectal cancer. His observations were derived from his study of western and traditional African communities. He observed that African diets were rich in fibre and low in refined carbohydrates. There have been many studies to date which have been inconclusive. In a large randomised US study, the Polyp Prevention Trial, the effect of increased fibre and reduced fat intakes in the diet was tested. No effects on adenoma recurrence were observed; although the general thought was that the change in dietary intakes in the intervention arm was not substantial (Rock 2007). Other risk factors are occupational asbestos exposure, reduced physical activity, environmental factors and reproductive history. Hereditary disorders like familial adenomatous polyposis, which occurs in 1:10000 to 1: 25000 of the population accounts for 1% of colorectal cancers (Järvinen 1992). It usually presents around the mean age of 40 years. Metabolic phenotype can predispose one to colorectal cancer. Studies show that 'fast' acetylators have an increased risk (Roberts-Thomson et al 1996). Reproductive factors have some association with the occurrence of colorectal cancers and use of OC can lower the risk in women (Lin et al 2007).

Epidemiological trends of cancer of the colon and rectum show rates at younger ages (15–34) have fallen in both sexes with a smaller decrease in older ages. Incidence trends are subject to consequences of screening programmes and classification. Overall mortality rates have fallen and survival rates have improved.

Conclusion: It is interesting to note that with life expectancy going up, there is an expansion of the ageing population. The consequences invariably will be a rise in cancer incidence rates. In the UK alone, the proportion of people over 50 has increased by 45% since 1951 and is projected to increase by a further 36% by the year 2031(Newby et al 2007). However, technological advances in medicine have led to better diagnosis and treatment. Incidence and mortality trends are subject to the influences of lifestyle changes, temporal trends in cancer reporting and public awareness. Public health studies in cancer epidemiology should be encouraged.

Many cancers in the reproductive age group are detected early. Immediate treatment is almost curative which increases the scope for reproductive future for these individuals. There is concern of damage to gametes due to surgery, chemo or radiotherapy. However, sperm preservation and oocyte recovery with in-vitro maturation and freezing prior to cancer treatment (Kelly et al 2003; Oktay et al 2008) has revolutionised the possibility of the affected individuals having children.

References

Alexander DD, PJ Mink, HO Adami et al. 2007. The non Hodgkin's lymphomas: A review of the epidemiologic literature. *Int J Cancer* 120 Suppl 12:1–39.

Anderson WF, MD Althuis, LA Brinton, SS Devesa. 2004. Is male breast cancer similar or different than female breast cancer? *Breast Cancer Res Treat* 83:77–86.

Arbyn M, A Raifu, P Autier and J Ferlay. 2007. Burden of cervical cancer in Europe: Estimates for 2004. *Ann Oncol* 18(10):1708–1715.

Barzilay J, GJ Heatley and GW Cushing. 1991. Benign and malignant tumors in patients with acromegaly. *Arch Intern Med* 151(8):1629–1632.

Baylis MS, WJ Henderson, CG Pierrepoint and K Griffiths. 1986. The aetiology of ovarian cancer. In: Morrow CP and Smart GE (eds). *Gynaecological Oncology*. Springer-Verlag, Heidelberg.

Beasley RP, LY Hwang, CC Lin and CS Chien. 1981. Hepatocellular carcinoma and hepatitis B virus. A prospective study of 22707 men in Taiwan. *Lancet* 2(8256):1129–1133.

Benshushan A and A Brzenzinski. 2002. Hormonal manipulations and breast cancer. *Obstet Gynecol Surv* 57: 314–323.

Beral V. 2003. Million Women Study Collaborators. Breast cancer and hormone-replacement therapy in the Million Women Study. *Lancet* 9; 362(9382): 419–427.

Breslow N, CW Chan, G Dhom, RA Drury et al. 1977. Latent carcinoma of prostate at autopsy in seven areas. The International Agency for Research on Cancer, Lyons, France. *Int J Cancer.* 20(5): 680–688.

Brinton LA. 1997. Hormone Replacement therapy and risk for breast cancer. *Endocrinol Metab Clin North Am* 26: 361–378.

Cancer Research Statistics. Mortality http://info.cancerresearchuk.org/cancerstats/mortality/ accessed 24th July 2007.

Capocaccia R, M Sant, F Berrino et al. 2007. Hepatocellular Carcinoma: Trends of Incidence and Survival in Europe and the United States at the end of the 20th Century. *Am J Gastroenterol* (Epub ahead of print).

Clemmensen J. 1955. The Danish Cancer Registry, under the National Anti-Cancer League. *Danish Medical Bulletin* 2: 124.

Collaborative Group on Hormonal Factors in Breast Cancer and Hormone Replacement Therapy. 1997. Combined reanalysis of 51 epidemiologic studies involving 52,705 women with breast cancer and 108,411 women without breast cancer. *Lancet* 350: 1947–1959.

Comber H and A Gavin. 2004. Recent trends in cervical cancer mortality in Britain and Ireland: The case for population-based cervical cancer screening. *Br J Cancer* 91(11): 1902–1904.

Corder EH, CG Chute, HA Guess et al. 1994. Prostate cancer in Rochester, Minnesota (USA), from 1935 to 1989: Increases in incidence related to more complete ascertainment. *Cancer Control* 5(3):207–214.

Coyle YM, AT Minahjuddin, LS Hynan, JD Minna. 2006. An ecological study of the association of metal air pollutants with lung cancer incidence in Texas. *J Thorac Oncol* 1(7): 654–661.

Doll R and AB Hill. 1950. A study of the etiology of the carcinoma of the lung. *British Medical Journal* ii: 740–748.

Doll R, P Payne and J Waterhouse.1966. *Cancer Incidence in Five Continents: A Technical Report*, Springer-Verlag, New York.

Dorn HF. 1944. Illness from cancer in the United States. *Public Health Reports*, 59; 35–48, 65–77, 97–115. US Department of Health, Education, and Welfare, Washington DC.

Filipovich AH, A Mathur, D Kamat and RS Shapiro. 1992. Primary immunodefeciencies: Genetic risk factors for lymphoma. *Cancer Research* 52:5465s–5467s.

Garcia-Closas M, N Malats, FX Real et al. 2006. Influence of common genetic variation in the Nucleotide Excision Repair (NER): Thought to protect damage from carcinogens in tobacco smoke. *Cancer Epidemiol Biomarkers Prev* 15:536–542.

Ghadirian P, P Maisonneuve, C Perret, et al. 1998. Epidemiology of sociodemographic characteristics, lifestyle, medical history, and colon cancer: A case-control study among French Canadians in Montreal. *Cancer Detect Prev.* 22:396–404.

Glattre E, T Haldorsen, JP Berg et al. 1993. Norwegian case-control study testing the hypothesis that seafood increases the risk of thyroid cancer. *Cancer Causes and Control* 4: 11–16.

Guo J, E Pukkala, P Kyyrönen et al. 2005. Testicular cancer, occupation and exposure to chemical agents among Finnish men in 1971–1995. *Cancer Causes Control* 16(2): 97–103.

Hochwald SN, NM Rofsky, Dobryansky et al. 1999. Magnetic resonance imaging with magnetic resonance cholangiopancraetography accurately predicts resectability of pancreatic carcinoma. *J Gastrointest Surg* 3(5):506–511.

International Agency for Research on Cancer. 1987. Overall Evaluations of Carcinogenicity: An updating of IARC Monographs 1-42 International agency for research on cancer monographs on evaluation of carcinogenic risks to humans. Supplement 7, 96–99, 272–309.

Järvinen HJ. 1992. Epidemiology of familial adenomatous polyposis in Finland: Impact of family screening on the colorectal cancer rate and survival. *Gut* 33(3):357–360.

Jensen OM. 1984. Different age and sex relationship for cancer of subsites of the large bowel. *British Journal of Cancer* 50:825–829.

Kazakov VS, EP Demidchik and LN Astakhova. 1992. Thyroid cancer after Chernobyl. *Nature* 359: 21–22.

Kelly SM, WM Buckett, AK Abdul-Jalil and SL Tan. 2003.The cryobiology of assisted reproduction. *Minerva Ginecol* 55:389–398.

Key TJA and MC Pike. 1988. The role of oestrogens and progestagens in the epidemiology and prevention of breast cancer. *Eur J Cancer Clin Oncol* 24:29–43.

La Vecchia C, F Levi, F Lucchini, E Negri and S Franceshi. 1992. Descriptive epidemiology of ovarian cancer in Europe. *Gynecol Oncol* 46(2):208–215.

Li LK, M Dai, GM Clifford et al. 2006. Human Papilloma Virus infection in Shenyang City, People's Republic of China. A population based study. *Br J Cancer* 95(11):1593–1597.

Lin J, SM Zhang, NR Cook et al. *2007*. Oral contraceptives, reproductive factors, and risk of colorectal cancer among women in a prospective cohort study. *Am J Epidemiol* 165(7):794–801.

Lubin JH and NE Caporaso. 2006. Cigarette smoking and lung cancer: Modelling total exposure and intensity. *Cancer Epidemiol Biomarkers Prev* 15(3): 517–523.

MacMahon B. 1957. Epidemiological evidence on the nature of Hodgkin's disease. *Cancer* 10:1045–1054.

McMichael AJ and JD Potter. 1980. Reproduction, endogenous and exogenous sex hormones and colon cancer: A review and hypothesis. *J Nat Cancer Inst* 65:1201–1207.

Molho-Pessach V and M Lotem. 2007. Ultraviolet radiation and cutaneous carcinogenesis. *Curr Prob Dermatol* 35:14–27.

Muscat JE, SD Stellman, D Hoffmann and EL Wynder. 1997. Smoking and pancreatic cancer in men and women. *Cancer Epidemiol Biomarkers Prev* 6(1):15–19.

Newby JA, CC Bushby, CV Howard and MJ Platt. 2007. The cancer incidence temporality index: An index to show temporal changes in the age of onset of overall and specific cancer (England and Wales, 1971-1999). *Biomed Pharmacother*; 61(10):623–630.

Oktay K, E Demirtas, WY Son et al. 2008. In vitro maturation of germinal vesicle oocytes recovered after premature leutinizing hormone surge: Description of a novel approach to fertility preservation. *Fertil Steril* 89(1):228.e19–22.

Pelucchi C, C Bosetti, E Negri et al. 2006. Mechanisms of disesase: The epidemiology of bladder cancer. *Nat Clin Prac Urol* 3(6):327–340.

Percy C and CS Muir. 1989.The international comparability of cancer mortality data: Results of an international death certificate study. *Am J Epidemiol* 129; 934–946.

Roberts-Thomson IC, P Ryan, KK Khoo. 1996. Diet, acetylator phenotype, and risk of colorectal neoplasia. *Lancet* 347(9012):1372–1374.

Rock CL. 2007. Primary dietary prevention: Is the fiber story over? Recent Results *Cancer Res*. 174:171–177.

Ronckers CM, P McCarron, E Ron. 2005. Thyroid cancer and multiple primary tumors in the SEER cancer registries. *Int J Cancer* 117(2):28128-8.

Sedio RL, T Byers, TR Levin et al. 2007. Change in body size and the risk of colorectal adenomas. *Epidemiol Biomarkers Prev* 16(3): 526–531.

Segi M. 1960. *Cancer Mortality for Selected Sites in 24 Countries (1950-57)*, Department of Public Health, Tohoku University School of Medicine, Sendai, Japan.

Smith HO, M Berwick, CF Verschraegen, C Wiggins et al. 2006. Incidence and survival rates for female malignant germ cell tumours. *Obstet Gynecol* 10(5):1075–10785.

Spicer DV and MC Pike. 1994. Epidemiology of breast cancer: In Lobo RA., ed. *Treatment of the postmenopausal woman: basic and clinical aspects*. New York: Raven Press.

Stanford JL and DB Thomas. 1993. Exogenous progestins and breast cancer. *Epidemiol Rev* 15:98–107.

Stocks P. 1936. Distribution in England and Wales of cancer of various organs.*13th Annual Report of the British Empire Cancer Campaign,* pp 240–280.

Swerdlow AJ and RG Skeet. 1988. Occupational associations of testicular cancer in South East England. *Brit J Ind Med* 45:225–230.

Thomas JO, R Herrero, AA Omigbodun et al. 2004. Prevalence of papilloma virus infection in women in Ibadan, Nigeria: A population based study. *Br J Cancer* 90(3):638–645.
Towler B, L Irwig, P Glasziou, et al. 1998. A systematic review of the effects of screening for colorectal cancer using the faecal occult blood test, hemoccult. *Br Med J* 317:559–565
Uauy R and N Solomons. 2005. Diet, nutrition and the life-course approach to cancer prevention. *J Nutr.* 135:2934s--2945s.
Ulcickas Yood M, CP Queensberry, D Guo *et al*, 2007. Incidence of non-Hodgkin's lymphoma among individuals with chronic hepatitis B virus infection. *Hepatology.* 46(1):107–112.
United Kingdom Testicular Cancer Study Group. 1994. Aetiology of testicular cancer: Association with congenital abnormalities, age at puberty, infertility, and exercise. *Br Med J* 308(6941):1393–1399.
Vercelli M, A Quaglia, E Marani, S Parodi. 2000. Prostate cancer incidence and mortality trends among elderly and adult Europeans. *Crit Rev Oncol Hematol* 35(2):133–144.
Wiseman RA. 2000. Breast cancer hypothesis: a single cause for the majority of cases. *J Epidemiol Comm Health* 54:851–858.
Wiseman RA. 2004. Breast Cancer: Critical data analysis concludes that estrogens are not the cause; however lifestyle changes can alter risk rapidly. *J Clin Epidemiol* 57:766–772.
Wu-Williams AH and JM Samet. 1994. Lung cancer and cigarette smoking In Samet JM (ed). *Epidemiology of Lung Cancer,* chapter 4 New York: Marcel Dekker Inc. 71–107
Zavitsanos X, A Hatzakis, E Kaklamani et al. 1992. Association between hepatitis C virus and hepatocellular carcinoma using assays based on structural and non-structural hepatitis C virus peptides. *Cancer Res* 52(19):5364–5367.

13

Hormone Replacement Therapy in Menopausal Women

Usha Krishna | Ajita Mandlekar

Hormone replacement therapy (HRT) is an important issue in the care of menopausal women especially for symptomatic women suffering from hot flushes, night sweats, insomia, fatigue and irritability as well as urogenital problems such as vulvovaginal infections and recurrent urinary infections. With increasing female life expectancy and heightened health awareness, it is necessary to have a holistic approach to health where medicines along with social and psychological support, physical exercise and appropriate lifestyle are important as the problems of menopause are complex and multi-dimensional.

With ageing, there is progressive loss of functional capacity due to senile changes. The ageing cells have poor capacity for nutrient uptake and repair of chromosomal damage. The decline of sex hormones as well as growth hormones has an effect on the reproductive and urogenital systems as well as on the skin, cardiovascular and nervous systems. Estrogen deprivation leads to atrophy of the vulva and vagina and the uterus as well as pelvic cellular tissue. Besides, deficiency of estrogen can lead to decrease in bone density, osteoporosis and increased risk of fractures. Although short-term use of HRT for relief of menopausal symptoms improves quality of life, the decision to continue HRT over a long period needs careful consideration of risks and benefits.

COMMON MENOPAUSAL PROBLEMS

Perimenopause is a period of transition, between 45 and 55 years, when decreased ovarian function leads to decreased estrogen levels. Studies comparing the relative frequency of climacteric symptoms reveal that Indian women seem to have a higher incidence of urogenital problems whereas women from the West have higher incidence of hot flushes, insomnia, depression and irritability (Table 13.1).

We note that a larger proportion of women attending the private clinics report climacteric symptoms compared to those attending general hospitals, as awareness and consciousness regarding menopause and stress are higher in the educated affluent group.

Examination and investigations: The diagnosis of estrogen deficiency is established by relevant history; a checklist approach helps to obtain detailed information about the previous therapy. Past as well as present medical problems should be recorded. It

TABLE 13.1: RELATIVE FREQUENCY OF CLIMACTERIC SYMPTOMS

Symptoms	*Indian Incidence**		*Western Average*
	Anklesaria	*Krishna*	*Studd and Barber*
Hot flushes	30%	33%	75%
Urinary complaints	74%	35%	20%
Vaginal symptoms	56%	50%	20%
Joint/muscle pain	20%	25%	48%
Psychological	36%	20%	92%
Insomnia	20%	10%	51%

*Due to an overlap of symptoms, the total of percentage exceeds 100.
(Adapted from Anklesaria 1995; Krishna 1996; Studd and Barber 1992)

is essential that perimenopausal women are checked for hypertension, diabetes and coronary insufficiency. Physical examination should include assessment of cardiovascular and respiratory systems and examination of the breasts. Thorough abdominal and pelvic examination is mandatory. A cervical smear will help screen for cervical pathological changes and lateral vaginal smear to determine the maturation index. Mammography is recommended especially in high-risk patients with family history of breast cancer or past history of breast disease. Ultrasonography is carried out to assess the ovarian size and volume as well as uterine and endometrial pathology. Hormone profiles are seldom necessary for diagnosis except when premature ovarian failure is suspected. Coagulation studies are necessary in women with previous deep vein thrombosis and pulmonary embolism. The lipid profile is helpful in planning diet and treatment of elderly women. Of late, there are elderly women's clinics, which offer ancillary services for dietary guidance, health education and group therapy programmes.

UROGENITAL PROBLEMS

These problems may be due to atrophy of the urogenital tract or loss of collagen from connective tissue. The symptoms are not self-limiting and tend to increase with time after menopause. About 10% of women complain of symptoms within three years of menopause which increases to 50% within eight years. There may be one or two significant problems related to lower urogenital atrophy even 20 years after menopause. Such patients are provided HRT till symptoms are alleviated; thereafter, the dose is tapered down or local vaginal estrogen cream recommended.

The problem associated with loss of collagen from connective tissue of the urogenital system include urinary incontinence, which may be urge incontinence in about 45%, stress incontinence in about 25% and mixed incontinence in about 30%. Urogenital prolapse is also noted after menopause, especially in women with genital tract injury during childbirth. HRT provides an effective treatment for urogenital problems as improvement is seen in one or two weeks; long-term therapy under closed monitoring is justified in some cases. Systemic HRT and local estrogen vaginal creams help to some extent in alleviating nocturia, dysuria and frequency. Patients with vaginal dryness, itching, irritation, dyspareunia and recurrent urinary infection show visible benefit. Local estrogen cream is advised for women unwilling to use systemic HRT or who cannot use it for medical reasons.

A study by Bachmann (1993) showed that of 329 healthy non-clinic attending women, aged between 18 and 73 years, over 50% of postmenopausal women reported a problematic lack of vaginal lubrication and frequent vaginal infections. An increasing number of studies show that even very low-dose estrogen therapy is effective against the characteristic vaginal symptoms of urogenital ageing.

The authors studied urogenital problems of 450 menopausal women in their clinic. The average age of natural menopause was 48.3 years: 35% had mainly urinary complaints and 50% had vulvovaginal problems. Of 308 women who required HRT, 39.93% continued the therapy satisfactorily: 11% had excellent relief, 71% good relief, 14% moderate relief and 4% could not give conclusive answers or had no relief (Krishna and Mandlekar 1998).

Vasomotor Symptoms

The hot flash is a sensation of intense heat felt on the face, arms and the upper body. This is followed by hot flush and profuse sweating, accompanied by palpitation, vertigo and anxiety due to vasomotor instability. Vasodilatation leads to flushing of the skin and elevation of luteinsing hormone which occurs about 9 minutes after initial increase in temperature. About 50%–70% of postmenopausal women have hot flushes. In 20%–25% symptoms persist for at least 5 years. Although the symptoms may appear trivial, hot flushes, insomnia, irritability and lethargy are sources of great discomfort. Oral HRT is highly effective in alleviating hot flushes and night sweats. Following the reduction of hot flushes and night sweating, insomnia is frequently improved, resulting in restored mood, functions and concentration.

HORMONE REPLACEMENT THERAPY

Hormone replacement therapy has to be individualised as the lifestyles and attitudes as well as the menopausal problems differ among women. No single product or regimen can be prescribed for all women and there are therapeutic choices that clinicians can offer. Pretreatment assessment and counselling are very essential. Encouraging optimum physical and mental fitness and providing ancillary services, health education and group therapy programmes are very useful. HRT can be administered by oral and non-oral routes and the choice of therapy depends on several factors such as age, symptomatology, presence of uterus and the purpose of the therapy. Treatment should be planned for about a year or less at a time, and tailored to the woman's needs. Hypertension and hyperlipidemia are not considered contraindications. Therapy should be withheld in patients with undiagnosed uterine bleeding and recent liver disease. Perimenopausal pregnancy though rare is possible and is of course a contraindication.

Therapies

HRT is used in various formulations, combinations, routes and duration of therapy and there are therapeutic choices that clinicians can offer to patients. Pre-treatment assessment and counselling is most essential.

Only estrogens: For many post-menopausal women who have undergone hysterectomy, daily estrogens are the preferred method of delivering HRT. The addition of progesterone is not necessary since the need for endometrial protection does not exist. This does not apply to patients who have undergone endometrial ablation since there may be endometrial glands which remain after surgery. In cases with severe progesterone intolerance, unopposed estrogens may be given for a short period in non-hysterectomised women. Transvaginal sonography to check for endometrial thickness and endometrial aspiration or biopsy and histopathology of the endometrium may be necessary. Estrogens have few side effects; weight gain, breast tenderness and nausea may occur and dosage may be reduced if the symptoms persist. In patients with fibromyomas, endometriosis or endometrial hyperplasia with irregular bleeding, removal of the uterus allows safe HRT use with no withdrawal bleeding. If bilateral oophorectomy has been performed, it must be followed by estrogen replacement therapy to avoid severe menopausal symptoms.

Cyclic estrogen–progesterone: This regimen is used frequently in postmenopausal women with intact uterus. Estrogen corrects the genitourinary and vasomotor disturbances and prevents osteoporosis and progestogen protects the endometrium from development of hyperplasia. Unopposed estrogens increase the risk of carcinoma of the endometrium. The progestogens are administered for 7 to 10 days or more. No hyperplasia was reported, when progestogens were used for 10 days or more. Based on a Medline search, Archer et al (1994) concluded that progestogens should be administered for 14 days per cycle. Besides, three weeks of treatment with norethisterone (5 mg) each month will reverse hyperplasia and 50% of the atypical changes. Cyclic estrogen and progestogen causes vaginal bleeding in about 50% of women. Though the bleeding is not heavy, it leads to poor compliance. Besides, progestogens cause symptoms similar to those in premenstrual syndrome—breast tenderness, bloatedness, nausea, edema, etc. Psychological complaints include depression, anxiety and irritability.

Continuous estrogen–progestogen: Since withdrawal bleeding is unacceptable to many patients, combined continuous regimens may improve the compliance and avoids withdrawal bleeding in a majority of cases. Studies by the Women's Health Initiatives (WHI 2002) are not particularly supportive of this treatment, as discussed later in this chapter.

Only progestogens: When estrogens are contraindicated, high doses of progestogens may be given. It acts on the hypothalamus to lower serum gonadotrophins and thus may control the vasomotor symptoms. Monthly injections of depot medroxy progesterone acetate (DMPA) provide reasonable relief with 50 mg dose, and significant relief with 100 mg or 150 mg, though the side effects are not entirely avoidable.

Estrogen–androgen: Androgens reduce vasomotor flushes and in women in whom estrogen therapy alone does not have sufficient benefits, testosterone may be added for a short duration. Preoperative short-term estrogen androgen therapy may improve the vaginal mucosa in women with atrophic vaginitis who have to undergo surgery for prolapse.

Formulations

Conjugated estrogens: These (e.g. Premarin) are a mixture of natural estrogens. The tablets are absorbed well orally and have a half-life of 12 hours. They relieve vasomotor and urogenital symptoms within a week and a daily dose of 0.625 mg also arrests bone loss in the majority of the cases. A lower dose may be used when HRT is required for longer periods. Vaginal application of conjugated estrogens is used for treating atrophic vaginitis and kraurosis valvae as it restores the vaginal cytology.

Estriol: (Evalon) is a natural estrogen, which is rapidly absorbed and achieves peak plasma level within an hour. It is administered as a dose of 2 mg per day for a few weeks and then a maintenance dose of 1 mg. Being short-acting with a short retention time in the nuclei of endometrial cells, no endometrial proliferation occurs at the recommended doses. Vaginal application of estriol cream also has satisfactory results..

Estradiol: One of the most potent estrogens available, 17β-estradiol, Progynova (estradiol valerate), is administered in a dosage of 1 or 2 mg cyclically and is titrated to a minimum effective dose. Continuous preparation using estrogens, progestogens in fixed dose are also available to avoid bleeding.

The authors studied the effectiveness of estradiol for vasomotor and urogenital problems in 75 patients for 18 months, in women between 40 to 55 years. The 24 hysterectomised women received estradiol valerate in 2 mg dose for 21 days with a 7 days break. All the women completed the study and were very satisfied. The rest had continuous combined estradiol valerate with norethisterone for 28 days, or sequential 21 days of estradiol valerate and 10 days of norethindrone. Eleven patients could not complete the study, and 78% were satisfied. There were 8 patients with premature ovarian failure who continued the treatment beyond 18 months with good compliance (unpublished).

Routes Of Administration

Besides the oral route, there are other routes with some benefits.

Transdermal delivery: Transdermal delivery by a skin patch (Estraderm TTS) has a sustained delivery of low dose estradiol controlled by rate limiting membrane covered by an adhesive that forms the skin of the patch. These are available in three doses delivering 25 μg, 50 μg and 100 μg per 24 hours. This method was particularly useful in women suffering from hypertriglyceidemia, hepatobiliary disorders, venous thrombosis and hypertension. It is an effective method but has not become popular in India. Skin reaction and local skin irritation with itching and redness are not uncommon.

Percutaneous gel: Percutaneous gel (Sandrena, Oestrogel) applications are convenient and are particularly suitable for women living in warm climates who wish to use the transdermal route. A metered dose has been developed in the form of sachets or measurement system. Cyclic progestogens are an essential adjunct to transdermal therapy in non-hysterectomised women.

Vaginal rings: These rings incorporating hormones have also been developed but are not used commonly.

Subcutaneous implants: The effectiveness of estradiol implants for HRT is well established (Magos and Studd 1990). The menopausal replacement dose with estradiol implants is 50 mg every six months. Testosterone implants (100 mg) may be used as adjuncts to estradiol therapy for associated psychosexual problems. Cyclic progestogen therapy is indicated in women with intact uteri. Though it has excellent bone protection effects, the incidence of breast cancer is considered higher with implants.

Intrauterine devices: Levonorgestrel intrauterine device (Mirena) releases 20 μg of the hormone over 24 hours. It has a local effect on the endometrium and is useful not only as contraceptive but also to control perimenopausal bleeding when used along with 2 mg of oral estradiol valerate for HRT. The levonorgestrel controls the endometrial proliferation and avoids erratic bleeding induced by estrogens (Anderson et al 1992).

The authors have used levonorgestrel IUCD in perimenopausal DUB in 59 cases. Of these, results of 20 patients were published (Krishna and Mandlekar 2002). After initial spotting and irregular bleeding for the first 3 months, 15 of them were satisfied with amenorrhea or scanty menstrual periods. The patients selected after 2002 had similar satisfactory results.

Tibolone: This is a 19-nortestosterone, a gonadomimetic preparation, which improves most of the menopausal symptoms, including mood and libido without inducing vaginal bleeding in most cases. The endogenic opioids (beta endorphins) come to premenopausal levels and prevent vasomotor and psychogenic symptoms as well as relieve urogenital problems. It has been given to prevent osteoporosis without endometrial stimulation (Greusens et al 1991)—there was an 8% increase in bone density two years after treatment compared to 2% annual bone loss in control cases. Its androgenic activity is too mild to cause acne, hirsutism or voice change. The combination of weak estrogenic, androgenic and progestogenic activity has satisfactory outcome and the effects on lipid metabolism are considered favourable. The daily dose is 2.5 mg and apart from improvement of vasomotor and psychogenic problems, there is definite improvement in vaginal cytology reducing dyspareunia and vulvovaginitis. As it is a tissue specific drug, it offers a special advantage by decreasing breast density.

The authors studied 70 patients enrolled on tibolone in their clinic (Krishna and Mandlekar 1997)—59 patients completed three cycles or more and 11 patients discontinued the treatment. Two of them had no relief and 2 had breakthrough bleeding; others discontinued medication for non-medical reasons. Thirty patients had excellent relief of urogenital and vasomotor symptoms, 10 had very good relief and 19 had satisfactorily relief.

Long-term HRT

Osteoporosis is a major health problem due to increasing life expectancy. It is characterised by age related reduction in bone mass, which compromises the mechanical competence of the skeleton to such an extent that even minimal trauma may result in fracture. The incidence is high in India due to nutritional, Vitamin D and calcium deficiency and the fractures are said to occur 10 to 20 years earlier in India compared to the West. Women of thin stature or having premature menopause, those with a sedentary lifestyle and with thyrotoxicosis, and those on steroids and using tobacco are more susceptible. Assessment of bone density by DEXA (dual energy x-ray absorptiometry) should be done in high-risk cases. HRT plays a definite role in preserving bone health, and decreases the hazard of a fracture, especially in women with premature, natural or surgical menopause. The basis of preventive therapy lies in correction of risk factors and effects of HRT on preservation of bone mineral density. It has been proved beyond doubt that long-term HRT prevents postmenopausal bone loss from both peripheral and axial sites of the skeleton. Bone resorption may be effectively reduced and bone mineral density maintained even by 1 mg of estradiol valerate. Marslew et al (1992) reported that 2 mg estradiol valerate given continuously or sequentially over 2 years, increased bone mineral density in the spine by 3%–4%. In the same study, biochemical estimates of bone turnover (serum alkaline phosphatase and fasting urinary calcium/creatinine) decreased significantly to premenopausal levels in the HRT groups, but remained unchanged in the placebo group. Data from many observational studies and clinical trials (Lutkin et al 1992) show that estrogen reduces the risk of hip fracture by about 30% and of spine fracture by about 50%.

From the authors' clinic, 206 women in the age group of 30 to 80 years were evaluated for bone mineral density (BMD) by DEXA for detection of osteoporosis: 48% of women were frankly osteoporotic, 39% were osteopenic and only 13% had normal bone density. The bone mineral density decreased with advancing age. There was a definite improvement in BMD in women who were on HRT and the improvement in bone density continued with the increased duration of HRT. However, it is essential to weigh the benefits against possible adverse effects of long term HRT (Krishna and Mehta 2000).

HRT AND BREAST CANCER

In earlier epidemiological studies of HRT-related risk of breast cancer, an RR of 1.1 was ascribed to all estrogen use, suggesting a 10% increase in risk relative to no estrogen use. Several meta-analyses have suggested either no significantly increased risk (that is, RR ~ 1.0) or a risk as high as 1.6 (Steinberg et al 1994).

Women's Health Initiative Study: This Study (2002) focused on defining the risks and benefits of strategies that could potentially influence the incidence of heart disease, breast and colorectal cancer, and fractures in postmenopausal women. This multicenter, randomised, placebo controlled, primary prevention trial enrolled 16,608 postmenopausal women aged 50 to 79 years with an intact uterus at baseline. The participants received conjugated equine estrogens (CEE), 0.625 mg/day, plus medroxyprogesterone acetate, 2.5 mg/day or placebo. Although the study had a planned duration of 8.5 years, the combination HRT arm was discontinued after a median follow-up period of 5.2 years. It was found that risks exceeded benefits. Mortality was not increased, but the risk of adverse events was significantly increased. Most adverse outcomes occurred within one to two years, except for breast cancer risk, which was not increased until four years. They reported that for every 10,000 women taking HRT for one year there would be an additional eight cases of invasive breast cancer, seven heart attacks, eight strokes and eight patients with pulmonary embolism. However, there would be six fewer bowel cancers and five fewer hip fractures. In the light of these findings, there is great apprehension regarding the use of HRT, especially combination HRT. The ERT arm in hysterectomised women has not shown a similar increase in breast cancer risk.

It is important to note that in the WHI study, two-thirds of the patients were above 60 years of age when the risk of breast cancer is already high. Second, in this study only one type of estrogen (CEE) was used and therefore the results cannot be extrapolated to other forms of estrogen and HRT. Significantly, this trial could not distinguish the effects of estrogen from those of progestin. The effects of progestin may be important for breast cancer and atherosclerotic diseases, including CHD and stroke. Addition of progestins may increase risk above that observed with estrogen alone, as mitotic activity in the breast during normal menstrual cycles is greatest when progesterone levels are highest However, breast cancer diagnosed in women who had ever used HRT, tend to be less advanced clinically than those diagnosed in never users. The increase in CHD may reflect prothrombotic and pro-inflammatory effects of progestins that outweigh any effects of estrogens on atherogenesis and vasodilatation. The WHI study did not include the most beneficial effects of HRT on vasomotor and urogenital problems in the overall benefit/ risk ratio evaluation.

Million Women Study: A cohort study of British women aged 50–64 years, the Million Women Study (2003) was set up chiefly to investigate the relation between various patterns of use of HRT and breast cancer incidence and mortality. The results are based on the follow-up of 1,084,110 women recruited between 1996 and 2001, who had not been registered as having had cancer before they joined the study. The average age of the women at recruitment was 55.9 years, and the average period of follow-up was 2.6 years for analyses of the cancer incidence and 4.1 years for analyses of mortality. During the follow-up period, there were 9364 cases of invasive breast cancers and 637 deaths from breast cancer as notified by the National Health Service Central Registers. For the women who died from breast cancer, the average time between diagnosis and death was 1.7 years. The magnitude of the relative risk of breast cancer was substantially greater in users of oestrogen–progestagen combinations than in other preparations. The relative risk of breast cancer in current users at baseline increased with increasing total duration of use of HRT. The results from the Million Women Study suggest little or no overall increase in the relative risk of breast cancer in past users of HRT. These findings are broadly in line with results from previous studies that had suggested that the effects of current use of HRT on the risk of breast cancer wore off largely, if not wholly, within 5 years of stopping use of HRT (MWS Collaborators 2003).

Study participants were more likely to report HRT use than the general population, and the ratio of current to previous users strongly suggests over-representation of women on long-term therapy. Since all patients recruited to the MWS were screened for breast cancer, their chances of being diagnosed with the disease were, overall, higher than those of the general population.

Such differences could be important, since the mean duration of follow-up was only 2.6 years, before most participants had attended for their next screening mammogram. Ascertainment bias might account in part for the observed increase in risk among HRT users, despite the potential adverse effect of HRT on sensitivity of mammographic screening (Chlebowski 2003).

Heart and Estrogen/Progestin Replacement Study (HERS): This too was a blinded, randomised controlled trial comparing the same regimen of estrogen plus progestin with placebo among women with intact uterus. However, in HERS, all 2763 participating women had documented CHD prior to randomisation. The HERS findings showed no overall effect on CHD but an apparent increased risk in the first year after randomisation (Grady et al 1992). It was speculated that any early adverse effect of hormones on CHD incidence was confined to women who have experienced prior CHD events (Grodstein et al 2001).

The **Iowa Women's Health Study** prospectively followed a cohort of women. After 6 years of follow-up, a statistically significant increase in the risk of breast cancer could not be detected in ever-users or current users of hormone therapy (Folsom et al 1995). Certainly the risk of breast cancer is not appreciably increased during the first four years, so women wishing to take this therapy for short-term relief of menopausal symptoms should be reassured (Stevenson and Whitehead 2002).

HRT AND LIPIDS

Within six months of the cessation of menstrual bleeding there is increase in serum concentrations of total cholesterol, low density lipoprotein (LDL) cholesterol, and triglycerides, with a gradual fall in the high density lipoprotein (HDL) cholesterol concentration. With the exception of triglycerides, this atherogenic profile is reversed by treatment with estrogens, with natural estrogens producing a more favourable response than ethinyl estradiol (Jensen 1992). In the WHI study, blood lipid levels showed greater reductions in LDL cholesterol and increases in HDL cholesterol and triglycerides with estrogen plus progestin relative to placebo, consistent with HERS and PEPI (Postmenopausal Estrogen/Progestin Intervention Trial) (Writing Group for PEPI Trial 2002).

Other effects of ERT: Six of 11 observational studies found that estrogen reduces the risk of colon cancer (Newcomb 1995). A meta-analysis of 10 observational studies showed significant protection from Alzheimer's dementia (Yaffe 1998). There may be some benefit in prevention of osteoarthritis, diabetes and Parkinson's disease, and in oral health, colon cancer and age related macular degeneration cataracts.

ALTERNATIVE THERAPIES

Phytoestrogens: These are important alternatives to HRT, though the extent of relief of menopausal symptoms is more effective with HRT. Phytoestrogens exert estrogenic and anti-estrogenic effects due to the similarity in the structure. Certain foods of plant origin such as soybeans have shown definite health benefits in cardiovascular disease, prevention of osteoporosis and even decreased risk of cancer. Of the five major classes of phytoestrogens, isoflavones are the most important. Though they appear to have a promising role, large clinical trials are required before evidence-based recommendations can be made.

The authors conducted a pilot study for 70 perimenopausal women to assess the efficacy of phytoestrogens on menopausal symptoms. Of 23 women, 17 were relieved of urogenital symptoms, and 9 of 11 were relieved from vasomotor symptoms. One patient who had severe hot flushes had no relief and required HRT. There was a feeling of well-being in most of the patients and tiredness and muscular pain decreased. There was no weight gain, no change in hemogram, blood sugar levels and lipid profile as well as liver function test. There was no change in vaginal cytology and maturation index (MI). There were no serious side effects (Krishna and Mandlekar 2005).

Bisphosphonates: Alendronate and Risedronate increase BMD at the spine and hip and reduce the risk of vertebral and non-vertebral fractures. Daily or once a week dosage have shown similar efficacy. The drug is available as Osteophos 70 or Risofoss 35. Bisphosphonates act by inhibiting bone resorption and conserving the bone even in established osteoporosis.

Selective estrogen receptor modulators (SERMS): These are synthetic compounds that have estrogen-like effects on bones and anti-estrogenic effect on breast and endometrium, thus preventing endometrial stimulation and bleeding. They may provide additional benefits such as possible reduction in incidence of breast cancer and cardiovascular risk. Benzothiophene (raloxifen) 60 mg per day is used for prevention and management of osteoporosis. Hot flushes, vaginal dryness and nausea are fairly common side effects.

Calcitonin: Nasal calcitonin spray (100 to 200 U/day) has been approved for prevention of osteoporosis. It is less effective than bisphosphonates and SERMS but has analgesic properties. It helps in preventing bone resorption. It is an expensive drug and is administered by intramuscular or subcutaneous injection or intranasal spray.

None of these alternative therapies are effective in controlling urogenital and vasomotor symptoms. Along with the drugs, a balanced diet, adequate intake of calcium, moderate exercise and change in lifestyle are beneficial.

To sum up, hormone replacement therapy has a definite place in the management of menopausal women and certainly relieves common menopausal problems such as vasomotor symptoms and urogenital problems. The gynecologist should prescribe for each patient a suitable appropriate preparation, dose, route and duration of therapy. However, it is necessary to monitor these patients to prevent complications. Understanding of the therapy and compliance are necessary on the part of the patient. Adequate counselling on the part of the doctor, positive attitude of the woman and emotional support from the family along with general physical fitness are essential to keep menopausal women in optimum health.

References

Andersson K, LA Mattsson, G Rybo and E Stadberg. 1992. Intrauterine release of levonorgestrel: A new way of adding progestogen in hormone replacement therapy. *Obstet Gynaecol* 79:963–967.

Anklesaria BS and RM Soneji. 1996. The climacteric. In *Menopause*. Ed Usha R Krishna and Duru Shah. Chennai: Orient Longman.

Archer DF, JH Pickar and F Bottiglioni. 1994. Bleeding patterns in postmenopausal women taking continuous, combined or sequential regimens of conjugated estrogens with medroxyprogesterone acetate. *Obstet Gynaecol* 83:686–692.

Bachmann GA. 1993. *J Am Geriatr Society* 4; 1:426–436.

Chlebowski RT, SL Hendrix, RD Langer et al. 2003. Influence of estrogen plus progestin on breast cancer and mammography in healthy postmenopausal women: The Women's Initiative Randomised Trial. *JAMA* 289:3243–3253.

Folsom AR, PJ Mink, TA Selers, CP Hong, W Zheng and JD Petter. 1995. Hormonal replacement therapy and morbidity and mortality in a prospective study of postmenopausal women. *Am J Public Health* 85:1128–1732.

Grady D, SM Rubin, DB Petitti, CS Fox, D Black, B Ettinger et al. 1992. Hormone Therapy to Prevent Disease and Prolong Life in Postmenopausal Women. *Ann Intern Med* 117:1016–1037.

Greusens P, J Deauckar, J Gelen and LPC Schot. 1991. Non-linear increase in vertebral density induced by a synthetic steroid (Org OD 14) in women with established osteoporosis. *Maturitas* 13:155–162.

Grodstein F, JE Manson, MJ Stampfer. 2001. Postmenopausal hormone use and secondary prevention of coronary events in the Nurses' Health Study. *Ann Intern Med* 135:1–8.

Jensen J. 1991. Effects of sex steroids on serum lipids and lipoproteins. *Bailiere's Clin Obstet Gynaecol*, Vol. 5:867–888.

Krishna UR and AV Mandlekar. 1997. Place of Livial (tibolone) for climacteric symptoms and urogenital problems. *Obstet Gynaecol Today* II(6):51–55.

Krishna UR and AV Mandlekar. 1998. Urogenital problems in menopausal women–Place of HRT. *J Obstet Gynaecol Ind* 48(6):54–59.

Krishna UR and AV Mandlekar. 2002. Levonorgestrel intrauterine system (LNG–IUS) for dysfunctional uterine bleeding and contraception. *Obstet Gynae col Today* 7(1):49–51.

Krishna UR and AV Mandlekar. 2005. Can phytoestrogens have a place as alternative to HRT–A pilot study. *Obstet Gynaecol Today* 10(7):407–409.

Krishna UR and RU Mehta. 2000. Osteoporosis–Incidence and implications. *Obstet Gynaecol Ind* 50(5):150–156.

Lutkin BG, HW Wahner, WM O'Fallon, SE Hodgson, MA Kotowicz, AW Lane et al. 1992. Treatment of postmenopausal osteoporosis with transdermal estrogen. *Ann Intern Med* 117:1–9.

Magos AL and JW Studd 1990. Hormone implants in gynaecology. In JW Studd (ed) *Progress in Obstetrics and Gynecology* Vol 8, 313–334.

Marslew U, K Overgaard, BJ Riis et al. 1992. Two new combinations of estrogen and progestogen for prevention of postmenopausal bone loss: Long-term effects on bone, calcium and lipid metabolism and climacteric symptoms and bleeding. *Obstet Gynaecol* 72(2):202–210.

Million Women Study Collaborators. 2003. Breast cancer and hormone replacement therapy in the Million Women Study. *Lancet* 362:419–427.

Newcomb PA, MP Longnecker, BE Storer et al. 1995. Long-term hormone replacement therapy and risk of breast cancer in postmenopausal women. *Am J Epidemiol* 142:788–795.

Rosen RC, Taylor JF, Leiblum SR, GA Bachmann. 1993. Prevalence of sexual dysfunction in women: Results of a survey study of 329 women in an outpatient gynaecological clinic. *J Sex Marital Ther* 19, 13: 171–188

Steinberg KK, SJ Smith, SB Thacker. 1994. Breast cancer risk and duration of estrogen use: The role of study design in meta-analysis. *Epidemiology* 5:415–421.

Stevenson JC and MI Whitehead. 2002. Hormone replacement therapy *BMJ*. 18:677–678.

Studd JWW and R Barber. 1992. The menopause. In *Shaw's Gynaecology* ed RW Shaw London: Churchill Livingstone.

Writing Group for PEPI Trial. 1995. Effects of estrogen or estrogen progestin regimens on heart disease risk factors in postmenopausal women. The postmenopausal estrogen/progestin interventions (Pepi Trial) *JAMA* 273:199–208.

Women's Health Initiative Randomised Trial. 2003. *JAMA* June 25; 289:3243–3253.

Writing Group for Women's Health Initiative Investigators Risk and Benefit for Estrogen and

Progestin in Healthy Postmenopausal Women. 1995. Principal results from the Women's Health Initiative randomized controlled trial. JAMA Jan 18; 273 (13):199–208.
Yaffe K, G Sawaya, J Lieberburg, D Grady. 1998. Estrogen therapy in postmenopausal women: Effects on cognitive function and dementia. *JAMA* 279:688–695.

14

Stress Urinary Incontinence

Pranathi Reddy

Stress incontinence is involuntary urine loss associated with sudden increase in intraabdominal pressure. The activities which usually produce a sudden increase in abdominal pressure are coughing, sneezing, jumping and running (Abrams et al 2002).

Terminology: The term, stress incontinence was coined by Sir Eadly Holland in 1928. It refers to either the patient's symptom or a sign demonstrated during clinical examination. This does not differentiate between rise in bladder pressure secondary to an increase in intraabdominal pressure or detrusor overactivity. Taking this into consideration, the ICS defined 'involuntary loss of urine occurring when intravesical pressure exceeds maximal urethral closure pressure in the absence of detrusor overactivity' as genuine stress incontinence. Since this is solely a uro-dynamic diagnosis, the term, genuine stress incontinence, has now been replaced with urodynamic stress incontinence (Abrams et al 2002).

Pathophysiology

The two major factors responsible for urinary stress incontinence are:

- Urethral hypermobilty due to loss of support of urethra and bladder neck
- Intrinsic sphincter deficiency

These involve the maintenance of the urethral closure mechanism and the transmission of abdominal pressure. If increases in intraabdominal pressure are sufficient to overcome urethral closing pressure, stress incontinence will occur. The proximal two-thirds of the urethra is normally an intraabdominal structure, increased intraabdominal pressure would normally be exerted against it as well as the bladder. The pubourethral ligaments and endopelvic fascia support the urethra and allow effective transmission of intraabdominal pressure (DeLancey 1989). This supporting tissue forms a hammock on which the bladder neck and proximal urethra rest. When this tissue is intact, in the presence of raised intraabdominal pressure, bladder neck and proximal urethra are forced to close and prevent leakage (DeLancey 1993). A structural or anatomic defect in the pelvic floor leading to weakness of this hammock causes urethral hypermobility. This leads the pelvic floor to move away from the intraabdominal force, rather than hold firmly against it, leading to incontinence (DeLancey 1989).

Urethral closure is maintained by coaptation of the urethral mucosal wall and depends on the intrinsic sphincter and urethral tone. The latter is maintained by the basic elasticity of the urethra, the presence of smooth and voluntary (striated) muscle, the vascular component supplying the urethra, and the presence of alpha receptors from the sympathetic nervous system, which when stimulated cause contraction of the urethral sphincter (DeLancey 1993). When there is loss of mucosal coaptation, the leakage is usually more severe.

Risk factors

Vaginal delivery: It has been well established that childbearing is a risk factor for urinary incontinence among young and middle-aged women. Irreversible trauma to the supporting pelvic muscles and nerves can result from excessive mechanical pressure, stretching, and shearing forces during the passage of the infant through the vaginal canal (Sampselle et al 2000). The neuromuscular effects are more pronounced in the case of larger infants and prolonged or protracted second stage of labour. Likewise, instrumentation (forceps or vacuum) or episiotomy can further increase the risk of pelvic floor dysfunction and incontinence (Klein et al 1997). The risk of persistent incontinence following a first delivery, however, has been noted to be as high as 30% at five years (Viktrup and Lose 2001). With additional pregnancies, the pelvic floor and bladder dysfunction may become more severe.

Pregnancy: Although vaginal delivery is believed to be the main contributing factor to a person developing SUI, the mechanical and hormonal changes associated with pregnancy itself pose a significant risk to the pelvic floor. Half of all women, pregnant for the first time, experience some degree of SUI, especially during the final trimester. Some suggest that the protective benefit of cesarean delivery on the development of pelvic floor dysfunction is maximised when it is performed on an elective basis before the onset of labour (Farrell et al 2001).

Prior pelvic surgery: Prior hysterectomy has been associated with a 40% risk of future incontinence (Brown et al 2000). Likewise, radical pelvic surgery, vaginal surgery, pelvic-perineal trauma, or radiation, disrupt the neuromuscular integrity of the pelvis. Pelvic muscle weakness leads to prolapse of the pelvic organs (cystocele, uterine or vaginal vault prolapse), which can increase the risk of bladder dysfunction and incontinence.

Obesity: Numerous studies have identified obesity as a risk factor for SUI. The additional weight results in higher pressures on the bladder, and causes greater mobility (hypermobility) of the urethra. Another hypothesis relates to pressure-induced pelvic nerve and vascular impairment to the bladder (Mommsen and Foldspang 1994).

Smoking and lung disease: The increased intraabdominal pressures associated with the frequent, harsh cough often seen with smoking or lung disease have been shown to promote the development of SUI (Bump and McClish 1994). The increased pressures cause repeated strain on the pelvic support structures. Nicotine acts as a direct irritant to the bladder wall, thereby inducing spontaneous detrusor contractions.

Menopause: The estrogen depletion associated with menopause results in atrophy of the mucosal lining of the urethra. Similarly, atrophy of the vaginal mucosa can be seen, which may serve as a marker for urethral atrophy. This mucosal deficiency can result in difficulties with urethral coaptation, predisposing the woman to urinary leakage.

In addition, the support provided by the pelvic musculature weakens more rapidly in the postmenopausal woman, leading to pelvic organ prolapse and, in some women, urinary incontinence.

Age: The incidence of SUI in women increases with age and is commonly believed to be related to the inherent age-related weakness of the supportive fascial tissues, ligaments, and muscles of the pelvic floor.

Physical activity: Physical activities associated with increased abdominal pressure or high impact jarring forces on the trunk can decrease the supporting strength of the pelvic floor. Such activities include gymnastics, jumping, running, horseback riding, martial arts and heavy weightlifting. Low-risk activities include swimming, bicycling, walking and rowing.

EVALUATION

The success of treatment in stress incontinence is intimately linked to appropriate patient selection. Appropriate selection of patients is entirely dependent on thorough evaluation.

Basic Testing

The basic evaluation of women with **stress urinary incontinence** includes a history, physical examination, cough stress test, voiding diary, post-void residual urine volume and urinalysis.

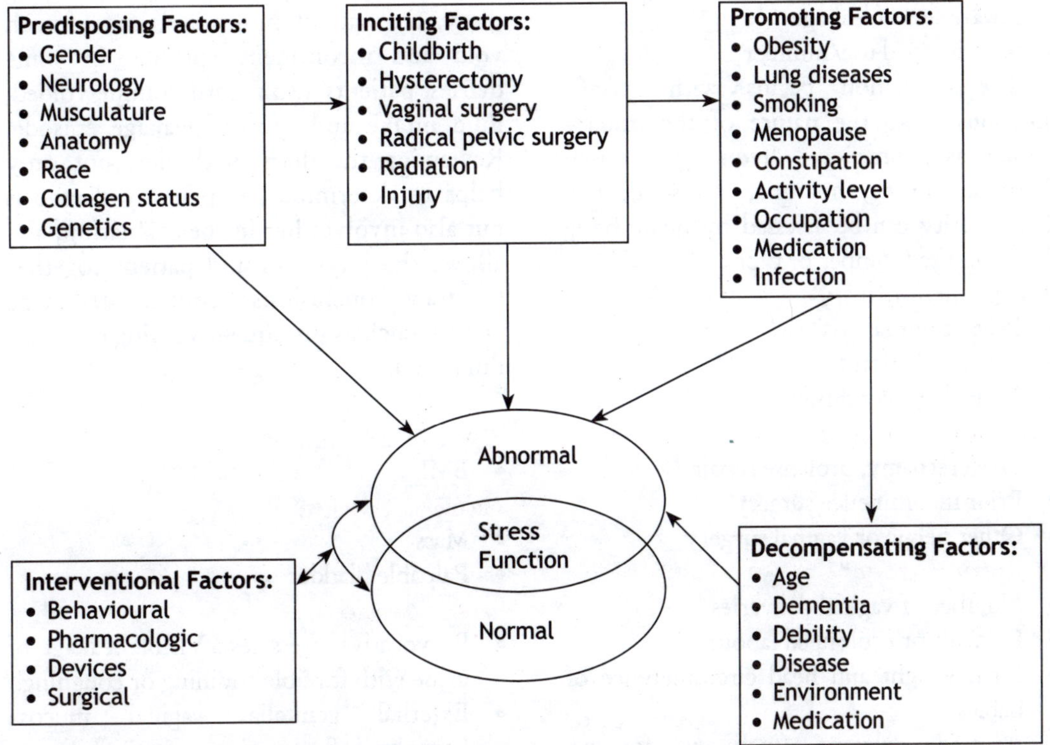

Figure 14.1: Risk factors for stress urinary incontinence

Table 14.1: Stress incontinence grading system	
Grade 0:	Continent
Grade I:	Patient loses urine with sudden increase in abdominal pressure but not supine
Grade II:	Patient loses urine with physical stress (walking; jogging, sneezing, coughing, changing from a reclining to a standing position; sitting up in bed)
Grade III:	Patient with total incontinence; urine loss unrelated to physical activity and/or position

History

Symptom-related history

- Leakage with maneuver (cough, sneeze, exercise)
- Frequency (>8 voids/day)
- Urgency
- Leakage with urgency
- Nocturia, enuresis
- Timing/duration of leakage
- Awareness of leakage
- Severity/pad use/number

The evaluation begins with specific questions as to the nature of the urinary symptoms (urgency, frequency, onset, duration, timing, nocturia, stress-induced). The severity can be assessed by quantifying daily pad use (number or type).

Past medical history

- Pelvic trauma
- Pelvic radiation
- Neurologic conditions

Past surgical history

- Hysterectomy, prolapse repair
- Prior incontinence surgery
- Other pelvic or vaginal surgery

Obstetric history

- Number of vaginal deliveries
- Difficult or prolonged labour
- Birth weight and head circumference of babies
- Assisted delivery (such as forceps, vacuum)

Social history

- Smoking

Voiding diary: A three-day voiding diary is an easy and reliable way to gain information about voiding habits (frequency, volumes per void) and the volume of fluid consumed or the intake of potential bladder irritants, such as caffeine or alcohol. In the voiding diary, the patient notes the time of each void and incontinent episode. In some diaries, patients also record volume voided, fluid intake and type of leakage episode. Reviewing the diary with her, not only helps to determine her primary diagnosis but also involves her in the evaluation, and allows the physician and patient together to draw conclusions about contributing factors, such as infrequent voiding or excess fluid intake.

Physical examination

- BMI

Abdominal examination

- Mass
- Palpable bladder

Pelvic examination

- Provocative stress test: Visible leakage of urine with forcible straining or coughing
- External genitalia, vaginal mucosa (atrophy, inflammation, irritation)
- Pelvic prolapse (such as cystocele)

- Urethral palpation (mass, tenderness, discharge)

EXAMINATION PROCEDURES: PVR (post-void residual): normal/50 ml. An important step in determining the possible cause of urinary leakage is to rule out overflow incontinence caused by inadequate bladder emptying and overdistention of the bladder. This can be evaluated easily by checking the post-void residual urine volume, or the urine remaining in the bladder following voiding. Catheterisation or bladder ultrasound should be performed within 15 minutes of voiding. Normal post-void residual urine volume is less than 50 ml (Abrams et al 2002). Patients at risk for urinary retention and overflow incontinence include women with severe pelvic organ prolapse (grade 3 to 4 cystocele); patients with neurologic disorders affecting spinal segments between C2 and S2; and patients with a prior history of urinary retention.

LABORATORY TESTS

- Urinalysis
- Urine culture if urinalysis is positive for nitrites, leukocyte, esterase, white blood cells, bacteria

COMPLEX TESTING: Indications for complex testing

- Failure of conservative measures
- When surgery is being contemplated
- Previous failed surgery
- Unclear history/mixed symptoms
- Significant SUI
- Significant pelvic prolapse

Urodynamic evaluation: Urodynamic testing refers to a combination of tests that involve simultaneous measurement of various physiologic parameters of urethral and bladder function during bladder filling and emptying. Urodynamic testing is a valuable adjunct to the rest of the evaluation.

To assess voiding function, urodynamic testing usually begins with **uroflowmetry,** in which the volume of urine passed is plotted over time. Flow time, peak flow rate and time to peak flow increase with the volume voided.

Next, a **cystometrogram** (also termed cystometry) is performed to assess bladder and urethral function during bladder filling. In **simple cystometry,** only bladder pressure is recorded and in **complex (or multichannel) cystometry,** both bladder and abdominal pressure (measured via a rectal or vaginal catheter) are recorded. It is easier to differentiate detrusor activity from abdominal activity with complex cystometry. Surface or needle electromyography is often done during filling and voiding to assess muscle activity of the urethral sphincter or pelvic floor.

Electromyography as generally performed has not been proven useful in neurologically intact women with symptoms of stress urinary incontinence alone and is not required in these patients. Multiple technical factors influence cystometry results, including the choice of distending medium, filling rate, patient position, and the type of catheter used to measure changes in bladder pressure.

Women with stress urinary incontinence have, on average, significantly lower maximal urethral closure pressures than those without. Leak-point pressure is a urodynamic measure of the minimum intraabdominal or intravesical pressure required to cause incontinence during abdominal strain or cough.

Results from this and other urodynamic tests must be evaluated as one piece of the patient's puzzle, and should be interpreted along with the history, physical examination, voiding diary and other tests.

Urodynamic testing usually concludes with an instrumented voiding study (also known as a **pressure flow study**), in which the vesical, abdominal and urethral pressures are measured simultaneously during bladder emptying. Various studies have identified Valsalva voiding, low preoperative flow rate and high preoperative detrusor pressures during voiding as risk factors for postoperative voiding dysfunction

Formal urodynamics testing may help guide clinical care, but whether urodynamics improves or predicts the outcome of incontinence treatment is not yet clear.

The distinction between urodynamic stress incontinence associated with hypermobility and urodynamic stress incontinence associated with intrinsic sphincter deficiency should be viewed as a continuum, rather than a dichotomy, of urethral function.

Normal Urodynamic Parameters

- Residual urine less than 50 ml
- First desire to void: 150 to 200 ml
- Strong desire to void not until after 250 ml
- Cystometric capacity: 400 ml to 600 ml
- No uninhibited detrusor contractions
- No demonstrable SUI despite provocation
- Voiding: Voluntary sustained detrusor contraction
- Flow rate: greater than 15 ml per second

Quality of Life Issues

Stress urinary incontinence rarely results in severe morbidity or mortality; rather it affects the quality of a person's life (Hunskaar and Visnes 1991). The WHO defines health as a state of complete physical, mental and social well-being and as not merely the absence of disease or infirmity. It defines 'quality of life' as an individual's perception of their position in life in the context of the culture and value system in which they live and in relation to their goals, expectations, standards and concerns. It is a broad-ranging concept affected in a complex way by the person's physical health, psychological state, personal beliefs, social relationships and their relationship to salient features of their environment.

Urinary incontinence undoubtedly has a significant negative impact on a woman's health-related quality of life. General health-related quality of life (HRQOL) instruments have the advantage of allowing comparisons across groups but may lack sensitivity to the unique aspects of a specific disease and how it affects the life of an affected patient (Hunskaar and Vinsnes 1991).

Given the importance of urinary incontinence on quality of life, there is increasing interest in the development and use of well-constructed questionnaires, which directly measure the quality of life in women with stress incontinence when evaluating the efficacy of a particular therapy or comparing symptom severity between patients or groups (Shumaker et al 1994).

This allows relatively easy collection of a woman's own assessment of subjective results in a standardised form. This form contains a series of questions which allows a woman to self-assess the impact of urinary incontinence on her everyday life For example; some of the questions that the King's Health Questionnaire would ask are as follows (Kelleher et al 1997).

1. To what extent does your bladder problem affect your household tasks? (for example, cleaning, shopping)
2. Does your bladder problem restrict your social life?
3. Does your problem affect your relationship with your partner?
4. Does your bladder problem make you feel depressed?

A score is obtained on completion of the questionnaire which allows objective assessment of the woman's impairment of quality of life. These can be issued from time to time to the same woman to assess improvement or effectiveness of therapy.

Every unit dealing with women with urinary incontinence should have a QOL assessment in place.

CONSERVATIVE MANAGEMENT OPTIONS

Initial treatment should include behavioural changes and pelvic floor muscle training. Estrogen is not indicated to treat stress urinary incontinence.

Lifestyle interventions: Lifestyle interventions can decrease stress urinary incontinence in many women (Wilson et al 2002). There is evidence that weight loss in both morbidly and moderately obese women decreases leakage; ongoing studies are evaluating optimisation of this intervention. Postural changes (such as crossing legs) often prevent stress urinary incontinence. There is some evidence that decreasing caffeine improves continence; however, fluid intake in general seems to play a minor role in the pathogenesis of incontinence. Although smokers are at greater risk for incontinence, no data have been reported on whether smoking cessation resolves incontinence.

Pelvic floor exercises: They were developed by Kegel in the 1940s and are still popularly known as Kegel Exercises. The initial idea of pelvic floor rehabilitation involved strengthening the striated musculature of the pelvis to increase muscle tone, pelvic support and urethral resistance, and thereby decrease episodes of incontinence. Successful PFEs begin with identification and isolation of the pelvic floor musculature. Direct clinician–patient biofeedback is generally required to ensure that the exercises are performed properly. The patient is instructed to contract or squeeze her vaginal muscles, as if she were attempting to stop the flow of urine during voiding. With the examiner's two fingers placed in the vaginal vault, gentle circumferential pressure should be observed, which elevates and moves the fingers toward the posterior vaginal vault, thereby indicating a successful pelvic floor contraction of adequate strength. Rehabilitation and strengthening of the levator muscles with PFEs have demonstrated a reduction in symptoms by 50%–75% in some women with SUI (Fantl et al 1996). When the objective is to strengthen the pelvic floor musculature, a daily exercise regimen is advised—a regimen of 24–36 contractions per day is adequate (Bo et al 1990). A practical strengthening regimen for PFEs involves two- to three-second contractions (squeezes), with 10–15 contractions per session, and three sessions per day. In a systematic literature review, the Cochrane Incontinence Group concluded that pelvic floor muscle training was consistently better than no treatment or placebo treatment for stress incontinence and should be offered as first-line conservative management to women. Intensive training sessions that include personal contact with a healthcare professional to teach and supervise pelvic floor muscle training may be more beneficial than standard care.

Occlusion devices: A variety of urethral support or occlusion devices are available for the patient who requires only intermittent treatment (that is, during strenuous activity). Vaginal pessaries provide anatomic support to the pelvic floor and inhibit downward descent of the urethra during times of abdominal straining (Thyssen et al 2001).

Urethral occlusion devices include disposable plugs, which directly block the urethra and prevent urinary leakage (FemSoft Insert). Although these cork-type devices sound attractive, in practice most women do not find them tolerable.

Pharmacological Treatment

Estrogens: In earlier uncontrolled studies, women using estrogen preparations reported less incontinence with estrogen use. However, more recently, in several large randomised trials, women assigned to receive estrogen and progesterone not only did not have less leakage, but in fact were more likely to experience the onset of incontinence or a worsening of baseline symptoms. Given that randomised controlled trials do not support using estrogen to treat stress incontinence and the recent limitations on estrogen use in general, initiating estrogen therapy specifically to treat stress urinary incontinence is not recommended.

Serotonin and norepinephrine reuptake inhibitors (duloxetine): These have been investigated for their role in treating stress urinary incontinence.

- Combined serotonin and noradrenaline re-uptake inhibitor duloxetine, increased synaptic concentrations of noradrenaline and 5HT within the pudendal nerve resulting in increased stimulation of the urethral sphincter
- Increases sphincter activity in the storage phase of the micturition cycle leading to continence with increases in intraabdominal pressure
- Recommended dose: 40 mg twice daily
- Nausea was the most common adverse event reported

Role of duloxetine (Cochrane database 2005)

- Long-term data are currently unavailable
- It is potentially useful in women awaiting surgery or women who have not completed their family. It is contraindicated in pregnancy
- It may be used in women who wish to avoid surgical intervention—physiotherapy remains a useful first-line option
- It cannot be considered as an alternative to surgery as long-term data is not available

SURGICAL MANAGEMENT

Conservative management should be offered to all women with stress urinary incontinence. Where conservative treatment has failed, surgical treatment can provide good results for the majority of women. Surgical procedures are more likely to cure stress urinary incontinence than nonsurgical procedures, but are associated with more adverse events.

Based on available evidence at this time, colposuspension (such as Burch colposuspension) and pubovaginal sling (including the newer midurethral synthetic slings) are the most effective surgical treatment (Cochrane database 2005).

For the last two decades, gynecologic surgeons have based surgical recommendations on the distinction between whether the patient had stress urinary incontinence resulting from 'intrinsic sphincter deficiency' or from 'hypermobility', recommending pubovaginal sling for the former and colposuspension for the latter (Enhorning 1961; DeLancey 1994). More recently, this dichotomy has been called into question, in that all women with stress incontinence have some degree of sphincter weakness, whether or not they have hypermobility.

Burch colposuspension: The urethra and bladder are supported by elevation of the paravaginal tissue to the ipsilateral ileopectineal ligament. Two to four sutures of no. 1 PDS (polyglycolic acid) or Ethibond are inserted into the paravaginal fascia. These are then inserted into the ipsilateral ileopectineal ligament. The initial suture is placed at the level of the bladder neck and subsequent sutures about 1 cm proximal. Once all the sutures have been positioned, each lateral fornix is elevated allowing the sutures to be tied without tension (Tanagho 1976).

Results of colposuspension

Laparoscopic colposuspension: In theory, laparoscopic colposuspension should provide the long-term success rates of an open colposuspension with low morbidity and short in-patient stay.

A number of variations in technique have been described using an extra-peritoneal approach or a transperitoneal approach. The use of standard suture materials or clips and prolene or mersilene mesh has also been described. The incidence of urinary tract injury is higher with the laparoscopic approach. Published across series are few, but two reports of ureteric injury, a very unusual occurrence at open surgery with only 15 cases reported in the literature (Virtaenen et al 1995), suggest that the risk of lower urinary tract injury may be much greater with a laparoscopic approach (Aslan and Woo 1997).

The major drawback of minimal access techniques is the relatively long time it takes to gain proficiency in laparoscopic Burch colposuspension. At present, although laparoscopic colposuspension appears to offer low morbidity and early return to work, the poorer long-term results and higher rate of urinary tract injury suggest that the open approach remains preferable.

Slings: The common feature of sling operations is the use of a strip of material, which is passed completely beneath the urethra or bladder neck and anchored to a point on the abdominal wall.

Sling insertion, utilising a combined vaginal and abdominal approach, a vaginal approach alone or a suprapubic technique alone, with blind dissection beneath the urethra and bladder base, have all been described. It is the choice of material and tension which appear to most influence the outcome of sling surgery.

Natural sling materials: Fascia lata can be obtained in an 18–20 cm long strip, with the use of fascial stripper and is thicker and stronger than abdominal aponeurosis. However, a second operative site is created with a concominant increase in operative morbidity. The operative time is also increased, as fascia must be first harvested and prepared before proceeding with colporrhaphy and sling insertion (Kaplan et al 1996). Allogenic fascia provides similar results to autologous grafts. There is additional advantage of no donor site morbidity and potential complications

Reference	*No. of patients*	*Continent (%)*	*Follow-up (months)*
Stanton et al 1979	25	84	4
Galloway et al 1987	50	84	6
Cardozo and Cutner 1992	100	80	6–12
Jarvis 1994	2300	84.3	>12

associated with intra-operative harvesting of the graft including a reduction in operative time (Wright et al 1998; Handa et al 1996). Allografts are either fresh-frozen or freeze-dried, both of which effectively destroy their antigenicity. As with human fascia lata, the process of preservation and sterilisation renders the tissue non-immunogenic and should destroy any viral particles.

Synthetic sling materials: While synthetic materials are easily available and circumvent the complications of graft harvesting, they may cause local tissue reaction leading to persistent local infection or erosion (Horbach 1991).

Mersilene was first used in vaginal sling surgery in 1962 in the form of a narrow ribbon, but this was discontinued as a result of high incidence of postoperative obstruction and urethral transaction (Williams and TeLinde 1985). The technique differs slightly from a standard sling in that a broad 'hammock' of mesh is placed beneath the bladder neck and urethra and anchored to Cooper's ligaments.

Gore-tex was introduced as a synthetic material for suburethral sling procedures as it was relatively inert and has been extensively used as a vascular prosthesis (Horbach et al 1998) with good results (Barabalias et al 1997). However, it is associated with the highest published erosion and infection rates of any synthetic sling material.

Results of sling surgery: Jarvis (1987) in a meta-analysis of all surgery for stress incontinence found an objective cure rate of 85.3% and a subjective cure rate of 82.4%. These figures agree closely with the results of the American Urological Association (Leach et al 1997) who report an overall subjective cure rate of 82%.

The tension free vaginal tape (TVT) procedure: This relatively new technique is based on the premise that stress incontinence results from failure of the pubo-urethral ligaments in the mid-urethra (Petros and Ulmsten 1990), which led to the proposal of 'an integrated theory for the maintenance of female stress incontinence' (Petros and Ulmsten 1995a, 1997a, 1997b). In this model, continence is maintained at the mid-urethra and not at the bladder neck.

The TVT procedure uses a knitted prolene mesh tape placed at the mid-urethra (Petros and Ulmsten 1995b). The tape is inserted via a small vaginal incision using two 6 mm trocars:, the weave of the tape is such that it is self-retaining. The procedure can be performed under local or regional anesthesia, allowing the position of the tape to be adjusted during a series of coughs. The aim is to have the tape lying free at rest (hence 'tension free') and to only exert sufficient pressure on the urethra during a cough to prevent leakage of urine. A multicentre study carried out in six centres in Sweden on women with no previous surgery for incontinence showed a 91% cure rate after one year (Ulmsten et al 1998). Recent results from Hilton and Ward show an 88% objective cure rate as a primary procedure and 75% as a secondary procedure (Ward and Hilton 1998).

Anterior colporrhaphy: Kelly described the excision of a portion of the anterior vaginal wall and plication of the paravesical tissue, at the bladder neck, and paravaginal fascia as a primary treatment for urodynamic stress incontinence (USI). Until recently, anterior colporrhaphy was widely used as primary treatment for USI. However, the relatively poor medium to long-term cure rates have lead increasingly to the use of alternative procedures (Van Geelen et al 1988). Anterior colporrhaphy should be reserved for treatment of prolapse alone. However, in a frail elderly woman whose main symptoms are of prolapse but with mild USI, insertion of 'Kelly' buttress sutures to the bladder neck may be appropriate. The procedure has a low morbidity and relatively little postoperative pain allowing early mobilisation and discharge from hospital.

Injectable peri-urethral bulking agents: The use of injectable peri-urethral bulking agents is gaining popularity. The mechanism of continence achieved after peri-urethral injection is not well defined. It is thought that peri-urethral bulking achieves better apposition of urethral epithelium without an increase in obstruction (Stricker and Haylen 1993). As peri-urethral injectables act by co-apting the urethral muscoa and increasing urethral closure pressure, it has been suggested that they would be particularly suitable for women with stress incontinence due to intrinsic sphincter deficiency.

Injections may be made either trans-urethrally via a cystoscope or peri-urethrally under cystoscopic control. It has also been suggested that peri-urethral bulking agents may have a place in the treatment of women who wish to have more children (Carr and Herschorn 1996). In general, the medium- to long-term results of this form of treatment are poor and, while it is claimed that injection has no effect on future surgery, it is possible that fibrosis, from repeated injections, may lead to a decline in intrinsic sphincter function. For this reason, this technique may be used as a primary procedure only with extreme caution.

A number of materials have been used for peri-urethral injection. The ideal material would be completely inert, cheap, easy-to-inject and free from long-term complications, yet provide long-lasting results.

Teflon was the first widely used peri-urethral injectable material. It was found to produce dense fibrous tissue and granulomatous reaction leading to urinary obstruction, urethral erosion and severe problems with any subsequent surgery. As a result of these problems, it is now rarely used. One of the most common materials used currently is glutaraldehyde cross-linked bovine collagen (GAX collagen). This has not been shown to have any side effects due to migration, but it does produce a local inflammatory response in which injected collagen is replaced with endogenous collagen (Kligman and Armstrong 1986). Due to the inflammatory response produced by GAX collagen and the resorption of this material, repeated injections may be necessary to sustain continence (Monga et al 1995).

Another injectable material that is used widely is micronised silicone rubber particles suspended in a non-silicone carrier gel (currently marketed as Macroplastique (Uroplasty, Reading, UK)) (Macroplastique Implants Technical Overview 1995). The larger particle size of this material makes migration and displacement less likely and, in addition, the inert nature of the material makes a local inflammatory reaction less problematic. The silicone particles are designed to act as a bulking agent with local inflammatory response removing the carrier gel, encapsulating the silicon in fibrin and replacing the gel with collagen fibres. Cure rates reported with Macroplastique are similar to those with GAX vary from 7% (Homer et al 1996) to 83% (Faerber 1996).

Injectable materials are expensive; however, they are invaluable in the treatment of secondary incontinence in women who have undergone multiple failed procedures or after radiotherapy where the urethra is fixed and scarred, a group of patients for whom other techniques have high morbidity and poor results.

Postoperative Complications

Voiding difficulties: This is a potential problem in all continence surgery. They are particularly common in patients with flow rates less than 15 ml/s or maximum voiding detrusor pressure below 15 cm H_2O on preoperative urodynamics (Stanton et al 1978). The relatively high incidence of voiding difficulties following sling surgery has been one of the most significant factors preventing more widespread use of this technique (Horbach 1991).

Of late, the importance of avoiding excess sling tension has been recognised (Blaivas and Jacobs 1991). As a result, slings are now placed under less tension, or even completely loose. This may reduce the incidence of voiding dysfunction.

Over-elevation of the urethra and bladder neck is associated with a high incidence of voiding difficulties. A number of techniques for avoiding and correcting excess sling tension have been advocated. Various intraoperative techniques to gauge correct sling tension have been described, including measurement of Q-tip angle, intraoperative UPP and cystoscopy, although there is no clear evidence that they accurately determine appropriate sling tension. Surgeons mainly rely on experience to judge what constitutes excess tension and how this could be avoided. When obstruction occurs postoperatively, simple urethral dilation has been suggested which may produce temporary relief but also progressive worsening of the obstruction due to peri-urethral fibrosis (Beck et al 1988).

De novo detrusor instability: It has been shown that detrusor instability arises de novo in 12%–18.5% of women postoperatively (Alcalay et al 1995). It occurs more commonly following previous continence surgery. It seems likely that a number of cases reflect pre-operatively. In addition, it has been suggested that damage to the autonomic nerve supply occurs during lateral displacement of the bladder at operation (Cardozo et al 1979).

Enterocele and rectocele formation: This occurs following Burch colposuspension and is believed to be the result of the elevation of the anterior vaginal wall creating a posterior defect and causing intraabdominal pressure to be transmitted directly to the posterior vaginal wall. The incidence of postoperative posterior compartment defects was estimated to be 7%–17% (Burch 1968). It is not clear whether these represent new defects or merely a pre-existing defect becoming symptomatic once the support of the anterior vaginal wall has been rectified.

Graft erosion: Problems related to erosion of the sling material, either through the vagina or the urethra, appear to be encountered almost exclusively with synthetic sling materials. Although the incidence of such problems is low, graft erosion can present with persistent vaginal discharge, vesicovaginal fistula formation and fibrosis and destruction of the urethral sphincter.

Factors Affecting Outcome of Surgery

1. **Age** appears to have an influence on the failure rate of continence procedures in general. Hilton showed that a decrease in success with increasing age was likely to be due to atrophic tissue changes with poorer healing, combined with the normal loss of urethral closure pressure that occurs with age. These changes may be partly reversible with preoperative estrogen replacement.
2. **The tensile strength of collagen** may also influence the results of surgery.

Patients with weaker collagen are likely to have earlier failure. Currently, interest in collagen status is growing, but it is not possible to predict results based on collagen biopsy at present.

3. **A well chosen primary procedure** ensures the highest success rates. There is an increased risk of postoperative detrusor instability with successive operations, presumably due to increased denervation. Complication rates rise, as with each successive operation, dissection becomes more difficult and wound infections and hematoma formation become more likely. Sphincter function may be adversely affected by denervation. This is not to say that secondary surgery cannot have reasonable success rates, but it is clear that a woman's best chance of long-term cure is with the first operation. Therefore, it is no longer appropriate to perform an operation with lower morbidity, such as an anterior colporrhaphy, first, then proceed to a needle suspension and finally, when this fails, to attempt a sling procedure.
4. **Preoperative assessment and appropriate patient selection:** Controversy still surrounds the need for urodynamic assessment prior to surgery and some gynecologists and urologists are prepared to undertake surgery without prior investigation. While it is reasonable to offer a short trial of conservative therapy based on clinical history and examination it would be unwise to undertake any major surgical interventions without thorough preoperative investigation and evaluation. Surgical treatment of USI should be no exception to this rule.

The symptom of stress incontinence may be produced by detrusor instability in the absence of anatomical disorder; bladder neck surgery will not lead to any improvement in symptoms and is in fact likely to worsen the underlying detrusor instability.

The presence of detrusor instability preoperatively has been shown to have a major impact on the success of colposuspension. Stanton et al demonstrated a significantly reduced cure rate in such patients compared to those with genuine stress incontinence (43% compared to 83%).

Where detrusor instability and urethral sphincter incompetence co-exist, it is recommended to treat detrusor instability, before surgery, using anticholinergic medication and to reassess urodynamics after irritative bladder symptoms are controlled, before considering surgical treatment of stress incontinence.

Pre-operative urodynamic studies also allow the assessment and prediction of voiding dysfunction. This allows adequate preparation of women at high risk of postoperative voiding difficulties; counselling can be provided and clean intermittent self-catheterisation (CISC), taught prior to surgery.

While clinical diagnosis may often be correct in detecting USI, the value of preoperative urodynamics in helping to predict outcome and prevent inappropriate surgery is undeniable. Both clinically and medicolegally, it is becoming increasingly difficult to justify surgical intervention without thorough urodynamic investigation.

Measurement Of Surgical Outcome

Assessment of the result of surgery for USI is complicated (Hilton 2002). What constitutes cure? Is it the absence of symptoms as reported by the patient? Is it the absence of signs as demonstrated by the clinician? Or is it a urodynamically demonstrated cure? One of the difficulties of assessing any continence procedure has been the choice of a suitable outcome measure. Simple cure of stress leakage is not sufficient as the occurrence of postoperative voiding problems and urinary urgency and frequency may have a profound influence on the outcome of surgery. Obtaining data on objective cure rates requires invasive investigations such as urodynamics which, although vital in clinical studies, are impractical in the majority of women undergoing routine surgery. A useful method of assessing outcomes, which has recently gained some popularity, is in measuring the effect of a procedure on quality of life before and after incontinence surgery with the means of validated and disease-specific quality of life questionnaires (Kelleher et al 1997).

This allows relatively easy collection of a women's own assessment of subjective results in a standardised form. There are a number of obvious flaws in this method of assessing subjective results. Women may feel inhibited discussing the outcome of recent surgery with the surgeon who undertook the operation and may report the absence of symptoms when this is not the case. Surgeons, on the other hand, may tend to interpret results with over-optimism.

Conclusion

- Quality of life issue: First do no harm
- Conservative options should be tried first
- Patient should be aware of all treatment options
- Knowledge of patient expectations from treatment
- Myth: Stress incontinence and surgery are synonymous
- Aim for a level of dryness with which patient is comfortable
- Complications of continence surgery may sometimes be worse than the original problem
- The decision to operate is patient driven

References

Abrams P, L Cardoze, M Fall, D Griffiths, P Rosier, U Ulmsten et al. 2002. The standardisation of terminology of lower urinary tract function: Report from the Standardisation Subcommittee of the International Continence Society. *Neurourol Urodyn* 21:167–178.

Alcalay M, A Monga, SL Stanton. 1995. Burch colposuspension: A 10–20 year follow up. *Br J Obstet Gynaecol* 102:740–745.

Aslan P and H Woo. 1997. Ureteric injury following laparoscopic colposuspension. *Br J Obstet Gynaecol* 104:266–268.

Barbalias GA, EN Liatsikos, A Athanasopoulos. 1997. Gore-tex sling urethral suspension in type III female urinary incontinence: Clinical results and urodynamic changes. *Int Urogynaecol J* 8:344–350.

Beck R, B McCormick, L Nordstrom. 1988. The fascia lata sling procedure for treating recurrent stress incontinence of urine. *Obstet Gynaecol* 72:699–703.

Blaivas G and B Jacobs. 1991. Pubovaginal fascial sling for the treatment of complicated stress urinary incontinence. *J Urol* 145:1214–1218

Bo K, R Hagen, B Kvarstein et al. 1990. Pelvic floor muscle exercise for the treatment of female stress urinary incontinence: III. Effects of two different degrees of pelvic floor muscle exercises. *Neurourol Urodyn* 9:489–502.

Brown JS, G Sawaya, DG Thom. 2000. Hysterectomy and urinary incontinence: A systematic review. *Lancet* 356:535–539.

Bump RC and DM McClish. 1994. Cigarette smoking and pure genuine stress incontinence of urine: A comparison of risk factors and determinants between smokers and nonsmokers. *Am J Obstet Gynecol* 170:579–582.

Burch JC. 1968. Cooper's ligament urethrovesical suspension for urinary stress incontinence. *Am J Obstet Gynaecol* 100:764–772.

Cardozo LD and A Cutner. 1992. Surgical management of stress incontinence. *Contemp Rev Obstet Gynaecol* 90:934–939.

Cardozo LD, SL Stanton, JE Williams. 1979. Detrusor instability following surgery for GSI. *Br J Urol* 58:138–142.

Carr LK and S Herschorn. 1996. Periurethral collagen injection and pregnancy. *J Urol* 155:1037.

DeLancey JO. 1989. Pubovesical ligament. A separate structure from the urethral supports: Pubourethral ligaments. *Neurourol Urodyn* 8:53–61.

DeLancey JO. 1993. Anatomy and biomechanics of genital prolapse. *Clin Obstet Gynecol* 36:897–909.

DeLancey J. 1994. Structural support of the urethra as it relates to stress urinary incontinence: The hammock hypothesis. *Am J Obstet Gynecol* 170:1713–1723.

Enhorning G. 1961. Simultaneous recording of intravesical and intraurethral pressure. *Acta Chir Scand* 276:1–68.

Faerber GJ. 1996. Endoscopic collagen injection therapy in elderly women with type one stress urinary incontinence. *J Urol* 155:512–514.

Fantl JA, DK Newman, J Colling et al. 1996. Urinary incontinence in adults: Acute and chronic management. Clinical Practice Guideline No. 2, 1996 Update (AHCPR Publication No. 96-0682). Rockville, MD: US Department of Health and Human Services, Public Health Service, Agency for Health Care Policy and Research. Available at www.ahrq.gov

Farrell SA, VM Allen, TF Baskett. 2001. Parturition and urinary incontinence in primiparous. *Obstet Gynecol* 97:350–356.

Galloway NTM, N Davies, TP Stephenson. 1987. The complications of colposuspension. *Br J Urol* 60: 122–124.

Handa V, J Jenssen, M Germain, D Ostergaard. 1996. Banked human fascia lata for the suburethral sling procedure: A preliminary report. *Obstet Gynaecol* 88:1045–1049.

Hilton P. 2002. Trials of surgery for Stress urinary Incontinence: Thoughts on Humpty Dumpty Principle. *Br J Obstet Gynaecol* 109:1081–1088.

Homer Y, K Kawabe, S Kageyama et al. 1996. Injection of glutaraldehyde cross-linked collagen for urinary incontinence. Two year efficacy by self assessment. *Int J Urol* 155:124–127.

Horbach NS, JS Blanco, DR Ostergard. 1988. A suburethral sling procedure with PTFE for the treatment of genuine stress incontinence in patients with low urethral closure pressure. *Obstet Gynaecol* 71:648–650.

Horbach NS. 1991. Suburethral sling procedures. In DR Ostegard, AE Bent (eds) *Urodynamics and urogynaecology: Theory and practice*, 3rd edn. Baltimore: Williams and Wilkins, 449–458.

Horbach NS. 1991. Suburethral sling procedures. In: Ostergard D R, Bent A E. (eds) *Urogynaecology and Urodynamics*, 3rd edn. Philadelphia: Williams and Wilkins, 413–421

Hunskaar S and A Vinsnes. 1991. The quality of life in women with urinary incontinence as measured by the sickness impact profile. *J Am Geriatr Soc* 39:378–382.

Jackson S, J Donovan, S Brookes, S Eckford, L Swithinbank, P Abrams. 1996. The Bristol Female Lower Urinary Tract Symptoms questionnaire: Development and psychometric testing. *Br J Urol* 77:805–812.

Jarvis GJ. 1987. Surgery for stress incontinence. *Br J Obstet Gynaecol* 69:399–402.

Kaplan SA, RP Santarosa, AE Te. 1996. Comparison of fascial and vaginal wall slings in the management of intrinsic sphincter deficiency. *Urology* 47: 885–889.

Kelleher CJ, LD Cardozo, V Khullar, S Salvatore. 1997. A new questionnaire to assess quality of life of urinary incontinent women. *Br J Obstet Gynaecol* 104:1374–1379.

Kelleher CJ, LD Cardozo, V Khullar, S Salvatore. 1997. A new questionnaire to assess the quality of life of urinary incontinent women. *Br J Obstet Gynaecol* 104:1374–1379.

Klein MC, PA Janssen, L MacWilliam et al. 1997. Determinants of vaginal-perineal integrity and pelvic floor functioning in childbirth. *Am J Obstet Gynecol* 176:403–410.

Kligman AM and Armstrong RC. 1986. Historical response to intra-dermal zyderm and zylapsy (gluteraldehyde cross linked) collagen in humans. *J Dermatol Surg Oncol* 12:351–357.

Kreder KJ. 2002. Managing incontinence: One size does not fit all. *Contemp Urol* 14 (suppl 9):S4–8.

Leach G, R Dmochowski, R Appell et al. 1997. Female stress urinary incontinence guidelines. Panel summary report on surgical management of female stress urinary incontinence. *J Urol* 158:875–880.

Macroplastique Implants Technical Overview. 1995. Maastricht, The Netherlands: Uroplasty BV.

Mariappan P, Z Ballantyne, JMO N'Dow, AA Alhasso. 2006. Serotonin and noradrenaline reuplake inhibitors (SNRI) for stress urinary incontinence in adults. (Cochrane Review) In *Cochrane Database of Systemic Reviews*, Issue 1, Oxford: Update Software.

Mommsen S and A Foldspang. 1994. Body mass index and adult female urinary incontinence. *World J Urol* 19:319–322.

Monga AK, D Robinson, SL Stanton. 1995. Peri-urethral collagen injections for genuine stress incontinence: A two year follow-up. *Br J Urol* 76:156–160.

Petros P and U Ulmsten. 1990. An integral theory on female urinary incontinence. Experimental and clinical considerations. *Acta Obstet Gynaecol Scand* 69 (suppl):153.

Petros P and U Ulmsten. 1995a. Urethral pressure increase on effort originates from within the urethra, and continence from muscolovaginal closure. *Neurourol Urodyn* 14:337–350.

Petros P and U Ulmsten. 1997a. Role of the pelvic floor in bladder neck opening and closure: I Muscle forces. *Int Urogynaecol J* 8:74–80.

Petros P and U Ulmsten. 1997b. Role of the pelvic floor in bladder neck opening and closure: II Vagina. *Int Urogynaecol J* 8:69–73.

Petros P and U Ulmsten. Intravaginal slingplasty. 1995b. An ambulatory surgical procedure for treatment of female urinary stress incontinence. *Scand J Urol Nephrol* 29:75–82.

Sampselle CM, JF Wyman, KK Thomas et al. 2000. Continence for women: A test of AWHONN's evidence-based protocol in clinical practice. *J Obstet Gynecol Neonatal Nurs* 29:18–26.

Shumaker SA, JF Wyman, JS Uebersax, D McClish, JA Fantl. 1994. Health-related quality of life measures for women with urinary incontinence: The Incontinence Impact Questionnaire and the Urogenital Distress Inventory. Continence Program in Women (CPW) Research Group. *Qual Life Res* 3:291–306.

Stanton SL, LD Cardozo, JE Williams, D Ritchie, V Allan. 1978. Clinical and urodynamic features of failed incontinence surgery in the female. *Obstet Gynaecol* 51:515–520.

Stricker P and B Haylen. 1993. Injectable collagen for type three female stress incontinence: The first 50 Australian patients. *Med J Aust* 158:89–91.

Tanagho EA. 1976. Colpocystourethropexy: The way we do it. *J Urol* 116:751–753.

Thyssen H, J Bidmead, G Lose et al. 2001. A new intravaginal device for stress incontinence in women. *Br J Urol Int* 88:889–892.

Ulmsten U, C Falconer, P Johnson et al. 1998. A multicentre study of tension-free vaginal tape (TVT) for surgical treatment of stress urinary incontinence. *Int Urogynaecol J* 9:210–213

Van Geelen J, A Theeuwes, T Eskes, C Martin. 1988. The clinical and urodynamic effects of anterior vaginal repair and colposuspension. *Am J Obstet Gynaecol* 159:137–144.

Viktrup L, G Lose. 2001. The risk of stress incontinence 5 years after first delivery. *Am J Obstet Gynecol* 185:82–87.

Virtanen HS, PJA Kiilholma, JI Makinen, MJ Nurmi, MB Chancellor. 1995. Ureteral injuries in conjunction with Burch colposuspension. *Int Urogynaecol J* 6:114–118.

Ward K and P Hilton. 1998. TVT early experience. *Int Urogynaecol J* 9:319

Williams TJ and RW Te Linde. 1985. The sling operation for urinary incontinence using Mersilene ribbon. *Obstet Gynaecol* 92:747–750.

Wilson PD, K Bo, J Hay-Smith, I Nygaard, D Staskin, J Wyman. 2002. Conservative treatment in women. In: P Abrams, L Cardozo, S Khoury, A Wein, eds. *Incontinence*. Plymouth: Plymbridge Distributors Ltd., 571–624.

Wright EJ, Iselin CE, Carr LK. 1998. Pubovaginal sling using cadaveric allograft. *J Urol* 169:1312–1316.

15

Urinary and Fecal Incontinence

Mala Vijayakrishnan | K Bhasker Rao

The most important cause of urinary incontinence in women in developing countries is indirect obstetric trauma due to obstructed labour. The estimated incidence is about 2% of all deliveries, though the hospital, incidence is reported to vary from 1% to 5% depending on healthcare and transport facilities. The fistula rate in most developing countries approaches the maternal mortality rates in the area (Danso et al 1996; Hilton and Ward 1998).

Obstructed labour resulting from neglected obstetrics is responsible for 8% of global maternal deaths (Lilejestrand 2000)—over 75% of spontaneous rupture of the uterus in labour and 80% of genital fistulas are seen in developing countries (Danso et al 1996). Maternal mortality and morbidity is usually due to hemorrhage and sepsis. Nahar (2000) from Bangladesh reported rupture of the uterus in 18%, VVF in 10% and vaginal stenosis in 6% of cases of obstructed labour, with a PMR of 64% and maternal mortality rate of 6%.

Incontinence is seen in all ages and becomes more prevalent with increasing age. It is a public health issue as it involves children, adults and elderly people and those with physical and neurological handicap. Involuntary escape of urine, feces or flatus is not only distressing, but at times an embarrassing disability. In the developing countries these commonly follow childbirth trauma, but may also be seen following infection, inflammation and neuropathy. Women may complain of either urinary or fecal incontinence depending on the nature of the injury; rarely, both may coexist. Urinary incontinence is seen more often than fecal incontinence in gynecological practice. Urinary incontinence is defined as the involuntary loss of urine which is objectively demonstrable and is a social or hygienic problem. It may be classified broadly as **extraurethral incontinence** or true incontinence (there is continuous involuntary passage of urine day and night due to a urinary fistula) and **transurethral incontinence**. The latter could be of different types: stress incontinence when there is intermittent escape of urine under conditions of stress when there is increased abdominal pressure, as during sneezing and coughing, or urge incontinence as in the presence of detrusor instability. Sometimes, both stress and urge incontinence may coexist in the same patient. Rarely, transurethral leak may be due to overflow incontinence.

URINARY FISTULA

Urinary fistula may be vesical, ureteric or urethral. Vesical fistula is the commonest of urinary fistulas. Excellent monographs on bladder fistula by Sims (1853), Mahfouz (1957) and Moir (1967) help us trace the course of the problem and its treatment.

Vesical Fistula

Incidence: Vesical fistula contributes to 0.5%–3% of gynecological admissions in the teaching hospitals of the developing countries of Asia (Bangladesh, India and Pakistan) and Africa (Nigeria, Kenya, Ethiopia, Sudan etc) (Table 15.1).

Etiopathology: The most common cause of vesical fistula is craniotomy (Tables 15.1 and 15.2). In Ethiopia, the mean age of fistula patients was 14.7 years at marriage and 17.7 years at first delivery; the mean duration of labour was 3.9 days. The mean maternal height was 149 cm and the mean weight was 44 kg. Primiparas formed 64% and multiparas 44% of these women with fistulas. Most of the patients who sought admission into the Fistula hospital in Addis Ababa, were poor and many of them were divorced (Muleta 2004). In most developing countries, fistula patients showed similar features.

In a review of 150 urinary fistulas reported by Danso et al (1996), 91.5% were due to obstetric trauma and 8.5% followed gynecological surgery. Of the patients with obstructed labour, 50% were primiparas and 25% were grand-multiparas (over para 5).

Of reported series, 76% to 97% of fistulas followed obstructed labour (Table 15.1).

Besides bladder injury, ureteric trauma may be the cause of urinary fistulas in those who had hysterectomy for obstetric or gynecological conditions.

In a series of 230 cases of vesico-vaginal fistula (VVF) reported from Thailand (Kochakarn et al 2000), there was a history of obstetric trauma in only 10 cases. Of the remaining, 164 were following abdominal hysterectomy, 23 after vaginal hysterectomy, eight after radical hysterectomy for carcinoma cervix, nine after radiation for carcinoma cervix and seven were patients with carcinoma cervix stage 4. Two cases each were due to suprapubic lithotomy and pelvic fracture.

In Nigeria, the tradition of the Gishiri cut causes bladder fistulas in 2% to 13%. In West Asia, the practice in certain communities of filling the vagina with rock salt in the puerperal period causes vaginal atresia with hematometra and fistula formation.

Table 15.1: Etiopathology, vaginal repair and success rates of bladder and fecal fistulas

Author/Year/Country	*Total Cases*	*Obst (%)*	*Gyn (%)*	*Fecal incontinence (%)*	*Vaginal Repair (%)*	*Success Rates (%)*
Devi 1965 (India)	500	95	05	08		
Moir 1973 (UK)	431	20	80	97	90–97	
Rao 1975 (India)	269	97	03	06	98	85–93
Gunaratne and Mati 1982 (Kenya)	254	92	08	07	60	
Tahzib 1983 (Nigeria)	1443	97	03	18		
Ahmed 1988 (Pakistan)	325	100	---	---	07	60
Lee and Simmonds 1988 (USA)	190	10	90			
Danso et al 1996 (Ghana)	150	91	05	08	05	

Pathology: Arrowsmith et al (1996) called the spectrum of injury seen following delivery the 'obstructed labour injury complex' and recommended treatment of the whole person; her bladder or the rectum alone should not form the basis of care. The site and size of the VVF largely depends on the level and duration of pelvic arrest in labour and the state of the cervix when impaction occurs. If it occurs prior to full dilatation, as would happen in a multipara, the cervix may be caught in the slough, with the resultant fistula being of a juxtacervical or uterovaginal type. If pelvic arrest occurs not at the brim but at mid-pelvis or at the outlet, after full dilatation, there is a risk of the urethra being partially or totally destroyed, avulsed or blocked as seen in 15% of cases. The site and duration of compression and the amount of tissue caught in it determine the site and size of the fistula formed, and may vary from a pinpoint to almost total destruction of the anterior vagina with a large fistula with bladder and ureteric orifices exposed. Rarely, there may be multiple fistulas. In about 3% vesical calculi may be present; sometimes these may be lodged in the scarred and sacculated vagina. Besides, in about 15% of patients there may be fecal fistulas and about 10% may have peroneal palsy.

In 6% to 24% of women with VVF, fecal incontinence along with vesical fistula or 'combined fistulas' are seen (Naidu 1962; Mustafa and Rushwan 1971; Hilton and Ward 1990; Kelly and Kwast 1993; Wall and Karisuma 2004). Among these one may find rectovaginal fistulas (RVF) in addition to complete perineal tear (in these cases one may find the RVF <3 cm from the anal verge, with a lax sphincter). In rectovaginal fistula with an intact sphincter, some of these were seen higher up in the post-vaginal wall and would need temporary colostomy prior to its closure.

Fecal incontinence may be seen in cases of complete perineal tear (CPT) or in cases of RVF with a lax sphincter. But in true RVF, the fistula is located at least over 3 cm from the anal verge and sphincter tone is good in these cases. Narrow subpubic arch and outlet contraction may be responsible for the high percentage of CPT/RVF seen in Ethiopian women.

Symptoms, signs and diagnosis: The diagnosis of a bladder fistula is easy. The history of continuous urinary incontinence following prolonged labour or gynecological surgery is suggestive. The vaginal examination helps in confirming it. The fistula may be visible, exposing the reddish bladder mucosa, or may be palpable. Often, it can be demonstrated by passing a metal catheter into the bladder. Incidentally, this is useful not only in determining the urethral patency but also in detecting an occasional vesical calculus. A urethrovaginal fistula could be visualised when urine spurts out through the fistulous opening on coughing with simultaneous blocking of the external urinary meatus with a finger. In this type, dribbling does not usually occur, but the patient splashes urine on her parts during micturition (Mahfouz 1957).

The diagnosis is easy in most cases when a woman, usually of a short build, complains of continuous dribbling of urine, 2 to 10 days after prolonged labour often ending in stillbirth, per vaginal examination shows excoriation of the vulva and dribbling of urine on separation of the labia. In most cases one could see the hole in the anterior vaginal wall. A catheter inserted through the urethra comes out through the defect in the anterior vagina. In other cases, the defect may vary in size as described earlier. In a tiny fistula or one at the vaginal vault, a methylene blue test may be useful to locate it. In obstetric hysterectomy cases, one may find the fistula in the anterior vaginal wall following a prolonged labour, but in gynecological cases, the fistula will be at the vaginal vault. Some patients may simultaneously complain of fecal incontinence and examination may reveal a vesicovaginal and rectovaginal fistula or retrovesical fistula. Constant change of pads with application of zinc oxide cream helps in healing of the vulval excoriation.

Management

Prevention: Preventive treatment consists of good antenatal care and risk screening of short stature women; delivery should be conducted at a referral centre. Partography will warn of obstructed labour so if there is lack of progress, she may be referred in time to an institution for abdominal delivery, if necessary. In all cases of obstructed labour, whether the delivery is abdominal or vaginal, the bladder should be drained for 7–10 days after the delivery.

Curative treatment: At least 12 weeks should elapse between delivery or gynecological surgery and surgical management of the fistula. In the meantime, the general and local condition of the patient has to improve. Preoperative intravenous pyelography is needed when

- The ureteric orifices are close to the fistulous margins,
- In those with vesical calculi and
- In large irreparable fistula which might require diversion of the urinary stream

The strategy for surgical closure of the fistula varies from case to case and, therefore, has to be planned in advance by examining the patient carefully as to the size, location, accessibility, amount of scarring, availability of tissues, mobility of the cervix and presence of any associated lesion. This examination is done in the theatre, if necessary under general anesthesia, with the patient in the Trendelenburg position so as to view the fistula properly. The first attempt should always be the best attempt as with each unsuccessful repair there is increased scarring.

Operative procedures: Almost all bladder fistulas can be repaired vaginally under regional or general anesthesia with the patient in the lithotomy position with a slight Trendelenburg position. In selected cases, a liberal episiotomy or a Schuchardt's incision may be needed to make the fistula more accessible. Continuous suction will help keep the operative field dry.

Standard method of repair, mid-vaginal fistula: The flap-splitting operation is the chosen method for repair. An incision is made around the vaginal margins of the fistula. The posterior margin and angles are dissected and mobilised first before proceeding to the anterior margin. After mobilising the bladder all round and ensuring hemostasis, the margins of the fistula are closed with interrupted chromic catgut No. 3-0 in two layers using a fine non-cutting curved needle taking care to seen that the stitches do not include the bladder mucosa. When there is excessive scar tissue or it is close to the periosteum, Mayo's cutting needle is useful. The edges of the fistula are not resected or freshened, as it would result in sacrificing some more bladder tissue. The direction of suture depends on the size and direction of the fistula, though at the bladder neck the longitudinal closure is preferred to reduce the risk of stress incontinence. The initial stay sutures must go well beyond the margins. The vaginal flaps are approximated with No. 2-0 chromic catgut though some prefer fine monofilament nylon which is removed two weeks later. The bladder is drained continuously for two weeks using a No. 14 Foley's catheter with a 5 ml bulb. In case the bulb of this catheter is likely to press on the suture lines at the bladder neck or in urethral repair, a No. 14 plastic catheter is used. After the removal of the catheter 14 days later, the patient is encouraged to pass urine frequently till the bladder tone is regained.

Repair of juxtacervical fistula: In juxtacervical or vesicocervical fistula, a transverse incision is made initially at the vaginocervical junction and the bladder is pushed up till the fistula is fully exposed. It may be necessary to use the scissors to release the scar tissue and mobilise the bladder all around, especially the upper margin. A stay suture here is helpful to prevent its retraction during the repair. There may be bleeding from the cervix requiring sutures. The vaginal flap could then be easily dissected away from the bladder anteriorly, before the fistulous margins are sutured in layers.

Repair of complicated vesicovaginal fistula

1. **Juxta-urethral fistula:** Vaginal cystotomy and drainage with a Foley's catheter is needed as the first step in the repair of fistula located at the bladder neck, in those with blocked or avulsed urethra and whenever urethral reconstruction is performed. During the repair, a fine urethral catheter is kept in position. The Foley's catheter is removed after two weeks in the theatre, and the bladder is drained for the next 4–5 days by a fine urethral catheter. Urethroplasty is indicated in all cases where the urethra is destroyed. The authors use a U-shaped flap of vaginal mucosa to form the urethra over a catheter, and by undermining the lateral margins the mucosa is approximated to cover the newly formed urethra, the bladder neck having been strengthened in the meanwhile. Moir (1964), and Hamlin and Nicholson (1969) who have used Martius graft or gracilis muscle to reinforce the repair have claimed a success rate of over 70%. In a series of 50 patients with total urinary incontinence due to loss of the urethra (40 of which followed vaginal surgery), Symmonds and Hill (1978) achieved a small caliber neourethra from the contractile tissue that remained in the urethral roof, supplemented in 22 cases by the myocutaneous labial skin flap or Martius graft. A second-stage retropubic urethrovesical suspension was necessary in two cases to remedy the stress incontinence. In their 15-year follow-up they claimed a 74% cure rate. The authors have found Martius graft useful when the fistula is on the vaginal fornix or close to the bone with a lot of scar tissue, and the vaginal flaps cannot cover it.
2. **Repair of large fistula and circumferential fistula:** In a large fistula, where most of the anterior vaginal wall is destroyed and the bladder mucosa is prolapsed exposing the ureteric orifices, the repair is technically difficult because of the considerable loss of tissue, associated scarring and hemorrhage during dissection of the bladder from the bone. It is always advisable to use the ureteric catheters before starting the repair in such cases, and keeping them in position till the end of the operation. In the circumferential fistula (Moir 1965), where there is all-round destruction of tissue and dense fibrosis, considerable experience is needed to repair it successfully. It is in these types of cases that supplemental grafts with muscle or labial fibro-fatty tissue are useful. In large fistula with excessive

scarring, where previous attempts at repair have failed, a combined abdominovaginal technique of closure has been described by Gogoi (1979).

In the Department of Urology, Sloan Kettering Institute, New York, during a 10-year period from 1991, 207 VVFs were repaired. Complex fistulas (larger than 2 cm diameter, radiation induced fistulas and failed previous repair) were repaired by tissue inter-position repair. In these cases, peritoneal flap for proximal fistulas, Martius graft for distal fistulas and labial graft for cases with insufficient vaginal flap were used in 83%, 34% and 3% of cases, respectively. The causes of fistula were hysterectomy in 91% (abdominal 83%, vaginal 8%); radiation in 4%; obstetric trauma and other causes in 5% each. In 58% of cases, tissue interposition surgery was performed. The cure rates with peritoneal, Martius and labial grafts were 96%, 97% and 33%, respectively. The conclusion of this study was that the peritoneal flap was as good as Martius graft and is useful in cases of proximal fistulas where previous repair had failed.

3. **Vesicocervical fistula (menouria):** Diversion of menstrual discharge via the bladder was first reported by Laffont and Ezes in 1947. Ten years later, Yousef (1975) coined the word 'menouria' for the high vesicocervical fistula. They may follow a classical cesarean section and, rarely, a difficult forceps delivery associated with cervical tear. The treatment of choice is abdominal repair (intraperitoneal extravesical).
4. **Vault fistula:** The bladder fistula seen at the vaginal vault following hysterectomy may be repaired by the flap-splitting method. If there is fixity of tissues, traction on Foley's catheter passed through the fistula helps surgery. A four-quadrant flap around the opening with adequate mobilisation is helpful in repairing it in layers. Sauterisation and repair do not yield satisfactory results. Modified Latzko's closure or high colpocleiesis is done, when there is dense scarring in the fistulous region. A drawback of this method is that the vagina is slightly shallow; however, urinary continence is fully restored.
5. **Vesical fistula with bladder calculi:** When vesical fistula is complicated with vesical calculi, the stones are first removed by suprapubic or vaginal cystolithotomy. Simultaneously, the scarring at the bladder neck or in the vagina is removed to promote free flow of urine. Eight weeks later, after the urinary infection is treated completely, the fistula can be repaired vaginally.
6. **Radiation fistula:** Repair of the radiation fistula requires patience and experience. To augment the blood supply, gracilis muscle graft is advocated by Moir (1967) and pedicled omentum by Kiricuta and Goldstein (1972).

Abdominal repair of a vesicovaginal fistula is very rarely indicated. Mahfouz (1957) after treating about 1000 such fistulas found that when it was not closed from below, the repair failed because of the dense scarring and relative inaccessibility. For high cervical fistula with fixed cervix or totally destroyed anterior lip and in few cases of surgically induced vault fistula, abdominal repair may be advocated. Of 320 bladder fistulas, only two were repaired by the author per abdomen.

Postoperative care: The postoperative care of these patients is very important. Urinary infection, slight hematuria and mild secondary hemorrhage are some of the complications. Prophylactic urinary antibiotics are always advisable. Care should be taken to see that the urinary sediment does not block the catheter or the drainage system. If secondary hemorrhage is moderate or persistent, the patient has to be examined in the theatre, the vagina viewed and the active bleeding vessels ligated. As far as possible, tight vaginal plugging should be avoided.

The remote complications are stress incontinence, vaginal stenosis and rarely, vesical calculus. Of these, urinary stress incontinence is seen in 5%–10% of cases. The risk is greater in bladder neck fistula and in those which extend from one pubic ramus to the other.

Secondary amenorrhea, a common complication is spontaneously corrected after the successful repair, as it is of hypothalamic origin.

Results: The cure rate following repair of bladder fistula varies from 61% (Ahmed 1988) to 96% (Lazarus 1959; Moir 1973). In the author's experience, 86% of repairs were successful in the first attempt; with subsequent attempts 94% were cured. Similarly, it is felt that no case should be considered irreparable at the initial examination and subjected to transplantation of the ureters. The reports of successful closure after 19–23 prior attempts are known (Sims 1853; Lazarus 1959; Moir 1965).

Urinary diversion: This is seldom indicated as a treatment of choice in bladder fistula. However, when repeated attempts at closure fail, especially in large fistula with urethral destruction, and there is scarring with practically no tissue available to close it and in a few cases of circumferential fistula, urinary diversion may be resorted to. In several large series of vesical fistula, diversion of the urinary stream was carried out in about 4% (Lazarus 1959; Devi 1965; Rao 1975) to 18% (Yennen and Babuna 1965; Das and Sengupta 1969) of patients.

Reproductive function following fistula repair: In multiparous women with live children, it is advisable to perform tubal ligation through the pouch of Douglas concurrently with the repair of the fistula. However, if they are short stature primiparas with bad obstetric history, careful supervision is needed during subsequent pregnancies. If the cervix is torn or damaged, there is a risk of mid-trimester abortions or premature labour; in such cases, Shirodkar's cerclage operation is advisable. Elective cesarean section at term is indicated in all cases following successful repair.

Pregnancy following urinary diversion (into the sigmoid or ileum) is safe, though the most common complication is asymptomatic bacteriuria and pyelonephritis. In these cases, cesarean section is indicated only for obstetric reasons (Barnett and Peters 1983).

Ureterovaginal Fistula

These form hardly 2% of urinary fistula in India compared to 16% reported in the US. They may be due to direct trauma, like ligation or section, or indirectly due to ischemia. The reported incidence is 0.5%–2.5% (Freda and Tacchid 1962) of the major gynecological operations for benign conditions. In some cases, the ureteric injuries are silent and may be discovered only during postoperative investigations. The chances of ureteric injuries are greater when surgery is done for broad ligament tumours, inflammatory adnexal masses, extensive pelvic endometriosis, etc. The risk of ureterovaginal fistula is 0.5%–1%, following total abdominal hysterectomy compared to 0.1% after vaginal hysterectomy (Thompson 1998). Rarely, it may follow a Manchester operation.

Following radical surgery for cervical carcinoma, there is an increased threat of ureteric fistula either due to direct injury or vascular necrosis. The incidence of such fistula after radical abdominal hysterectomy was reported to be 7.2%–10% (Meigs 1954); but with improved techniques and postoperative bladder drainage, it has been reduced to 1.4% according to Macasaet and co-workers (1976). With radical vaginal hysterectomy, ureterovaginal fistulas are seen only in about 1.5% (Ghosh 1960; Inguila and Cosmi 1967). The risk of damage to the ureter in radical pelvic surgery increases with the stage of the malignancy, the thoroughness with which the ureters are stripped of the surrounding tissues and with preoperative pelvic irradiation.

The ureterovaginal fistula may rarely follow lower segment cesarean section when the incision extends to the uterine artery resulting in hemorrhage or hematoma (Lawson 1967). Two cases of ureterocervical fistula of obstetric origin were reported by Sen and Chaudhury (1976). Oumachigui et al (1982) found ureteric injuries in 0.09% due to transection, extension of incision or hemostasis. However, bladder injury was more common (0.03%), especially in repeat sections.

The diagnosis of this type of fistula could be arrived at from the history of recent pelvic surgery, location of the fistula at the vault by methylene blue testing, and confirmed by chromocystoscopy (using indigo carmine) and by passing a ureteric catheter through the fistulous opening. Intravenous pyelography is always necessary to determine the state of renal function in such cases before surgery is planned.

Even when the injury has been detected during surgery, prompt steps should be taken to repair the ureter or reimplant it. When a fistula is noticed, an interval of eight weeks is allowed before corrective surgery is undertaken. The commonest site of injury is where the ureter is crossed by the uterine artery. The ideal treatment is submucosal tunnel uretero-neocystostomy. The bladder often requires some mobilisation to avoid tension at the site of anastomosis. If the level of injury is slightly higher, the bladder flap is used as in Boari operation rather than by resorting to end-to-end anastomosis. The bladder is drained postoperatively for two weeks.

STRESS INCONTINENCE

Transurethral incontinence may be due to stress incontinence or due to urge incontinence, (detrusor instability). In stress incontinence there is involuntary escape of urine whenever there is an increase in the intraabdominal pressure. Urge incontinence is due to detrusor instability which causes increased bladder contractility and is associated with the urge to pass urine.

Incidence: It is seen in about 60% of the population, especially in women who have urinary incontinence of sufficient severity to interfere with their quality of life (Cheater and Castleden 2000). For a proper understanding of stress incontinence, knowledge of physiology of micturition is necessary.

Anatomy and pathophysiology of micturition: The smooth muscle of the bladder, like that of the ureters, is arranged in spiral, longitudinal and circular bundles. Contraction of this muscle (detrusor muscle) is mainly responsible for emptying the bladder during micturition. These muscle bundles pass on either side of the urethra and are called the internal urethral sphincter. Further down along the urethra is the sphincter urethra (external urethral sphincter) composed of skeletal muscle. The bladder is lined by transitional epithelium. The bladder is innervated by parasympathetic (S2, S3 and S4) and sympathetic ganglia (hypogastric nerve L1, L2 and L3). Somatic supply is from the pudendal nerve (S2, S3 and S4) which mainly supplies the urethra and part of the base of the bladder. Micturition is fundamentally a spinal reflex under the control of higher centres in the brain—the pons (facilitatory area) and mid-brain (inhibitory area). It is subject to voluntary facilitation and inhibition.

Urine enters the bladder without producing much increase in the intravesical pressure (IVP) till the viscus is well filled. The involuntary muscle of the bladder has the property of plasticity, that is, when it is stretched, the tension initially produced is not maintained. This follows the law of Laplace, which states that the pressure in a spherical viscus is twice the wall tension (T) divided by radius (R). So the intravesical pressure is 2T/R. As further increments of volume are produced, the sharp rise in pressure leads to an urge to micturate—this occurs when there is about 400 cc of urine. During the act of micturition, the perineal muscles, the urethral and external urethral sphincter relax, the detrusor contracts and urine passes out through the urethra. The perineal muscles and external urethral sphincter are under voluntary control. After urination, the female urethra empties by gravity (Ganong 1999).

Normally, during the filling phase, the detrusor muscle is relaxed due to sympathetic stimulation of β-adrenergic receptors in the bladder wall. Sympathetic stimulation of α-adrenergic receptors in the internal sphincter causes constriction and rise in intraurethral pressure. Once the bladder reaches functional capacity (400–600 cc), receptors in the detrusor send a signal to cortical centres in the brain to initiate the emptying phase of the bladder. Activation of parasympathetic cholinergic receptors in the detrusor stimulates bladder contraction to commence micturition. Simultaneously, the pudendal nerve produces relaxation of voluntary sphincters and the levators facilitating urination.

As the intravesical pressure (IVP) is normally 10–15 cm H_2O and the urethral pressure is 30 cm H_2O (due to contraction of sphincter urethra), escape of urine is prevented. The continence of urine is also normally maintained by the tone of the internal urethral sphincter, integrity and tone of external sphincter and the pubocervical fascia which supports the bladder neck at the vesicourethral junction and connects it to the back of the symphysis pubis to maintain the posterior urethrovesical (PUV) angle. When there is an increase in the intraabdominal pressure, escape of urine is prevented by the contraction of the sphincter urethra and the angulation of the vesicourethral junction and the transmission of raised intraabdominal pressure to proximal urethra above the pelvic diaphragm.

Predisposing causes of urinary stress incontinence:

1. The most common cause is childbirth trauma. In the terminal part of the second stage of labour, downward pressure by the presenting part can cause injury to the sphincter urethra, the levators and the pudendal nerves. The tears in the pubocervical fascia are produced by the shearing force of uterine contractions during delivery of the head. This neuromuscular injury (to the pudendal nerve, pelvic floor muscle and urethra) is one of the key factors in the pathophysiology of urinary stress incontinence, as it interferes with the proper contraction of the internal and

external sphincters and leads to lowered urethral pressure. The proximal part of the urethra is above the pelvic diaphragm and during stress, the increase in intra-abdominal pressure is equally conveyed to the bladder and proximal urethra. With laxity of pelvic floor musculature due to injury, hormone deficiency and age, the proximal urethra descends below the pelvic diaphragm. In this situation, the increase in intraabdominal pressure is conveyed to the bladder and not to the proximal urethra, leading to stress incontinence. The weakness of the internal sphincter and the external sphincter urethra further contribute to the escape of urine.

2. With menopause and fall in estradiol level, there is atrophy of the vaginal mucosa and lack of coaptation of the urethral mucosa. This results in stress incontinence which can be corrected with estrogen replacement, preferably by local application of estrogen cream.
3. Disease/injury to the higher centres in the brain causes involuntary contraction of detrusor with escape of urine due to loss of control by higher centres as in Alzheimer's disease, multiple sclerosis and Parkinson's disease

Causes of transurethral incontinence

Stress incontinence: It is anatomically due to hypermobility of the urethra with descent of proximal urethra below the pelvic diaphragm and/or incompetence of the internal urethral sphincter or both.

Detrusor instability or overactivity: It is due to neuropathies (detrusor hyperreflexia) or may be idiopathic, when there is no neurological cause.

Mixed incontinence: It is a combination of genuine stress and urge incontinence.

Other causes: It includes incontinence with overflow, urethral diverticulum, pyelitis, pyelonephritis, etc.

Diagnosis of genuine stress incontinence (GSI): As stress incontinence is a symptom, a sign and a diagnosis, it is extremely important to establish the diagnosis of stress incontinence prior to its management.

Initially, a detailed obstetric history is taken including of previous childbirth trauma, duration of labour (especially of the second stage), weight of baby and nature of the delivery. History regarding duration and nature of urinary symptoms like urgency, dysuria, pain, fever and precipitating factors for stress incontinence should be analysed. Also, the drug history, and investigation and treatment protocols undertaken previously for this complaint, and the effect of urinary incontinence on her lifestyle should be enquired into.

A detailed physical examination including neurological examination should be conducted. Next, the patient should be examined with a full bladder, while standing and in dorsal positions, to determine the amount of urine escaping when she coughs, to confirm the diagnosis. According to Ingleman-Sundberg, the severity of GSI is graded as

- Incontinence only with cough
- Incontinence during daily activity such as rising from chair or walking
- Dripping in upright position

Local examination helps to find out excoriation of vulva, presence of cystocele, urethrocele, myoma/ovarian tumour and estrogen status. If there is spurting of urine on coughing, the vesicourethral junction is supported by two fingers (with a finger on either side of the urethra), and she is asked to cough again: if there is no spurting, a diagnosis of stress incontinence can be made (Bonney's test). If Bonney's test is positive, the Q-tip test is done next by inserting a cotton bud into a urethra and observing the angulation at the rest and when patient coughs. If the angulation is more than the normal 30°, the Q-tip test is positive and the cause of stress incontinence is hypermobility of the urethra and loss of PUV angle.

Investigations include:

1. Urine microscopy and culture; renal function tests, if necessary
2. Measurement of residual bladder volume by ultrasonography
3. Urodynamic studies like cystometry, uroflowmetry
4. In those cases with complex history, cystoscopy, urethrocystoscopy and voiding cystourethrography may be required.

Indications for cystometry are:

1. Failure to respond to empirical treatment
2. Previous continence surgery
3. Prior to definitive continence surgery
4. Prior to prolapse repair associated with incontinence
5. Symptoms suggestive of voiding difficulty
6. Presence of neurological disease

Cysto-urethrograph: The vertical axis shows the pressure changes and the horizontal axis indicates the rate and volume of water let into the bladder.

Causes of genuine urinary stress incontinence

i. Childbirth trauma to the levator ani (the most important cause)
ii. Menopausal atrophy
iii. Neurological disorders

In some cases, the urethra is like a 'rigid patent tube' surrounded by scar tissue and further corrective surgery is not possible.

In stress incontinence, there is involuntary escape of urine whenever there is increased intraabdominal pressure as during laughing, coughing or sneezing. In detrusor instability there is increased contractility of bladder resulting in an irresistible urge to pass urine.

Management of transurethral urinary stress incontinence: After the investigations, cases diagnosed as stress incontinence and mixed type of incontinence are considered for conservative management and those not responding to it are taken up for surgery.

Those with detrusor instability are treated conservatively. Conservative therapy for detrusor instability consists of bladder drill, step-by-step bladder training, pelvic floor exercises, transcutaneous electrical nerve stimulation (TENS) and drugs. Surgery is of limited value in these cases.

All cases of genuine stress incontinence (GSI) as well as mixed incontinence should receive conservative therapy before deciding on surgery. Associated conditions like obesity, chronic cough or constipation, estrogen deficiency and urinary tract infection require treatment.

The conservative treatment consisting of exercises to strengthen pelvic floor muscles under the guidance of a physiotherapist or a nurse gives better results than if the patient is asked to do it at home. Exercises carried out for about 3–6 months offer relief in about 25% of cases. In those who do not respond to physiotherapy or cannot contract the pelvic floor muscle, adjunctive therapy with biofeedback, cones or electrostimulation may provide benefit. Those with missed (GSI/DI) type of urinary incontinence, not responding to conservative therapy or unsuitable for surgery or with multiple failed operations can be treated with vaginal or urethral devices. Vaginal device of silastic material with two prongs to fit behind the symphysis and cradle the urethra during cough have been tried with 50% success. A plastic urethral device can also be inserted into the urethra and retained at the urethrovesical junction. However, both these devices have not been tested in a large series (Moore 2000).

Menouria-Youssef coined the word 'menouria' for the high vesicocervical fistula following a classical cesarean section or a difficult forceps delivery or cervical tear. As in most of these cases there is good control, patients refuse surgery since they also save on sanitary pads.

Surgical management of genuine urinary stress incontinence: More than 100 surgical procedures for stress incontinence have been tried during the last ten decades. However, the choice of the surgical procedure depends on the age of the patient, associated conditions like prolapse, hypermobility of the urethra, incompetent internal sphincter, scarring due to previous surgery, any other associated pathological conditions (like DUB, myoma), the degree to which her social life is affected by the disability and the patient's choice of surgical treatment.

Surgical procedures for urinary stress incontinence can be grouped under the following basic surgical methods:

1. Cases with hypermobility of urethra:
   a. Vaginal methods: Bladder buttressing with Kelly's/Pacey's sutures
   b. Abdominal methods: Retropubic—bladder-neck suspension
      i. Marshall–Marchetti–Krantz (MMK) cystourethropexy
      ii. Colposuspension of Burch and its modification (e.g. Stanton's)
      iii. Colposuspension by non-endoscopic needle method (Pereyra's)
      iv. Colposuspension by endoscopic needle method (Stamey's)
2. Cases with internal urethral sphincter deficiency:
   a. Sling procedures
   b. Periurethral injections
3. Artificial urinary sphincter

Surgical method: Besides the urodynamic factor, one has to consider the success rates and complications of each method. Most procedures yield good short-term results whereas long-term follow-up (over 10 years) revealed diminishing success rates.

Vaginal method

Kelly's operation: The vaginal method of repair for stress incontinence consists of approximation of endopelvic fascia with interrupted sutures using vicryl to strengthen the bladder neck. This form of bladder buttressing supports the bladder neck and restores the PUV angle (Kelly and Dumm 1914). It is indicated in those cases of bladder prolapse with urinary stress incontinence and can be done with or without hysterectomy. On follow-up, the success rate was found to vary from 50% to 70% (Thompson et al 1998).

Abdominal methods

MMK cystourethropexy: In this operation, the paraurethral tissue on either side of the bladder neck is fixed by two pairs of sutures to the back of the pubic bone. It carries success rates of 90% in primary and 85% in recurrent cases. However, it carries a risk of osteitis pubis in 2.5% of the cases and does not correct the cystocele and therefore is not the preferred procedure.

Burch colposuspension: This was first described by Burch in 1961. In a comprehensive review of over 3500 cases who underwent the Burch procedure, Dainer et al (1999) concluded that the Burch procedure has withstood the test of time and is considered by most gynecologists and urogynecologists as the gold standard. As a primary procedure,

Table 15.2: Drugs used in the treatment of bladder hyperactivity (based on the evaluation made by the ICI, 1998)

Drug Group	*Quality of Trial*	*Recommendation*	*Drug Dose*
Antimuscarines (or anticholinergics)			
Propantheline	A	R	15–30 mg qid
Tolterodine	A	R	1–4 mg/day
Antispasmodics			
Oxybutynin	A	R	2.5 mg tds
Flavoxate	A		400 mg tds
Antidepressant			
Imipramine	A	RR	30 mg tds
Antidiuretics			
Desmopressin intranasally at bedtime	A	R	20 μg
Calcium channel blocker	-	-	Under trial

A–Good quality; R–Recommended; RR–Recommended with reservation

long-term success rate of 90% has been claimed, whereas, for recurrent cases the success rates varied from 62% to 80%.

The operation consists of a suprapubic transverse abdominal incision for access to the space of Retzius. The bladder neck is identified with Foley's catheter in the bladder, and the paravaginal tissue is exposed. Three pairs of sutures with chromic catgut, the most caudal suture placed opposite the bladder neck, and the next two more proximally along the base of the bladder are placed through the perivaginal tissue and vaginal wall, except the mucosa, and approximated with the closest point on Cooper's ligament without tension. A Penrose drain is kept in the space of Retzius and the bladder drained with a Foley's catheter. In partial modification of this method, Tanagho (1976) and Stanton (1984) have used dexon and vicryl sutures respectively. Currently, most gynecologists use delayed absorbable sutures like vicryl, though a few use non-absorbable suture like mersilene or proline. However, no difference was noticed in the success rates related to the number of sutures, their placement or adjunctive procedures like culdoplasty or hysterectomy (Dainer et al 1999). A prospective study in which 289 women were randomly selected to undergo Kelly plication, Pereyra needle or Burch retropubic colposuspension showed five-year cure rates of 37%, 43% and 82% respectively confirming the superior results with the Burch colposuspension (Bergman et al 1989; Bergman and Elia 1995).

The significant complications of Burch colposuspension are urinary retention or delayed voiding (12%), de novo detrusor instability (5%–10%) and rarely hemorrhage, wound infections and enterocele (2%–10%) (Dainer et al 1999). The open versus laparoscopic Burch gave 93% versus 90% cure at the end of one year (Ross 1995), though long-term results are awaited.

1. In the last 10 years from 1991, 24 girls (Age 1–16 yrs) with spina bifida, who were treated for urinary incontinence with transvaginal sling suspension with rectus abdominis were evaluated. Of the 24, 19 remained dry after the procedure

after injection of a bulking agent into the bladder neck. This procedure reported by Dik et al (2003) at Utrecht, the Netherlands seems to be encouraging.

2. A randomised trial of Burch colposuspension with laparoscopic colposuspension using a mesh and staples for urinary stress incontinence was reported from Sweden. From the results, it appears that the open Burch procedure gave better results, with less operative time but with greater blood loss and longer hospital stay than the laparascopic method (Ankardal et al 2004).
3. A three-arm study conducted in the same institution comparing the open Burch colposuspension, laparoscopic suture and laparoscopic method using the mesh and staples has also been reported. It again demonstrated that the open Burch procedure with sutures was less time consuming than the laparoscopic suture placement, with better results, albeit with greater blood loss. The patients with laparoscopic mesh repair (the third group) had the shortest stay in hospital and least use of catheter postoperatively (Ankardal et al 2005).

Sling Procedures For Stress Incontinence

In sling operations, a strip of material is passed completely beneath the urethra or bladder neck and anchored to some point on the abdominal wall. The material used may be natural (fascia lata or muscle flaps like the Gracilis or Martius graft), or synthetic (mersilene ribbon, polypropylene prolene mesh tapes). These operations may be vaginal, abdominal or abdominovaginal. Sometimes the vaginal wall sling surgery is performed with needle suspension techniques. The relatively new transvaginal tape (TVT) procedure uses a knitted prolene mesh tape placed at the mid-urethra and not at the bladder neck as in other techniques. Ulmsten et al (1999) have reported a 3-year follow-up of 50 women after TVT procedure with the objective cure rate of 86% and with no long-term voiding difficulties, de novo detrusor instability or graft erosion. Results of a large-scale randomised trial comparing the TVT and open colposuspension are awaited.

Based on an extensive 30-year review of the literature on sling procedures for stress incontinence, Bidmead and Cardozo (2000) opine that sling procedures are indicated mainly for women with intrinsic sphincter deficiency and those who have had one or more failed incontinence operations, with a fixed scarred urethra leading to poor urethral sphincter function and low maximum urethral closure pressure. In their analysis, the objective cure rates ranged from 61% to 100% and subjective cure from 73% to 93% (with a follow-up for 1–5 years). According to the survey by Jarvis (1994) however, the overall objective cure rates were 85.5%. It was 93% for the primary procedures and 86% for recurrent cases.

Complications of sling operations: Sling operations are reported to be more obstructive than other operations for stress incontinence, with voiding difficulties in 12% of the cases requiring catheterisation for 12–60 days, de novo detrusor instability in 16%, erosion of the graft material with vaginal discharge, injury to lower urinary tract in 4% and destruction of urethral sphincter and fibrosis. To prevent postoperative voiding difficulties, the trend now is to place the sling under less tension or completely loose (Blaivas and Jacobs 1991).

Periurethral injection: Periurethral injection of collagen and other material like fat, polytetrafluoroethylene and silicon have been used in cases of recurrent incontinence and in older women. Injection made around proximal urethra produces a cushion of tissue increasing the urethral closure pressure. Injections are made under local anesthesia as daycare treatment. The success rate was 60%; however, follow-up showed 40% cure rates and some required repeated injections. There are complications in 20% of cases like urinary urgency in 12.6% and hematuria in 5% (Duckett 1998). After injections of polytetrafluoroethylene, the chemical was seen in the regional lymph nodes and therefore this substance should be avoided. Those patients who have had some improvements with previous surgery for stress incontinence but are unwilling to undergo further surgery could benefit by periurethral implantation of collagen (Eckford and Abrams 1991).

Artificial sphincter appears to be the final choice in patients with previous surgery and low urethral closure pressure. Though success has been claimed in 92%, 17% required an average of two revisions in an eight-year follow-up for malfunction or erosion of the cuff (Webster et al 1992).

Detrusor Instability

It is usually treated conservatively. A limited number of surgical procedures have been described for the unstable bladder and not all have stood the test of time or have been found to be superior to placebo. The various procedures include urethral dilatation (empirical, 23% relief of symptoms), bladder denervation, prolonged cystodistension and augmentation cystoplasty.

Following successful repair of stress incontinence, subsequent delivery should be with cesarean section to avoid recurrence.

According to Jarvis (1994), there is no single operation for stress incontinence for all women as the first choice because of morphological and urodynamic variables. The surgical procedures should therefore be individualised. The aim should be to obtain a long-term cure rate in at least 90% of the cases after surgery.

FECAL INCONTINENCE IN WOMEN

Fecal incontinence is the involuntary loss of feces or flatus. Although the definition varies, one consensus report defined it as continuous or recurrent uncontrolled passage of feces for at least one month in an individual over three years of age (Drossman et al 1998). The exact incidence of the condition is unknown, as it is a cause of social embarrassment and mild cases are rarely volunteered as a complaint (Johanson and Lafferty 1996). Fecal incontinence predominantly affects parous women, with 7%–11% of women affected in the childbearing age group, and as high as 33%–47% of inmates of old age homes suffering from the condition (Borrie and Davidson 1992). Poor physical health and advancing age contribute to the severity. It may be of minor grade (partial incontinence), where there is only loss of control of flatus or liquid stool, or major grade (complete incontinence) as in fistulas resulting in involuntary passage of feces.

Anatomy and physiology of continence:

Continence is achieved by maintenance of higher pressure in the anal canal than that in the rectum, and this is achieved by the involuntary actions of the rectum and the internal anal sphincter and voluntary control by the external anal sphincter, the puborectalis muscle and the pelvic floor muscles (Fig. 15.1). The rectum contains three distinct semilunar mucosal folds which help to maintain capacitance and, by coaptation to form a hermetic seal preventing seepage of discharge. Up to 300 cc contents can be

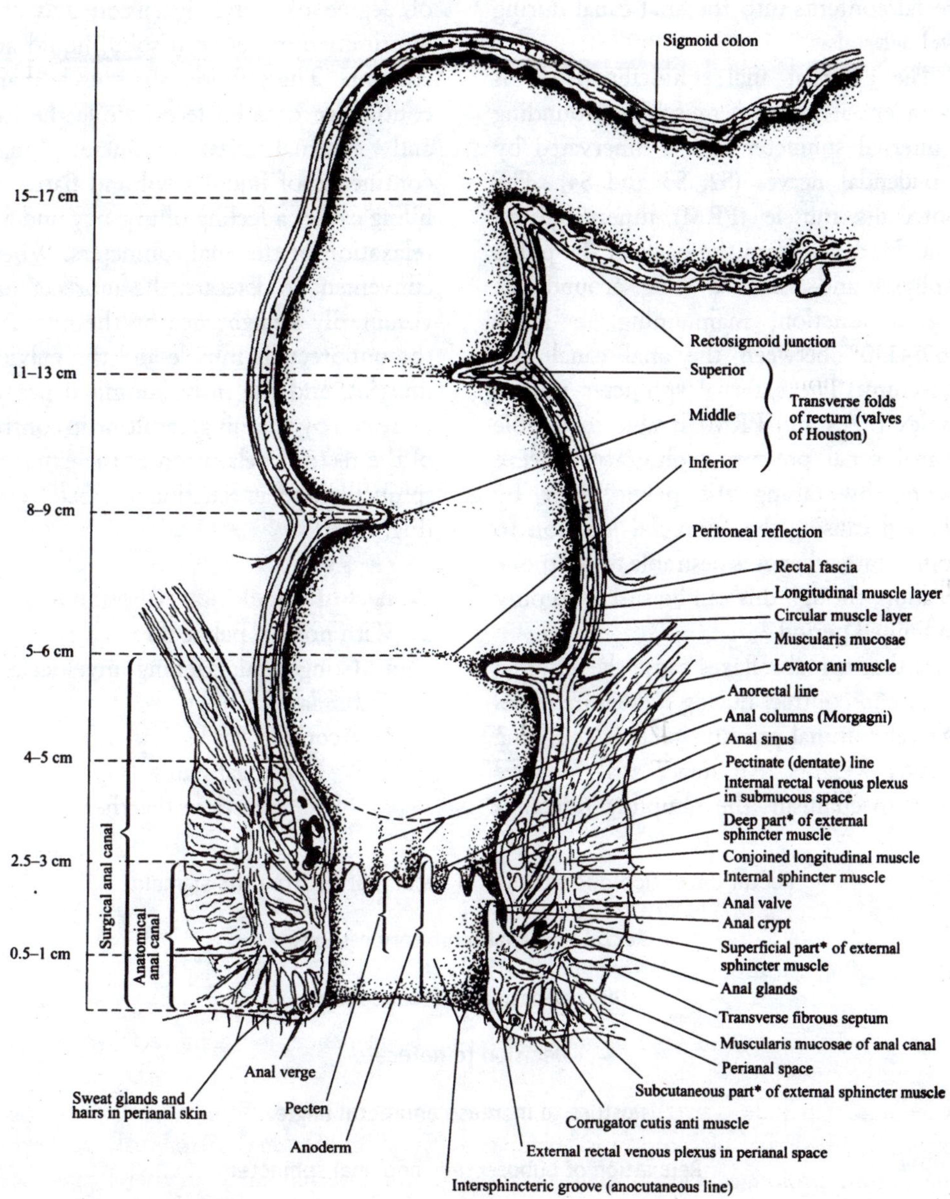

FIGURE 15.1: ANATOMY OF THE RECTUM AND ANAL CANAL

accommodated in the rectum without rise in intraluminal pressure, but filling beyond this causes a feeling of urgency.

The internal anal sphincter (IAS) is a thickening at the top of the anal canal of the circular smooth muscle from the rectal wall. This is under autonomic control and is usually tonically contracted, accounting for 75%–80%

of anal resting pressure and preventing escape of rectal contents into the anal canal during bowel peristalsis.

The external anal sphincter (EAS) is a cylinder of striated muscle surrounding the internal sphincter and is innervated by the pudendal nerves (S2, S3 and S4). The puborectalis muscle (PRM) innervated by S2 and S3, arises from the back of the pubic symphysis and forms a sling around the anorectal junction, maintaining an angle of 60°–130° between the anal canal and the rectum. The external sphincter muscle complex (EAS and PRM) is able to double the anal canal pressure (voluntary squeeze pressure) by raising the pelvic floor by 1 cm and causing the anorectal junction to become acute when it is desirable to postpone defecation, though this can be sustained only for a limited period.

Further spinal reflexes cause the external sphincter to contract during sudden increases in intraabdominal pressure such as coughing or lifting weights. An intact anal mucosal sensory mechanism (the sampling reflex) is also important for continence, for awareness of degree of rectal distension and also for discrimination between solid, liquid and gas contents. The puborectalis muscle maintains continence of solid feces, while the internal and external anal sphincters maintain continence of liquid stool and flatus. Rectal filling causes a feeling of urgency and a reflex relaxation of the anal sphincters. When it is convenient to defecate, the anorectal angle is voluntarily straightened by the relaxation of the puborectalis muscle and the pelvic floor muscles, and the intraabdominal pressure is increased by straining, resulting in contraction of the rectum, relaxation of the external anal sphincter and evacuation of rectal contents (Fig. 15.2).

Causes of Fecal Incontinence

1. With normal pelvic floor
   a. Congenital: Meningomyelocele, spina bifida
   b. Acquired
      i. Diarrheal states
         - Infectious diarrhea

Rectal distention due to entry of fecal matter from the sigmoid
↓
Rectal and anal inhibitary response
↓
Discrimination of fecal contents
↓
Decision to defecate
↓
Posture to increase anorectal angle
↓
Relaxation of puborectalis and anal sphincters
↓
Defecation (with or without strain) due to mass peristalsis
↓
External anal sphincter and puborectalis contract
↓
Closure reflex

FIGURE 15.2: MECHANISM OF FECAL EXPULSION

- Inflammatory bowel disease (ulcerative colitis, diverticulitis, TB, LGV, granulomatous disease, STD, perirectal abscess)
- Laxative abuse
- Radiation enteritis/proctitis
- Short gut syndrome

ii. Overflow
- Rectal neoplasms
- Secondary to cancer of the cervix, vagina or vulva
- Impactions

iii. Neurologic conditions (poor involuntary nervous control)
- Multiple sclerosis
- Dementia, stroke, tabes dorsalis
- Neuropathies (diabetes)
- Neoplasms of brain, spinal cord, cauda equina
- Injuries to brain, spinal cord, cauda equina

2. Abnormal pelvic floor
 a. Congenital: Anorectal malformations, vestibular anus
 b. Acquired
  i. Trauma
  - Obstetric injury (third or fourth degree perineal tear, instrumental delivery, breakdown of episiotomy)
  - Injury during operative procedures (fistulectomy, lateral internal anal sphincterotomy for chronic anal fissures or other anorectal surgery, colpoperineorrhaphy, radical vulvectomy, radical or difficult hysterectomies, hemorrhoidectomy, colpotomy and drainage of pelvic abscess)
  - Accidental injury (impalement, pelvic fractures)

 c. Pelvic floor denervation (idiopathic neurogenic incontinence)
  - Vaginal delivery
  - Chronic straining at stool
  - Rectal prolapse
  - Descending perineum syndrome

3. Ageing
4. Sexual abuse

Pathophysiology of incontinence: Fecal incontinence most commonly results from dysfunction of anal sphincters due to childbirth, operative trauma and occasionally from neurologic disorders or infiltrative disease. It may also be caused by higher rectal pressure (as in impaction of feces or neoplasms in the rectum), or active propulsion of contents into the rectum (as in small gut disease). Decrease in rectal compliance as in ulcerative or radiation proctitis and impaired rectal sensation as in multiple sclerosis, dementia, meningomyelocele and spinal cord injuries also result in incontinence in spite of intact sphincter function. Idiopathic incontinence occurs most commonly in elderly or middle-aged women and is probably due to pelvic floor denervation due to chronic straining at stool or prolonged vaginal delivery. Inflammatory conditions of the rectal mucosa as in Crohn's colitis lead to fecal incontinence because of the extreme urgency caused by the inflammation and not due to anatomic sphincter abnormality (Rao et al 1987). Incontinence due to rectovaginal fistula is seen most commonly after radiotherapy, trauma due to instrumentation during labour, at difficult hysterectomies and in granulomatous infections. Loss of mucosal co-aptation as in full thickness rectal prolapse or prolapse of internal hemorrhoids may cause loss of mucus or liquid stool.

Childbirth and fecal incontinence: Obstetric trauma is one of the commonest causes of fecal incontinence (Malouf et al 2000a). A prospective study with anal endosonography showed that a third of vaginal deliveries had obstetric anal sphincter trauma and a third of these (11%) complained of bowel symptoms (Sultan et al 1993b). Although some degree of incontinence is common in the first six weeks postpartum, about 4% of patients still suffer from the problem even after two years (Sultan et al 1993a). The most common injuries are anal sphincter tears which may be incomplete and therefore occult or missed, or injury to the pudendal nerve. The risk factors are prolonged second stage of labour, forceps/vacuum delivery, vaginal delivery in a full term primipara, birth weight of more than 4 kg and occipitoposterior delivery as these may cause damage to the internal anal sphincter even though the perineum remains intact. Instrumentation during labour such as a difficult mid-cavity forceps application or destructive procedures like craniotomy may occasionally result in a rectovaginal fistula. Third degree perineal tears resulting in obvious anal sphincter damage occur in 0.5% of vaginal deliveries (Sultan et al 1993b). Improper repair of such third or fourth degree tears may result in the patient presenting with fecal incontinence due to an anovaginal or rectovaginal fistula. The risk of sphincter damage is maximal in the first delivery. Episiotomy does not protect the mother from anal injury, although a midline episiotomy tends to extend into the anal sphincter more commonly than a mediolateral episiotomy (Coats et al 1980). The use of forceps or vaccum during delivery is also associated with a higher risk of anal sphincter injury (Johansen et al 1993). Damage to the pelvic floor also occurs due to stretching at the time of perineal descent with pudendal nerve damage and denervation as well as direct pelvic muscle injury (Snooks et al 1985). This progressive denervation may be the cause for persistent and worsening fecal incontinence even 5 years after vaginal delivery. This may be further aggravated by chronic constipation or by the descending perineum syndrome.

Evaluation of fecal incontinence: This begins with a careful history, followed by a thorough physical examination, which together often reveal a probable cause for the incontinence, thus enabling focused diagnostic testing.

History: A complete history usually reveals the cause of the problem and the type of intervention required. Severity of the incontinence may be judged by the frequency of incontinent episodes, the number of pads used and restriction of normal activity. The nature of stool is important—if small amounts of watery stools are passed between normal defecatory episodes, IAS damage is suggested, while if the patient is not able to hold solid feces till convenient time or place is available, EAS or voluntary muscle weakness is the cause. Details of previous anorectal or bowel surgery, medical disease and drugs used, as well as history of childbirth should be elicited—instrumentation at the time of delivery (and injury if any) prolonged or difficult labour and number of deliveries. Sexual history should also form part of routine history taking, to screen for history of sexual abuse or anal intercourse (Novi and Mulvihill 2005).

Physical examination: External examination of the perineum reveals fecal soiling or dermatitis if the incontinence is chronic, fistula and scars of previous sepsis, episiotomies or presence of complete perineal tears. Perineal sensation is tested by gently stroking the skin to the side of the anus. Failure of reflex contraction of the external sphincter suggests S3 and S4 nerve damage or interruption of spinal reflex arc. Digital examination may reveal fecal impaction or rectal neoplasms. It also provides a crude assessment of anal resting tone. When the patient is asked to bear down or squeeze against the finger, anal sphincter tone, PRM function, pelvic floor descent and squeeze pressure may be estimated. Per rectum examination is also useful for palpation of the torn and retracted ends of the sphincter in cases of complete perineal tear.

Rectovaginal fistula (RVF): Defects more than 3 cm away from the anal verge are called rectovaginal fistula and those within 3 cm are termed anovaginal fistula. Most commonly, these follow obstetric trauma. Following obstructed labour, rectovaginal fistula have been reported in 7%–18% of cases in addition to bladder fistula (Tahzib 1983). Occasionally, they may be due to a difficult total or radical hysterectomy. In a series of 1000 cases of Schauta's operation for cancer of cervix, Inguila and Cosmi (1967) reported 2.4% of bladder fistula, 1.6% of ureterovaginal and 2% of rectovaginal fistula. These fistulas may vary in size from a pinpoint to one which may admit a finger easily on rectal examination. They may be surrounded by scarring or may be associated with a defective sphincter. Occasionally, very small rectovaginal fistulas may require instillation of methylene blue into the rectum for exact localisation in the vagina.

Special tests: Detailed anorectal physiological studies and radiological examination may be used to confirm the clinical diagnosis or the studies repeated to reassess efficacy of treatment, but all patients will not need all the tests available. Careful history and clinical examination enable the physician to advise individualised investigations. The outcome of these tests is reproducible and hence they may be used for medicolegal reasons.

Anorectal manometry: This may be performed using water-perfused catheters, air and water filled balloons or by microtransducer pressure catheters and are best used to determine the amplitude and duration of voluntary squeeze pressure (normal range 75–250 cm H_2O). It can also be used to record maximal anal resting pressure (45–95 cm H_2O), rectal compliance, and rectal and anal pressure during straining. Low resting anal pressure suggests IAS defects while low squeeze pressure suggests weakness of the EAS. Rectal sensation and compliance can be assessed to predict surgical outcome (Young et al 1998).

Anorectal ultrasonography: This is performed using a rectal probe of 7 mHz and 10 mHz, either vaginally or anally and is rotated through 360° inside a plastic cone of 15 mm diameter. Withdrawal of the probe provides good images of the IAS which is seen as a dark homogenous ring and the EAS seen as a white heterogeneous ring surrounding this (Peschers et al 1997). Structural abnormalities of the anal sphincters such as disruption, the size and locations of such defects, rectal wall and PRM abnormalities can be understood in detail by this method. Anorectal ultrasonography findings correlate well with manometry and EMG results. It is the simplest, most reliable and least invasive test for diagnosis of anatomic defects and allows for correct selection of patients for surgical repair as well as postoperative assessment of treatment efficacy (Meyenberger et al 1996; Ternent et al 1997).

Pudendal nerve terminal latency (PTNL): This is measured using a rubber finger stall with electrodes for stimulating the pudendal nerve as it passes the ischial spine and for recording the time taken for the stimulated nerve to contract the external sphincter muscle, which is normally 2 ms (Tetzschner et al 1997). Prolongation of PNTL suggests damage to the pudendal nerve; however, this does not always negatively affect surgical results (Gilliland et al 1998), even though normal conduction is a predictor of favorable outcome (Suilleabhain et al 2001).

Electromyography: It is performed by inserting fine needles into the EAS surface or in concentric fashion and can be used to detect neurogenic or myogenic damage. However, ultrasonography has made EMG obsolete in sphincter mapping.

Defecography: Photography or videography performed after instillation of barium paste into the rectum, at rest and while straining can be used to measure anorectal angle, pelvic descent, anal canal length and to demonstrate occult or overt rectal prolapse.

Other investigations: Selected patients may need inspection of the distal colon and anus by colonoscopy, sigmoidoscopy, proctoscopy, or by barium studies to determine upper bowel causes of diarrhea and fecal incontinence. Stool culture may be necessary to rule out an infectious cause. Magnetic resonance imaging (MRI) is currently being investigated as a diagnostic tool for incontinence as it is more accurate than ultrasound at identifying external sphincter abnormalities and pelvic floor muscle movement (Rociu et al 1999). Availability and cost are major deterrents to its routine use.

Management of Fecal Incontinence

Prevention: As vaginal delivery is the major cause of fecal incontinence in women, care should be taken during delivery to avoid this complication especially in nullipara or patients with high infant weight, occipitoposterior position, prolonged active phase of second stage, perineal edema or instrumental delivery (Hagberg et al 2000). A mediolateral episiotomy is associated with fewer extensions into the anal sphincter and rectum than a midline one. Sufficient perineal support should be provided during delivery of the head as well as the shoulders. A digital rectal examination should be performed after all deliveries to diagnose third or fourth degree perineal injury. Repair of such injuries should be performed preferably by a senior or experienced surgeon and with good visualisation of the perineum to ensure correct identification of tissue layers and optimum results (Sultan et al 1995). The first suture in the repair of a third or fourth degree tear should be taken well above the apex of the mucosal or sphincteric tear to avoid nonclosure of an anorectal wall defect which may result in the patient presenting with a fistula later.

Treatment

Medical: The causes of diarrheal states such as inflammatory bowel disease are ascertained and treated. Methylcellulose or other bulk laxatives to convert liquid stool may be given. Frequency of stool can be reduced by gut motility slowing anti-diarrheals such as loperamide, codeine phosphate or diphenoxylate. Dis-impaction of impacted stool and treatment to prevent recurrence may help selected patients. A regular bowel programme or scheduled toileting benefits patients with incontinence related to mental or physical disability. Food and liquid diary may reveal excessive caffeine intake or lactose intolerance to be the source of fecal urgency and incontinence and restriction of these substances may offer relief (Choi et al 2003). Early studies demonstrate presence of estrogen, androgen and progesterone receptors in the anal canal and sphincters and suggest a positive role for hormone replacement therapy in postmenopausal women with fecal incontinence (Oettling and Franz 1998).

Biofeedback therapy: This is an established method of treating urinary incontinence and may be used in patients with fecal incontinence. Patients with intact sphincter mechanisms and mild to moderate decrease in rectal sensations are the best candidates for this treatment, with 80%–90% of them showing good results (Norton and Kamm 1999). Biofeedback also improves outcomes after sphincteroplasty (Palsson et al 2004). In this, patients are guided to recognise rectal distension and retrain their pelvic floor and abdominal muscles to contract with maximum effect when this occurs. Success depends on improvement of rectal sensation. The benefit of biofeedback may begin to decline after 6–8 months, requiring repeat therapy. The treatment is time-consuming and requires dedication from both patient and therapist (Hill and Kiff 1999).

Surgical management: Depending on the lesion, various surgical procedures may be performed to improve fecal incontinence.

1. *Complete perineal tear and direct sphincter repair:* Even after overt third degree tear (involving anal sphincters) and fourth degree tear (extension of tear into anal mucosa) are recognised and repaired at childbirth, the outcome is often unfavourable, with 30%–50% of these patients still suffering from chronic incontinence, fecal urgency, chronic pelvic pain and dyspareunia (Hagberg et al 2000). The primary repair usually fails because of faulty technique, and improper approximation of the cut edges of the sphincter, sepsis or unrecognised injury and symptoms develop 7–10 days after delivery. A second attempt to repair this tear should be undertaken only three to six months after the primary repair in order to ensure good vascularisation and reinnervation of tissue and freedom from inflammation and sepsis. Complete perineal tear may be repaired by the layered method where the rectovaginal septum is dissected into layers recreating the fourth degree tear which is then repaired by suturing in layers. Dimples on either side of the anal opening denote the two edges of the torn sphincter, and these should be picked up by Allis' forceps, mobilised and approximated. Vaginal mucosa and superficial perineal muscles are then closed like an episiotomy.
2. *Warren flap method*: This method, while providing a better cosmetic result due to better perineal body formation, offers no advantage over the layer method in providing better muscular control. It involves formation of a vaginal pedicle graft to form the anterior wall of the lower end of the anal canal avoiding direct anal wall incision. The torn ends of the sphincter are approximated over it and layered closure is performed.
3. *Direct sphincteroplasty*: When primary repair has failed to provide continence and a persistent sphincter injury is demonstrable clinically or by endosonography, direct sphincter repair may be undertaken. In these cases, a wide lateral mobilisation of the sphincter tissue is made along its entire length of 3–4 cm, scar tissue at the site of previous injury identified and divided, and edges sutured either end to end or overlapping, without tension, using delayed absorbable interrupted sutures (Sultan et al 1999). The sphincter tissue is then closed in a layered manner to ensure non occurrence of fistula. Results are good in 80% of patients unless associated with

severe pelvic floor denervation due to pudendal nerve neuropathy.

4. *Overlapping anterior anal sphincter repair*: This is the standard treatment for anterior structural damage to anal sphincter as shown by anal endosonography. Short-term follow-up showed 60%–97% success rates. However, on long-term follow-up of over 5 years only 50% were fully continent (Malouf et al 2000b).

RECTOVAGINAL FISTULA

Transvaginal Repair

1. **Anovaginal fistula** These are fistulas within 3 cm of sphincter. They may be treated by simply laying open the fistula without interfering with the sphincter, especially if the patient has good sphincter tone. Where the sphincter is suspected to be partially torn, conversion of the fistula into a fourth degree perineal tear should be followed by the classical layered repair, taking care to refashion the external sphincter.
2. **Very small rectovaginal fistula:** This may be closed by two or more simple purse string sutures.
3. **Larger rectovaginal fistula:** Larger fistulas in this region will require layered closure of rectal and vaginal walls after wide mobilisation of the posterior vaginal and anterior rectal walls and excision of the fistula.
4. **High fistula:** A Latzko repair or saucerisation may be performed for high fistula (sigmoido-vaginal) seen in the vaginal vault following hysterectomy. A circular incision is taken around the fistula in the vaginal wall which is then dissected off the underlying rectal tissue up to the margins of the fistula. This vaginal flap is then closed transversely with interrupted sutures enclosing the fistula and reinforced by the surrounding vaginal epithelium forming a second layer. A gracilis muscle flap or labial flap may be interposed in correction of previous unsuccessful fistula surgery where excessive scar tissue may be present.
5. **Rectovaginal fistula:** Any underlying cause of RVF such as tuberculosis, veneral disease, foreign body injury or other granulomatous condition have to be treated first. An RVF following radiotherapy and active Crohn's disease are difficult to treat due to poor tissue healing, and a permanent or temporary colostomy may prove to be more beneficial to the patient. Surgery is advocated only 10–12 weeks after occurrence after ensuring that the patient is in good physical condition, tissues are free of sepsis, bowel is prepared preoperatively and prophylactic antibiotic therapy is instituted.

Trans-abdominal Repair

Complicated high rectovaginal fistulas require a trans-abdominal approach (especially with primary bowel disease), which while removing the fistula preserves the sphincteric mechanism. However, care must be taken to ensure that the underlying disease (such as tuberculosis, granulomatous conditions), is treated before embarking on repair, and a temporary colostomy may be required Where poor healing is expected, as in fistula caused by radiotherapy or inflammatory granulomatous lesions, temporary colostomy may be required.

Closure of fistula is successful if the basic principles of adequate mobilisation, excision of tract, hemostasis, meticulous approximation and closure with no tension on suture lines are followed. In all these cases, a preliminary temporary colostomy will be necessary.

RECTAL PROLAPSE

Incontinence is reported in approximately half the number of patients with rectal prolapse (Madoff et al 1992). It may be due to a weakened internal anal sphincter as a result of the prolapse or due to loss of half of the external anal sphincter due to constant dilatation by prolapsed tissue. Mucosal prolapse which results from a disruption of the submucosa from the underlying muscularis propria is considered to be part of the spectrum of hemorrhoidal disease and is treated by excision, injection of sclerosant or by rubber band ligation. Complete or full-thickness prolapse of the rectum through the anal orifice can be corrected, either by the perineal approach where excision of the prolapsed mucosa is followed by plication of the muscularis or by abdominal rectopexy where the rectum is mobilised and fixed to the back of the sacrum by sutures or mesh. Both procedures are safe, even for elderly patients, in whom the condition is most common, and the marked improvement in symptoms after the surgery greatly facilitates their nursing care.

Neosphincters: Artificial anal sphincters were introduced in 1996 for the treatment of patients with severe fecal incontinence who are not responsive to conventional therapy. These consist of silastic inflatable cuffs which can occlude the anal canal, and can be deflated by a pump placed in the labium majus when defecation is desired. On deflation, the fluid in the cuff is transferred to a reservoir placed in the retroperitoneal space superior to the bladder. Success rates range from 33% to 76%. Infection, cuff erosion through the perineum and poor wound healing are the common causes of failure (Malouf et al 2000b). Neosphincters made of the gracilis muscle encircling the anal canal increase the anal canal resting tone. This involves transposing the gracilis muscle from the inner thigh to wrap around the anal canal and attaching the tendon to the opposite ischial tuberosity. The muscle is stimulated by a stimulator placed subcutaneously in the abdominal wall to maintain constant tone. Although 70% to 80% success rates have been reported (Niriella and Deen 2000), only 16% had normal continence on follow-up 5 years later (Thornton et al 2003).

Sacral nerve stimulation: This involves stimulation of the nerves passing through the S2, S3 and S4 sacral foramen which innervate the pelvic floor muscles. These are suitable for patients with intact but functionally deficient anal sphincters. Although the exact mechanism of action is not known, stimulation of the sensory and motor afferents and modulation of neural reflexes are likely causes (Madoff 2004).

Radiofrequency ablation: This newer modality of incontinence treatment involves delivery of temperature controlled radiofrequency energy to create thermal lesions deep to the anal mucosa, creating scarring and thus narrowing of the anal canal and retraction of the anal sphincter complex (Takahashi et al 2002).

Post-anal repair: If all methods fail, a patient with intractable incontinence would be better off with a colostomy or ileostomy—this would considerably improve her quality of life.

All obstetricians and gynecologists will have patients with fecal incontinence, minor degrees of which will never be volunteered by the patient. The majority are due to obstetric trauma, overt or occult, especially to the anal sphincters, and respond very well to surgical correction provided extensive nerve denervation and muscle damage do not coexist.

Care should be taken in subsequent deliveries to prevent a recurrence by avoiding a prolonged second stage, providing good perineal support to the fetal head and shoulders and the use of adequate mediolateral episiotomy.

The role of cesarean section for women with occult injuries is controversial because studies have shown that further tearing of the sphincter in subsequent deliveries is rare; however, there is an increased risk of development of fecal incontinence with subsequent vaginal deliveries (Faltin et al 2001). Although a recent study (MacArthur et al 2005) failed to show conclusive evidence of benefit in maintaining long-term fecal continence following a planned cesarean in subsequent pregnancies, if the patient is still troubled by persistent symptoms, or has sustained a major tear necessitating repeated operative repair and is currently continent, cesarean section is strongly recommended (Wattchow and Rieger 1999; McKenna et al 2003).

Although literature focuses mainly on surgical management for continence of both urine and feces, these must be seen only as anatomic closure and not as cure. A cure following fistula surgery occurs not only when the patient is continent, but is able to have coitus without dyspareunia and is able to have children (Coetzee and Lithgow 1966). This means that a more holistic approach to the problem is required, which would also include psychosexual and emotional counselling in order to restore her quality of life to as near normal as possible.

References

Ahmed S. 1988. *Urinary fistulas in gynecological practice in North West Frontier Province.* Paper presented in Lahore, December 1988. Unpublished. Cited in Report of the Technical Working Committee for the prevention and treatment of obstetric fistulae. Geneva: World Health Organization, p 15.

Ankardal M, A Ekerydh, K Crafoord, I Milsom, J-H Stjerndahl, ME Engh. 2004. A randomized trial comparing open Burch colposuspension with lap.colposuspension with mesh staples for women with stress urinary incontinence. *Br J Obstet Gynaecol* 111:974–981.

Ankardal M, I Milsom, J-H Stjerndahl, ME Engh. 2005. A three-armed trial comparing open Burch colposuspension with laparoscopic colposuspension and with laparoscopic colposuspension using mesh and staples. *Acta Obstet Gynec Scand* 84:773–779.

Arrowsmith S, EC Hamlin and LL Wall. 1996. Obstructed labor injury complex: Obstetric fistula formation and the multifacted morbidity of maternal birth trauma in the developing world. *Obstet Gynecol Surv.* Sept; 51(9):568–574.

Barnett RG and WA Peters. 1983. Pregnancy following urinary diversion. *Obstet Gynecol* 62:582–586.

Bergman A, KM Ballard and PP Koonings 1989. Comparison of three different surgical procedures for genuine stress incontinence: A prospective randomized study. *Am J Obstet Gynecol* 110:1102–1106.

Bergman A and G Elia. 1995. Three surgical procedures for genuine stress incontinence. Five-year follow up of a prospective randomized study. *Am J Obstet Gynecol* 173:66–71.

Bidmead J and L Cardozo. 2000. Sling techniques in the treatment of genuine stress incontinence. *Br J Obstet Gynecol* 107(2):147–156.

Blaivas G and B Jacobs. 1991. Pubovaginal fascial sling for the treatment of complicated stress urinary incontinence. *J Urol* 145:1214–1218.

Borrie MJ and HA Davidson. 1992. Incontinence in institutions; costs and contributing factors. *Can Med Assoc* 147–322.

Burch JC. 1961. Urethrovaginal fixation of Cooper's ligament for correction of stress incontinence, cystocele and prolapse. *Am J Obstet Gynecol* 81:281–290.

Cheater FM and CM Castleden. 2000. Epidemiology and classification of urinary incontinence. *Bailliere's Clin Obstet Gynecol* 14:183–206.

Choi YK, FC Johlin Jr, RW Summers et al. 2003. Fructose intolerance: An under recognized problem. *Am J Gastroenterol* 98:1348–1353.

Coats PM, KK Chan, M Wilkins et al 1980. A comparison between midline and mediolateral episiotomies. *Br J Obstet Gynecol* 87:408–412.

Coetzee T and DM Lithgow. 1966. Obstetric fistulae of the urinary tract. *J Obstet Gynaecol Br Cwlth* 73:837–844.

Dainer M, CD Hall, GA Choe et al. 1999. Burch procedure: A comprehensive review. *Obstet Gynecol Surv* 54: 49–60.

Danso KA, JO Martey, LL Wall, TE Elkins. 1996. Epidemiology of genitourinary fistulae in Kumasi, Ghana. *Int Urogyn J* 7:117–120.

Das RK and SK Sengupta. 1969. Treatment of vesicovaginal fistulae. *J Obstet Gynecol India* 19:383.

Devi NS. 1965. A study of 500 cases of urinary fistulae. *Obstet Gynecol India* 15:632.

Dik P, AJ Klijn, JD vanGool et al. 2003. Transvaginal sling suspension of bladder neck for neurogenic sphincter incontinence. *J Urol* 170:580–581.

Drossman DA, GW Thompson, NJ Talley, P Funch-Jensen, J Janssens, WE Whitehead. 1998. Identification of subgroups of functional gastroenterological disorders. *Gastro Enterol Intl* 3:159.

Duckett JDA. 1998. Use of periurethral injectables in the treatment of genuine stress incontinence. *Br J Obstet Gynaecol* 105(4):390–396.

Eckford SD and P Abrams. 1991. Paraurethral collagen implantation for stress incontinence. *Br J Urol* 68:576–581.

Faltin DL, MR Sangalli, B Roche et al. 2001. Does a second delivery increase the risk of fecal incontinence? *Br J Obstet Gynaecol* 108:684–688.

Freda VC and D Tacchid. 1962. Ureteral injury discovered after pelvic surgery. *Am J Obstet Gynecol* 83(3):406–409.

Ganong WF 1999. Renal function and micturition. In *Review of Medical Physiology*. WF Ganong Ed. 19th edn, New York: Simon and Schuster, 693–694.

Ghosh TK 1960. *J Obstet Gynecol India* 10:287.

Gilliland R, DF Altomare, H Moreira et al. 1998. Pudendal nerve neuropathy is predictive of failure following anterior sphincteroplasty. *Dis Colon Rectum* 41:1516–1522.

Gogoi MP 1979. Abdominovaginal method of repair of difficult bladder fistulae. *J Obstet Gynecol India* 29:843.

Gunaratne M and JKG Mati. 1982. Acquired fistulae of the female lower genital tract: A comprehensive five year review. *J Obstet Gynecol Eastern and Central Africa* 1:11–115.

Hagberg H, E Samuelsson, L Ladfors et al. 2000. Anal sphincter tears: Prospective study of obstetric risk factors. *Br J Obstet Gynecol* 107:926–931.

Hamlin RH and EC Nicholson. 1969. Reconstruction of urethra totally destroyed in labour. *Br Med J* 2:147.

Hill J and ES Kiff. 1995. Investigations and management of faecal incontinence. *Rec Adv Obstet Gynecol* 19:175–189.

Hiton P and A Ward. 1998. Epidemiological and surgical aspects of urogenital fistulae: A review of 25 years' experience in southeast Nigeria. *Int Urogynecol J Pelvic Floor Dysfunct.* 9(4):189–194.

ICI Scientific Committee of 1st International Consultation on Incontinence. 2000. Assessment and treatment of urinary incontinence. *Lancet* 355:2153–2158.

Inguila W and EV Cosmi. 1967. Radical vaginal surgery for cancer cervix. *Am J Obstet Gynecol* 99:1078.

Jarvis GJ. 1994. Surgery for GSI–Review. *Br J Obstet Gynaecol* 101:371–374.

Johansen RB, C Rice, M Doyle et al. 1993. A randomized prospective study comparing the new vacuum extractor policy with forceps delivery. *Br J Obstet Gynecol* 100:524–530.

Johanson JF and J Lafferty. 1996. Epidemiology of fecal incontinence: The silent affliction. *Am J Gastroenterol* 91:33–36.

Kelly HA and W Dumm 1914. Urinary incontinence in women without manifest injury to the bladder. *Surg Gynecol Obstet* 18:444–450.

Kelly J and BE Kwast. 1993. Epidemiology of VVF in Ethiopia. *Int Urogyn J* 4:278–281.

Kiricuta I and AM Goldstein. 1972. The repair of extensive vesicovaginal fistulas with pedicted omentum: a review of 27 cases. *J Urol* Nov; 108(5):724–727.

Kochakarn W, K Ratana-Olarn, V Viseshsindh, V Muangman and P Gojaseni. 2000. Vesico-vaginal fistula: experience of 230 cases. *J Med Assoc Thai.* Oct; 83(10):1129–1132.

Lazarus HM. 1959. Urinary fistulae in women with reference to operative techniques. *J Obstet Gynecol India* 10:1.

Laffont A and H Ezes. 1947. May–Sept; 17(5):120–123.

Lee CA and RS Simmonds. 1988. Etiology of bladder fistulae. *Obstet Gynecol* 72:313.

MacArthur C, C Glazener, R Lancahire, Herbison et al. 2005. Fecal incontinence and mode of first and subsequent delivery: A six-year longitudinal study *Br J Obstet Gynaecol* 112:1075–1082.

Macasaet MA, T Lu and GH Nelson. 1976. Uterovaginal fistula as a complication of radical pelvic surgery. *Am J Obstet Gynecol* 124:757–760.

Madoff RD, JD Watts, DA Rothenberger et al 1992. Rectal prolapse: In MM Henry and M Swash (eds) *Coloproctology and the pelvic floor.* London: Butterworth, p. 2.

Madoff RD. 2004. Surgical treatment options for fecal incontinence. *Gastroenterology* 126:S48–S54.

Mahfouz N. 1957. Bladder fistulae of obstetric origin. *J Obstet Gynecol Br Emp* 64:23.

Malouf AJ, CS Norton, AK Engel et al. 2000a. Long term results of overlapping anterior anal-sphincter repair for obstetric trauma. *Lancet* 355:260–265.

Malouf AJ, CJ Vaizey, MA Kamm, RJ Nicholls. 2000b. Reassessing artificial bowel sphincters. *Lancet* 355:2219.

McKenna DS, JB Ester and JR Fischer. 2003. Elective cesarean delivery for women with a previous anal sphincter rupture. *Am J Obstet Gynecol* 189:1251–1256.

Meigs GV. 1954. *Surgical treatment of carcinoma cervix.* London: Grune and Stratton.

Meyenberger C, P Batschinger, GF Zala and P Buchmann. 1996. Anal sphincter defects in faecal incontinence: correlation between endosonography and surgery. *Endoscopy* 28(2):217–224.

Moir JC. 1964. Reconstruction of the urethra. *J Obstet Gynecol Br Emp* 71:349.

Moir JC. 1965. Circumferential vesicovaginal fistula. *J Obstet Gynecol India* 15:44.

Moir JC. 1967. *The vesicovaginal fistula.* London: Bailliere Tindall.

Moir JC. 1973. Vesicovaginal fistula as seen in Great Britain. *J Obstet Gynecol Br Cmwlth* 80:598.

Moore KH. 2000. Conservative management for urinary incontinence. *Bailliere's Clin Obstet Gynecol* 14:251–290.

Muleta M. 2004. Socio-demographic profile and obstetric experience of fistulae at Addis Ababa fistula hospital. *Ethiop Med J* 42:9–16.

Mustafa AZ and BME Rushwan. 1971. Acquired genito-urinary fistula in Sudan. *J Obstet Gynecol Br Cmwlth* 74:1039.

Naidu PM. 1962. A study of 208 cases of VVF. *J Obstet Gynecol Br Cmwlth* 69:211–218.

Niriella DA and Deen KI. 2000. Neosphincters in the management of faecal incontinence: A review. *Br J Surg* 87:1617–628.

Norton C and MA Kamm. 1999. Outcome of biofeedback for faecal incontinence. *Br J Surg* 90(9):1159–1163.

Novi JM and BHK Mulvihill. 2005. Fecal incontinence in women: A review of evaluation and management. *Obstet Gynecol Surv* 60(4):261–269.

Oettling G and HB Franz. 1998. Mapping of adrogen, estrogen and progesterone receptors in the anal continence organ. *Eur J Obstet Gynecol Reprod Biol* 77(2):211–216.

Oumachigui A, SB Sen, PN Nayak. 1980. Utero-urinary fistula in obstetrics: report of three cases. *Int J Obstet Gynecol* 18:258–263.

Palsson OS, S Heyman, WE Whitehead. 2004. Biofeedback treatment for functional anorectal disorders: A comprehensive efficacy review. *App Psychophysiol Biofeedback* 29:153–174.

Peschers UM, Delansing JO, Scaer GN, Schuessler B. 1997. Exoanal ultrasound of the anal sphincter: Normal anatomy and sphincter defects. *Br J Obstet Gynecol* 104(9):999–1003.

Rao KB. 1972. Vesicovaginal fistulae. *J Obstet Gynecol India* 22:536–541.

Rao KB. 1975. Bladder fistulae. *J Obstet Gynecol India* 25:58.

Rao KB. 1989. Genital fistulae. In MKK Menon, PK Devi and KB Rao (eds) *Postgraduate Obstetrics and Gynecology*, 4th edn. Madras: Orient Longman, 526–534.

Rao SSC, NW Read, P Davison et al. 1987. Anorectal sensitivity and responses to rectal distension in patients with ulcerative colitis. *Gastroenterology*. 93:1020–1026.

Rociu E, J Stoler, MJ Eijkemans et al. 1999. Fecal incontinence: Endoanal US versus endoanal MR imaging. *Radiology* 212 (2):453–458.

Ross JW. 1992. Laparoscopic Burch repair compared with laparotomy Burch to cure urinary stress incontinence. *J Am Assoc Gynecol Laprosc* 2 (Suppl.):S47–S48.

Sen NK and NN Chowdhury 1976. *J Obstet Gynecol India* 26:921.

Sims JM. 1853. *On the treatment of VVF*. Philadelphia: Clanchard and Lea.

Snooks SJ, MM Henry, M Swash. 1985. Faecal incontinence due to external anal sphincter division in child birth is associated with damage to the innervation of the pelvic floor musculature: A double pathology. *Br J Obstet Gynaecol* 92:824–828.

Stanton SL. 1984. The Burch colposuspension procedure. *Acta Urol Belg* 52:280–282.

Suilleabhain CB, AF Horgan and L McEnroe. 2001. The relationship of pudendal nerve terminal motor latency to squeeze pressure in patients with idiopathic fecal incontinence. *Dis Colon Rectum* 44:666–671.

Sultan AH, MA Kamm, CN Hudson 1995. Obstetric perineal tears: An audit of training. *J Obstet Gynecol* 15:19–23.

Sultan AH, MA Kamm, CL Bartram et al. 1993a. Anal sphincter trauma during instrumental delivery. *Int J Gynecol Obstet* 43:263–270.

Sultan AH, MA Kamm, CN Hudson et al. 1993b. Anal sphincter disruption during vaginal delivery. *N Engl J Med* 329:1904–1911.

Sultan AH, AK Monga, SL Stanton, D Kumar. 1999. Primary repair of obstetric anal sphincter rupture using the overlap technique. *Br J Obstet Gynecol* 106:318–323.

Symmonds RE, HN Hill 1978. Loss of the urethra. Report of 50 patients. *Am J Obstet Gynecol* 130:131.

Tahzib F. 1983. Epidemiological determinants of vesicovaginal fistulae. *Br J Obstet Gynaecol* 90:387–391.

Takahashi T, S Garcia-Osogobio, MA Valdovinos et al. 2002. Radiofrequency energy delivery to the anal canal for the treatment of fecal incontinence. *Dis Colon Rectum* 445:915–922.

Tanagho EA. 1976. Colpocystourethropexy: The way we do it. *J Urol.* Dec; 116(6):751–753.

Ternent CA, M Shashidharan, GJ Blatchford et al 1997. Transanal ultrasound and anorectal physiology findings affecting continence after sphincteroplasty. *Dis Colon Rectum* 160(4):324–331.

Tetzschner T, M Sorenson, G Lose and J Christiansen. 1997. Pudendal nerve function during pregnancy and after delivery. *Int Urogynecol J Pelvic Floor Dysfunct* 8(2):66–68.

Thompson JD. 1998. Repair of vesicovaginal fistula. In JA Rock and JD Thompson (Eds) *TeLinde's Operative Gynecology*. 8th edn, Boston: Lippincott-Raven, p. 1197.

Thornton MJ, ML Kennedy, DZ Lubowski et al. 2004. Long-term follow-up of dynamic graciloplasty for fecal incontinence. *Colorectal Dis* 46:470–476.

Ulmsten U, P Johnson, MA Ruzapour. 1999. A three-year follow-up for surgical treatment of female stress urinary incontinence. *Br J Obstet Gynecol* 106:345–350.

Wall LL and JA Karisuma. 2004. A study of 869 cases of VVF from Jos, Nigeria. *Am J Obst Gynec* 190:1011–1019.

Wattchow DA and N Rieger. 1999. Faecal incontinence after vaginal delivery. *Lancet* 354:965.

Webster SD, LM Perez, JM Khoury et al. 1992. Management of stress urinary incontinence using artificial urinary sphincter. *Urology* 39:499–503.

Yennen E and C Babuna 1965. Genital fistula: A study based on 197 consecutive cases. *Obstet Gynecol* 26:219–224.

Young CJ, MN Mathur, AA Eyers et al. 1998. Successful overlapping anal sphincter repair: relationship to patient age, neuropathy, and colostomy formation. *Dis Colon Rectum* 41:344–399.

16

Gestational Trophoblastic Disease

P K Sekharan

Gestational trophoblastic disease (GTD) is the term now used to describe the spectrum of cellular proliferation ranging from the various forms of hydatidiform mole, through invasive mole and choriocarcinoma to placental site trophoblastic tumours. The screening programmes for persistent trophoblastic disease following evacuation of hydatidiform mole have been instrumental in the near elimination of fatalities from sequelae to mole (Bagshawe 2003). It is now well recognised that molar pregnancy comprises two distinct entities, complete hydatidiform mole (CHM) and partial hydatidiform mole (PHM), which differ on the bases of chromosomal pattern, gross and microscopic pathology and clinical presentation. Placental site trophoblastic tumour is a rare neoplastic subtype of gestational trophoblastic disease. Epithelioid trophoblastic tumour (ETT) is the most recently described and rarest of the trophoblastic tumours.

Gestational trophoblastic diseases are:

- Complete hydatidiform mole (CHM)
- Partial hydatidiform mole (PHM)
- Invasive mole (IM)
- Gestational choriocarcinoma (CC)
- Placental site trophoblastic tumour (PSTT)
- Epithelioid trophoblastic tumour (ETT)

Complete and partial hydatidiform mole (PHM) differ in their invasive potential and propensity for malignant transformation. Approximately 8% to 20% of patients with CHM may be expected to develop persistent trophoblastic disease following molar evacuation (Curry et al 1975; Bagshawe et al 1990; Lawler et al 1991)· PHM gives rise to persistent trophoblastic disease in less than 3% of cases (Goto et al 1993)·

Normal trophoblast: Trophoblast populations of normal placenta are composed of cytotrophoblast, syncytiotrophoblast and intermediate trophoblast (Shih and Kurman 2001). Cytotrophoblast and syncytiotrophoblast form the villous trophoblast that covers the chorionic villi. The cytotrophoblast is the trophoblastic stem cell. In the villi which are in contact with the placental bed, the cytotrophoblast merges imperceptibly with the trophoblastic columns. They usually express cytokeratins but produce little or no hormones. Syncytiotrophoblast is formed from the fusion of cytotrophoblasts and is composed of multinucleated cells with abundant dense cytoplasm. It secretes large amounts of hCG, some human placental lactogen (hPL) and placental alkaline phosphatase (PLAP) but has little capacity for further proliferation. After 8 weeks, production of hCG decreases while hPL and PLAP increase as pregnancy advances (Kurman et al 1984). Syncytiotrophoblast also synthesises estrogen and progesterone (Pattilo et al 1983). Intermediate trophoblast can be further subdivided into villous intermediate trophoblast located in the villous columns, implantation site intermediate trophoblast located in the placental site and chorionic type intermediate trophoblast located in the chorionic laeve of the fetal membranes (Shih and Kurman 2001).

Studies using monoclonal antibodies with high sensitivity and specificity for measuring hCG and its free subunits suggest that trophoblastic cells in complete and partial moles differ significantly in the manner in which they secrete the free subunits of hCG. Complete moles have higher serum levels of free α hCG whereas partial moles have higher levels of β hCG.

Genetics of Hydatidiform Moles

The male and female gametes are unique in having a haploid set of chromosomes. At fertilisation the complete complement of 23 pairs is restored. The fertilised egg before division duplicates its chromosome so that each daughter cell has a complete set of 23 pairs.

Vassilakos, Szulman, Surti and Fisher (Vassilakos and Kaiji 1976; Vassilakos et al 1977; Szulman and Surti 1978; Lawler et al 1979; Lawler et al 1982; Fisher et al 1997) have clearly demonstrated that CHM and PHM are separate syndromes with different genetic backgrounds.

Complete hydatidiform mole (CHM): Chromosomes in CHM are entirely paternally derived. The ovum loses its maternal haploid set of 23X by an obscure mechanism and is fertilised by a sperm containing paternal haploid set of 23X. Further development takes place by duplication of the 23X to form 46XX without simultaneous cell division (monospermic—homozygous) Nearly 95%

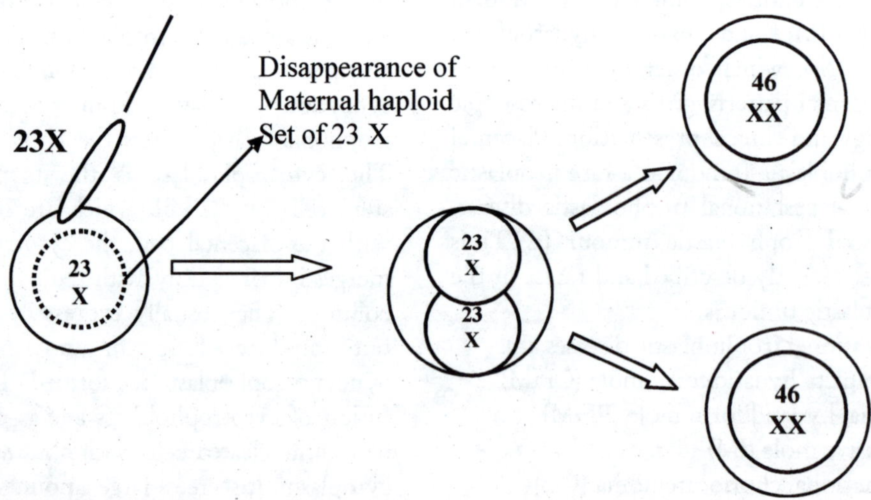

Figure 16.1: The origin of complete mole. The maternal haploid set of 23X chromosome is extruded by some obscure mechanism and fertilisation is effected by a single sperm containing 23X which duplicates (without concomitant cell division) to provide 46XX chromosomes, all of paternal origin.

of complete moles are formed in this manner and rarely, 46XY moles are found as a result of fertilisation of an 'empty egg' by two sperms carrying X and Y chromosomes (dispermic diploidy—heterozygous). The resulting moles are totally androgenetic and therefore total allografts in the mother instead of being hemi-allografts, as in normal pregnancy. It has been suggested that heterozygous moles are more prone to turn into invasive mole and choriocarcinoma, but this is not supported by conclusive evidence.

Partial hydatidiform mole (PHM): Partial hydatidiform mole is a product of a fertilisation error. An apparently normal ovum containing 23X haploid set of maternal chromosome is fertilised by two spermatozoa, commonly one with 23X and other with 23Y paternal haploid set of chromosomes, resulting in 69XXY karyotype. Partial moles are thus diandric triploid. A diploid ovum of 46XX if combined with a paternal haploid set 23X/Y does not result in molar pregnancy. Thus in both complete mole and partial mole, there is a dominance of the zygote by paternally derived chromosomes.

Clinical pathology of gestational trophoblastic diseases: All types of gestational trophoblastic diseases exhibit proliferation of both syncytiotrophoblast and cytotrophoblast cells which maintain secretion of hCG. Placental-site trophoblastic tumour arising from the intermediate trophoblast cells produces low levels of hCG and hPL.

Complete hydatidiform mole: The classical histologic features of complete mole are generalised diffuse hyperplasia of both cytotrophoblast and syncytiotrophoblast often associated with cytological atypia, generalised edema of chorionic villi which distend to form central cisterns giving the macroscopic appearance of 'bunch of grapes',

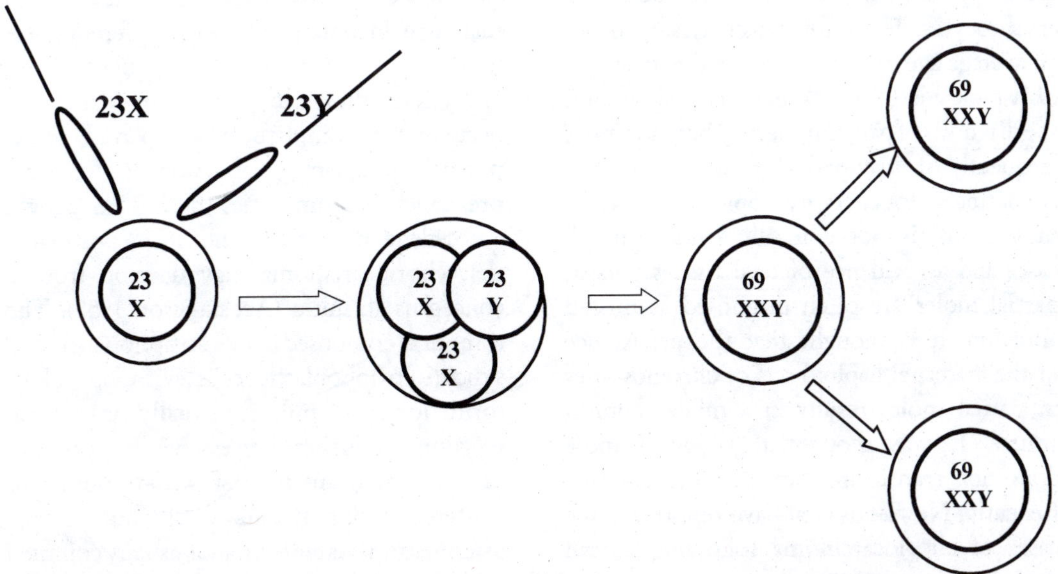

Figure 16.2: Origin of a partial mole. Two sperms, usually one with 23X and the other with 23Y sets of chromosomes, enter an apparently normal ovum to have a total of 69 chromosomes.

and the absence of an embryo which perishes before attaining a size of 1 mm, embryonic death and resorption occurring before the formation of fetal erythrocytes. Fisher and others in 1997 reported the presence of fetal blood cells in seven complete hydatidiform moles by polymerase chain reaction amplification of DNA. Their conclusion was that fetal blood cells may be present in the villi of complete hydatidiform moles and the presence of fetal erythrocytes alone should not be considered indicative of a diagnosis of partial hydatidiform mole. Even though hyperplasia of the trophoblast is the important factor in molar disease, this does not provide a reliable guide to the subsequent development of persistent disease.

Partial hydatidiform mole: Partial hydatidiform mole is formed by diandric triploidy; the placenta is characterised by focal, variable hydropic villi and usually by focal, mild trophoblastic hyperplasia predominantly confined to the syncytium. Fetal vessels are usually present and contain nucleated fetal erythrocytes. The embryo usually survives to an average age of 9 weeks. Since the incidence of triploidy is 1% to 2% in clinical abortions, the diagnosis of partial mole may be made more frequently if histopathological examination is routinely done. As hydropic degeneration of the villi is not clinically evident in all cases and as evidence of fetal tissues persist, partial moles are often diagnosed as missed abortion. It is thought that the persistence of the maternal haploid sets of chromosomes in partial moles results in a milder clinical course. It was thought that partial mole does not transform into choriocarcinoma. Recently, Newlands et al have reported three cases of choriocarcinoma following partial mole (Seckl et al 2000).

Invasive mole: An invasive mole is the presence of molar villi in places other than the original implantation site (usually in the myometrium, but could even be present in the vagina or lungs). It is a locally invasive, rarely metastatic lesion characterised microscopically by trophoblastic invasion of the myometrium with identifiable villous structures. Most invasive moles show moderate to marked trophoblastic activity and persistence of villous structures. It behaves like blood-borne deposits of a malignant neoplasm. The histological diagnosis of invasive mole is rarely made, as hysterectomy is seldom done and it is difficult to identify from curettings. It is associated with uterine sub-involution, post-molar bleeding and rising hCG level. Deep penetration into the myometrium can lead to perforation of the uterus and massive intra-peritoneal hemorrhage. Chemotherapy may be started on the basis of rising hCG level and it is not necessary to confirm the histopathological diagnosis of invasive mole or choriocarcinoma.

Gestational choriocarcinoma: This is a malignant neoplasm in which differentiation towards villous cytotrophoblast and syncytiotrophoblast is seen. It can occur after complete mole, partial mole, normal pregnancy, abortion or ectopic pregnancy. In some cases there is no known antecedent pregnancy and it is postulated that choriocarcinoma may develop from a conceptus ab initio (Acosta-Sison 1959). The tumour is composed of cyto-trophoblastic and syncytio-trophoblastic cells without villous formation. It stimulates virtually no stromal reaction and is therefore essentially a mixture of hemorrhage and necrosis with tumour cells scattered within the mass. On microscopic examination, viable tumour is usually confined to the rim of the neoplasm as choriocarcinoma lacks an intrinsic vasculature, the tumour cells deriving nutrition by invasion of maternal blood vessels. Widespread intravascular dissemination to lungs, brain and other sites is common. The metastatic sites have a tendency to rapidly outgrow their blood supply resulting in necrosis and hemorrhage.

Placental site trophoblastic tumour (PSTT): The name placental site trophoblastic tumour (PSTT) was proposed by Scully and others two decades ago to describe a variant of gestational trophoblastic tumour (Scully and Young 1981). It is a rare type of gestational trophoblastic neoplasia (GTN) and is composed mainly of intermediate cyto-trophoblastic cells arising from the placental implantation site. These tumours can result from any type of antecedent pregnancy and are locally invasive and less widely metastatic. Placental site trophoblastic tumour produces more hPL than hCG as it contains less syncytiotrophoblast and hence hCG may not serve as a reliable tumour marker for follow-up. However, clinically the diagnosis should be suspected when hCG levels are low relative to the tumour burden. Necrosis is more prominent in PSTT as opposed to hemorrhage in GTN and vascular invasion is not as common as in GTN. The tumour invades the myometrium by dissecting between the smooth muscle fibres. Treatment of this condition is primarily surgical with multi-agent chemotherapy if indicated. In a series of 13 patients following hysterectomy for PSTT, a 43% recurrence was reported (Feltmate et al 2001).

Epithelioid trophoblastic tumour (ETT): This is a rare form of trophoblastic tumour described recently. It is composed of chorionic-type intermediate trophoblast and is distinct from choriocarcinoma and PSTT. The tumour is composed of sheets and nests of mononuclear trophoblast with clear, eosinophilic and vacuolated cytoplasm resembling 'chorionic type' intermediate trophoblast. ETT usually presents as a discrete uterine mass and its biological behaviour appears similar to PSTT (Shih and Kurman 1998).

Epidemiology: The earlier report of an increased incidence of hydatidiform mole among Asian countries was probably a result of hospital-based rather than population-based studies. The incidence of hydatidiform mole is around 1 per 1000 pregnancies in most parts of the world and perhaps as high as 2 per 1000 in Japan (Palmer 1994). The hospital based data in the author's series from Calicut Medical College is 5 per 1000 deliveries (Sekharan et al 2003). Many studies have documented an increased incidence of hydatidiform mole among women over 35 and an even greater increase in women over 40 years of age. Some of the studies showed a modest increase in risk in teenagers.

The history of a previous mole imparts nearly ten times risk for subsequent molar pregnancy. For those with two previous moles, the risk reported by Bagshawe et al (1986) was 1 in 6.5 pregnancies. An increased risk has been observed among women whose partners were above 45 years. The age-related differences in the incidence of hydatidiform mole may be due to the defective gametogenesis at the extremes of reproductive life. No maternal or paternal age-related risk was seen in partial moles. There is some evidence to suggest that the deficiency of beta-carotene and animal fat in the diet may increase the risk of hydatidiform mole. Studies from Vietnam suggest a possible link with exposure to the chemical, Agent Orange.

The most important risk factor for choriocarcinoma is a history of hydatidiform mole, accounting for a 1000- to 2000-fold increased risk of subsequent choriocarcinoma. Estimates of proportion of women who develop choriocarcinoma after a molar pregnancy have ranged from 2% to 19% (Matalon et al 1972). Persistent Trophoblastic Disease or Gestational Trophoblastic Tumour (GTT) may follow complete and partial mole with an incidence of approximately 8% and 0.5% respectively. Nearly 50%–60% of choriocarcinoma patients have a history of hydatidiform mole. The risk of developing GTT after a normal delivery is 1 in 40,000 to 50,000. In a series from Charing Cross Hospital, 13% of the patients treated for choriocarcinoma had developed GTT following normal delivery (Tidy et al 1995). GTT following normal delivery tends to be a highly aggressive variant with widespread metastases. GTT may also follow spontaneous abortion or ectopic pregnancy. Maternal age above 40 is a strong risk factor and there is some evidence to suggest that teenage patients are also at a higher risk.

Presentation of Molar Pregnancy

Vaginal bleeding: This is the most common presenting symptom in patients with complete mole, occurring in nearly 95% of cases (Curry et al 1975; Kohorn 1984; Berkowitz and Goldstein 2003). Molar chorionic villi may disrupt maternal vessels by separating from the decidua resulting in large amounts of retained blood in the endometrial cavity. Retained blood may undergo oxidation and prune juice-like fluid may leak from the uterine cavity. Sudden and profuse bleeding can also occur in patients with complete mole. The majority of the patients will be anemic.

Excessive uterine enlargement: The uterine size on palpation tends to be larger than the size corresponding to gestational age in nearly 50% of the cases. Excessive uterine size is usually associated with markedly elevated hCG from trophoblastic overgrowth. In the rest of the cases the size may correspond to the period of gestation and in some, it may even be small for age.

Theca Lutein Cysts: Clinically evident theca lutein cyst is seen in 20%–25% of cases along with marked elevation of hCG. While theca lutein cysts are generally noted at the time of presentation, they may enlarge substantially after evacuation. The mean regression time for the lutein cyst is 8 weeks (Montz et al 1988). Acute ovarian torsion and rupture needing emergency laparotomy has been noted in patients with large lutein cysts. Ultrasound-guided aspiration is recommended to avoid such complications. During hysterectomy, ovaries may be retained, after aspiration of the cyst.

Pre-eclampsia: With the routine use of ultrasound in early pregnancy, especially in patients with first trimester bleeding, the diagnosis of hydatidiform mole is made at an early stage resulting in a dramatic reduction in the incidence of pre-eclampsia. About 10% of women with molar pregnancies develop pre-eclampsia, which is associated with hyperemesis and an unduly enlarged uterus.

Hyperemesis gravidarum: Hyperemesis requiring anti-emetic treatment and hospitalisation for correction of electrolyte disturbances may be seen in 15%–20% of cases.

Hyperthyroidism: Clinically evident hyperthyroidism with elevation of serum free thyroxine (fT_4) is seen in about 5% of cases. The thyroid function tests will rapidly return to normal after evacuation. It is proposed that high levels of hCG has TSH-like activity (Kenimer et al 1975). Patients with uncontrolled hyperthyroidism may develop 'thyroid storm' at the time of induction of anesthesia and evacuation. Thyroid storm is characterised by hyperthermia, delirium, atrial arrhythmias including atrial fibrillation, cardiovascular collapse and coma. Administration of β-adrenergic blocking agents prevents or rapidly reverses many of the cardiovascular and metabolic complications of thyroid storm. Antithyroid drugs and high dose hydrocortisone are also used in treating these patients.

Respiratory insufficiency: About 2% of patients may develop respiratory insufficiency. The patient may present with tachycardia, tachypnea, anxiety or confusion immediately after evacuation. While embolisation of molar tissue to the pulmonary vasculature may contribute to respiratory distress, it may also result from cardiovascular complication of toxemia, thyroid storm or overzealous fluid replacement. Some patients may require intubation and mechanical ventilation.

With the availability and use of ultrasound for the diagnosis and evaluation of early pregnancy, diagnosis of complete hydatidiform mole is currently made before the patients develop the classic signs and symptoms. Investigation of first trimester bleeding by ultrasound is routine now and it may diagnose an abnormal pregnancy like hydatidiform mole at the earliest. In some cases, routine ultrasound examinations for confirming gestational age or for antenatal screening will lead to the diagnosis of asymptomatic molar pregnancy.

Presentation of partial mole: Patients with partial mole usually do not present with the classical features of complete mole. The vaginal bleeding is slight and occurs late. The clinical diagnosis before evacuation is incomplete or missed abortion in more than 90% of cases. The diagnosis of partial mole is made after histological review of products of conception from presumed incomplete or missed abortion.

Diagnosis: Ultrasonography has proved to be an accurate and sensitive technique for the diagnosis of complete mole. Complete mole produces a characteristic vesicular pattern due to generalised swelling of the chorionic villi. In the first trimester complete moles tend to be smaller and have less cavitations. However, the majority of first trimester, complete moles still demonstrate the typical ultrasound appearance of a complex, echogenic intrauterine mass containing multiple small cystic spaces (Benson et al 2000). Ultrasonography may also help detect partial hydatidiform mole: the ultrasound findings observed in these cases are an excessively enlarged placenta, cystic spaces within the placenta, gestational sac which is either empty or containing amorphous echoes or a growth retarded fetus.

hCG measurement: Markedly elevated hCG levels are commonly seen in patients with complete mole. Genest et al (1991) reviewed the clinical and pathological characteristics of 153 cases of complete mole managed at the NETDC between 1980 and 1990 and suggested that pre-evacuation hCG levels were greater than 100,000 U/l in 46% of the patients. The measurement of a high hCG level (> 100,000 U/L) may therefore suggest a complete molar pregnancy, particularly when associated with vaginal bleeding and uterine enlargement. In contrast, partial hydatidiform mole is less commonly associated with markedly elevated hCG values. Studies using monoclonal antibodies with high sensitivity and specificity for measuring hCG and its free subunits suggest that trophoblastic cells in complete and partial moles differ significantly in the manner in which they secrete the free subunits of hCG (Ozturk et al 1988; Berkowitz et al 1989). Complete moles have higher serum levels of percentage free α hCG fraction than do partial moles (2.4 versus 1.0, $p < 0.005$). In contrast, partial moles have higher serum levels of percentage free β hCG than do complete moles (0.85 versus 0.17, $p < 0.0005$).

Management of hydatidiform mole: When a diagnosis of complete or partial molar pregnancy is made, the most appropriate method of evacuation should be decided. Assessment of the patient for the presence of medical complications including anemia, pre-eclampsia, hyperthyroidism and respiratory insufficiency is essential. It is appropriate to have a baseline hCG estimation in addition to routine blood and urinalysis.

The primary management of hydatidiform mole is evacuation of the mole. Cross-matched blood for transfusion and appropriate fluid resuscitation measures should be kept ready at the time of evacuation. Evacuation is done under anesthesia by suction curettage and intravenous oxytocin is given to promote uterine contraction. When the uterus is empty, the uterine cavity is gently curetted with a sharp curette to ensure complete evacuation; the specimen is sent for histopathological examination. Big theca lutein cysts if present are managed by ultrasound guided aspiration to avoid torsion. It may take 6 to 8 weeks for the lutein cysts to disappear. An ultrasound examination after one week of suction curettage will ensure completeness of evacuation. A repeat curettage is done if the pre-evacuation size of the uterus is >14 weeks and if there is evidence of incomplete evacuation.

Hysterectomy with mole in situ may be attempted in patients who are above 40 years and who desire no further childbearing. Hysterectomy reduces the risk of subsequent development of choriocarcinoma (Bahar et al 1989) and completely eliminates the risk of invasive mole. It does not eliminate the potential for malignant sequelae and monitoring with β hCG levels is mandatory. Theca lutein cysts if present are left alone after reducing the size with multiple needle pricks. Hysterotomy is not to be considered as a method of evacuation of the mole. Patients who are Rh negative should receive Rh immune globulin at the time of evacuation as the Rh D factor is expressed on trophoblast (Kenimer et al 1975) and also due to the reported presence of fetal RBCs in complete mole (Fisher et al 1997).

Chemoprophylaxis: The use of chemoprophylaxis during evacuation of hydatidiform mole remains controversial. However, several investigators have reported that chemoprophylaxis reduced the incidence of post-molar tumour (Berkowitz et al 1981; Kohorn 1982; Kim et al 1986). In a prospective randomised trial, Kim et al (1986) observed that in patients with high-risk complete mole, prophylactic chemotherapy reduced the incidence of post-molar tumour from 47% to 14% and among patients with low-risk complete mole, prophylactic chemotherapy did not influence the incidence of persistent disease (7.7% versus 5.6%). However, patients who developed persistent tumour after prophylactic chemotherapy required more courses of chemotherapy. Prophylactic chemotherapy may be useful in patients with high-risk complete mole when hormonal follow up is either unavailable or unreliable. The main objection to exposing all patients with molar pregnancy to chemotherapeutic agents is that only a small percentage are at risk for developing persistent disease, who are readily identified by proper follow-up.

Follow-up: Patients with complete and partial mole should be monitored with serial hCG values after evacuation to assure that they achieve complete and sustained remission. The expected fall in serum β hCG per week follows a log linear fashion. Patients must be encouraged to use reliable contraception during the period of follow-up. There is no conclusive evidence to suggest that oral contraceptives increase the risk of development of choriocarcinoma (Berkowitz et al 1981). Low dose oral contraceptive pills may be safely prescribed without increasing the risk of persistent disease. With the controversy surrounding this issue, it may be prudent to advise them on barrier contraceptives till the hCG is normal and then start OC pills. Intrauterine devices are avoided due to the risk of perforation.

On an average, 20% of patients undergoing evacuation of complete hydatidiform mole develop post-molar GTD, with a range of 6% to 36% as reported by various authors (Lurain et al 1983; Bagshawe 1993; Morrow et al 1997). In our own series of 1569 cases of hydatidiform moles diagnosed and treated over a period of 15 years from June 1990, the incidence of persistent GTD was 20.5% (Sekharan et al 2005).

Diagnostic evaluation: The optimal management of GTN requires through evaluation of the extent of the disease prior to initiation of chemotherapy. All patients should undergo a careful pre-treatment evaluation including physical examination, hCG measurement, hepatic, renal and thyroid function tests and complete blood count. The metastatic work-up should include chest x-ray, ultrasonography or CT scan of abdomen and pelvis, CT or MRI scan of the head. Extensive work-up with CT and MRI is not required in patients diagnosed on the basis of serum hCG levels following molar evacuation unless they show resistance to chemotherapy.

Classification of the Malignant Gestational Trophoblastic Disease

Hammonds Clinical Classification of GTT (Hammonds et al 1973)

I. Non-metastatic GTD: No evidence of disease outside of uterus not assigned to prognostic category.

II. Metastatic disease: Any metastasis

A. Low-risk metastatic GTD
1. Short duration (<4 months)
2. Low hCG level (<40,000 mIU/ml)
3. No metastasis to brain or liver
4. No antecedent term pregnancy
5. No prior chemotherapy

B. High-risk metastatic GTD
1. Long duration (>4 months since last pregnancy)
2. High pre-treatment hCG level (>40,000 mIU/ml)
3. Brain or liver metastasis
4. Antecedent term pregnancy

Suggested regimen for follow-up (Newlands 2003)

Serum β-hCG	Once in 2 weeks, till negative for 4 weeks
Serum β-hCG	Monthly, until one year post evacuation
Urine sample for hCG	Once in 3 months, until 2 years post evacuation.

1. hCG follow-up may range from 6 months to 2 years after evacuation
2. If the hCG values become negative within 8 weeks after evacuation, follow-up will be limited to 6 months post-evacuation
3. Patients who do not have normal hCG 8 weeks post-evacuation should be followed-up for 2 years
4. Estimation of hCG is recommended at 6 weeks and 10 weeks postpartum or after termination of subsequent pregnancies as there is a small increase in choriocarcinoma in these patients

Criteria for the Diagnosis of Post-Molar Trophoblastic Neoplasia (GTN) (Newlands 2003)

Serum hCG	>20,000 IU/l 4 weeks after evacuation
Plateau of hCG	Four measurements over a period of 3 weeks
Rise of hCG	
Level of hCG	Remains elevated 6 months post mole*
Histological evidence of choriocarcinoma	

*(*Author recommends treatment after 16 weeks if positive)*

5. Prior chemotherapy

All cases of non-metastatic disease can be cured by single-agent chemotherapy. Many patients with low-risk metastatic cases can also be treated initially with single agent chemotherapy to get a cure but some of them may require multi-agent chemotherapy. High-risk metastatic disease should always be started on combination chemotherapy.

FIGO Staging and Risk Factor Scoring for Gestational Trophoblastic Neoplasia 2002 (Kohorn 2003) Placental site trophoblastic tumour will be categorised separately from other gestational trophoblastic neoplasia.

Criteria for the Diagnosis of Post-Hydatidiform Mole Trophoblastic Neoplasia (GTN)

1. GTN may be diagnosed* when the plateau of human chorionic gonadotropin (hCG) lasts for four measurements over a period of 3 weeks or longer, that is days 1, 7, 14, 21.
2. GTN may be diagnosed* when there is a rise of hCG on three consecutive weekly measurements, over a period of two weeks or longer, days 1, 7, 14.
3. GTN is diagnosed if there is histologic diagnosis of choriocarcinoma.
4. GTN is diagnosed when the hCG level remains elevated for 6 months or more.†

**The actual level of hCG or the amount of rise will be determined by the individual investigator*

†This may not apply to patients with unexplained low hCG levels without clinical or imaging evidence of GTN (Kohorn 2002).

Criteria for Methods Used to Diagnose Metastases in Trophoblastic Neoplasia

1. Chest x-ray is appropriate for diagnosing lung metastases and is used to evaluate the risk factor score according to the number and size of lung metastases (CT scanning is preferable).
2. Liver metastases may be diagnosed by CT scanning or by ultrasound.
3. Brain metastases may be diagnosed by MRI or CT scanning.
4. To diagnose intraabdominal metastases CT scanning is preferable.

The FIGO 2002 staging and risk factor scoring system for gestational trophoblastic neoplasia

Stage I	Disease confined to the uterus.
Stage II	GTN extends outside the uterus but is limited to the genital structures (adnexa, vagina, broad ligament).
Stage III	GTN extends to the lungs with or without genital tract involvement.
Stage IV	All other metastatic sites.

FIGO Risk Factor Scoring Values

In order to stage and allot a risk factor score a patient's diagnosis is allocated to a stage as represented by roman numerals I, II, III and IV. This is then separated by a colon from the actual risk factor score expressed in arabic numerals. For purposes of reporting, patients are divided into low-risk (score 0–6) and high-risk (score ≥7) groups. Bagshawe's risk scoring system (Bagshawe 1976) which was modified and adopted by WHO (1983) was further modified in the FIGO risk scoring system. From the WHO scoring, ABO blood grouping has been omitted and liver metastasis has been given a score of 4. Placental site trophoblastic tumour has been classed separately.

Examples of low-risk and high-risk staging/scoring are as follows:

Example 1: A 45-year-old lady has a hydatidiform mole evacuated uneventfully. The hCG decreases from a pre-evacuation value of 80,000 mIU/ml to 1000 mIU/ml 4 weeks after the D&C but then persists between 800 and 1000 mIU/ml for 4 weeks. Clinical examination shows no abnormality or evidence of metastases. Ultrasound of the uterus shows a 2 cm lesion in the myometrium. Chest x-ray is negative.

This patient is staged FIGO stage I:2. The two risk factors are the patient's age and the hCG of 1000, that is, 10^3–10^4. Each risk factor has a score of one.

Example 2: A 41-year-old woman has bleeding after her third successful pregnancy. Histology of curettings are suggestive of choriocarcinoma. Ultrasound shows a 5 cm lesion in the myometrium and the chest x-ray shows multiple (more than 8) lung nodules, 1 to 2 cm in size. Brain MRI shows a 3 cm lesion in the right frontal lobe of the brain.

This patient is staged FIGO IV:13 as she is 41 years old (1) and is post–full-term pregnancy (2), has a brain metastasis (4), has more than eight metastases to the lung (4) and has a 5 cm lesion in the uterus (2). The histologic confirmation of choriocarcinoma does not add to the risk score by the FIGO System.

Management of non-metastatic GTD: Patients in this category are diagnosed essentially by regular post-molar serum β hCG assays. A sustained 100% remission can be achieved in these patients after primary treatment with single-agent chemotherapy. Methotrexate and actinomycin-D are the primary drugs used in the management of non-metastatic disease. 5-fluorouracil and oral etoposide give excellent results.

Methotrexate: This has been used in the management of malignant GTD since the 1950s and achieves up to 100% cure rates in non-metastatic disease. It is given at a dose of 0.4 mg/kg intramuscularly for five days and repeated every two weeks. Pre-treatment evaluation of liver function and renal function along with complete hemogram should be done. Total WBC count and platelet count are monitored twice a week. Toxicity includes ulceration of the GI tract, bone marrow depression, alopecia and photosensitivity reaction of the skin. Anemia and infections increase the risk of toxicity. Methotrexate should not be given if there is impairment of renal or liver function. Mild to moderate toxicity is experienced by 25%–30% of patients.

Methotrexate-Folinic Acid regimen: Bagshawe and Wilde proposed the use of folinic acid along with methotrexate to rescue normal tissues from the dihydrofolate reductase block of methotrexate, allowing safe use of high methotrexate doses (Berkowitz et al 1986; Bagshawe et al 1989). The regimen used is inj. methotrexate 1 mg/kg body weight on days 1, 3, 5 and 7 and inj. folinic acid 0.1 mg/kg body weight on days 2, 4, 6 and 8. The cycle can be repeated depending on the serum β hCG level every 10 to 14 days to achieve complete remission in non-metastatic and low-risk metastatic GTD. More than 80% of non-metastatic disease will attain remission with one course of MTX-FA regimen (Bagshawe et al 1989).

In a series of 321 cases of non-metastatic disease treated by the author (2005) using MTX-FA regimen, complete remission could be achieved in 88% of cases with 20% responding to a single course. Additional therapy with EMACO regimen and/or hysterectomy was required in 10% of cases. No serious side effects were noticed with this regimen.

Actinomycin-D: Given as intravenous infusion at a dose of 9–13 μg/kg for 5 days, Actinomycin-D is an equally effective therapy. The cycle can be repeated every 14 days. Nausea, vomiting, alopecia and transient marrow depression is seen in 30%–40% of patients. Local extravasation of the drug may cause sloughing of the tissues and extreme care should be taken in administering the drug, preferably as a diluted infusion via a large peripheral vein. Actinomycin-D can also be given in alternating cycles with methotrexate to improve the remission rate and to reduce the toxicity.

Management of low-risk metastatic disease: Patients categorised as low-risk metastatic disease group should be treated with single-agent chemotherapy with methotrexate or actinomycin-D according to one of the protocols described below.

Methotrexate should be avoided if there is an abnormality in hepatic or renal function. Patients who develop resistance to sequential single-agent chemotherapy are then treated with combination chemotherapy as for high-risk disease. Several studies have demonstrated the high curability of low-risk metastatic GTD when appropriate therapy is administered. Ross and co-workers were the first investigators to identify the highly favorable prognosis in this group of patients (curing 20 of 21 patients—a rate of 95%) with relatively non-toxic sequential methotrexate and actinomycin-D chemotherapy (Ross et al 1965). Subsequent reports by Brewer et al (1971), Hammond et al (1973, 1980), Goldstein and coworkers (1972, 1982, 1986), Bagshawe (1976), Jones and Lewis (1974), Jones (1981) and Lurain et al (1982) documented virtually 100% cure rates in low-risk metastatic disease using initial single-agent chemotherapy.

Chemotherapy for low-risk metastatic gestational trophoblastic tumours

Methotrexate 0.4 mg/kg IV or IM QD x 5 days; repeat every 12–14 days (7–9 day window)
Actinomycin D 10–13 μg/kg IV QD x 5 days; repeat every 12–14 days (7–9 day window)

FIGO risk factor scoring system

FIGO scoring	0	1	2	4
Age	<40	>40		
Antecedent pregnancy	Mole	Abortion	Term	
Months from index pregnancy	<4	4 to <7	7 to <13	≥13
Pre-treatment serum hCG (IU/l)	$<10^3$	10^3 to $<10^4$	10^4 to $<10^5$	$\geq 10^5$
Largest tumour size (cm)	<3	3 to <5	≥5	
Site of metastasis	Lung	Spleen, kidney	GIT	Liver, brain
Number of metastasis	--	1–4	5–8	>8
Previous failed chemotherapy	--	--	Single drug	2 or more drugs

Methotrexate 1 mg/kg IM on days 1, 3, 5, 7;
folinic acid 0.1 mg/kg IM on days 2, 4, 6, 8;
Repeat every 15–18 days (7–10 day window)

Single-agent chemotherapy is safe, highly effective and avoids the greater morbidity associated with multi-agent chemotherapy. With appropriate initial classification and selection of patients as well as proper administration of treatment, cure rates approach 100%. It is apparent however, that 30%–50% of patients in this category will develop resistance to the first chemotherapeutic agent and require alternative treatment. It is therefore very important to carefully monitor patients undergoing treatment for evidence of drug resistance (plateau or rise in hCG level and/or development of new metastases), so that a change to a second agent can be made at the earliest possible time. Approximately 5%–15% of patients treated for low-risk metastatic disease with sequential single-agent chemotherapy will require multi-agent chemotherapy with or without surgery to achieve complete remission.

Surgery may be necessary to eradicate persistent disease in the uterus, if all evidence of metastatic disease has disappeared and if the hCG remains elevated despite repeated courses of chemotherapy or rarely to excise isolated pulmonary metastases (Hammond et al 1980). Hysterectomy may also be incorporated into the initial management of the patient with low-risk metastatic disease resulting in greater likelihood of single-agent chemotherapy success, fewer courses of chemotherapy and a shorter duration of treatment (Hammond et al 1980).

Management of high-risk metastatic GTD: The association of the following prognostic factors place the patient in the high-risk category and will require multi-agent chemotherapy for cure:

- Duration more than four months from the antecedent pregnancy
- Pre-treatment serum hCG level >40,000 U/l
- Metastasis to sites other than the lung and vagina
- Antecedent term gestation
- Previous failed therapy

These patients should be treated initially with multi-agent chemotherapy, with or without adjuvant radiotherapy or surgery. Until the mid-1980s, the primary multi-agent regimen used was MAC: methotrexate, actinomycin-D, and cyclophosphamide and reported cure rates ranged from 63% to 71% (Berkowitz et al 1984; Lurain and Brewer 1985). Bagshawe and colleagues at Charing Cross Hospital, London developed the seven-drug CHAMOCA protocol in the mid-1970s using cyclophosphamide, hydroxyurea, actinomycin-D, methotrexate with folinic acid, vincristine and doxorubicin and reported a primary remission rate of 82% (Begent and Bagshawe 1982).

After the discovery of etoposide in the late 1970s as a very effective chemotherapeutic agent for gestational trophoblastic tumours, Newlands et al (1991) formulated the EMA-CO regimen employing etoposide, high-dose methotrexate with folinic acid, actinomycin-D, cyclophosphamide and vincristine with a complete clinical response of 80%.

Bower et al (1997) updated the Charing Cross experience using EMA-CO to treat 272 women with high-risk disease. There were 11 (4%) early deaths, 214 (78%) complete remission and an additional 33 (12%) complete response to subsequent cisplatin-based chemotherapy and surgery with an overall survival rate of 88%. Kim et al (1998) from Korea treated 165 high-risk patients with EMA-CO regimen with an overall survival rate of 84%.

The high response rates, good long-term survival and the minimal acute and cumulative toxicity associated with EMA-CO protocol make it the current initial treatment of choice for high-risk metastatic gestational trophoblastic tumours. Colony stimulating factors should be used when necessary to avoid treatment delays, as the success of the EMA-CO regimen seems to depend on treatment given at short intervals without interruption. Granulocyte Colony Stimulating Factor (G-CSF), 300 μg subcutaneously, may be given on days 9 to 14 of each subsequent treatment cycles in patients who develop neutropenia. Chemotherapy should be continued until three consecutive weekly hCG values are normal. Two to four courses of EMA-CO regimen are given after the first normal hCG level.

The EMA-EP regimen, substituting etoposide and cisplatin for cyclophosphamide and vincristine in the EMA-CO regimen seems to be the most appropriate therapy for patients showing incomplete remission. The BEP (bleomycin, etoposide, cisplatin), VIP (Etoposide, ifosfamide, cisplatin) and ICE (ifosfamide, carboplatin, etoposide) protocols were also successful in patients who failed to respond to EMA-CO regimen.

When CNS metastasis is present, whole brain irradiation (3000 cGy in 200 cGy fractions) is given simultaneously with initiation of chemotherapy. Brain irradiation has the dual purpose of being both tumouricidal and hemostatic. During radiotherapy, the methotrexate infusion dose in the EMA-CO protocol is increased to one g/m^2 and 30 mg folinic acid is given every 12 hours for three days, starting 32 hours after the infusion begins. As an alternative to brain irradiation, the Charing Cross hospital group recommended intrathecal as well as high-dose intravenous methotrexate.

Liver metastases from choriocarcinoma are ominous as they tend to be extensive disease at multiple sites. There is a significant risk of serious hepatic bleeding, especially during the first course of chemotherapy. Whole-liver irradiation with 2000 cGy over two weeks combined with chemotherapy is recommended to reduce the risk of bleeding.

Intensive multi-modality therapy with appropriate combination chemotherapy, adjuvant radiotherapy and surgery has resulted in cure rates of 80%–90% in patients with high-risk metastatic gestational trophoblastic tumours.

Role of surgery in the management of trophoblastic disease: Surgery has an important role in the management of GTD. Molar pregnancies should be evacuated by suction curettage and medical methods are best avoided. Hysterectomy may be considered as part of primary evacuation if other gynecological morbidity is present. Additional surgical procedures, especially hysterectomy and thoracotomy can remove known foci of chemo-resistant cases with persistent or recurrent high-risk metastatic disease (Hammond et al 1980; Soper 1994). Prompt hCG regression within one or two weeks of surgical resection indicates a favorable outcome. In women with excessive vaginal bleeding, arterial embolisation should be considered if fertility is to be maintained. Hysterectomy may be required for the management of excessive uterine bleeding either at presentation or after the onset of chemotherapy and in the management of chemo-resistant disease localised to the pelvis. Hysterectomy is the treatment of choice for the management of placental site tumours confined to the uterus. In cases of intra-peritoneal bleeding as a result of perforation of the uterus by invasive mole, resection and closure or even hysterectomy may be required.

Pregnancy following gestational trophoblastic disease: Patients with gestational trophoblastic disease may be assured that they may expect a normal reproductive outcome. However, patients with GTD are at an increased risk of developing recurrent molar pregnancy, the reported risk being 1% (Sand et al 1984; Newlands et al 1998). Some of the series have reported a higher incidence of abortion. The risk of congenital anomalies is not increased by chemotherapy for malignant GTD. An increased risk of placenta accreta was reported by some authors. All patients should have an ultrasound at 8–10 weeks in the subsequent pregnancy to rule out molar changes.

In our own series, out of the 262 pregnancies following hydatidiform mole, 224 women had full-term normal delivery, 17 had cesarean section, 16 ended in abortion, two developed ectopic pregnancy and three developed recurrent mole.

Recurrent molar pregnancy: The risk of recurrent molar pregnancy following one molar pregnancy is approximately 1%, which is an increased risk as compared to that in the general population (1:1000 pregnancies) (Bagshawe et al 1986; Rice et al 1989). In a series of 34 patients who had at least two molar pregnancies between 1965 and 2001 at the New England Trophoblastic Disease Centre (Newlands et al 1998), four patients with an initial partial mole had a subsequent complete mole, and six patients with initial complete mole had a subsequent partial mole. Ten patients had repeat partial mole and fourteen had repeat complete mole.

The risk of recurrent mole after two molar pregnancies was reported as 15% and 28% respectively by Bagshawe et al (1986) and Sand et al (1984).

In patients with recurrent mole, there is an increased risk of persistent Gestational Trophoblastic Tumour (GTT). Parazinni et al (1988) reported a threefold increase in persistent GTT in subsequent molar pregnancies in patients with repeat mole. Among 34 patients with repeat mole, reported by Garner et al (2002), 4 (20%) out of 20 complete moles and none out of 14 partial moles were treated for

EMA-CO Regimen for high-risk metastatic gestational trophoblastic tumours

Day	*Drug*	*Dose*
1	Etoposide	100 mg/m ^{2} IV over 30 min
	Actinomycin D	0.5mg IV bolus
	Methotrexate	100 mg/m^2 bolus and 200 mg/m^2 IV infusion 1000 ml 5% dextrose over 12 hours.
2	Etoposide	100 mg/m^2 IV infusion over 30 min
	Actinomycin D	0.5 mg IV bolus
	Folinic acid	15 mg IM every 12 h, for 4 doses beginning 24 h after start of methotrexate
8	Cyclophosphamide	600 mg/m^2 IV
	Vincristine	1 mg/m^2 IV bolus

Repeat cycles on days 15, 16 and 22 (every 2 weeks)

persistent GTT following their first molar pregnancy. In contrast, persistent GTT developed following the second mole in 8 of 18 (44.4%) complete moles and 2 of 16 (12.5%) partial moles. Therefore, the risk of persistent GTT after one molar pregnancy is reported to be 11.8% and after two molar pregnancies is 29.4%.

Repeat Molar Pregnancies with Different Partners: Tuncer et al (1999) reported that six of their patients developed a molar pregnancy with at least two different partners and one patient with three different partners. Similarly, Magili et al (1993) described a patient who had two molar pregnancies with one partner and developed a third mole following donor insemination. Repeat molar pregnancy with different partners suggests that the abnormality of the oocyte may be contributing to the development of molar pregnancy. Ovum donation may be an option for patients with repeat moles. Garner et al (2002) reported a normal term delivery after ovum donation in a patient who had recurrent mole with different partners.

In vitro fertilisation and recurrent mole: Recurrent hydatidiform mole following in vitro fertilisation and embryo transfer has been reported by Barash et al (1993) and by Tanos et al (1992). In vitro fertilisation with embryo selection does not guarantee the prevention of molar pregnancy (Pal et al 1996). As most complete moles develop by monospermic fertilisation, with replication of the paternal chromosomes, attempted prevention of triploid embryos by intracytoplasmic sperm injection alone may not be successful in the prevention of molar disease. The use of IVF with fluorescence in situ hybridisations (FISH) for male sex selection or with DNA typing has been described as a technique for identification of those abnormal conceptuses (Reubinoff et al 1997).

Multiple pregnancies with mole and coexisting fetus: This is a rare condition estimated to be 1 per 22,000 to 100,000 pregnancies (Vejerslev 1991). Patients present with what appears to be hydatidiform mole or twin gestation with rapid enlargement of uterus. Careful ultrasound examination will reveal a normal fetus, amniotic sac and placenta with separate molar tissue elsewhere. Partial moles may have a fetus, but have diffuse molar changes throughout the single placenta. However, the diagnostic accuracy of this condition is only 70%. These cases are often diagnosed late, are associated with a live birth rate of around 25%, and are at a higher risk of developing pre-eclampsia and hemorrhage (Newlands 1999). The subsequent need for chemotherapy for persistent disease is greater than in other molar pregnancies (Steller et al 1994; Goldstein and Berkowitz 1999). The present policy is to allow the pregnancy to proceed to term depending on the patient's choice. Patients are counselled regarding a substantial risk of fetal loss and are registered for follow-up. Conservative management of these patients allowing the pregnancy to go ahead unless there are clear-cut medical grounds for termination such as pre-eclampsia or hemorrhage appears to be the treatment of choice.

Management of PSTT: For patients with disease localised to the uterus, the treatment of choice is hysterectomy followed by adjuvant chemotherapy in selected cases. Women with metastatic PSTT at the time of diagnosis cannot be cured by surgery alone and treatment with multi-agent systemic chemotherapy is required. Initially there were fears that PSTT was unresponsive to chemotherapy (Lathrop 1988). However, more recently there have been a number of reports demonstrating success of various different multi-agent chemotherapeutic regimens in treating metastatic PSTT, particularly pulmonary metastases. Data from Charing Cross Hospital, London suggest that EMA-EP (Etoposide, Methotrexate Actinomycin-D –Etoposide, Cisplatin) is the preferred adjuvant chemotherapeutic regimen (Newlands et al 2000). However, the effectiveness of newer anticancer agents such as the taxanes (paclitaxel, docetaxel) and camptothecins (topotecan and irinotecan) need to be evaluated for their effectiveness in GTN.

False positive hCG: False-positive or 'phantom hCG' is now recognised as a problem where patients are treated inappropriately by curettage, laparoscopy, single-agent and multi-agent chemotherapy, and even hysterectomy assuming they have trophoblastic tumour. These false positive tests are due to heterophilic antibodies in the blood mimicking hCG in hCG tests. In spite of treatment, the hCG will remain high in such cases. To distinguish false positive from true hCG rise, it is necessary to do the following tests:

1. The finding of more than fivefold differences in serum hCG results with alternative immunoassays (critical criterion).
2. The presence of hCG in serum and absence of detectable hCG or hCG related molecule immunoreactivity in a parallel urine hCG assay sample (critical criterion).
3. The observation of false positive results in other tests for molecules not normally present in serum, such as urine b-core fragment (confirmatory criterion)
4. The finding that a heterophilic antibody blocking agent (Scantibodies Inc HBR) prevented or limited false detection (confirmatory criterion).

DPC Immulite assay and Roche Elecsys hCG assays are reported not to have false positive results (Cole 2005).

Quiescent gestational trophoblastic disease: Highly differentiated trophoblastic tissue remains in the body following mole, normal pregnancy or abortion producing low levels of real hCG. This is slow growing tissue that does not respond to chemotherapy. These cases should be followed-up as they may become active and metastatic disease may develop later. Presence of hyperglycosylated hCG (hCG-H) is an indication to start treatment. Low levels of hCG is seen in PSTT. An increase in free β-sub unit is associated with PSTT (Cole 2005).

Conclusion: The outcome of GTD depends on the early detection of persistent disease by regular follow-up of patients after evacuation of hydatidiform mole. The regional and national referral centres in UK and USA have resulted in very high cure rates and elimination of fatality from GTT. In developing countries, including India, there is no such programme. It is up to the practising physicians to organise follow-up clinics in regional tertiary care centres and start a GTD registry for scientific analysis. The authors started such a centre 15 years ago at Calicut in the northern region of Kerala in India, and have so far followed-up more than 1500 cases with excellent results.

One of the fascinating aspects of GTD is the ability of the disease to exist in a quiescent form without producing clinical problems for long periods of time. Clearly, there must a small amount of abnormal tissue present but not producing enough hCG to be detected by currently available assays. These rests of GTD are important since they can be reactivated by the hormonal surge of subsequent pregnancies. The dilemma of false positive hCG versus low persistent levels of real hCG has to be addressed by refining the hCG assay methods.

References

Acosta-Sison H. 1959. Ab initio choriocarcinoma: Two unusual cases. *Obstet Gynecol* 13:350–352.

Bagshawe KD. 1976. Risk and prognostic factors in trophoblastic neoplasia. *Cancer* 38:1373–1385.

Bagshawe KD, J Dent, J Webb. 1986. Hydatidiform mole in England and Wales. *Lancet* 2:673.

Bagshawe KD, ES Newlands et al. 1989. The role of low dose methotrexate and folinic acid in gestational trophoblastic tumours. *Br J Obstet Gynecol* 96:795

Bagshawe KD, SD Lawler, FJ Paradinas et al. 1990. Gestational trophoblastic tumours following initial diagnosis of partial hydatidiform mole. *Lancet* 335:1074–1076.

Bagshawe KD. 1993. Trophoblastic neoplasia. In *Cancer Medicine,* eds. JF Holland Frei III, R Bast Jr et al, 3rd edition, Baltimore: Williams & Wilkins.

Bagshawe KD. 2003. Introduction. In *Gestational Trophoblastic Disease*, eds BW Hancock, ES Newlands, RS Berkowitz, LA Cole. 2nd edition, London: Chapman and Hall, 1–5

Bahar AM, MS el-Ashnehi, A Senthilselvan et al. 1989. Hydatidiform in the elderly: Hysterectomy or evacuation. *Int J Obstet Gynecol* 29:233.

Barash A, Y Zalel, et al. 1993. A partial hydatidiform mole following in vitro fertilization and embryo transfer. *J Assist Reprod Genet* 10:171–173.

Begent RHJ and KD Bagshawe. 1982. The management of high-risk choriocarcinoma. *Semin Oncol* 9:198–203.

Benson CB, DR Genest, MR Bernstein V Soto-Wright, RS Berkowitz. 2000. Sonographic appearance of first trimester complete hydatidiform moles. *Ultrasound Obstet Gynecol* 16:188–191.

Berkowitz RS, DP Goldstien et al. 1981. Oral contraceptivesand postmolar trophoblastic disease. *Obstet Gynecol* 58:474.

Berkowitz RS, DP Goldstein, MR Bernstein. 1984. Modified triple therapy in the management of high-risk metastatic gestational trophoblastic tumours. *Gynecol Oncol* 19:173–181.

Berkowitz RS, DP Goldstein and MR Bernstein. 1986. Ten years experience with methotrexate and folinic acid as primary therapy for gestational trophoblastic disease. *Gynecol Oncol* 23:111–118.

Berkowitz R, M Ozturk, D Goldstein et al. 1989. Human chorionic gonadotropin and free subunit's serum levels in patients with partial and complete hydatidiform moles. *Obstet Gynecol* 74:212–216.

Berkowitz RS and DP Goldstein. 2003. Presentation and management of molar pregnancy. In *Gestational Trophoblastic Disease*, eds BW Hancock, ES Newlands, RS Berkowitz, LA Cole. 2nd edition, London: Chapman and Hall, 206–228.

Bower M, ES Newlands, L Holden et al. 1997. EMA-CO for high-risk gestational trophoblastic tumors: Result from a cohort of 272 patients. *J Clin Oncol* 15:2636–2643.

Brewer JL, TR Eckman, RE Dolkart et al. 1971. Gestational trophoblastic disease: A comparative study of the results of therapy in patients with invasive mole and with choriocarcinoma. *Am J Obstet Gynecol* 109:335–340.

Cole LA. 2005. Choosing a test for monitoring gestational trophoblastic disease. *Proceedings of the XIII World Congress on gestational trophoblastic disease, Hong Kong.* Abstract 10.3.

Curry SL, CB Hammond, L Tyrey et al. 1975. Hydatidiform mole: Diagnosis, management and long-term follow up of 347 patients. *Obstet Gynaecol* 45:1–8.

Feltmate CM, DP Goldstein, RS Berkowitz. 2001. Placental site trophoblastic tumour. *Gynecol Oncol* 82(3):415–419.

Fisher RA, ES Newlands et al. 1997. Diploid hydatidiform moles with foetal blood cells in molar villi. 2—genetics. *J Pathol* 181(2):189–195.

Garner EIO, E Lipson, MR Bernstein et al. 2002. Subsequent pregnancy experience in patients with molar pregnancy and gestational trophoblastic tumors. *J Reprod Med* 47:380–386. Pub Med.

Genest D, 0 Laborde, RS Berkowitz et al. 1991. A clinico-pathologic study of 153 cases of complete Hydatidiform mole (1980–1990): Histologic grade lacks prognostic significance. *Obstet Gynecol* 78:402–409.

Goldstein DP. 1972. The chemotherapy of gestational trophoblastic disease: Principles of clinical management. *JAMA* 220:209–213.

Goldstein DP and RS Berkowitz. 1982. Non-metastatic and low-risk metastatic gestational trophoblastic neoplasms. *Semin Oncol* 9:191–197.

Goldstein DP and RS Berkowitz. 1999. *J Int Soc Study Troph Dis* 3.

Goto S, A Yamada, T Ishizuka *et al.* 1993. Development of postmolar trophoblastic disease after partial molar pregnancy. *Gynecol Oncol* 48:165–170.

Hammond CB, LG Borchert, L Tyrey et al. 1973. Treatment of metastatic trophoblastic disease: Good and poor prognosis. *Am J Obstet Gynecol* 115:451–457.

Hammond CB, Weed JC Jr and Currie JL. 1980. The role of operation in the current therapy of gestational trophoblastic disease. *Am J Obstet Gynecol* 136:844–856.

Jones WB and JL Lewis Jr. 1974. Treatment of gestational trophoblastic disease. *Am J Obstet Gynecol* 120:14–20.

Jones WB. 1981. Management of low-risk metastatic gestational trophoblastic disease. *J Reprod Med* 26:213–217.

Julie R. Palmer. 1994. Advances in the epidemiology of trophoblastic disease. *J Reprod Med* 39:158.

Kenimer JG, JM Hershman, HP Higgins. 1975. The thyrotropin in hydatidiform moles is hCG. *J Clin Endocrinol Metab* 40:482–91.

Kim O, I Moon, KT Kim et al. 1986. Effects of prophylactic chemotherapy for persistent trophoblastic disease in patients with complete hydatidiform mole. *Obstet Gynecol* 67:690–694.

Kim SJ, SN Bae, JH Kim et al. 1998. Risk factors for the prediction of treatment failure in gestational trophoblastic tumors treated with EMA-CO regimen. *Gynecol Oncol* 71:247–253.

Kohorn EI. 1982. Hydatidiform mole and gestational trophoblastic disease in Southern Connecticut. *Obstet Gynecol* 59:78–84.

Kohorn EI. 1984. Molar pregnancy: Presentation and diagnosis. *Clin Obstet. Gynecol* 27:181–191.

Kohorn EI. 2002. Persistent low level real human chorionic gonadotropin: A clinical challenge and a therapeutic dilemma. *Gynecol Oncol* 85:315–320.

Kohorn EI. 2003. The FIGO 2000 Staging and risk factor scoring system for Gestational Trophoblastic Neoplasia. In *Gestational Trophoblastic Disease*, eds BW Hancock, ES Newlands, RS Berkowitz, LA Cole. 2nd edition, London: Chapman and Hall, 175–181.

Kurman RJ, RH Young, HJ Norris et al. 1984. Immunocytochemical localization of plascental lactogen and chorionic gonadotropin in the normal placenta and trophoblastic tumors with emphasis on intermediate trophoblast and placental site trophoblastic tumor. *Int J Gynaecol Pathol* 3:101–121.

Lathrop JC, S Lauchlan, N Ramakrishna, M Ambler. 1988. Clinical characteristics of placental site trophoblastic tumour. PSTT. *Gynecol Oncol* 31:32–42.

Lawler SD, RA Fisher, VJ Pickthall, S Povey, MW Evans. 1982. Genetic studies on hydatidiform moles. I.The origin of partial moles. *Cancer Genet Cytogenet* 5:309–320.

Lawler SD, RA Fisher, J Dent. 1991. A prospective genetic study of complete and partial hydatidiform moles. *Am J Obstet Gynecol* 164:1270–1277.

Lawler SD, VJ Pickthall, RA Fisher, S Povey, MW Evans, AE Szulman. 1979. Genetic studies of complete and partial hydatidiform moles. *Lancet* ii:58.

Lurain JR, JL Brewer, FE Torok et al. 1982. Gestational trophoblastic disease: Treatment results at the Brewer Trophoblastic Disease Center. *Obstet Gynecol* 60, 354–360.

Lurain JR, JI Brewer, FE Torok, B Halpern. 1983. Natural history of hydatidiform mole after primary evacuation. *Am J Obstet Gynecol* 145: 591–595.

Lurain JR and JI Brewer. 1985. Treatment of high-risk gestational trophoblastic disease with methotrexate, actinimycin D and cyclophosphamice chemotherapy. *Obstet Gynecol* 65:8304.

Magili G, F Parazzini, R Maggi. 1993. Repeated gestational trophoblastic disease after natural and heterologous assisted conception. *J Reprod Med* 38:405–406.

Matalon M, B Paz, L Modan et al. 1972. Malignant trophoblastic disorders, epidemiologic aspects and relationship to hydatidiform mole. *Am J Obstet Gynecol* 112:101.

Montz FJ, JB Schlaerth, CP Morrow. 1988. The natural history of theca lutein cysts. *Obstet Gynecol* 72: 247–251.

Morrow CP, OA Kletzky, PT DiSaia et al. 1977. Clinical and laboratory correlates of molar pregnancy and trophoblastic disease. *Am J Obstet Gynecol* 128:424–430.

Newlands ES et al. 1998. Influence of Chemotherapy for gestational trophoblastic disease on subsequent pregnancy outcome. *Br J Obstet Gynaecol* 105:1032–1035.

Newlands ES. 1999. Opinion: Twin gestation comprising mole in concert with normal foetus: Test, Treat, Abort or let go to term. *J Int Soc Study Troph Dis* 3.

Newlands ES, KD Bagshawe, RHJ Begent et al. 1991. Results with EMA-O REGIMEN in high-risk gestational trophoblastic tumours. *Br J Obstet Gynaecol* 98:550–557.

Newlands ES, PJ Mulholland, L Holden et al. 2000. Etoposide and cisplatin/etoposide, methotrexate and Actinomycin-D chemotherapy for patients with high-risk gestational trophoblastic tumours refractory to EMA/cyclophosphamide and vincristine chemotherapy and patients presenting with metastatic placental site trophoblastic tumours. *J Clin Oncol* 18:854–859.

Newlands ES. 2003. Investigation and treatment of patients with persistent gestational trophoblastic disease and gestational trophoblastic tumours in the United Kingdom. In *Gestational Trophoblastic Disease*, eds BW Hancock, ES Newlands, RS Berkowitz, LA Cole. 2nd edition, London: Chapman and Hall, 268–292.

Ozturk M, R Berkowitz, D Goldstein et al. 1988. Differential production of human chorionic gonadotropin and free subunits in gestational trophoblastic disease. *Am J Obstet Gynecol* 158:193–198.

Pal L, TL Toth, L Leykin. 1996. High incidence of triploidy in in vitro fertilized oocytes from a patient with a previous history of recurrent gestational trophoblastic disease. *Hum Reprod* 11:1529–1532.

Parazzini F, G Mangili, C Belloni. 1988. The problem of identification of prognostic factors for persistent trophoblastic disease. *Gynecol Oncol* 30:57–62.

Pattilo RA, RO Hussa, DE Yorde, LA Cole. 1983. Hormone synthesis by normal and neoplastic human trophoblast. In *Biology of Trophoblast*, eds YW Loke and A White. New York: Elsevier, 283–316.

Reubinoff BE, A Lewin, M Verner. 1997. Intracytoplasmic sperm injection combined with preimplantation genetic diagnosis for the prevention of recurrent gestational trophoblastic disease. *Hum Reprod* 12:805–808.

Rice LW, JM Lage, RS Berkowitz et al. 1989. Repetitive complete and partial hydatidiform mole. *Obstet Gynecol* 74:217–219.

Ross GT, DP Goldstein, R Hertz et al. 1965. Sequential use of methotrexate and actinomycin-D in the treatment of metastatic choriocarcinoma and related trophoblastic diseases in women. *Am J Obstet Gynecol* 93:223–229.

Sand PK, JR Lurain, JI Brewer. 1984. Repeat gestational trophoblastic disease. *Obstet Gynecol* 63:140–144.

Scully R and R Young. 1981. Trophoblastic pseudotumour: A reappraisal. *Am J Surg Pathol* 5:75–76.

Seckl MJ, RA Fisher, ES Newlands et al. 2000. Choriocarcinoma and partial hydatidiform mole. *Lancet* 356:36–39

Sekharan PK, NS Sreedevi, VP Radhadevi et al. 2003. Hydatidiform mole in Calicut, India. *Proceedings of XII World Congress on Gestational Trophoblastic Diseases,* Boston.

Sekharan PK, NS Sreedevi, VP Radhadevi et al. 2005. Incidence and management of PTD following hydatidiform mole. *Proceedings of the XIII World Congress on gestational trophoblastic diseases,* Hong Kong.

Shih IM and R Kurman. 2001. The pathology of intermediate trophoblast, tumours and tumour-like lesions. *Int J Gynaecol Pathol* 20:31–47.

Shih IM and RJ Kurman. 1998. Epithelioid trophoblastic tumour: A neoplasm distinct from choriocarcinoma and placental site trophoblastic tumour simulating carcinoma. *Am J Surg Pathol* 22:1393–1403.

Soper JT. 1994. Surgical therapy for gestational trophoblastic disease. *J Reprod Med* 39:168–174.

Steller MA, DR Genest, MR Bernstein. 1994. Clinical features of multiple conception with partial or complete molar pregnancy and coexisting foetus. *J Reprod Med* 39:147–154.

Szulman AE and U Surti. 1978. The syndromes of hydatidiform mole. I. Cytogenetic and morphologic correlations. *Am J Obstet Gynecol* 131: 665–671.

Tanos V, D Meirow, BE Reubinoff et al. 1992. Recurrent gestational trophoblastic disease following in vitro fertilization. *Hum Reprod* 9:2010–2013.

Tidy JA, GJ Rustin, ES Newlands. 1995. Presentation and management of choriocarcinoma after nonmolar pregnancy. *Br J Obstet Gynecol* 102(9):715–719.

Tuncer ZS, MR Burnstein, J Wang. 1999. Repetitive hydatidiform mole with different male partners. *Gynecol Oncol* 75:224–226.

Vassilakos P and T Kajii. 1976. Hydatidiform mole: Two Genetics entities. *Lancet* i:259.

Vassilakos P, G Riotton, T Kajii. 1977. Hydatidiform mole: Two entities. A morphological and cytogenetic study with some clinical considerations. *Am J Obstet Gynecol* 127:167–170.

Vejerslev LO. 1991. Clinical management and diagnostic possibilities in hydatidiform mole with co-existent fetus. *Obstet Gynecol Surv* 46:577–588.

World Health Organization. 1983. Scientific Group: Gestational trophoblastic diseases. *Tech Rep* 692. Geneva: WHO.

17

Benign Lesions of the Cervix and Uterus

Barun Sarkar

Anatomical considerations: The cervix is constantly exposed to insults. This is because the squamocolumnar junction or transformation zone is extremely susceptible due to rapid cell division. Moreover, the endocervical glands are of the tubuloracemose type, so any infection becomes deep-seated in the crypts; a block in the opening can lead to nabothian cysts.

Classification: Benign lesions of the cervix can be classified into

1. Cervical erosion
2. Cervical stenosis
3. Cervical polyp
4. Ectropion
5. Nabothian cyst
6. Cervicitis
7. Cervical tuberculosis

Cervical Erosion

Cervical erosion can be defined as a raised red velvety area on the cervix which is better seen than felt. Although the term erosion suggests the image of an ulcer, there is no ulcer in this case

Types: Cervical erosion can be of two types

1. Congenital
2. Acquired

Incidence: It is one of the commonest lesions of the cervix due to a high incidence of cervicitis in India. It is a disease of the reproductive age group. There is no genetic predisposition.

Etiopathogenesis

Congenital erosion: It is a condition observed in neonates which may be due to maternal estrogen exposure during pregnancy. It is self-limiting, but may sometimes persist into puberty.

Acquired erosion: It is invariably a sequel to cervicitis. There are three stages of the disease.

Stage 1: Stage of ulceration. There is a denudation of the squamous epithelium leading to ulceration.

Stage 2: Stage of overgrowth of columnar epithelium from the endocervical canal to cover the ulcer as a process of repair.

Stage 3: Growth of squamous epithelium of the portiovaginalis under the columnar epithelium raising the area; this provides the final picture.

Clinical features: The patient is usually a multipara in the reproductive age group. There is usually a history of abortions and home deliveries which points to infections

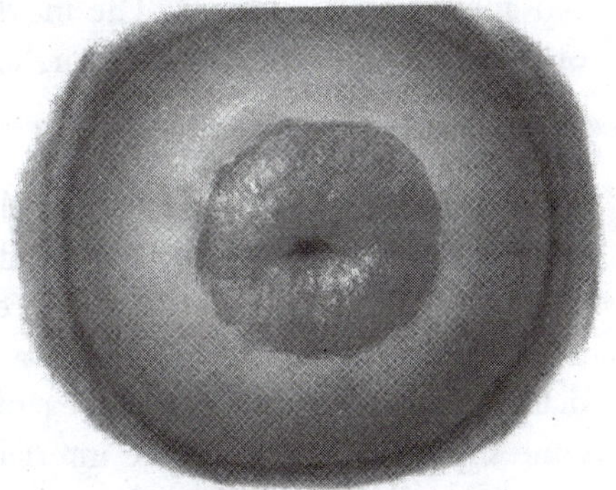
Congenital erosion in nulliparous cervix

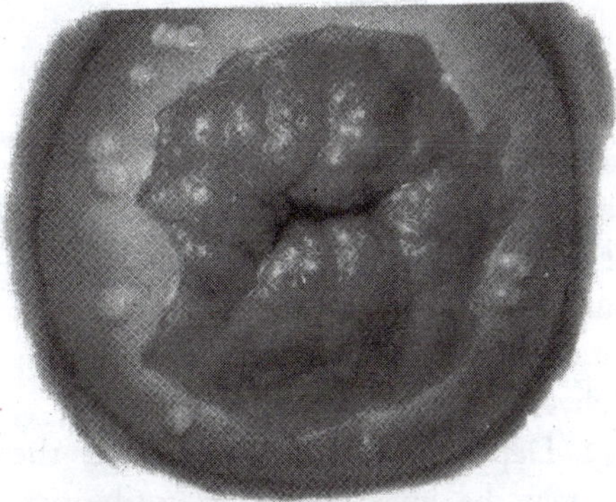
Extensive erosion with proliferation (papillary erosion); also nabothian cysts

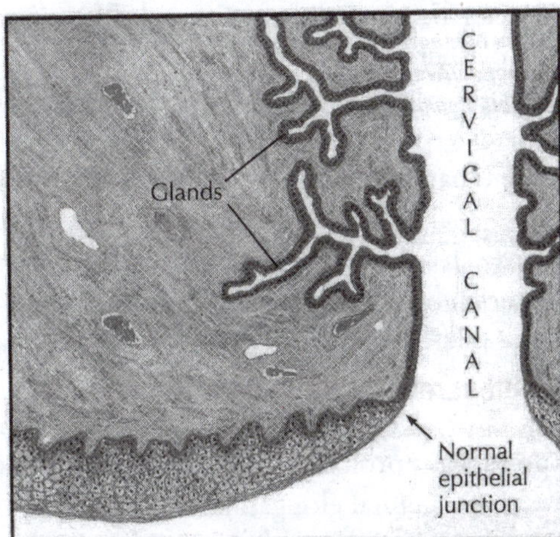

Section through normal portico vaginalis (schematic)

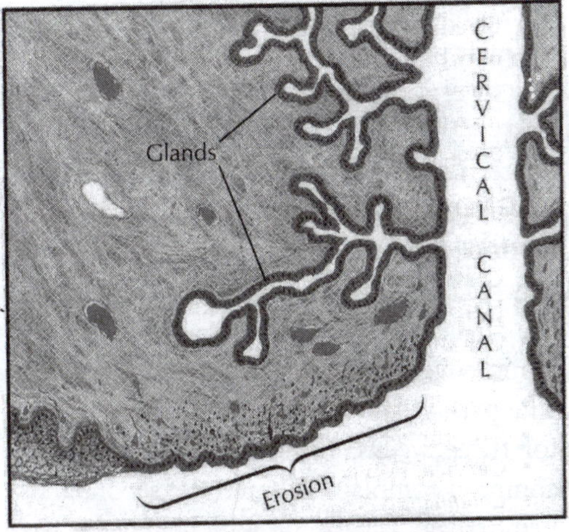

Section through portico vaginalis showing erosion (schematic)

Figure 17.1: Cervical erosions (Adapted from: Smith, Roger P. 2003. Netter's Obstetrics, Gynaecology and Women's Health. USA: Icon Learning Systems (permission awaited)

during previous labours and puerperium.

Symptoms: The most common complaint is excessive discharge per vaginum; in relatively chronic cases, there may be a history of contact bleeding.

Signs: Speculum examination must always precede a bimanual examination. One can observe a raised red area on the cervix which may be extensive enough to cover a major part of the ectocervix. It may bleed on touch.

Investigations: Both Pap smear and Gram stain must be done to pinpoint the causative organism. Colposcopy is indicated in extensive erosions and in those with a history of contact bleeding. Biopsy, usually colposcopy-directed, should be a part of the work-up especially in non-healing erosions.

Differential diagnosis: Cervical erosion has to be differentiated from carcinoma cervix, tuberculosis, syphilis, viral infections such as HSV, HPV.

Treatment

Expectant: Most erosions may be asymptomatic and are detected on a routine gynecological examination. They may require no treatment other than reassurance and regular follow-up. In erosions detected during pregnancy, treatment is deferred till delivery. The patient is reassessed around three months after delivery.

Medical: Depending on smear report, the patient may be given systemic antibiotics, antifungals (fluconazole), metronidazole or its derivatives.

Local treatment with antibiotics, pessaries or ointments can be used in conjunction with cautery or cryotherapy.

Surgical

1. Cauterisation

- Electrocautery or thermal cautery: It is done in the postmenstrual period and usually no anesthesia is required. Cauterisation is done to a depth of 2 mm covering the whole area of erosion. The patient should be advised abstinence for three weeks. Excessive discharge is a common complaint. Sometimes secondary hemorrhage can occur which may be so severe as to require hospitalisation. It is best treated by packing using betadine. The pack is removed after 24 hours; in some cases repacking may be required. The use of systemic and local antibiotics are said to reduce the chances of secondary hemorrhage.
- Cryosurgery with carbon dioxide or nitrogen: Special probes are used with nitrous oxide or carbon dioxide as the cooling agent. The freezing is done for two minutes to ensure proper iceball formation. The probe should not be pulled forcibly but one must wait for defrosting when the probe comes away easily without pulling. No anesthesia is required. The incidence of infection and secondary hemorrhage is said to be lower with cryo.

2. Conisation

- This procedure is being replaced by alternative methods which have incidence of complications. A cone-shaped area of the cervix is removed which has a base diameter of 2.5 mm and the apex of the cone should fall short of the internal os. General, spinal or epidural is required for the procedure. It is the procedure of choice in suspicious cases. The procedure can be carried out with a knife, surgical diathermy or laser.

Cervical Stenosis

It is a narrowing of the cervical canal leading to partial or total obstruction of the cervical canal. It usually occurs at the level of the internal os.

Etiopathogenesis

Congenital: It is usually rare and may sometimes present as a prolapse. It is sometimes associated with congenital elongation of cervix.

Acquired: This is much more common

1. After surgery
   - Cauterisation
   - Conisation
   - Fothergill repair
   - Cervical tear repair
2. After radiation
3. In postmenopausal women
4. In women with carcinoma cervix
5. In those with infection

Clinical features: The patient of congenital cervical stenosis is young, nulliparous. Acquired cervical stenosis can occur any time between 25 to 65 years. There is a history of badly managed obstetrics in the form of forceps application or cervical tear repair. Postmenopausal cervical stenosis is usually seen in untreated cases.

Symptoms: The young infertile patient may present with menstrual problems like dysmenorrhea (spasmodic) and amenorrhea. The condition may be diagnosed during a routine infertility work-up. In patients who have an associated pyometra, hematometra or lochiometra, the presentation may be in the form of a suprapubic lump. Some patients may be asymptomatic (especially postmenopausal patients) and may be diagnosed on a routine pelvic ultrasound.

Signs: On bimanual examination, one may detect uterine enlargement (boggy), possibly due to hematometra, pyometra or lochiometra. The cervical os may be pinpointed, but it may be difficult to pass a sound or probe.

Investigations: Ultrasonography may reveal uterine enlargement and presence of fluid in the cavity.

Differential diagnosis: It is absolutely mandatory to rule out carcinoma cervix and carcinoma endometrium, especially in an elderly patient.

Treatment: Dilatation of cervix is with serial dilators (ultrasound guided). Alternatively, one may prescribe prostaglandin gel (cerviprime) or misoprostol tablets (vaginally).

Cervical Polyps

Polyps are one of the commonest lesions of the cervix with an incidence of about 4%. They usually arise from the columnar epithelium of the endocervical canal but can also sometimes arise from the ectocervix.

Types: Cervical polyps are of three types—fibroid, fibro-adenomatous and mucous. In the present context, we will restrict our discussion to mucous polyps

Etiopathogenesis: Most polyps are presumably a result of inflammation leading to hyperplasia and proliferation of the endocervical mucosa. Histologically therefore, they are of the adenomatous type.

Clinical features: The disease is commonly observed in patients around age 40 to 60 years. They are usually multiparous. Postmenopausal patients can sometimes present with mucous polyps. It is usually an incidental finding in patients presenting with postmenopausal bleeding. Cervical polyps are sometimes observed in oral contraceptive users.

Symptoms: A fair number of patients with cervical polyps can be asymptomatic. The most common symptom is as contact bleeding in the young patient. Menorrhagia or irregular bleeding can also be observed in these patients. Excessive discharge per vaginum, usually serous but sometimes mixed with blood, is also common.

Signs: Typically, a cervical polyp on a speculum examination appears as a cherry red mass at the cervical os, in later stages due to secondary infection it becomes friable. This is the stage where it bleeds to touch.

A fibroid polyp has a thick pedicle, a fibro-adenomatous polyp has a thin pedicle and a mucous polyp has no pedicle

Investigations: A Pap smear is mandatory, especially in the postmenopausal patient and in patients with secondary infection where the polyp is friable since it may be difficult to rule out malignancy.

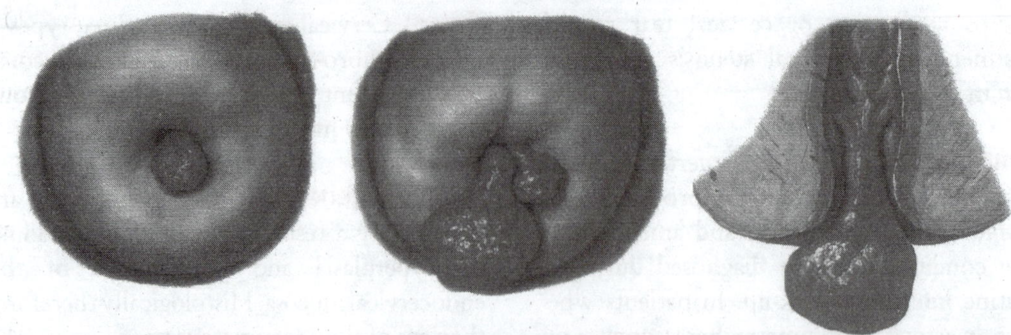

Figure 17.2: Cervical polyps
(Adapted from: Smith, Roger P. 2003. Netter's Obstetrics, Gynaecology and Women's Health. USA: Icon Learning Systems (permission awaited)

Differential diagnosis: A mucous polyp has to be differentiated from cervical erosion, carcinoma cervix, products of conception and ectropion.

Treatment: Surgical removal is the treatment of choice in cervical polyps. Usually, the polyp may be held with a sponge-holding forceps and twisted till it detaches easily. The polyps are usually pedunculated but the base does not usually bleed. Sometimes, however, the bleeding may require packing. If the pedicle is big it may sometimes require cauterisation of the base of the pedicle or cryocautery to stop the bleeding.

Endocervical and endometrial curettage is absolutely mandatory to rule out malignancy and endometrial hyperplasia and must be carried out concurrently with polypectomy.

Histology: Six histological types have been described

- Adenomatous
- Cystic
- Vascular
- Fibrous
- Fibromyomatous
- Inflammatory

Ectropion

Ectropion of the cervix (as the name suggests) is an eversion of the endocervical canal. It appears as a red inflamed mass at the cervical opening.

Etiopathogenesis: Ectropion is usually associated with chronic cervicitis and bilateral cervical tear.

Clinical features: The patient is usually a multipara with a history of badly managed obstetrics (cervical tear which has not been repaired). The patient is usually in the reproductive age group.

Symptoms: A majority of these patients may be asymptomatic but some may present with postcoital bleeding or intermenstrual bleeding. There is invariably a history of discharge per vaginum. In case of extensive spread it may cause cervical incompetence leading to recurrent abortions.

Signs: On speculum examination one can observe an everted hypertrophic red congested cervix which can sometimes bleed on touch.

Investigations: Colposcopy is required to rule out cervical malignancy. A cervical biopsy may be necessary in suspicious cases.

Differential diagnosis: An ectropion has to be diferrentiated from endocervical cancer, polyp and prolapse.

Treatment: It usually requires no treatment. However, in patients with a history of recurrent abortion, trachelorrhaphy may be required to correct the incompetence.

Nabothian Cysts

Nabothian cysts are retention cysts of the cervix. They are formed by blockage of the crypt of endocervical glands. Once the mouth of the gland is blocked, the pent up secretions cause single or multiple cysts, ranging from 3 mm to 3 cm, translucent to opaque; the colour may be yellow or blue. They are invariably a sequel to chronic cervicitis and are therefore common. Because of their innocuous nature they usually do not require treatment. Sometimes however, they may have to be differentiated from barrel-shaped carcinoma of the cervix.

Cervicitis

It is an inflammation of the endocervical glands or ectocervix. It is the most common cervical lesion afflicting 20%–40% of women in the reproductive age group.

Etiopathogenesis

Endocervical: The common organisms responsible are *Chlamydia trachomatis* and *Neisseria gonorrhoeae.*

Ectocervical: The usual causative organisms are herpes simplex, human papilloma virus, *Mycoplasma hominis*, *Ureaplasma urealyticum* and *Trichomonas vaginalis.*

Clinical features: The patient is around 20 to 40 years (it is a disease of the reproductive age group). There is usually a history of exposure to multiple sexual partners. A past history of abortion or infection during delivery or postpartum is commonly observed. History of contraceptive use, particularly IUCD, can be elicited

Symptoms: Patients may be asymptomatic (about 50%). The most common symptom is discharge per vaginum. It may be plenty, pale, frothy with pruritus in trichomonaisis. Mucopurulent discharge is usually observed in gonococcal infection. Fungal infection (monilial) is associated with a thick, curdy discharge accompanied by intense pruritus. If the discharge is thin with burning the cause is usually viral.

The patient may also experience dyspareunia. Toxic symptoms like fever and malaise are common in the acute stage. There is invariably pain in the lower abdomen which may be so intense as to mimic an acute abdomen. Backache is commonly observed in chronic cases.

Signs: On speculum examination, the cervix appears red, congested, ulcerated and friable and there is a discharge from the os.

The primary sites of infection in gonorrhea are the urethra and Skene's tubules, Bartholin's glands and the cervix. These sites must be checked for concurrent infection

Investigations

High vaginal swab
Cervical swab

- Pap stain
- Gram stain
- Culture and sensitivity
- Hanging drop

For Chlamydia

- ELISA
- Fluorescent monoclonal antibody testing

Serum testing for other STD

Management: This is primarily medical:

WITH GONORRHEA

- Ceftriaxone125 mg im or
- Cefixime 400 mg or
- Ciprofloxacin 500 mg or
- Ofloxacin 400 mg as single dose
- Plus doxycycline 100 mg twice daily for 7 days

WITHOUT GONORRHEA

- Doxycycline 100 mg twice daily for 7 days or
- Azithromycin 1 g as single dose

SURGICAL TREATMENT

1. Cauterisation or cryocautery: In resistant cases, by these methods, the cystic glands are punctured and erosion or ectropion coincidentally treated. It is always better to coincidentally carry out cervical dilatation to facilitate drainage of the glands and avoid subsequent cyanosis. General anesthesia is therefore better to carry out the procedure.
2. Conisation: It is the procedure of choice in the young patient who has completed her family and particularly if there is associated erosion.
3. Hysterectomy: Most chronic cases do not respond to conservative surgical procedures. In fact, in the perimenopausal patient it is the procedure of choice because the associated pelvic cellulitis does not respond unless the basic trigger of infection is removed.

CERVICAL TUBERCULOSIS

It is a rare lesion of the cervix but has to be kept in mind in both exfoliative and ulcerative lesions of the cervix

Etiopathogenesis: It is invariably secondary to tubercular endometritis or tubercular salpingo-oophoritis. In rare instances, it can be transmitted sexually from a partner with tubercular epididymitis.

Clinical features: The patient is 20 to 40 years of age, usually infertile.

SYMPTOMS: The presentation is very similar to cervicitis and erosion. The common symptoms are contact bleeding, discharge per vaginum or systemic symptoms like low grade fever and malaise.

SIGNS: Speculum examination reveals either an ulcerative lesion or an exfoliative lesion.

Investigations: Pap smear can lead to a suspicion of the disease. Cervical excisional biopsy is mandatory to confirm the diagnosis. PCR or ELISA can also be used as diagnostic aids.

Treatment: Medical treatment is systemic antitubercular drugs. Surgery is rarely required in resistant cases.

BENIGN LESIONS OF THE UTERUS

The common benign lesions found in the uterus are

- Fibromyoma
- Adenomyosis
- Endometrial polyp
- Rare conditions like hemangioma, osteoma, chondroma and glioma

FIBROMYOMA

It is the commonest tumour of the genital tract. It is also called fibroid, leiomyoma, fibroleiomyoma or simply myoma.

Etiology: The exact cause is unknown though many theories have been proposed.

1. Growth energy view: It is said that the

normal function of the uterus is to grow during pregnancy. Since this function is not fulfilled in infertility, fibroids are an exhibition of abnormal growth. It is a known fact that fibroids and infertility are closely associated.

2. Infertility: The association of infertility with fibroids is a known fact, whether it is the cause or the effect is debatable.
3. Hyperestrogenemia: The association of hyperestronemia is clearly documented. Whether it can cause fibroids is debatable. Hyperestronemia is associated with a number of conditions in the genital tract—endometriosis, endometrial polyps, endometrial carcinoma, cervical erosion, clear cell carcinoma of the vagina following maternal estrogen exposure and follicular cysts of the ovary to name a few. However, in rats exposed to estrogens, uterine tumours did develop but they were purely composed of fibrous tissue.

Types of fibroids: Fibroids may be uterine or extrauterine. Uterine fibroids are interstitial or intramural; when they grow outwards, they are called subserous. Those growing inwards are called submucous.

Extrauterine fibroids may locate in the following sites

- Cervix
- Broad ligament: Can be primary when they grow from the tissue in the broad ligament or secondary when a uterine fibroid grows between the leaves of the broad ligament. It is important to clearly distinguish between the two because of the relation of the ureter. In primary, the ureter lies medially and upwards, while in the secondary it lies laterally and downwards.
- Round ligament
- In relation to the uterosacral ligament.

Pathology: On gross appearance, fibroids appear as circumscribed spherical tumours surrounded by a pseudocapsule. They may be single or multiple (as many as 200 have been reported). They vary in size from a pinhead to as large as weighing 50 to 70 lb (Beacham et al 1971). It is surprising that even with modern diagnostic aids, fairly huge tumours can be encountered. The author has had the experience of removing a uterus weighing 24 kg from a woman who had been presuming she was pregnant!

The fibroids are hard and the cut surface presents a whorled, white appearance unless modified by degeneration. They are composed essentially of muscle tissue admixed with fibrous tissue.

Secondary changes: Fibroids can undergo various secondary changes:

- Atrophy
- Hypertrophy
- Fatty changes
- Hyaline degeneration
- Cystic degeneration
- Red degeneration
- Calcareous degeneration
- Sarcomatous change
- Myxomatous degeneration
- Telangiectasis
- Lymphangiectasis
- Torsion
- Infection

Atrophy usually occurs in postmenopausal women and with the use of GnRH therapy. Hypertrophy is usually associated with pregnancy or the use of estrogen progesterone preparations. Fatty changes can be in the form of fatty degeneration. Hyaline degeneration occurs due to compromise in the blood supply. This is the commonest type. The fibromuscular tissue is replaced by a homogenous substance staining pink with eosin.

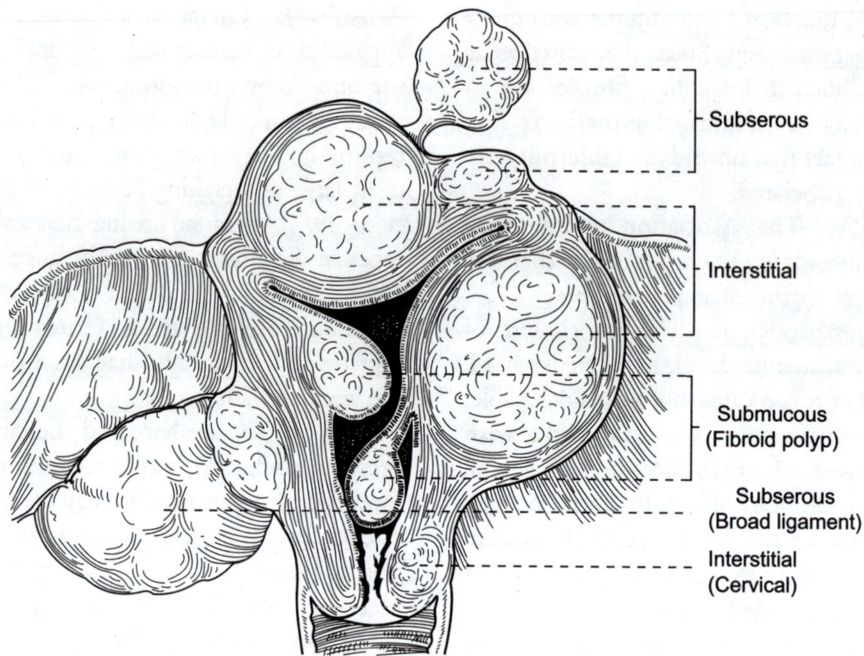

FIGURE 17.3: TYPES OF FIBROIDS

Cystic degeneration is usually secondary to hyaline degeneration, red degeneration, sarcomatous change, lymphangiectasis or telangiectasis. Red degeneration is a necrobiosis in the fibroid. It is observed during pregnancy, puerperium or menopause. The patient presents with fever, malaise and acute pain in the abdomen. On examination, there is acute tenderness and an increase in the size of the fibroid. The gross appearance is of a soft, red tumour with a fishy odour. Histologically, there is a degenerated area in the centre which is structureless and poorly stained.

There is thrombosis of the blood vessels. The basic change is an alteration in the vascularity. The blood vessel walls which are already weak and fragile due to degeneration rupture leading to extravasation of blood in the substance of the tumour. Some workers have talked of a lipid toxin being released from the degenerating tumour leading to thrombosis of the blood vessels.

The management is primarily conservative comprising rest, analgesics and prophylactic antibiotics. Surgery may be required in patients who do not respond to conservative treatment.

Calcareous degeneration is usually a sequel to fatty degeneration. Sometimes, calcium may be deposited in the periphery of the tumour leading to an avascular tumour which if subserous may detach from the uterus and form what is colloquially termed a 'womb stone.'

Sarcomatous change usually occurs in postmenopausal women. The incidence is around 0.2%. The condition is suspected when a known case of fibroid presents with postmenopausal bleeding and acute pain in the abdomen. On examination, there is an increase in the size of the tumour and tenderness.

Myxomatous degeneration, telangiectasis and lymphangiectasis are rare. Torsion can occur in a subserous pedunculated fibroid. It is usually an acute condition. Sometimes it may occur as a subacute process, in which case the tumour tends to acquire a secondary blood supply from the omentum or bowel to which it may become adherent. Such a tumour is called a 'parasitic fibroid.'

Infection most commonly affects submucous fibroids. In other fibroids, it is usually secondary to necrosis, most commonly red degeneration.

Clinical features: The patient is in the reproductive age group usually between the ages of 20 to 40 years. She is usually infertile or may have a small family. She may have a hyperestrogenemic profile. It is more commonly observed in people of African origin. There is a familial predisposition.

1. Asympomatic symptoms: It is remarkable that even large fibroids may be asymptomatic while the smallest of tumours may cause symptoms necessitating intervention.

2. Menstrual irregularities: These include menorrhagia, metrorrhagia, dysmenorrhea, irregular bleeding, amenorrhea and postmenopausal bleeding. Menorrhagia or increased menstrual bleeding in duration and amount is most commonly associated with interstitial and subserous fibroids. The causes of menorrhagia are

- An increase in the surface area of bleeding due to myohyperplasia
- Increased vascularity of the uterus
- Venous congestion
- Endometrial hyperplasia
- Muscular distortion leading to interference in the contractibility and 'physiological hemostatic mechanism' which would normally stop the bleeding.
- Metrorrhagia or intermenstrual bleeding is seen in submucous fibroids. Because the apex is the most avascular portion, there is necrosis, ulceration and infection at the tip which can bleed irregularly.

3. Dysmenorrhea: This is usually spasmodic in association with submucous fibroids. It can also be congestive in association with interstitial and subserous types.

4. Amenorrhea: This can occur due to

- Pregnancy
- Menopause
- Bilateral ovarian destruction due to associated tubo-ovarian masses (in 15%–20%, there is associated salpingo-oophoritis)
- Large submucous fibroids causing pressure atrophy of the endometrium
- Cryptomenorrhea with large cervical fibroids.

5. Lump in the Abdomen (Mass in the abdomen)

- Pressure symptoms: Anteriorly, pressure can cause bladder symptoms like frequency, dysuria, and rarely, retention of urine which may be associated with fibroids incarcerated in the pouch of Douglas or cervical fibroids. Laterally, pressure on the ureters can cause hydroureters and hydronephrosis. Posteriorly, pressure on the veins and lymphatics can cause edema and varicosities, while pressure on the nerves of the sacral plexus or obturator nerve can rarely cause referred pain. Pressure on the bowel leading to constipation or subacute intestinal obstruction is rare; however, dyspepsia can occur.
- Abdominal pain

  Pain is associated with torsion, infection, red degeneration, sarcomatous change, adhesions with surrounding organs, extrusion of a polyp

Systemic effects include:

1. Effects of anemia like lassitude, malaise, palpitation, loss of weight

2. Polycythemia: In rare cases, large broad ligament fibroids may form; these disappear on removal of the fibroid. The cause could be
- Respiratory embarrassment with large tumours leading to compensatory erythropoieisis
- Pressure on the ureter affecting the erythropoietic function of the kidney
- The fibroid may itself be erythropoietic

3. Hypoglycemia: This rare symptom may be associated with large fibroids which are retroperitoneal; pressure on the pancreas has been postulated as the cause.

6. **Infertility:** It can be the effect as well as the cause of fibroids. Common reasons are
- Anovulation
- Interference with ascent of sperms
- Due to associated salpingo-oophoritis, tubal blockage can occur
- Interference with implantation of the fertilised zygote

7. **Pregnancy and fibroids:** A fair number of patients with fibroids do conceive. The effects of pregnancy on fibroids are hypertrophy, red degeneration, torsion and infection. The effects of fibroids on pregnancy are abortions, placenta previa, abruptio placentae, malpresentations and malpositions, preterm labour, uterine inertia, obstructed labour, increased incidence of operative delivery, postpartum hemorrhage, subinvolution of the uterus and retained placenta.

Abdominal examination: Uterus size of above 12 weeks is palpable as firm, round mobile mass. Bimanual examination may reveal tumours which are single or multiple, firm, non-tender unless undergoing degeneration. If there is a cystic change or if the tumour is pedunculated, it can be difficult to distinguish it from an ovarian cyst.

Differential diagnosis: All conditions causing enlargement of the uterus or suprapubic lump have to be distinguished. It is surprising how frequently pregnancy is mistaken for fibroids. The common conditions to be considered are
- Full bladder
- Pregnancy
- Adenomyosis
- Ovarian tumors
- Tubo-ovarian masses
- Bicornuate uterus

Investigations

Ultrasound: Ultrasound has revolutionised the diagnosis of pelvic tumours. Abdominal as well as transvaginal scans are used, although the former are less accurate.

However, since the tumours may appear hyperechoic, hypoechoic and even anecoic, it requires a highly skilled sonologist to ensure that the diagnosis is not missed. An accurate scan for fibroids should ideally have a diagram drawn by the sonologist depicting the exact sites of the tumours. The ovaries have to be scanned for any pathology. Evidence of pressure on the surrounding structures should be documented.

Colour doppler studies: They help in distinguishing uterine from adenexal tumours. More importantly, they are useful in the diagnosis of leiomyosarcoma.

CT scan and MRI: They are important investigations in complex tumours and where the diagnosis is unclear.

Hysterosalpingograhy: This is the procedure of choice for the detection of submucous fibroids and concurrent tubal assessment. However, Emanuel et al (1995) found transvaginal sonography to be accurate in the detection of intracavitary pathology.

Endoscopy: Laparoscopy and hysteroscopy are currently an integral part of the work-up in patients of fibroid, especially if associated with infertility.

Treatment: The various factors to consider in deciding the treatment modalities for fibroids are

- Age of the patient
- Fertility status
- Patient's wishes
- Size, location, number and growth of the tumours
- Symptoms
- Associated pathology

Most small asymptomatic tumours only require close observation. Asymptomatic tumours require intervention if

- The size of the uterus exceeds 12 weeks
- It is likely to cause infertility
- It can interfere with labour
- It is growing rapidly
- It is a pedunculated subserous fibroid prone to torsion
- The nature of the tumour is doubtful
- The patient is postmenopausal

Since most patients with fibroids are anemic, it is imperative that anemia be corrected before undertaking surgery. This may sometimes require blood or packed cell transfusion. Any concurrent infection must be treated.

Medical treatment: This is indicated as a temporary measure:

- In patients being prepared for myomectomy, especially laparoscopic and vaginal
- To temporarily relieve symptoms
- In cases of recurrence following surgery
- The drug of choice is GnRH agonists, although Danazol has also been tried with limited success. GnRH acts by inducing hypoestrogenism and a decrease in the size of fibroid (Filicori et al 1983) and endometrial atrophy leading to amenorrhea which is especially beneficial in anemic women as a significant rise in hemoglobin occurs (Candiani et al 1990). The injection is given monthly for three months. The main disadvantage is postmenopausal side effects.

Preoperative GnRH:

- Reduces menorrhagia
- Improves hemoglobin level
- Facilitates elective surgery
- Reduces incision size
- May help convert open procedures to laparoscopic or vaginal procedures
- Reduces arterial flow to myoma thus reducing operative blood loss (Rees 1985; Lumsden et al 1987; West et al 1987, 1992; Ravina 1997).

Surgical treatment: The basic treatment of fibroids is surgery. It can be performed abdominally, vaginally or more recently, endoscopically (laparoscopic or hysteroscopic).

The various procedures being carried out are polypectomy, myomectomy and hysterectomy.

1. *Polypectomy*: Most cervical polyps or even endometrial polyps presenting through the cervix can be removed easily by twisting or diathermy coagulation or cryo if the pedicle is large. Endometrial polyps which are sessile can be removed hysteroscopically rather than abdominally as was the previous practice.
2. *Myomectomy*: It is the treatment of choice in the young infertile woman or in women desirous of conserving the uterus. The number of fibroids is theoretically not a deterrent to myomectomy, but one has to ensure that the uterus is not left functionless. As many as 200 myomas have been removed in a patient in one sitting!

Previously, it was considered imperative to ensure that all other factors like seminogram, tubal function were normal before proceeding to do a myomectomy. With advances in ART techniques, this is now an obsolete consideration.

a. Vaginal myomectomy: This has been discussed above.
b. Abdominal myomectomy is the preferred route, although endoscopy is gaining popularity.

Myomectomy is a more difficult procedure than hysterectomy because there is much more bleeding. It is best avoided during pregnancy and at the time of cesarean section unless it is a pedunculated subserous fibroid. Although each myomectomy procedure is different, testing surgical skills to the fullest, one has to keep certain basic principles in mind:

- The number of incisions on the uterus is kept to a minimum employing methods like tunneling to access the tumours.
- The incisions are best made in the relatively avascular midline
- Posterior wall incisions are best avoided to prevent adhesions by approaching intracavitary or using Bonney's hood technique (1931).
- Hemostasis is the key: This can be done using myomectomy clamps and tourniquets, obliterating the base of the bed after enucleation, strictly adhering to the planes

The morbidity is slightly higher than hysterectomy (about 0.3%). It is essential to arrange for blood to be available preoperatively. The recurrence rate is 5%–10%. Pregnancy following myomectomy is usually uneventful although some people have reported a higher incidence of abortion. Rupture of the scar is more of a theoretical possibility. Most deliveries are by cesarean section because the patients are elderly and the pregnancy precious.

c. Laparoscopic myomectomy: With increasing experience, laparoscopic myomectomy is gaining popularity as more physicians use it. Usually, danazol or GnRH is given to reduce the size and vascularity of the tumour before myomectomy. The availability of morcellators has allowed the endoscopic surgeon to tackle bigger fibroids.

3. *Hysterectomy*: In patients above the age of 40 years who have completed their family, it is the best form of treatment. Most operations are carried out abdominally.

However, vaginal hysterectomy is gaining popularity. The various debulking procedures are:

- Bisection of the uterus
- Morcellation
- Circumferential incision
- Spiral incision and traction
- Wedge excision
- Myomecyomy: internal and external
- Cervical wedge

Laparoscopic assisted vaginal hysterectomy is also being performed. Hysteroscopically, smaller submucous myomas can be removed during transcervical resection of the endometrium (TCRE).

Newer therapeutic procedures are drugs, myolysis and uterine artery embolisation. Laparoscopic myolysis entails destruction of the stroma and vascular supply of a subserous or interstitial fibroid. This leads to a reduction in size or even disappearance of the tumour. More importantly, the symptoms are relieved. The following procedures are used for myolysis

- Monopolar coagulation needle (Wood et al 1994)
- Bipolar coagulation needle (Goldfarb 1992, 1994, 1995, 1996; Emanuel et al 1995; Philips et al 1995, 1997)

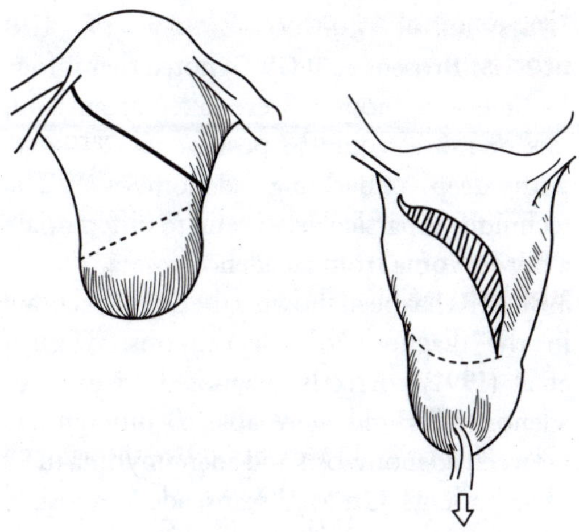

FIGURE 17.4: SPIRAL INCISION

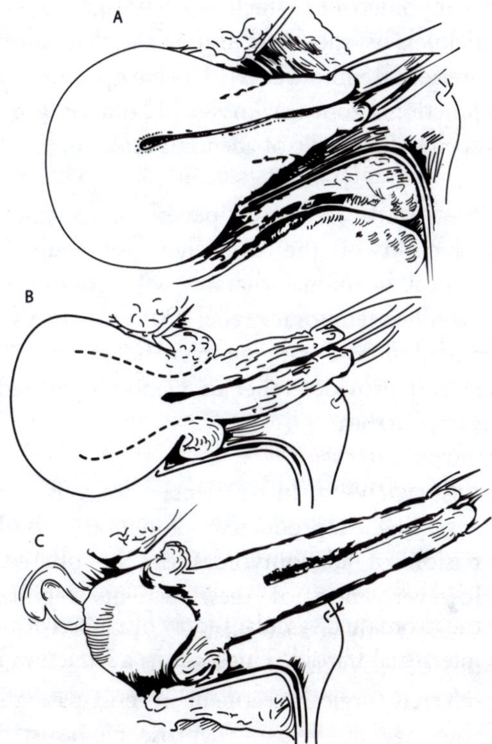

FIGURE 17.5: CIRCUMFERENTIAL INCISION

- Hyperthermia electrode (diathermy) (Chapman et al 1993)
- Laser (Nd:YAG) (Goldfarb et al 1992, 1994, 1995, 1996; Emanuel et al 1995; Philips et al 1995, 1997; Nisolle et al 1993)

Uterine artery embolisation (unilateral or bilateral) has been practised for the control of acute pelvic hemorrhage, postpartum hemorrhage and hemorrhage in association with malignancy.

According to Ravina et al (1997), bilateral or unilateral transcatheter embolisation of the uterine arteries is an effective alternative to surgery in the treatment of fibroids. There is not only symptomatic relief but a definite reduction in the size of myomas.

ADENOMYOSIS

Adenomyosis is defined as the presence of endometrial foci in the myometrium. Although a minor amount of microscopic endometrial invasion is fairly common, to be labelled as adenomyosis, the invasion has to be so extensive that it is visible to the naked eye (Jeffcoate 1975). It is also called endometriosis interna but the preferred term is adenomyosis since colloquially, the term endometriosis is reserved for endometriosis externa.

Etiology: The factors responsible are very similar to those for fibroids. In fact, the two are commonly known to coexist. The exact cause of myometrial invasion is not known, although hyperestronemia is known to be associated.

Pathology: There is a uniform enlargement of the uterus. There is no capsule and that is the most important distinguishing feature between fibroids and adenomyosis. The cut surface shows cystic areas filled with menstrual blood. The surrounding areas are discoloured due to deposition of hemosiderin. Microscopic examination shows myometrial invasion of endometrial glands.

Diagnosis: The disease afflicts women around the age of 40 years. They are usually multiparous. There is a familial predilection.

Symptoms: Menorrhagia is the commonest symptom. Dysmenorrhea is of the classically progressive or crescendo type. It starts in the premenstrual phase and gradually peaks in the postmenstrual period. Associated symptoms such as breathlessness and pallor, related to anemia as a result of excessive bleeding, are fairly common.

Signs: There is uniform enlargement of the uterus, usually corresponding to a pregnancy of 8 to 12 weeks. Rarely, the size of the uterus may be as large as 16 to 20 weeks. The uterus is freely mobile. The consistency is neither hard nor soft.

In localised adenomyomas, the findings are similar to fibroids of localised masses. They can be distinguished only during surgery by the presence or absence of capsule during surgery.

Investigations: It is usually difficult to differentiate adenomyosis from fibroid.

Transvaginal sonography: This is the procedure of choice in detecting adenomyosis since transabdominal ultrasound of the uterus provides insufficient resolution to detect the small and subtle architectural disturbances produced by adenomyosis.

The more diffuse form of adenomyosis produces areas of mild echoic heterogenecity and the presence of anechoic areas of less than 4 mm diameter. Reinhold et al (1996) felt that these anechoic areas appeared to be due to cystic dilatation of ectopic endometrial glands or hemorrhagic foci. In a study of 119 patients, they found a positive predictive value of 71% for ultrasound and 61% for MRI.

Transvaginal guided biopsy of the uterus: Brosens et al (1995) noted that if four 14 Fr needle biopsies were taken at random, one or more would be positive in 70% uteri with deep underlying adenomyosis. The technique is particularly useful to differentiate a fibromyoma from an adenomyoma.

MRI: MRI has been shown to be highly accurate in the diagnosis of adenomyosis. Togashi et al (1991) correctly diagnosed 15 cases of adenomyosis and were able to differentiate between adenomyosis and adenomyoma in 92 of 93 patients. On MRI scans, adenomyosis is best diagnosed on T2-weighted images.

The junctional zone (the innermost area of the myometrium which is a low signal area) thickness is the most important diagnostic criterion. Reinhold et al (1996) have postulated a junctional zone thickness of 12 mm or more as being diagnostic of adenomyosis.

Treatment: Since most patients are anemic, correction of the deficiency is required. Cyclical hormonal therapy with combined pills offers temporary relief. Danazol can also be used in doses ranging from 100 mg to 600 mg and provides relief in menorrhagia and dysmenorrhea.

Surgical Treatment

Conservative: In patients desirous of conserving reproductive function, local excision of adenomyomas can be offered. However, most of these patients require hysterectomy at a later date.

Radical: Vaginal hysterectomy is the preferred surgical treatment in most patients about age 40 years. Laproscopic assisted vaginal hysterectomy (LAVH) or abdominal hysterectomy offers equally good results.

Uterine Polyps

The common benign polyps in the uterus are adenoma, fibromyoma and placental polyp.

Adenoma: It is called an endometrial polyp or a mucous polyp. They can be single or multiple; in the latter case it is also designated as multiple polyposis.

Pathology: They are usually the size of a grape or pea. On section they show endometrial glands and stroma. There is an association with hyperestronemia. Because of the associated endometrial hyperplasia, multiple polyps show a strong tendency for recurrence.

Clinical features: The patient is usually postmenopausal with a hyperestronemic tendency.

Symptoms: The patient may be asymptomatic and it may be a chance finding. The most common presentation is as menstrual abnormality, commonly menorrhagia, which is observed in 12% of women with endometrial polyps (Van Bogaert 1988), intermenstrual bleeding or postmenopausal bleeding; rarely postcoital bleeding may also be the presenting symptom. Sometimes, dysmenorrhea may be observed.

Signs: Usually except for a generalised enlargement of the uterus, there may be no other clinical finding. Often, the diagnosis is incidentally detected on an ultrasound, hysteroscopy, hysterography or on opening the specimen after hysterectomy.

Investigations

1. Ultrasonography: Small polyps may be missed even on transvaginal ultrasonography. The injection of fluid in the cavity can help detect small polyps better. On colour doppler, vascularity of the pedicle can be observed.
2. Diagnostic curettage: It is mandatory in all women suspected to be suffering from endometrial polyp, particularly because of endometrial hyperplasia.
3. Hysteroscopy: It not only helps in targeting the endometrial sample but helps visualise the endometrial lining in totality, especially the uterotubal junction.

Treatment: Dilatation and curettage usually resolves the problem. Hysteroscopy is particularly useful in the postmenopausal woman. Hysterectomy is advisable in case of recurrence especially in multiple polyps and associated endometrial hyperplasia.

Hemangioma

This is a rare condition which is also called angioma, hamartoma, circoid aneurysm or more currently, arteriovenous malformation of the uterus (AVM). It is usually a benign condition restricted to the endometrium but may, in rare cases, involve the myometrium or extrauterine pelvis as well.

In a review of literature, Fleming et al (1989) identified 15 idiopathic and 14 cases secondary to trophoblastic disease, DES syndrome and endometrial carcinoma. Histologically, they comprise a localised network of blood vessels (venous, capillary and arterial), but there may be arteriovenous shunts, fistulas and aneurysms.

The main presenting symptom is severe intractable menorrhagia not responding to conventional treatment and requiring blood transfusion. Advances in imaging techniques have revolutionised the diagnosis of arteriovenous malformation. AVM is well demonstrated by angiography, CT (Fakhri et al 1987), Doppler (Jain et al 1991; Huang et al 1998) and MRI (Amparo et al 1984).

The most common diagnostic modality used is colour doppler. Huang et al observed adjacent blue and red components due to the intimate proximity of arterial and venous channels, and yellow and white components related to very high peak systolic velocities (96–201 cm/s) as opposed to peak systolic velocities of spiral arteries (9–44 cm/s). Similar findings are observed in missed abortion, trophoblastic disease and ectopic pregnancy which can be eliminated by beta hCG estimation.

MRI is useful not only in demonstrating AVM but in determining the extent of the lesion (presence of signal voids within the lesion). The evaluation of exact spread is vital in cases that may be undergoing uterine artery embolisation. The procedure may be hazardous if AVM is present.

Rare Tumours of the Uterus

They are usually remnants of fetal tissue left after termination of pregnancy. They can be cartilagenous, gliomatous or osseus. They are the outcome of endometrial metaplasia. On ultrasound, they are detected as areas of ossification in the endometrial cavity.

References

Amparo EG, CB Higgins, H Hricack. 1984. Primary diagnosis of abdominal arteriovenous fistula by MR imaging. *J Comput Assist Tomogr* 8:1140–1142

Beacham WD, HD Webster, EH Lawson, LM Roth. 1971. Uterine and/or ovarian tumors weighing 25 pounds or more. A review of the literature in English since 1946. *Am J Obstet Gynecol* 1153–1161.

Bonney V. 1931. The technique and results of myomectomy. *Lancet* 220:171–173

Brosens JJ, NM de Souza, FG Barker, T Paraschos, RM Winston. 1995. Endovaginal ultrasonography in the diagnosis of adenomyosis uteri: Identifying the predictive characteristics. *Br J Obstet Gynaecol* 102(6):471–474

Candiani GB, Vercellini P and Fedele L. 1990. Use of goserelin depot, a gonadotropin-releasing hormone agonist, for the treatment of menorrhagia and severe anemia in women with leiomyomata uteri. *Acta Obstetrica et Gynaecologica Scandanavia* 69 (5):413–415

Chapman R. 1993. Treatment of uterine myomas by interstitial hyperthermia *Gynaecol Endosc* 2:425-433

Emanuel MH, MJC Verdel, H Stas et al. 1995. A prospective comparison of transvaginal ultrasonography and diagnostic hysteroscopy in the evaluation of patients with abnormal uterine bleeding: Clinical implications. *Am.J Obstet Gynecol.* 172:547–552

Fakhri A, EK Fishman, SE Mitchell, SS Siegelman, RJ White. 1987. The role of CT in the management of pelvic arteriovenous malformations. *Cardiovasc Intervent Radiol* 10:96–99

Filicori M, DA Hall, JS Loughlin, J Rivier, W Vale, WF Crowley. 1983. A conservative approach to the management of uterine leiomyoma: pituitary desensitization by a luteinizing hormone-releasing hormone analogue. *American Journal of Obstetrics and Gynecology* 147:726–727.

Fleming H, AG Ostör, H Pickel, DW Fortune.1989. Arteriovenous malformations of the uterus. *Obstet Gynecol* 73(2):209–213

Goldfarb HA. 1992. Nd:Yag laser laparoscopic coagulation of symptomatic myomas. *J Reprod Med* 36:636–638

Goldfarb HA.1994. Removing uterine fibroids laparoscopically. *Contemp Ob/Gyn* 39:50–72

Goldfarb HA. 1995. Bipolar laparoscopic needles for myoma coagulation. *J Am Assoc Gynecol Laprosc* 2:175–179

Goldfarb HA. 1996. Laparoscopic coagulation of myoma (myolysis). *Infertil Reprod Med Clin North Am* 7(1) 129–141

Huang MW, D Muradali, WA Thurston, PN Burns, SR Wilson. 1998. Uterine arteriovenous malformations: Gray-scale and Doppler US features with MR imaging correlation. *Radiology* 206 (1): 115–123

Jain KA, RB Jeffrey Jr, FG Sommer. 1991. Gynecologic vascular abnormalities: Diagnosis with Doppler US. *Radiology* 178: 549–551

Jeffcoate, Thomas Norman Sir. 1975. *Principles of Gynaecology*, Fourth edition. London, Boston: Butterworths.

Lumsden MA, CP West and DT Baird. 1987. Goserelin therapy before surgery for uterine fibroids *Lancet* 1(8523):36–37

Nisolle M, M Smets and V Malvaux. 1993. Laparoscopic myolysis with the Nd: YAG laser. *J Gynecol Surg*. 9:95–99

Phillips DR.1995. Laparoscopic leiomyoma coagulation. *Gynaecol Endosc*. 4 (2):5–12

Phillips DR, SJ Millim, HG Nathanson, JS Haselkorn. 1997. Experience with laparoscopic leiomyoma coagulation and concomitant operative hysteroscopy *J Am Assoc Gynecol Laprosc* 4:425–433

Ravina JH, JM Bouret, N Ciraru-Vigneron et al. 1997. Recourse to particular arterial embolization in the treatment of some uterine leiomyoma. *Bull Acad Natl Med* (Paris) 181:233–243

Rees MCP. 1985 Prostaglandins *Leukol Med*. 18:65–68

Reinhold C, S McCarthy, PM Bret, A Mehio, M Atri, et al. 1996. Diffuse adenomyosis: comparison of endovaginal US and MR imaging with histopathologic correlation. *Radiol* 199 (1):151–158

Togashi K, K Nishimura, I Kimura, Y Tsuda, K Yamashita, T Shibata, Y Nakano, J Konishi, I Konishi, T Mori. 1991. Endometrial cysts: Diagnosis with MR imaging. *Radiology* 180 (1):73–78

Van Bogaert LJ. 1988. Clinicopathologic findings in endometrial polyps. *Obstet. Gynecol* 71 (5):771–773

West CP, MA Lumsden, S. Lawson, J Williamson and DT Baird. 1987 Shrinkage of uterine fibroids during therapy with goserelin (Zoladex): a luteinizing hormone-releasing hormone agonist administered as a monthly subcutaneous depot. *Fertility and Sterility* 48:45–51

West CP, MA Lumsden and DT Baird. 1992. Goserelin (Zoladex) in the treatment of fibroids. *Br Journal Obstet Gynaecol* 99(Supplement 7):27-30

Wood C, P Maher and D Hill. 1994. Myoma reduction by electrocautery *Gynaecol Endosc* 3:163–165

18

Pathology and Management of CIN Lesions of the Cervix

Virochana Kaul

Worldwide, cervical cancer is the most common cause of mortality from gynecologic malignancy, the second most common cancer in women, and the third most frequent cause of death (IARC 2002). Since the introduction of cervical cytology screening with the Papanicolaou test (Pap test), a marked reduction in the incidence and mortality of cervical cancer has followed. This is because the natural history of cervical cancer lends itself well to screening programmes, and as a rule, decades pass from the introduction of the human papillomavirus (the causative agent of cervical cancer) to the basal layer of the cervical epithelium via sexual intercourse until the development of invasive cancer—during this long latent period, HPV infections may be cleared or cytological abnormalities (covering a broad range from reactive changes to intraepithelial low- and high-grade lesions) picked up for intervention and prevention of cancer. The use of screening tests is further justified by the low cost, non-invasive nature and its wide acceptance. Studies by Agency for Health Care and Policy Research (AFHCPR 1999) concluded that the sensitivity of a Pap smear was 51% (against previous 80%) which increased with three annual smears to 86.8% (previously 99.2%); the American College of Obstetrics and Gynecology Guidelines (ACOG 2003) and the US Preventive Services Task Force Guidelines (USPSTF 2003), reiterate the need for more frequent and regular screening.

The Bethesda System (TBS) (2001) has divided epithelial cell abnormalities based on Pap smear into two groups, squamous cell and glandular cell (Table 18.1), reflecting the current understanding of the development of the pre-invasive changes leading to cervical cancer (Solomon et al 2002). Broadly, LSIL includes reactive changes and CIN I, while HSIL includes CIN II and CIN III, on confirmation by biopsy.

In this chapter, we will review the incidence, histology, management and follow-up required for atypical cervical cytology and cervical intraepithelial neoplasia since the available data requires us to be alert regarding the possible methods for diagnosis and management, their sensitivity and specificity, economic considerations and application.

Risk Factors

1. HPV infection—the persistence of high-risk HPV infection is the most important factor.
2. Smoking

TABLE 18.1: EPITHELIAL CELL ABNORMALITIES (PAP SMEAR DIAGNOSIS)

A. Squamous cell
Atypical squamous cells (ASC)
i. Of undetermined significance (ASC-US)
ii. Cannot exclude HSIL (ASC-H)
Low-grade squamous intraepithelial lesion (LSIL)
High-grade squamous intraepithelial lesion (HSIL)
Squamous cell carcinoma (SCC)
B. Glandular cell
Atypical glandular cells of undetermined significance (AGUS)
i. Endocervical
ii. Endometrial
iii. Glandular (NOS)
Atypical
i. Endocervical favouring neoplasia
ii. Glandular favouring neoplasia
Endocervical adenocarcinoma in situ (AIS)
Adenocarcinoma

3. Multiparity
4. Oral contraceptives intake for prolonged period
5. History of sexually transmitted diseases
6. Multiple sexual partners
7. Immunocompromised state

TESTING MODALITIES

1. **Pap smear:** the earliest method, sensitivity is low.
2. **Liquid based cytology** has increased sensitivity (60%). It is considered better because it picks up more CIN II and III, infection, and the results are not obscured by blood. Repeat liquid cytology increased sensitivity to 85% and is one of the options in follow up.
3. **Visual inspection of the cervix after application of acetic acid (VIAA)** is an inexpensive, widely applicable, easy to learn method and if practised correctly has 82% sensitivity. This is a very viable option in developing countries and rural settings.
4. HPV DNA testing: Although common in the reproductive age group, the presence of high-risk strains can help in triage.
5. Colposcopy (magnification and visualisation under high-power lens).
6. Biopsy (direct or colposcopy guided).

   Since Pap smear is a frequently and routinely used modality, it is important to be aware of the terminology used, the relative frequency of diagnosis of such Pap smears (Table 18.2), the categorisation and basis of diagnosis. The physician should also be aware of the recommended guidelines for the treatment of such smears and the follow-up in such situations.

ASCUS (atypical squamous cells of undetermined significance): These cells are characterised by:

a. Nuclear enlargement 2½ to 3 times that of normal intermediate squamous cells
b. Slight increase in nuclear/cytoplasmic ratio
c. Variation in nuclear size and shape or binucleation

It usually forms 3%–5% of cases (Table 18.2).

Studies have revealed that the possibility of having a high-grade lesion (HSIL) (that is, CIN II or III) is found in 5%–10% in such smears and the risk of progression to invasive disease is 1%–2%. Conversely, although most women with biopsy diagnosis of moderate dysplasia or worse may present with ASCUS, in those with a Pap diagnosis of ASCUS, immediate referral to colposcopy may not be cost-effective because the majority have no significant cervical abnormalities. Also, the risk of presence of HSIL or invasion depends on patient's age (risk is greater in younger women), previous history of abnormal Pap smear or dysplasia etc.

The modalities recommended by ASCCP

Table 18.2: Relative incidence of Pap smear diagnosis in a screening population

Cytological diagnosis	*%*
ASCUS	3.5
AGUS	0.5
LSIL	0.9
MSIL	0.3

(American Society for Colposcopy and Cervical Pathology) are:

1. Follow-up and repeat testing
2. HPV DNA testing
3. Colposcopy

The ASCCP states that all three options are safe and effective (Wright et al 2002).

Follow-up and repeat testing: The easiest and probably the best way of follow-up would be to give a course of antibiotics (since inflammatory changes can also cause similar picture) and repeat a pap smear after 4–6 months

Follow-up testing can also be done by:

a. Liquid based cytology: Instead of fixation on a slide, the exfoliated cells are collected on the spatula and transferred onto a liquid medium. The advantage is that adequate specimen is collected and hence better quality of specimen is available for diagnosis.
b. Visual inspection of the cervix after application of acetic acid (VIAA): Usually an alternative employed in the periphery where the routine Pap smear is not feasible or economically rational. The use of acetic acid causes the abnormal areas to appear as thick curdy acetowhite—it can be identified with the naked eye, is economical, easily available and can be used by the paramedical staff.

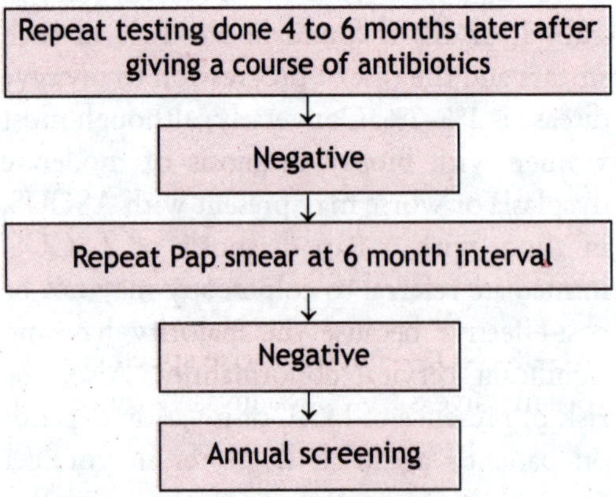

Repeat testing done 4 to 6 months later after giving a course of antibiotics
↓
Negative
↓
Repeat Pap smear at 6 month interval
↓
Negative
↓
Annual screening

Algorithm 1: Follow up and repeat testing regimen

The advantages and disadvantages of the follow-up method are:

Advantages

Over-diagnosis is avoided

Even if HSIL is present, no progression expected in 4–6 months

Economical

Infection present will subside

Disadvantages

Delay in diagnosis

20% will be lost to follow-up

HPV DNA testing: Here, the residual cells that are collected in the liquid fixative medium are analysed for HPV DNA for identification of the possibility of the presence of high-risk HPV types, so that the risk can be assessed. It is preferred if liquid-based cytology or co-collection is available (since residual cells are available).

The ALTS trial (Solomon et al 2001) concluded that HPV triage is highly sensitive in identifying CIN II and CIN III, with an acceptable rate of referral for colposcopy (56.1%).

Randomised controlled trials comparing simple follow-up with HPV testing show 90%–95% sensitivity in the latter method for identifying CIN III or greater (Mannos et al 1999; Schiffman et al 2000). Even more importantly, a negative screen for high-risk HPV has 98% probability that CIN II to III will not be present. Such patients can be kept on follow-up and hence the colposcopy load will be reduced.

The advantages and disadvantages of the HPV DNA testing method are:

Advantages

Sensitivity for CIN II-III

Decreases colposcopy load

Single office visit (testing done from residual fluid of cervical sample)

Disadvantages

Variability of results depending on the generation of Hybrid capture test

Increased cost

Colposcopy: The use of magnification and visualisation of the cervix to identify abnormal areas and diagnose malignancy either directly (using scores), or by use of colposcopy-guided biopsy for histological diagnosis which is confirmatory, is probably the safest route of action, though not the most economical. It can be done:

a. Routinely as a triage method
b. At repeat cytology for ASC or higher
c. For HPV DNA (high-risk) positive patients

The advantages and disadvantages of the direct routine colposcopy method are:

Advantages

All lesions picked up

Patient satisfaction

Disadvantage

More expensive (by 3–4 times)

After colposcopy, either alone, with HPV or guided biopsy, the further course of action is as follows:

Urgent Colposcopy: These conditions are considered as direct indications for colposcopy since there is a higher risk of presence of serious abnormalities.

- HIV positive with ASCUS
- ASC-H (25%–95% will have CIN II to to III)
- Poorly compliant patient
- Previous history of pre-invasive smear
- Repeat ASCUS abnormal

Special Circumstances: Some circumstances that warrant special attention are:

1. Postmenopausal: Treat with topical estrogen for two months. Then repeat smear after 1 week of stopping therapy.
2. Pregnancy: Colposcopy and directed biopsy is mandatory to rule out invasive cancer. However, there are risks of
   a. Bleeding
   b. Cervical trauma may cause labour
   ECC (endocervical curettage) is contraindicated in pregnancy.
   Cone is contraindicated because it causes >500 cc blood loss; has a 30% risk of PPH; and in 10% causes fetal loss.
3. Adolescence: Colposcopy is indicated.

ASC-H (atypical squamous cells: cannot exclude high-grade): This is a subset which carries much more risk of high-grade disease. It is reported in 0.27% to 0.6% of all Pap tests and the risk of CIN II or CIN III is about 40% (Solomon et al 2001). The ASCCP recommends direct colposcopy and management as outlined above in all cases.

AGUS (atypical glandular cells of unknown significance): Usually constitute 0.1%–0.7% of diagnosis and has been associated with invasive cancer in 5.7% as outlined below:

AGUS associated changes: 25% pre-invasive disease* (usually with reactive squamous) 2% invasive cancer.

AGUS (NOS—not otherwise specified): 26% pre-invasive cancer* 6% invasive cancer

AGUS favouring neoplasm: 40% pre-invasive cancer* 25% invasive cancer

**Pre-invasive usually means adenocarcinoma in situ (AIS)*

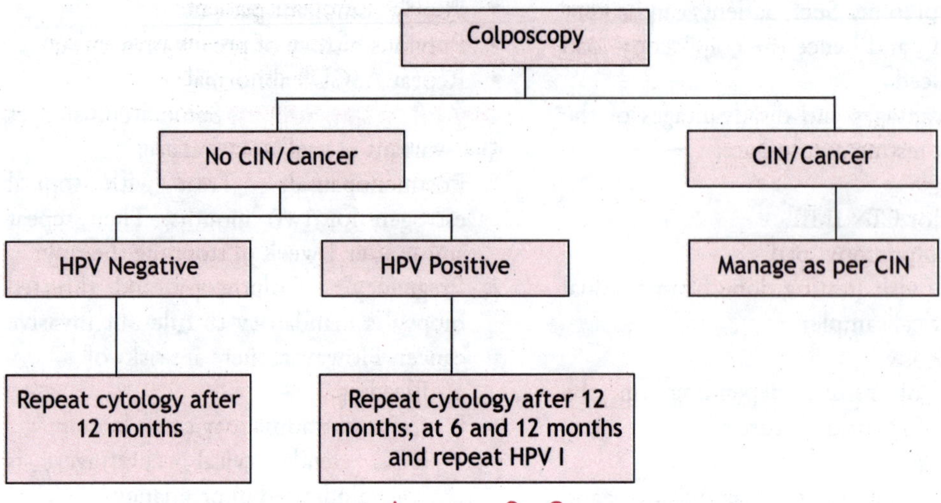

ALGORITHM 2: COLPOSCOPY

The formal definition of atypical glandular cells is endometrial or endocervical cells showing nuclear atypia that exceeds obvious reactive or reparative changes but lack unequivocal features of invasive adenoma carcinoma.

Overall, between 17% and 52% of AGUS cytology will have a significant cervical lesion indicating complete evaluation. Usually, the lesion associated is squamous and not glandular. The sensitivity of the Pap test for diagnosing glandular dysplasia and malignancy is 50%–72%; hence repeat cytology does not improve the detection of disease (Kim et al 2000).

TRIAGE SCHEME IN AGUS: In all cases of AGUS, colposcopy with endocervical sampling and endometrial sampling is mandatory, except where atypical endometrial cells are reported, in which case only endometrial sampling may suffice. Also, HPV testing can be included to rule out the presence of high-risk HPV types. The further course of action is outlined:

1. Colposcopy and ECC (endocervical curettage and biopsy of visible lesion)
2. HPV testing: Endocervical glandular neoplasia is also related to HPV, especially type 18, so HPV testing may be included.

Women with AGUS with HPV Positive status and negative ECC will require follow-up and cone biopsy or large-loop excision.

Cone biopsy is indicated if ECC is positive

LSIL (low-grade squamous intraepithelial lesion): Of all Pap smears, 1.5% to 2.0% are LSIL and of these 15%–30% will have moderate dysplasia or worse and 1%–2% may have invasive cancer. Although the risk of a significant lesion is lower in these women, referral for colposcopic evaluation is recommended. Further follow-up is outlined below.

HPV triage in LSIL is not recommended because of positivity (the presence of high-risk HPV is 82%); hence it is not a valid discriminator in determining the presence of disease.

HSIL (high-grade squamous intra-epithelial lesion): This lesion is quite significant and constitutes 0.5% of all Pap smears. Specifically, 70% will have CIN II or III and 1%–2% will have invasive carcinoma. This means that immediate action is warranted.

Colposcopy is necessary in HSIL to rule out invasion, delineate the lesion, decision regarding mode of treatment, to take biopsy and ECC.

It is clear from the management schemes outlined above that a biopsy (either colposcopy directed or direct visual biopsy) is mandatory and further treatment is usually always carried out after confirmation by a histological diagnosis, that is, the diagnosis of cervical intraepithelial neoplasia.

CERVICAL INTRAEPITHELIAL NEOPLASIA (BIOPSY DIAGNOSIS)

Cervical Intraepithelial Neoplasia I (CIN I)

Referred to earlier as mild dysplasia, it includes lesions with abnormal cells in the upper third of the epithelium. It is a heterogeneous group, with high levels of inter/intra-observer variation, and in the ALTS trial (Solomon et al 2001), only 43% of biopsies initially diagnosed as CIN I were repeat CIN I, out of which 41% were downgraded to normal, only 13% upgraded to CIN II or III. The poor reproducibility and uncertain biological potential makes the management problematic.

The usual course hence has been spontaneous regression in 57% (Oster 1993), progression to CIN II–III in 11%, risk of invasive cancer in 0.3%.

Management of CIN I

Management of CIN II to III

Earlier, these were referred to as moderate to severe dysplasia, the abnormal cells are present in two-thirds to full thickness of the epithelium, and the basement membrane is intact.

The course of the disease is:

43% CIN II and 32% CIN III will regress (Shafi and Luesley 1995)

35% CIN II and 56% CIN III will persist

22% CIN II and 14% CIN III will progress

Hence, the management becomes more definitive in these situations.

Both excision and ablation are acceptable but only if colposcopy is satisfactory. If the colposcopy is unsatisfactory, or if CIN II or III recurs, excision is recommended.

Follow-up of cases is with either cytology or colposcopy at 4–6 months till three consecutive results are negative after which annual screening can be followed.

Treatment options: The various treatment options available are:

Ablative methods:

1. Cryotherapy: This is a destructive technique using nitrous oxide or carbon dioxide as a refrigerant to lower tissue temperature to –22°C to produce cell death by intra- and extracellular crystallisation of water, dehydration of cell and cell death due to release of lysosomal enzymes. Cryo-destruction is effective for 5 mm and the application is by a special probe through which the gas is circulated for a cycle of 3 minutes with break of 2 minutes. Such cycles are repeated till the required destruction is achieved. Such therapy is reserved for the lesions on ectocervix and usually low-grade lesions.
2. Laser treatment: Carbon dioxide laser is used to generate a high intensity columnar beam directed to the tissue to produce high intensity power, causing dehydration of the cell and cell explosion and death. The CO_2 laser can be used for either excision or ablation depending on the beam strength, power intensity and the spot size used.
3. Electrocautery: Burning with electrical

TABLE 18.3: ADVANTAGES AND DISADVANTAGES OF ABLATIVE AND EXCISION TREATMENT METHODS FOR CIN

Procedure	*Indications*	*Advantages*	*Disadvantages*	*Side effects*
Punch biopsy	Small lesion at SCJ in young nulliparous women	Minimal trauma, under local anesthetic	Lesion may be missed	Bleeding, discharge, pain
Cryo-surgery	• Low grade lesions 1 and 2 • Single or two quadrants • Young, reproductively active women. • Small cervix • Microinvasion ruled out • Whole lesion can be seen and usually comes under probe contact. If multiple probes are used, then probably not the right choice	• Maximum precision • Ability to continue superficially to include any extension to vaginal fornices • Healing swift • Little necrotic debris and post treatment	• Discharge • After 15 days slight bleeding because of separation of eschar. • Stenosis	Same as dis-advantages
Laser	• Large lesion (3 or > quadrants) • Isolated to ectocervix. • Extension to vagina • Laser is used here because it allows removal of underlying tissues and for an acceptable cosmetic and fine outcome • Irregular cervix • Extension to glandular tissue in which deep treatment is required	• Control of depth and width ablation up to 7 mm • Rapid healing (3–4 weeks)	• Expensive • Difficult to maintain • Difficult to learn • No specimen in vaporisation • Extent of damage not known	• Discharge • Spotting • Fever/rarely TSS • Stenosis
LEEP/ LETTZ	Same as above	• Cost-effective • Easy to learn • Safe • Tailor according to lesion • Less bleeding • Rapid healing • History, review of specimen • See and treat • Rapid procedure • OPD procedure		• Potential for excessive discharge • Injury to vagina • Bleeding • Infection

Cold knife	• At places where invasive needs to be ruled out • Adenocarcinoma or ECC +ve • Large lesion HSIL • Loop cannot be used e.g., vaginal extension • Discrepancy between reports • Unsatisfactory colposcopy		• Under general anesthesia • More bleeding	

current. This is neither very effective nor popular.

EXCISION METHODS:

1. Laser (see above)
2. LEEP (Large loop excision procedure): Electro-surgical generators coupled with loop electrodes, made of thin tungsten or steel wire, or ball electrodes are used to either cauterise or excise the abnormal tissue.
3. Cold knife excision: It requires the use of a surgical blade to excise the abnormal area, and is both diagnostic and therapeutic. Cold knife excision is associated with higher morbidity and hence is not warranted in CIN I or LSIL.

Treatment: Treatment for all three grades of CIN depend on

1. Grade of lesion
2. Size of lesion (I–IV quadrant)
3. Site of lesion
4. Type of cervix
5. Age of patient and reproduction status
6. Surgeon's skill
7. Availability of modality

Before an ablative procedure, it is mandatory to

a. To rule out invasion
b. Rule out endocervical disease (glandular disease)
c. No ectocervical lesion

Hence, the use of cryosurgery and electrocautery in high-grade lesions is not recommended (CIN II to III).

In a study by Follen-Mitchell et al (1998), the capacity of cryotherapy, laser and LEEP for treatment of LSIL/CIN was evaluated. Regardless of the therapy used, the risk of persistence is greater with older women, larger lesions, repeated treatment and HPV, types 16 and 18 positive. In all methods, persistence following treatment is 4% and recurrence usually 10%.

A brief overview of the advantages and disadvantages of the various methods is given in Table 18.3.

SUMMARY

1. Cancer cervix is amenable to early detection by means of simple tests.
2. The Pap smear is widely used, easily available and universally acceptable as a screening test for pre-cancerous cervical lesions.
3. In countries with economic constraints, visual inspection with acetic acid (VIAA), Lugol's iodine (VILI) is an acceptable method of screening.
4. In the developed countries, liquid-based cytology is preferred since it is a more sensitive tool for detection of abnormalities.
5. The Bethesda classification should be followed in reporting abnormalities in

order to have a uniform reporting system for management and follow-up.

6. The ASCCP (American Society for Colposcopy and Cervical Pathology) and the ALTS Trial are the basis of guidelines for the management of abnormal smear.
7. ASCUS can be managed by wait and watch policy and repeat Pap taken after 4–6 months.
8. ASC-H, LSIL and HSIL require follow-up with colposcopic examination and, if available, HPV typing.
9. Follow-up of all cases can be by Pap smear after appropriate action is taken.
10. Treatment modalities can be either ablative or excisional; ablative methods should only be used if invasion is ruled out and the lesions are low-grade.

References

American College of Obstetrics and Gynecologists. 2003. Cervical cytology screening. ACOG Practice Bulletin No.45. *Obstet Gynecol* 102:417–427.

Evidence report/technology assessment. 1999. Maryland: Agency for Health Policy and Research, January. No. 5.

Follen-Mitchell M, Tortolevo Luna G, Cook E et al. 1998. A randomized clinical trial of cryotherapy, laser vaporisation and loop electrosurgical excision for treatment of squamous intraepithelial lesions of the cervix. *Obstet Gynecol* 92:737–744.

International Agency for Research on Cancer. Globocan 2000 database: Cancer incidence, mortality and prevalence worldwide. World Health Organization. 2002. http://www-dep.iarc.fr/globocan/globocan. html. Accessed 20 June 2004.

Kim TJ, Kim HS, Park CT et al. 2000. Clinical evaluation of follow-up methods and results of atypical glandular cells of undetermined significance (AGUS) detected on cervico-vaginal pap smears. *Gynecol Oncol* 73:292–298.

Mannos MM, Kenney WK, Hurley LB, et al. 1999. Identifying women with cervical neoplasia: Using HPV DNA listing for equivocal Papanicolaou results. *JAMA* 281:1605–1610.

Oster AG. 1993. Natural history of cervical intra-epithelial neoplasia: A critical review. *Int J Gynecol Pathol* 12:186–192.

Schiffman M, Hervero R, Hildesheim A, et al. 2000. HPV DNA testing in cervical cancer screening: results from women in a high-risk province of Costa Rica. JAMA 283:87–93.

Shafi ML, Luesley DM. 1995. Management of low-grade lesions: Follow up or treat? *Baillere's Clin Obstet Gynecol* 9:121–131.

Solomon D, Davery D, Kurman R, Moriarty A, O'Connor D, Prey M, et al. 2002. The 2001 Bethesda System: terminology for reporting results of cervical cytology. *JAMA* 287:2214–2219.

Solomon D, Schiffman M, Tarone R. 2001. Comparison of three management strategies for patients with atypical squamous cells of undetermined significance, baseline results from a randomized trial. *J Natl Cancer Inst* 93(4):293–318.

U.S. Preventive Services Task Force. 2003. Screening for cervical cancer. Agency for Healthcare Research and Quality. http://www.ahrq.gov/clinic/3rduspstf/cervcan/cervcanwh.pdf. Accessed 19 June 2004.

Wright TC Jr, Cox JT, Massad LS et al. 2002. The 2001 Consensus Guidelines for the management of women with cervical cytological abnormalities. *JAMA* 287:2120–2129.

19

Diagnosis and Management of Early Cervical Cancer

AP Manjunath | Girija S

The uterine cervix is of interest and importance to almost every obstetrician and gynecologist. To the gynecologic oncologist, it represents a common focus of cancer. To the obstetrician, it represents the primary barometer for the progress of labour and delivery. No other organ is as accessible in terms of both diagnosis and therapy. Its easy accessibility led to the great strides made possible by the Pap smear, resulting in complete reversal of the prognosis in cancer of this organ. Easy access to the cervix leads to skillful application of radiation techniques, which have resulted in some of the best overall cure rates for any malignancy found in humans. Cervical cancer is a common malignant disease and it remains one of the main causes of death in women worldwide, with about half a million new cases a year, 80% of which arise in less-developed countries (Greenlee et al 2000; Parkin 2001). In this chapter, the clinical profile, current screening and diagnostic scenario for cervical cancer is addressed initially. Staging work-up and standard surgical management of early cervical cancer will be discussed. Recent advances in the field are highlighted.

EARLY CERVICAL CANCER

Definition: Traditionally, International Federation of Gynecologists and Obstetricians (FIGO) Stages IA, IB and IIA cervical cancers have been regarded as early disease. This allowed for different prognostic groupings, as well as a convenient way of deciding and applying uniform treatment policies for the different stages.

Clinical profile

Symptoms: Typically, the patient with early cervical cancer is a multiparous woman between 45 and 55 years, who married and delivered her first child at an early age. Preinvasive and early invasive cervical cancer may not produce any symptoms. Cytological screening may discover the disease. As the disease progresses, symptoms start appearing which is related to the disruption of the cervical mucosa. Probably, the first symptom of early cancer of the cervix is a thin, watery, blood-tinged vaginal discharge. The classic symptom is intermittent, painless metrorrhagia or postcoital spotting or spotting after douching. As the malignancy enlarges, the bleeding episodes become heavier, more frequent and of longer duration. The patient may also describe an increase in the amount and duration of her regular menstrual flow; ultimately, the bleeding becomes essentially continuous. Postmenopausal bleeding is frequently seen in these patients. The triad of sciatic pain, leg edema and hydronephrosis is almost always associated with extensive pelvic wall involvement by tumour.

Physical examination: In general physical examination, particular attention is given to pallor, pedal edema and lymphadenopathy. Supraclavicular and inguinal nodes can be sites of metastases. The patient's height and weight is recorded to calculate the body surface area to administer chemoradiation, or neoadjuvant chemotherapy is planned. A speculum examination should be performed with care so as not to traumatise the friable cervical growth to initiate bleeding. Look for evidence of growth and type of growth. Primary tumours can be exophytic. Endophytic tumours can result in massive expansion of the endocervix, with no visible tumour. Fixity and friability of cervix are suggestive of malignancy.

When the speculum examination has been completed, a digital bimanual exam is performed, to determine the full extent and spread within the pelvis. Insert both fingers in the vagina and palpate the cervix. Detect if there is spread to the fornices or the vagina that was missed on speculum examination. Try to detect any endocervical expansion. With these findings in mind, perform a rectovaginal examination. The vaginal examination is not of great value in assessing the extent of spread towards the pelvic side walls. However, rectal examination must be performed in a patient with cervical cancer—estimate the size of the tumour; palpate the parametrium and the uterosacral ligaments for tumour infiltration. These findings can be quite subtle, even for experienced examiners. With the fingers, sweep along the pelvic sidewall as laterally as possible.

Screening and diagnosis

Cervical cytology: The Pap smear has been the cornerstone of screening for cervical neoplasm for the last fifty years (Papanicolaou and Traut 1941). The success of cervical cancer control is because of the long natural history of the disease and easy accessibility of the cervix for screening. The recommendations for cervical cancer screening vary, not only internationally, but among professional organisations. The American Cancer Society (ACS) and the American College of Obstetricians and Gynecologists (ACOG 2003) recommends that annual screening for cervical cancer should begin approximately three years after the onset of vaginal intercourse, or by age 21 years, which ever comes first. For women younger than 30 years, ACS recommends annual screening with conventional cytology or every two years using liquid-based cytology (Smith et al 2006). ACS guidelines for cervical cancer screening are sumarised in Table 19.1. The World Health Organization (WHO) suggested that in countries where resources are limited, the aim should be to screen every woman once in her lifetime between 35 and 40 years of age. When more resources are available, the frequency of screening should be increased to once in every ten or fifteen years for the age group 35 to 55 (WHO 1986). There is evidence that even once-in-a-lifetime screening can result in a 19% reduction in the incidence of cervical cancer (Goldie et al 2001).

The mean sensitivity and specificity of cervical cytology were 60% and 75%, respectively (Fahey et al 1995; Nanda et al 2000). With such a low sensitivity for a single cervical cytology test, the reduction in cervical cancer incidence is dependent on regular screening. The false negative rate of

Table 19.1: American Cancer Society recommendations for cervical cancer screening

1. **When to start screening?** Cervical cancer screening should begin approximately three years after a woman begins having vaginal intercourse, but no later than 21 years of age
2. **Screening intervals and screening tests:**
   - Screening should be done every year with conventional Pap tests or every 2 years using liquid-based Pap tests
   - At or after age 30 years
     - Women who have had three normal test results in a row may get screened every two to three years with cervical cytology (either conventional or liquid-based Pap test) alone or
     - Every three years with a HPV DNA test plus cervical cytology
3. **When to discontinue screening?** Women aged 70 years who have had three or more normal Pap tests and no abnormal Pap tests in the last 10 years
4. **Screening of women who have had a hysterectomy:** Women who have had a total hysterectomy for benign cause may choose to stop cervical cancer screening

cervical cytology is about 20% and it is mainly due to sampling errors. The false positive rate is about 5% and this is mostly due to interpretation errors.

Liquid-based cytology (LBC): It is a new technique for the preparation of cervical cytology specimens. The basic principle is that the sample from the cervix is removed from a broomstick type of device (Fig. 19.1) and rinsed into a cell-preserving transport fluid which is centrifuged and passed through a filter and then transferred by machine in a thin monolayer of cells on the slide. Thus, cervical cytology obtained has well-preserved cellular morphology without any air-drying, cell crowding and obscuring cells, with minimal cell overlapping. It is also suitable for additional testing procedures, such as Human Papilloma Virus (HPV) testing. LBC is more expensive than conventional cytology and requires additional instrumentation to prepare the smears. It is not feasible to implement LBC in many low-resource settings. There is no evidence that liquid based cytology is more accurate than conventional cytology at detecting high-grade disease (Davey et al 2006).

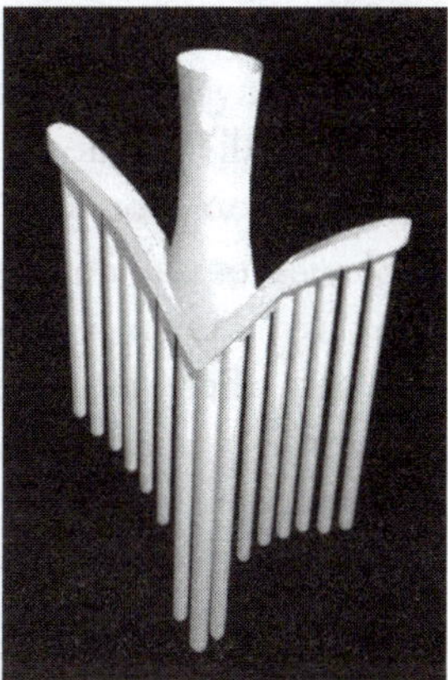

Figure 19.1: Device used to remove cytology sample from the cervix

Colposcopy: In current practice, colposcopy is reserved in women with abnormal Pap smear to identify the location of the lesion to target the site for biopsy. It is a low-powered binocular microscope which provides a stereoscopic vision of the female lower genital tract under bright illumination. The image in the colposcope can be magnified from four to forty times. A comprehensive colposcopic examination involves three steps—inspection of the unprepared cervix followed by saline colposcopy, colposcopy after dilute acetic acid application and inspection after application of Lugol's iodine. Once the tumour has reached a certain size, colposcopy is no longer required. After colposcopy, it is important to document the findings and care must be taken to ascertain that the abnormal area seen through the colposcope is actually biopsied. If there is no source of abnormal Pap test on colposcopy, before labelling it as a false positive smear, endocervical curettage should be performed to rule out endocervical lesion.

The International Federation for Cervical Pathology and Colposcopy has designated colposcopic features suggestive of various levels of disease. These features are listed in Table 19.2. In experienced hands, the sensitivity and specificity of colposcopy is over 90%. Unfortunately, there are no pathognomomic colposcopic patterns that distinguish microinvasive lesions from their precursors. All diagnosis based on colposcopic impression should be confirmed by histopathological examination.

Table 19.2: Colposcopic features suggestive of abnormalities (Walker 2003)

Features suggestive of low-grade disease
- Smooth surface with irregular outer border
- Slight acetowhite change, quick to disappear
- Mild, speckled iodine partial positivity
- Fine punctation or fine regular mosaic pattern

Features suggestive of high-grade disease
- Generally smooth surface with sharp outer border
- Dense acetowhite change; slow to resolve
- Iodine negativity; yellow appearance in previously densely white epithelium
- Coarse punctation; wide irregular mosaic pattern
- Dense acetowhite changes in columnar epithelium may indicate glandular disease

Features suggestive of invasive cancer
- Irregular surface, erosion or ulceration
- Dense acetowhite change
- Wide irregular punctation or mosaic pattern
- Atypical vessels

Cervical biopsy: This is most commonly carried out where there is a suspicion on clinical, cytological or colposcopic grounds of cancer or precancer of the cervix. There are four main techniques for obtaining specimens—punch biopsy, cone biopsy, loop electrosurgical excision procedure (LEEP) and endocervical curettage.

Punch biopsy: A Pap smear in a patient with a visible lesion not only causes delays but can also produce false-negative smears in up to 40% of patients. A biopsy sample taken from the periphery of a tumour is more likely to represent the tumour pathologically. Specimen size should be greater than 5 mm. Even though the most commonly used fixative is formalin, the Susa solution gives superior nuclear details. The biopsy forceps should be sharp; it should not crush the specimen. For taking biopsy of lesions of external os, the fixed part of the forceps should be introduced inside the cervical canal while the mobile part lies outside. When more than one sample is required, the posterior part of the cervix should be biopsied first, to prevent the impairment of vision related to bleeding.

Conisation biopsy: Conisation may be both diagnostic and therapeutic. Indications of cone biopsy are summarised in Table 19.3. The cone biopsy must be performed if no gross lesion of the cervix is observed and an endocervical tumour is suspected. When a large visible lesion is present on the cervix, large cone biopsies add little to the diagnosis. It induces an inflammatory response and compromises the assessment of tumour size by both histology and preoperative MRI, and can cause delay in definitive treatment.

TABLE 19.3: INDICATIONS FOR CONE BIOPSY

- Minimal or quiescent microinvasion suspected on colposcopic directed biopsy to rule out deep invasion
- Major grade lesion extending into the cervical canal outside the range of colposcopic examination
- Major grade lesions which are focal but extensive in area
- Suspected adenocarcinoma
- Abnormal or inconclusive findings on ECC
- Repeated abnormal smear suggestive of significant lesion in the absence of colposcopic lesion
- Transformation zone is not seen colposcopically (unsatisfactory colposcopy)
- Absence of satisfactory correlation between colposcopy, cytology and histology

LOOP ELECTROSURGICAL EXCISION PROCEDURE (LEEP): It is sometimes referred to as large-loop excision of the transformation zone (LLETZ) which allows the physician to 'see and treat' in an outpatient setting. Bleeding and thermal artifacts of margins are of main concern. Sound electrosurgical principles can result in excellent specimens with minimal complications.

ENDOCERVICAL CURETTAGE (ECC): This is most important in patients with abnormal cytology to prevent unnecessary conisation, and when the entire transformation zone is not visible colposcopically, to exclude the possibility of glandular abnormalities. ECC is obtained by short and firm strokes to scrape the entire length and circumference of cervical canal at least twice to obtain an adequate specimen through the undilated cervix. The Kelly curette (Fig. 19.2) or Novak endometrial biopsy curette can be used to obtain ECC (Fig. 19.3). There is no need to use a tenaculum to catch the cervix. It has been shown that ECC misses nearly 50% of all endocervical lesions compared to only 8% for the cytobrush (Andersen 1988).

Screening and diagnosis in resource-poor settings: The success of cervical cytology in organised screening programmes in developed countries seems to be due to repeated testing at frequent intervals (1–5 years), high population coverage and quality-control procedures. Cytology is not a viable option in many low-resource countries because of an inability to meet requirements. Simpler alternatives to cytologic screening for low resource settings have been evaluated.

DOWNSTAGING: The WHO defines the downstaging of cervical cancer as the detection of disease in an earlier stage (when still curable), by nurses and paramedical workers using a simple per speculum examination of the cervix. This method of screening is not

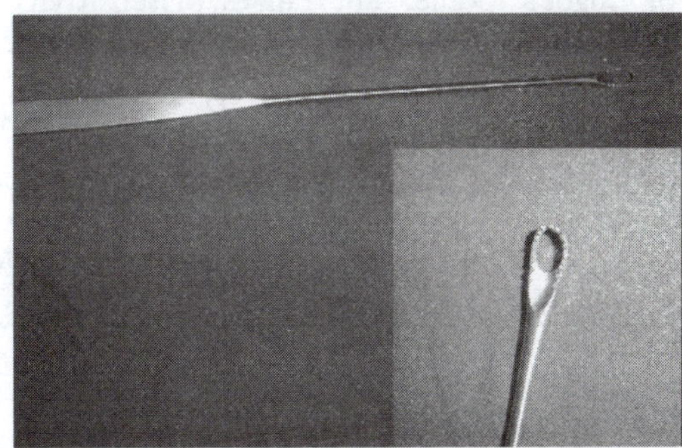

FIGURE 19.2: THE KELLY CURETTE

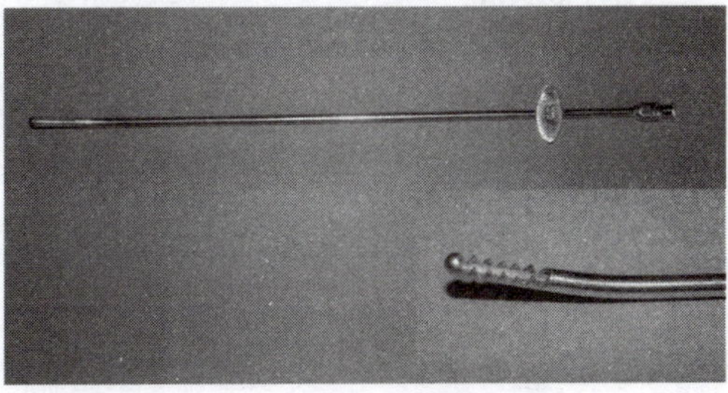

FIGURE 19.3: NOVAK ENDOMETRIAL BIOPSY CURETTE

expected to decrease the incidence of disease, but it will decrease mortality through early detection.

Visual inspection with acetic acid (VIA) is looking for acetowhite areas on the cervix after the application of 3%–5% dilute acetic acid. A wide range of healthcare providers can perform VIA. The immediate availability of results after VIA is a major advantage. The sensitivity varies from 67% to 79% and the specificity ranges from 49% to 86% (Cronjé 2003; Sankaranarayanan 2004).

In visual inspection with acetic acid with magnification (VIAM), the added value of low-level magnification (2–4 X) to inspect acetowhite changes of cervix has not been shown to improve the performance (Sankaranarayanan 2004).

Visual inspection with Lugol's iodine (VILI) is the examination of the cervix to identify iodine-non uptake areas after the application of Lugol's iodine. The ranges of sensitivity and specificity for VILI were 77.8% to 98.0% and 73.0% to 91.3%, respectively. Recent data suggest that VILI is as specific as and more sensitive than VIA (Sankaranarayanan 2003, 2004).

Human papilloma virus (HPV) testing: The sensitivity of HPV testing in detecting CIN II–III lesions and invasive cancer varied from 66% to 100% and the specificity varied from 61% to 96% (Womack 2000; Sankaranarayanan 2004). In comparison with cytology, HPV testing is highly sensitive and much more reliable and also has better sensitivity and specificity than visual screening. The downside of HPV testing is its mediocre specificity. Since HPV infection is common and transient among young women, HPV testing is not recommended as part of primary cervical screening for women younger than 30 years of age (ACOG 2005). Detailed information about HPV can be obtained at www.hpvtoday.com.

Combination of tests: The high sensitivity and long-term predictive value of the combination of HPV testing and cytology prompted the ACS and ACOG to recommend this combination as an option for the primary cervical screening of women above 30 years and to lengthen the screening interval for these women to three years. The sensitivity of cytology was improved from 57.4% to 83.3% by adding VIA to cytology as an adjunctive

TABLE 19.4: METHODS OF CERVICAL CANCER SCREENING AND DIAGNOSIS

Screening	Diagnosis
Papanicolaou smear (Pap test)	Biopsy
Colposcopy and biopsy	Punch biopsy
Liquid based cytology	Excision biopsy
HPV testing	Directed biopsy
Low resource settings	Conisation
Downstaging	Loop electrosurgical excision procedure (LEEP)
Visual inspection with acetic acid (VIA)	Endocervical curettage (ECC)
Visual inspection with acetic acid and magnification (VIAM)	Fluorescent spectroscopy
Visual inspection with Lugal's iodine (VILI)	
Combination	
Cytology and VIA	
Cytology & VILI	
Cytology and HPV	

TABLE 19.5: ACCURACY OF SCREENING TEST FOR CERVICAL CANCER

Test	Cytology	VIA	VIAM	VILI	HPV testing
Sensitivity	30%–87%	71%–74%	64.9%	77.8%–98.0%	80%–90%
Specificity	86%–92%	64%–74%	86.3%	73.0%–91.3%	57%–89%

test. The combination of cytology and VILI significantly improved test sensitivity to 88.9% (Shastri 2005). Various methods available for cervical cancer screening and diagnosis are summarised in Table 19.4. The accuracy of different screening tests for cervical cancer is highlighted in Table 19.5.

INNOVATIONS IN SCREENING AND DIAGNOSIS

Fluorescence spectroscopy: Optical diagnosis of cervical cancer by fluorescence spectroscopy is a promising new technique which has been developed recently. These techniques are based on biophysical properties of light and tissue that can be manipulated to predict diagnosis (Fig. 19.4) (Chidanand et al 2006). It is a near real-time measurement that is fully automated and does not require the expertise needed for colposcopy. It is completely noninvasive and involves the application of white light at different wavelengths to the surface of the cervix. The higher the grade of dysplasia, the more the absorption, the less the emitted fluorescence, and therefore, the lower the signal from the tissue (Ramanujam et al 1994, 1996). Preliminary data and cost analysis of this technique show that fluorescence spectroscopy of the cervix has a higher sensitivity than the Pap smear and a higher specificity than colposcopy. Figure 19.4 illustrates the fluorescence spectroscopy technique to identify carcinoma cervix. If the positive predictive value for high-grade CIN were sufficiently high, spectroscopic classification could serve as an 'optical biopsy,' obviating the need for traditional histologic sampling prior to treatment. This would be particularly useful in underserved settings with a high prevalence of disease (Parker 2005).

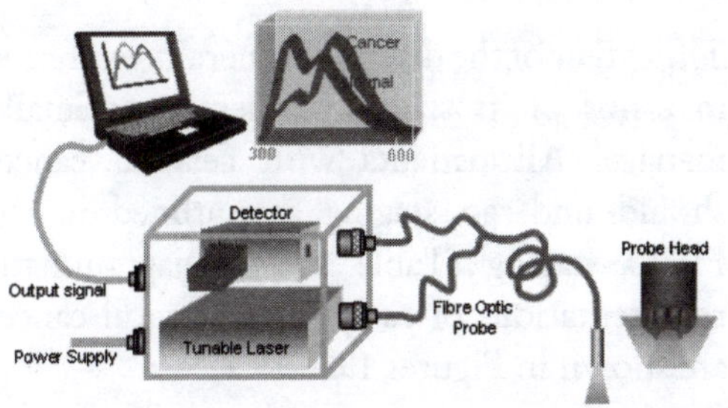

FIGURE 19.4: FLUORESCENT SPECTROSCOPY

PATHOLOGY OF CERVICAL CANCER

Carcinomas of the cervix may be classified into four groups—squamous carcinomas (80%-90%); adenocarcinoma (10%-15%) which is a miscellaneous group including adenosquamous carcinomas; and neuro-endocrine tumours. The recent WHO classification of cervical tumours is shown in Table 19.6 (Tavassoli and Devilee 2003). Squamous neoplasms are categorised as large cell keratinising, large cell non-keratinising or small cell carcinoma. Verrucous carcinoma is a form of low-grade carcinoma; the tumour does not respond to radiation therapy. Adenoma malignum is a very low-grade malignancy and metastases are very rare. Mixed histology is common in the cervix. Adenosquamous carcinomas are the most common mixture.

There is a recent change in the nomenclature of neuroendocrine and small-cell tumours of the cervix which is subdivided into typical carcinoid, atypical carcinoid, large cell neuroendocrine carcinoma, and small cell carcinoma (SCC) (Albores-Saavedra 1997). These 'small cell' tumours have a high proliferation rate and marked propensity to regional lymph node and distant metastases and death from even the smallest tumour. Therefore, work-up may include bone marrow aspiration and other tests to detect the metastatic spread characteristic of this histology. In view of its systemic disease and failure rates, the combination chemotherapy is advocated as part of standard therapy in all stages of the disease.

Adenocarcinoma of the cervix shows a wide range of biologic activity. Poorly differentiated adenocarcinomas are highly malignant, and regional and distant metastases are common. In addition, high-grade adenocarcinomas can have a neuroendocrine component. Even though adenocarcinomas are generally considered to have a poorer prognosis than squamous carcinomas, early stage invasive adenocarcinoma appears to be similar in outcome to its squamous equivalents (Davy et al 2003).

Table 19.6: World Health Organization classification of cervical cancer

Squamous cell carcinoma
- Keratinising
- Nonkeratinising
- Verrucous
- Papillary transitional
- Lymphoepithelioma-like

Adenocarcinoma (glandular)
- Mucinous:
  - Cervical-type
  - Intestinal-type
  - ***Signet-ring***
- Endometrioid
- Clear-cell
- Minimal deviation (adenoma malignum)
- Well-differentiated villoglandular (papillary)
- Serous
- Mesonephric

Other epithelial
- Adenosquamous
- Glassy-cell
- Adenoid cystic
- Adenoid basal
- Carcinoid tumour (adenocarcinoma with features of carcinoid)
- Small-cell
- Undifferentiated

Histopathological prognostic indicators: In general, prognosis of cervical carcinomas depends on the clinical stage. The most important independent histopathological indicators of prognosis are size of tumour, depth of invasion and the presence or absence of lymph node metastases. The lymphovascular space invasion is not an independent indicator, but an essential part of the histology report. Small cell carcinomas, large cell neuroendocrine carcinomas and possibly adenoid cystic carcinomas are aggressive. Tumour grade is currently not believed to be of significant value.

The main role of immunohistochemistry is to distinguish adenocarcinomas of endocervical origin from endometrial origin (endocervical adenocarcinomas are CK7 and CEA positive, Vimentin negative; endometrial carcinomas are CK7 and Vimentin positive, CEA negative).

Staging

The extent of the disease is generally expressed in terms of its stage in order to optimally manage. All patients with cervical cancer should undergo staging as outlined in the FIGO staging (Table 19.7). Diagrammatic representations of early stage cervical cancer are shown in Figures 19.5–19.7.

Principles of cancer staging: The major purpose of staging is to provide a uniform system for reporting the clinical experience and comparison of treatment methods without confusion. A good staging system must have three basic characteristics. It must be valid, reliable, and above all, practical. It must be suitable for day to day use and must not require diagnostic procedures that are not readily available.

Rules for classification: Staging of cervical cancer is based on clinical evaluation and it is the only gynecologic malignancy at present staged clinically. The single most important clinical examination in a case of cervical cancer is per rectum examination. Rectal examination will reveal whether the parametrium is completely free (Stage I) or involved medially (Stage IIB) or up to pelvic wall (Stage IIIB) and also if the rectal mucosa is involved (Stage VIA). When there is doubt as to which stage a particular cancer should be allocated, the earlier stage is mandatory. The following examinations are permitted: inspection, palpation, colposcopy, endocervical curettage, hysteroscopy. Additional studies such as cystoscopy, proctosigmoidoscopy, intravenous pyelogram, x-ray examination of the lungs and skeleton, bone scan, CT scan, or MRI should be considered only in patients with symptoms and with more advanced disease (Benedet 2000). Suspected bladder or

Table 19.7: International Federation of Gynecology and Obstetrics (FIGO) Clinical Staging of Cervical Cancer

Stage	Substage		Description
Stage 0	Carcinoma in situ		
Stage I	Carcinoma is confined to the cervix		
	Stage IA	Stage IA1	Microscopic lesion; invasion of the stroma ≤3.0 mm in depth and ≤7.0 mm in width
		Stage IA2	Microscopic lesion; invasion of the stroma >3.0 mm and ≤5.0 mm in depth and ≤7.0 mm in width
	Stage IB	Stage IB1	Clinical (visible) lesion confined to the cervix and not >4.0 cm in size
		Stage IB2	Similar, but clinical lesion >4.0 cm in size
Stage II	Carcinoma extends beyond the cervix but not to the pelvic sidewall, or carcinoma involves the vagina but not the lower third		
	Stage IIA	No obvious parametrial involvement	
	Stage IIB	Obvious parametrial involvement	
Stage III	Carcinoma extends to the pelvic sidewall or to the lower third of the vagina. All cases with hydronephrosis or nonfunctioning kidney should be included, unless known to be due to another cause		
	Stage IIIA	No extension to the pelvic sidewall, but involvement of the lower third of the vagina	
	Stage IIIB	Extension to the pelvic sidewall and/or hydronephrosis or nonfunctioning kidney	
Stage IV	Carcinoma extends beyond the true pelvis and involves the bladder or rectal mucosa		
	Stage IVA	Involves the bladder or rectal mucosa	
	Stage IVB	Distant metastasis	

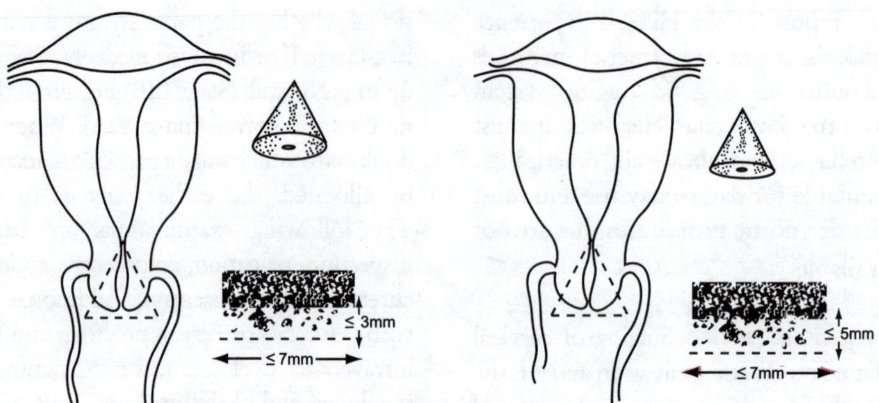

FIGURE 19.5: FIGO STAGE 1A

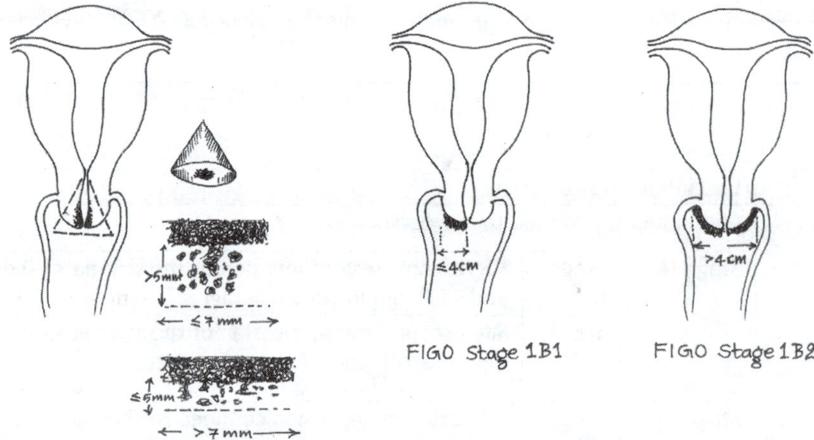

FIGURE 19.6: FIGO STAGE 1B

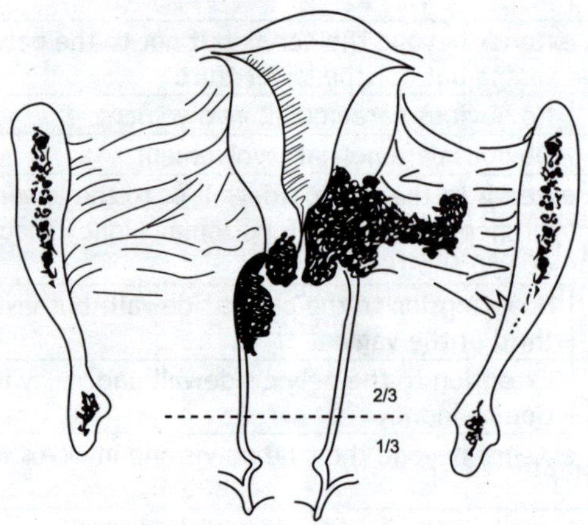

FIGURE 19.7: FIGO STAGES 2A AND 2B

rectal involvement should be confirmed by biopsy. Conisation or amputation of the cervix is regarded as a clinical examination. Staging is determined at the time of the primary diagnosis and the clinical staging must not be changed on discovery of more extensive disease during surgery or even at recurrence. If unsuspected extensive invasive cervical carcinoma is detected after a simple hysterectomy, it cannot be clinically staged or included in therapeutic statistics, but it should be reported separately.

Notes about the staging: Stage 0 comprises patients with full-thickness, involvement of the epithelium with atypical cells, but with no signs of invasion into the stroma. The diagnosis of both Stage IAl and IA2 should be based on microscopic examination of removed tissue, preferably a cone biopsy or LEEP, which must include the entire lesion. The depth of invasion should not exceed 5 mm taken from the base of the epithelium, either surface or glandular, from which it originates. The second dimension, the horizontal spread, must not exceed 7 mm. Vascular space involvement, either venous or lymphatic, should not alter the staging, but should be specifically recorded because it may affect treatment decisions in the future.

Larger lesions should be staged as IB. As a rule, it is impossible to clinically estimate if a cancer of the cervix has extended to the corpus. Extension to the corpus should therefore be disregarded.

A growth fixed to the pelvic wall by a short and indurated, but not nodular parametrium should be allotted to Stage IIB. A case should be classified as Stage III only if the parametrium is nodular to the pelvic wall or if the growth itself extends to the pelvic wall.

The presence of hydronephrosis or non-functioning kidney resulting from stenosis of the ureter by cancer permits a case to be allotted to Stage III even if the parametrium is free or medially involved. The presence of bullous edema, as such, should not permit a case to be allotted to Stage IV. Finding malignant cells in cytologic washings from the urinary bladder requires further histological confirmation in order to be considered for Stage IVA. FIGO staging rules are summarised in Table 19.8.

TABLE 19.8: FIGO STAGING RULES FOR CERVICAL CANCER

- Clinically staged
- Clinical examination include: Inspection and palpation of the pelvic organs with bimanual and rectovaginal examinations, per speculum, per vaginal and per rectal examination
- Investigations permitted: Colposcopy, endocervical curettage, hysteroscopy, cystoscopy, proctoscopy, intravenous urography and X-ray examination of the lungs and skeleton
- Other rules: If there is doubt regarding the stage, the earlier stage is chosen
- Staging is done at the time of primary diagnosis, it cannot be changed subsequently
- Histopathological confirmation is mandatory for primary as well as metastasis

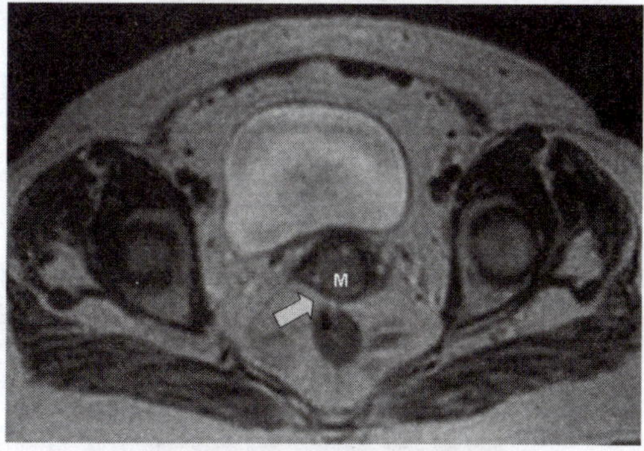

FIGURE 19.8: MRI STAGING OF EARLY CERVICAL CANCER: T2 weighted axial image shows preservation of low signal intensity cervical rim in stage IB cervical cancer (M: mass lesion which appears hyperintense)

Recently, a noninvasive MRI-assisted FIGO staging system for cervical cancer providing greater prognostically homogeneous groupings for selecting patients appropriately for a given treatment package has been devised (Narayan 2005). The MRI staging of early cervical cancer is shown in Fig. 19.8–19.9.

Cervical Cancer Imaging

Magnetic resonance imaging (MRI) has the widest application in cervical carcinoma. It plays an important role in staging, surgical and radiotherapy planning, monitoring treatment and detecting recurrence. In the early stage of cervical cancer, there is a good correlation between MRI and FIGO staging (Renju and Rai 2005). The advantages of MRI scanning are soft tissue definition, a larger field of view and the potential benefit of multiplanar imaging. MRI can provide useful information about the distribution and depth of invasion of tumours in the cervix but tends to yield less accurate assessments of the parametrium. MRI scanning does not differentiate tissue edema from tumour invasion, which may lead to an overestimation of tumour size. Bipat et al showed that overall tumour staging accuracy was 86% by MRI, compared to 47% by clinical FIGO staging (Bipat et al 2003). One of the main uses of MRI is the prediction of the proximal extension of the tumour which helps in planning radical trachelectomy, a fertility sparing radical surgical treatment of early stage cervical cancer. An important criterion for surgery is that the proximal end of the tumour should be at least 1 cm away from the internal cervical os. The sensitivity of the MRI to detect tumour extension beyond the internal os was 100% (Peppercorn et al 1999). Recently, De Souza et al demonstrated an alternative technique using an endovaginal coil to magnetic resonance imaging in order to assess tumour volume and also identification of early parametrial spread. This technique has high sensitivity even for cervical lesions less than 1 cm^3 (De Souza et al 2006).

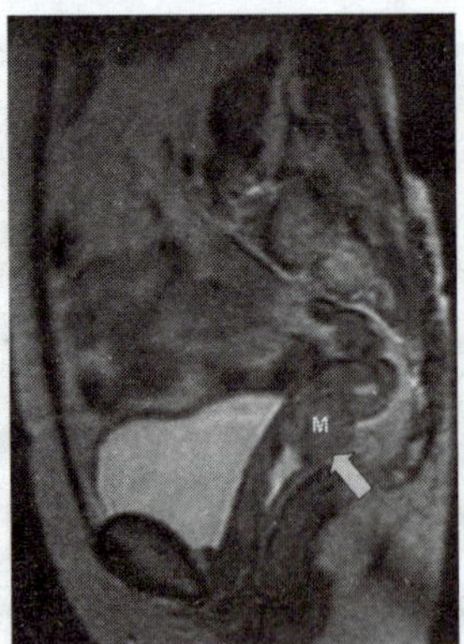

Figure 19.9: MRI stage 2A: T2 weighted sagittal image depicting the hypertensive mass lesion (M) and loss of low signal intensity wall of the vagina in the postero-superior aspect suggestive of stage IIA cervical carcinoma

CT and MRI help detect abnormal masses or enlarged organs, but they do not provide information on the functional or metabolic status of lesions. A promising new technology for cervical cancer imaging is the positron emission tomography (PET) scan which is based on increased glucose utilisation in malignant cells; however, it does not provide anatomic landmarks (Rose et al 1999). Hence, hybrid PET/CT which combines metabolic and structural information is of value in planning irradiation therapy. Using this modality may reduce unnecessary surgical interventions, help modify radiation fields and change therapeutic approaches. However, this examination is less accurate in detecting microscopic diseases and lesions smaller than 1.5 cm (Amit et al 2006), but it is a very sensitive noninvasive method of evaluating the regional nodes of patients with cervical cancer (Grigsby et al 2001).

Currently, on MRI, metastasis to the lymph nodes is thought to have occurred mainly by virtue of the nodes being enlarged to 8 mm or more. However, work is currently being undertaken using lymph node-specific MRI contrast agents known as ultra-small iron oxide particles, which are taken up by normal lymph nodes but not by nodes involved by tumour.

Pretreatment Assessment And Preparation

These have been mentioned while discussing staging. Standard laboratory studies for fitness to undergo surgery or radiotherapy should be undertaken. Routine tests include a complete blood cell count and renal function and liver function tests. Routine cystoscopy is uninformative for most small tumours less than 4 cm and it is reserved for large tumours and for small tumours encroaching on the anterior vaginal fornix. Table 19.9 gives the work-up for a case of visible cervical cancer.

For surgical therapy the abdomen, perineum and vagina should be prepared in the usual way with antiseptic toileting and douches. Antibiotic prophylaxis is given. The bowel should be emptied using suitable laxatives and an enema should be given the night before surgery, so that a loaded colon does not obstruct adequate access to the pelvis. It will also prevent the severe constipation problems occurring postoperatively. Any medical condition, like anemia, diabetes, hypertension, bronchial asthma should be corrected before surgery. Preoperative physiotherapy and mobilisation is vital. The use of low molecular weight heparins and compression elastic stockings is advisable for prevention of deep vein thrombosis and pulmonary embolism. Bleeding may occur during surgery hence adequate blood should be cross matched and should be available. Consent, especially for inoperability, should be obtained.

Table 19.9: Work-up of patients with visible cervical cancer

All patients	Common optional studies
• History, physical examination • Cervical biopsy • Routine blood studies, hemoglobin, blood grouping cross matching, renal function tests and liver function tests, complete blood count • Chest X-ray	• Examination under anesthesia • CT or MRI of abdomen and pelvis • Intravenous pyelogram • Lymphangiogram • Cystoscopy • Barium enema/ rectosigmoidoscopy • Skeletal X rays • CT or MRI of brain • PET scan

Treatment

Patient management always needs to be individualised, taking into account a patient's general medical condition, her cultural environment, availability of resources, expertise and technology. Before treatment commences, a histological diagnosis is a must. Specific therapeutic measures are usually governed by the age and general health of the patient, extent of the cancer, tumour volume, nodal status, histological parameters, technical factors, and the surgeon's ability. It is desirable to have multidisciplinary meetings where possible and patients should be informed about therapeutic alternatives, including their toxicity and the expected outcomes. Risk factors for complications of surgery or radiotherapy also need to be considered. The appropriate choice of therapy should be based on the patient's preference and desire for ovarian (or even fertility) preservation.

Microinvasive carcinoma of the cervix: The society of gynecologic oncologists (SGO) and FIGO define microinvasive carcinoma differently. The most practical and clinically useful definition of microinvasion was adopted by the SGO. This includes tumour invasion to a depth no greater than 3 mm below the base of the epithelium with no confluent tongues and no areas of lymphatic or vascular invasion (Creasman et al 1985). The FIGO definition does not include the evaluation of lymphovascular invasion. It divides microinvasive carcinoma into stage IA1 (depth of invasion less than 3 mm and horizontal dimension less than 7 mm) and stage IA2 (depth of invasion more than 3 mm but less than 5 mm and horizontal dimension less than 7 mm). There is a consensus that depth of stromal invasion is the major factor in determining the outcome of patients with microinvasive carcinoma.

Stage IA: Simple hysterectomy is more commonly accepted therapy. Abdominal, vaginal or laparoscopic procedure produces excellent results. If fertility is desired, lesions up to 3 mm that meet the other criteria of the SGO definition may be excised (conisation of the cervix, or loop excision).

Stage IA2: Management of lesions between 3 mm and 5 mm depth of invasion should be individualised. There is a definite risk of nodal metastases of approximately 5%, so pelvic lymphadenectomy should be included in the treatment protocol (Webb et al 2001). The recommended treatment is modified radical hysterectomy (Type 2) and pelvic lymphadenectomy. If there is no lymphovascular space invasion, consideration may be given to extrafascial hysterectomy and pelvic lymphadenectomy. If fertility is desired, options are

- Large cone biopsy plus extraperitoneal or laparoscopic pelvic lymphadenectomy, or
- Radical trachelectomy and extraperitoneal or laparoscopic pelvic lymphadenectomy (Shepherd et al 2006).

Although surgical treatment is standard for microinvasive cancer, patients with severe medical problems or other contraindications to surgical treatment can be successfully treated with intracavitary brachytherapy alone (65 to 75 Gy to point A in one or two insertions) with excellent results (Hamberger et al 1978).

Stages IB and IIA: Radiation therapy is equivalent to radical hysterectomy for definitive treatment of early-stage cervical carcinoma (Landoni et al 1997). However, morbidity is usually higher when surgery and radiation are combined. Patients who are treated with radical hysterectomy whose tumours are found to have high-risk features may benefit from postoperative radiotherapy or chemoradiation. However, in order to minimise treatment-related sequelae and increased cost, primary therapy should avoid the planned use of both radical surgery and radiation therapy.

Surgery offers primary tumour removal with potential to preserve ovarian function, coital function, and in certain cases, the potential to maintain reproductive function. It has other advantages such as a shorter treatment time, more limited tissue injury, a specimen for pathological evaluation. For patients with similar tumours, the overall rate of major complications is similar with surgery and radiotherapy, although urinary tract complications tend to be more frequent after surgical treatment and bowel complications are more common after radiotherapy. With surgical treatment, complications are acute and treatable and with radiotherapy, it is delayed and more difficult to treat. Radiation cystitis or proctitis may occur periodically for years following radiotherapy and are difficult

TABLE 19.10: RADIATION VS SURGERY FOR EARLY CERVICAL CANCER

Radiotherapy	*Surgery*
Advantages	
▪ May be given on an outpatient basis ▪ Survival rates are similar to surgery	▪ Psychological effect of removal of the tumour ▪ Conservation of ovaries in the young ▪ Coincidental adnexal masses or pyosalpinges with infected adnexa may be removed ▪ Accurate surgical staging ▪ A more pliable, although shortened, vagina remains for coital function
Disadvantages	
▪ Vaginal stenosis with consequent dryness and rigidity with a lack of sensation ▪ Urinary tract complications hemorrhagic cystitis urinary frequency contracted bladder chronic hematuria ureteric stricture fistulas (urethro-vaginal and vesico-vaginal) ▪ Bowel complications chronic diarrhea flatulence procto-colitis rectal stricture malabsorption from the terminal ileum fistulae (entero-vaginal and recto-vaginal) ▪ Avascular necrosis of the femoral head ▪ Pyometra from cervical stenosis ▪ Ovarian ablation with consequent enforced Menopause ▪ Risk of secondary malignancy	▪ Complications from a prolonged operation (anesthetic complications and hemorrhage). ▪ Infection in the chest, wound, urinary tract and pelvis ▪ Urological complications: atonic blader, frequency. ▪ Reduced bladder capacity, fistulae (urethro-vaginal and vesico-vaginal ▪ Lymphocyst formation with subsequent lymphedema ▪ Obturator nerve damage during lymphadenectomy ▪ Paralytic ileus ▪ Thromboembolism ▪ Sexual dysfunction from shortened vagina ▪ Patient may still require postoperative radiotherapy/chemotherapy depending on the final findings at laparotomy

to repair in view of the inevitable endarteritis, reducing the blood supply. Surgical treatment tends to be preferred for young women with small tumours. Radiotherapy is often chosen for older, postmenopausal women. The relative merits and demerits of surgery and radiotherapy are highlighted in Table 19.10.

The patient with stage IB2 bulky cervical carcinoma has three treatment options:

- Chemoradiation therapy
- Radical hysterectomy (followed by tailored postoperative treatment, when indicated, on the basis of high-risk factors for recurrence)
- Neoadjuvant chemotherapy followed by radical hysterectomy.

Radical radiotherapy: The unique accessibility of the cervix for radiation therapy makes it one of the few internal cancers that can be cured by radiation therapy alone. To sterilise disease, the combination of external-beam irradiation to the whole pelvis to treat regional nodes and shrink primary tumour is followed by a central intracavitary application (brachytherapy) to boost the central tumour. However, brachytherapy is a critical element in the curative radiation treatment of all carcinomas of the cervix. Concurrent chemoradiotherapy is the current standard of practice for patients with advanced-stage cervical cancer. It is used both for primary treatment and after hysterectomy in women at high risk. A meta-analysis of trials demonstrated an absolute improvement in survival of 10% and progression free survival of 13% with chemoradiotherapy (Green et al 2005). The details of the principles, techniques and complications of radiotherapy are discussed in more detail in chapter 24 on 'Radiotherapy in Gynecology'.

Current Surgical Treatment

Radical abdominal hysterectomy and pelvic lymphadenectomy has been the standard of care for surgical management of early stage cervical cancer. Many technical modifications of the initial radical hysterectomy have been described.

Radical hysterectomy: This procedure involves en bloc removal of the uterus, cervix, and paracervical, parametrial and paravaginal tissues up to the pelvic sidewalls bilaterally, with removal of as much of the uterosacral ligaments as possible. The uterine vessels are ligated at their origin, and the proximal third of the vagina and paracolpium are resected. Pelvic node dissection involves the four major lymph node chains—ureteral, obturator, hypogastric and iliac. Metastatic lesions to ovaries are rare; hence, they may be preserved in young women and suspended outside the pelvis if postoperative radiation is likely to be given.

Radical hysterectomy is a procedure that must be performed by a skilled person with sufficient experience to make the morbidity acceptable (1%–5%). Radical hysterectomy is complex because the tissues removed are in close proximity to many vital structures such as the bowels, bladder, ureters and great vessels of the pelvis.

Extent of radical hysterectomy: The complications of surgery for cervical cancer are strongly related to the extent of tissue removed. Thus, the extent of surgery should be tailored to the disease. Variations in techniques exist while performing radical hysterectomy. The term radical hysterectomy is not adequate to record the extent of excision. The five classes of extended hysterectomy described by Piver et al are of practical value (Piver et al 1974). The extent of resection for surgical procedures to treat early stage cervical cancer is sumarised in Table 19.11. The main difference between Type II and. Type III is the amount of parametrial tissue taken and degree of ureteral dissection (Fig. 19.10). Class III hysterectomy is most commonly performed.

Aiming to decrease the local recurrence rates, a more extensive radical surgery has been introduced for the lymph node positive Stage IB and in Stage IIB cases. This extended Wertheim's procedure is called the 'laterally extended parametrectomy' (LEP), has been proposed. It involves the removal of all the lymphatic tissue from the pelvic side wall. The long-term disease free interval seems to be better than that obtained with conventional surgery plus radiation or irradiation alone (Ungar and Palfalvi 2003).

Technique of radical hysterectomy Radical hysterectomy can be performed by the following techniques.

- Radical abdominal hysterectomy with pelvic lymphadenectomy
- Radical vaginal hysterectomy with

TABLE 19.11: COMPARISON OF EXTENT OF RESECTION FOR SURGICAL PROCEDURES TO TREAT EARLY STAGE CERVICAL CANCER

Type of surgery	*Intrafascial Hysterectomy*	*Extrafascial type I hysterectomy*	*Modified radical type II hysterectomy*	*Radical type III hysterectomy*	*Radical vaginal trachelectomy*
Cervical fascia	Partially removed	Completely removed	Completely removed	Completely removed	Completely removed
Vaginal cuff removal	None	Small rim	Proximal 1-2 cm	Upper 1/3 to 1/2	1-2 cm removed
Bladder	Partially mobilised	Partially mobilised	Partially mobilised	Mobilised	Mobilised
Rectum	Not mobilised	Partially mobilised	Partially mobilised	Mobilised	Mobilised
Uterine vessels	Ligated at level of internal cervical os	Ligated at level of internal cervical os	Ligated at level of ureter	Ligated at origin of internal iliac artery	Ligated at level of ureter
Ureters	Not mobilised	Not mobilised	Unroofed in ureteric tunnel	Completely dissected to bladder entry	Unroofed in ureteric tunnel
Cardinal ligaments	Resected medial to ureters	Resected medial to ureters	Resected at level of ureters	Resected at pelvic side wall	Partially removed
Uterosacral ligamnets	Resected at level of cervix	Resected at level of cervix	Partially resected	Resected at post pelvic insertion	Partially removed
Cervix	Partially removed	Completely removed	Completely removed	Completely removed	Majority removed
Parametria and paracolpos	Preserved	Preserved	Removed at level of ureter	Removed lateral to ureter	Partially removed

extraperitoneal pelvic lymphadenectomy (Schauta–Mitra)

- Laparoscopic assisted radical vaginal hysterectomy (Celio Schauta)
- Total laparoscopic radical hysterectomy

Basic surgical technique: The key steps of radical hysterectomy are summarised here. The two most crucial initial steps of radical hysterectomy are

- Development of the pelvic spaces permits inspection and palpation of the parametria to assess resectability (Fig. 19.11).
- Mobilisation of the bladder confirms that disease has not penetrated anteriorly through the cervix and that an adequate parametrial and vaginal resection should be possible.

Bladder dissection is accomplished by sharp dissection. Indications to abandon the procedure are unresectable parametrial disease, inability to sufficiently mobilise the bladder and gross para-aortic nodal disease. Involved pelvic nodes are not an absolute contraindication to the procedure if they can

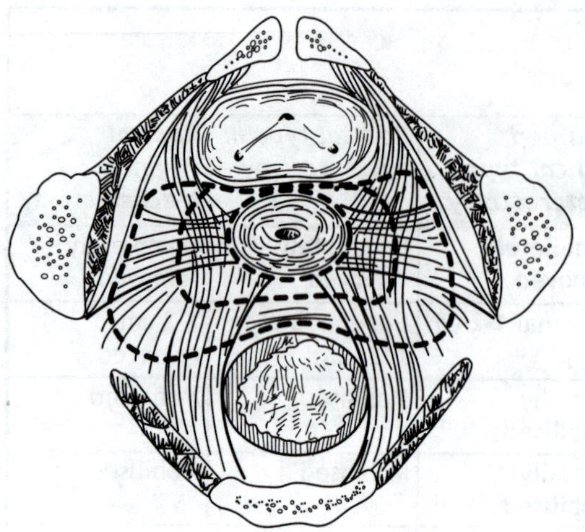

FIGURE 19.10: SURGICAL PROCEDURE IN EARLY CERVICAL CANCER, TYPES II AND III

be completely resected. The intraperitoneal cytology is of limited value. Hence, it should not be performed routinely (Estape et al 1998). Ureteric dissection is done by deroofing the ureter for resection of the entire parametrial tissue (Fig. 19.12). The uterine artery is divided at its origin from the anterior division of the internal iliac artery to allow the parametrium to be completely dissected (Fig. 19.13). In posterior dissection, the rectovaginal space is developed which allows development of and resection of uterosacral ligaments and the upper third of the vagina (Fig. 19.14). Currently, peritoneal closure is not performed. Pelvic drains are also not required if pelvic peritoneum is not closed. However, they are necessary in some patients to assess postoperative blood loss (Franchi et al 1997). Since ovarian metastasis occurred more frequently among patients with adenocarcinoma than among those with squamous cell carcinoma (5.31% vs. 0.79%) (Shimada et al 2006), it is recommended that the ovaries be preserved and transposed

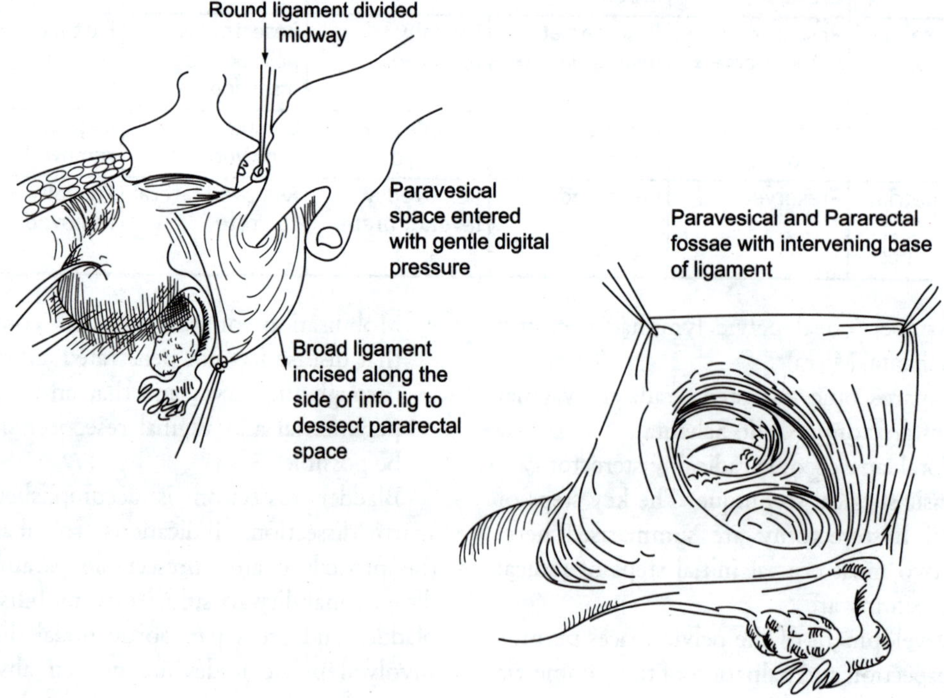

FIGURE 19.11: PELVIC SPACES

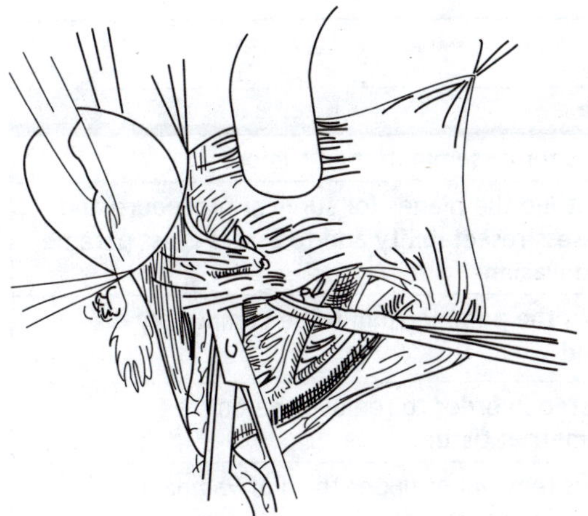

Figure 19.12: Deroofing the ureter

in Stage IB and IIA patients with squamous cell carcinoma, but removed in all patients with adenocarcinoma. The technical steps for performing radical hysterectomy is summarised in Table 19.12.

Systematic pelvic lymphadenectomy: All visible nodal tissue is removed from the mid-portion of the common iliac artery down to the distal portion of the external iliac artery, where the deep circumflex iliac vein crosses the external iliac artery, which includes complete skeletonisation of all blood vessels. Laterally, the resection extends from the mid-portion of the psoas muscle to the ureter medially. The lymph nodes removed were the external and internal iliac, obturator and common iliac group on both sides (Fig. 19.15). The five-year overall survival of patients with stage IA and IB1 cervical carcinoma approaches 90%–95% with radical abdominal hysterectomy (RAH) (Benedet et al 2001).

Landmarks for radical abdominal hysterectomy

1. Removal of uterus, cervix and upper third of vagina with contiguous parametrium and paravaginal tissue
2. Development of paravesical and pararectal spaces
3. Division of the uterine artery at its origin

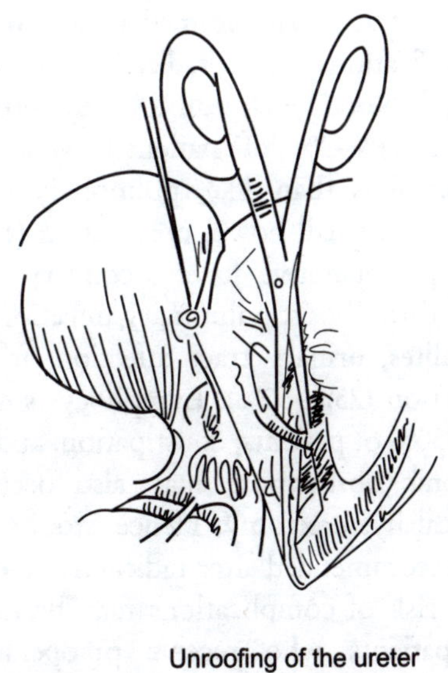

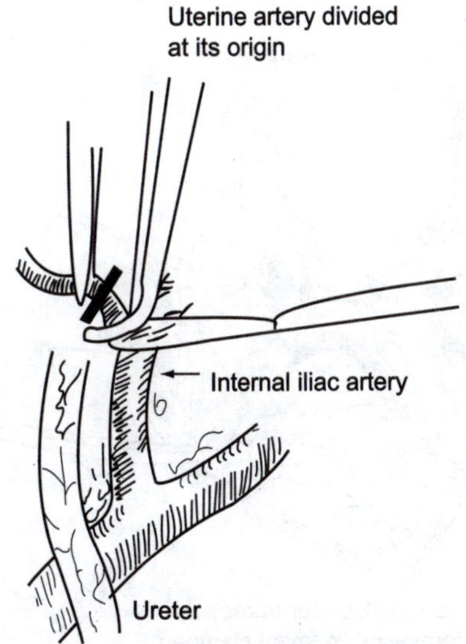

Figure 19.13: Uterine artery ligation at origin

Table 19.12: Technical steps for performing radical hysterectomy	
Step	***Comment***
Exploration of abdomen	Assess for dissemination of tumour
Development of pelvic spaces	To outline the planes for surgical procedure and to assess resectability and to assess gross parametrial invasion
Division of the uterine artery at its origin from internal iliac artery	Allows the parametrium to be completely dissected
Mobilisation of bladder and ureteric dissection	Key step in order to remove the entire parametrial tissue
Posterior dissection in rectovaginal space	Allows removal of upper third of vagina and uterosacral ligaments
Pelvic lymphadenectomy	All pelvic nodes are removed
Specimen removal and closure	En bloc removal of specimen with 2 cm clear margin

from the internal iliac artery

4. Ureteric dissection: Deroofing of the ureter to its entry into the cardinal ligament
5. Posterior dissection on cul de sac to develop rectovaginal space

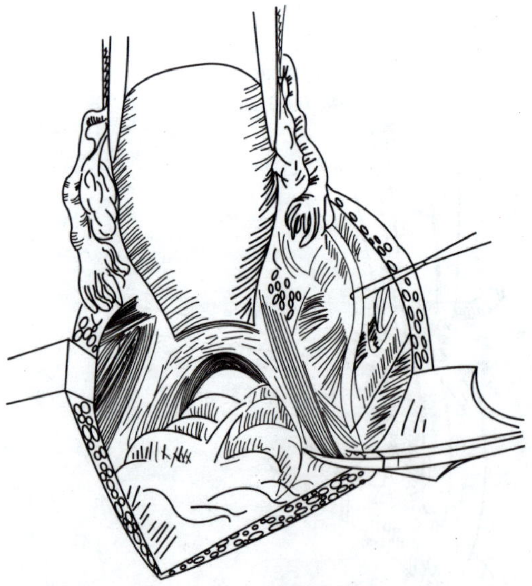
Cul-de-sac opened, ureter retracted laterally, uterosacral ligament clamped

Figure 19.14: Post dissection

6. Resection of uterosacral ligament near its sacral attachment

Complications of radical hysterectomy and pelvic node dissection: The need to dissect widely the ureters and the bladder gives rise to most of the common complications. Intraoperative and immediate postoperative complications of radical hysterectomy include blood loss (mean 0.8 l), ureterovaginal fistula (1%–2% of patients), vesicovaginal fistula (less than 1%), pulmonary embolus (1%–2%), small bowel obstruction (1%–2%), and postoperative fever secondary to deep vein thrombosis, pulmonary infection, pelvic cellulites, urinary tract infection or wound infection (25%–50%). Lymphocysts occur in 1%–30% of patients; constipation, and rarely, chronic obstipation, may also occur after radical hysterectomy. Hence, stool softeners are recommended after radical hysterectomy. The risk of complications may be increased in patients who receive preoperative or postoperative irradiation. The list of potential complications due to extensive and complex surgery is enumerated in Table 19.13.

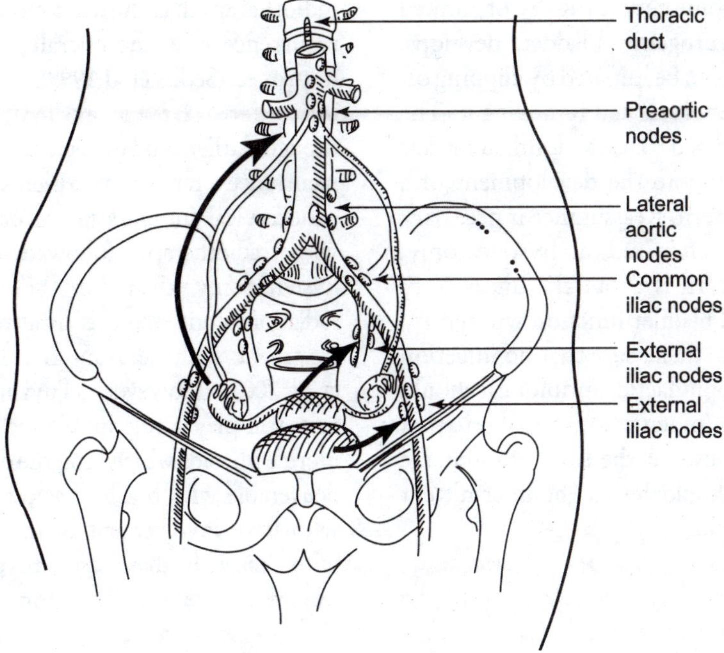

FIGURE 19.15: LYMPH NODES

During ureteric tunnel dissection, troublesome hemorrhage can occur. One of the most dangerous places in the pelvis is bifurcation of the common iliac artery and vein. This is called the axilla of the pelvis where severe life-threatening hemorrhage can occur due to laceration of the internal iliac vein and its branches. This area deserves its reputation as the corona mortis of the pelvis or 'suicide corner'. Another major complication following radical hysterectomy is post-operative bladder dysfunction. It manifests as difficulty in initiating micturition and in fully emptying the bladder. This is due to sympathetic nerve damage during radical hysterectomy resulting in parasympathetic dominance which leads to an increase in resting bladder pressure. Catheterisation is essential for only 6–8 days postoperatively. If the residual urine volume is greater than 150 ml, then another period of 48 hours of catheterisation should be instituted. The use

TABLE 19.13: COMPLICATIONS OF RADICAL HYSTERECTOMY

Intraoperative	*Postoperative*	*Long term*
Hemorrhage and vascular trauma Ureteric and bladder trauma Bowel trauma Nerve trauma	Ileus Infection Thromboembolic disease Lymphocyst Vascular, ureteric, bladder and bowel fistulas Acute rectal dysfunction	Lymphocyst and leg edema Bladder dysfunction Ureteric and bladder fistulas Chronic rectal dysfunction

of parasympathomimetic drugs is of limited value. If a neurogenic bladder develops, bladder training can be initiated by clipping off the catheter at intervals and removing it. The patient is encouraged to use abdominal muscle assistance to promote the development of a new voiding pattern. Reassurance is necessary for all patients after radical hysterectomy. The major concern is about the uncertainty of when normal bladder function will return. It is important to make sure that no infection occurs and prophylactic antibiotics should always be used. Women who are unable to pass urine spontaneously at the time of discharge from hospital should be taught intermittent self-catheterisation.

Radiotherapy after radical hysterectomy: Radical hysterectomy will frequently be sufficient therapy for early-stage cervical cancer, but a number of risk factors have been identified by pathological assessment of the radical hysterectomy specimen that can predict which patients are at increased risk of local recurrence. Indication for adjuvant therapy is summarised in Table 19.14. The existing evidence suggests that concurrent chemotherapy is beneficial in high-risk patients following hysterectomy (Peters 2000). Even though the addition of adjuvant radiotherapy has shown a reduction of pelvic recurrence rate, the overall survival has not improved (Sedlis et al 1999).

Table 19.14: Risk factors for pelvic recurrence in cervical cancer

High-risk factors—absolute indication for adjuvant therapy

- Multiple positive lymph nodes
- Parametrial involvement
- Positive surgical margins

Intermediate-risk factors—indication for adjuvant therapy when more than one factor present

- Lymphovascular space invasion
- Deep stromal invasion
- Tumour size >4 cm

Irradiation followed by hysterectomy: Even though earlier studies reported a lower pelvic recurrence rate for patients with bulky endocervical tumours (6 cm or larger) treated with radiotherapy followed by extrafascial hysterectomy than for those treated with radiation alone, there is little role for routine treatment with adjuvant hysterectomy (Keys et al 2003). However, adjuvant hysterectomy may still play a role in selected cases in which uterine fibroids which limit the dose of radiation deliverable with brachytherapy and in patients who have involvement of the uterine fundus with cancer. In these cases, a type I extrafascial hysterectomy is usually performed.

Chemotherapy followed by radical surgery: There are theoretical advantages to administering neoadjuvant chemotherapy (NACT) or 'upfront' chemotherapy or induction chemotherapy. It may be more effective if given before tumour blood flow is disturbed by surgery or radiation therapy. It may be less toxic when given before the bone marrow is affected by radiation therapy. Chemo debulking could improve the effectiveness of local radiotherapy or could facilitate tumour resection. Moreover, larger tumours at risk for harboring subclinical metastases, may be eradicated earlier, while the secretion of antiangiogenic factors by the primary tumour might be in circulation and neoadjuvant chemotherapy may more effectively address this risk for distant failure. The use of NACT may also decrease the risk of intraoperative dissemination of tumour cells. The use of neoadjuvant chemotherapy prior to surgery for bulky stage IB2 and IIB tumours is currently being evaluated with cisplatin and bleomycin.

INVASIVE CANCER FOUND INCIDENTALLY AFTER SIMPLE HYSTERECTOMY: Patients who undergo simple hysterectomy for presumed benign disease and are found to have invasive cervical cancer (greater than stage IAI) are considered candidates for postoperative radiation therapy. Surgical therapy in the form of radical parametrectomy, upper vaginectomy and lymphadenectomy can also be offered.

Routine post-treatment surveillance for asymptomatic patients: There is no universally accepted follow-up surveillance for asymptomatic patients. Routine follow-up should include a detailed history, general and pelvic examination. At rectovaginal examination, it is important to distinguish between radiotherapy-induced smooth and firm parametrial changes and recurrence that usually has a nodular growth pattern. Biopsy is indicated when there is suspicion of recurrence. Even though vaginal vault cytology has been used for patients who were treated with radical surgery without radiotherapy, recently, the cytology has been shown to be of limited value in the identification of recurrent disease in asymptomatic patients (Duyn et al 2002). On the other hand, patients who have isolated pulmonary metastasis identified on chest x-ray have several treatment options and longer survival prognosis than patients with recurrences at other locations. Hence, chest x-ray is of great value. The typical post-treatment surveillance of patients of cervical cancer is shown in Table 19.15.

NEW DEVELOPMENTS IN THE MANAGEMENT OF CERVICAL CANCER

Radical trachelectomy: A fertility sparing surgery for cervical cancer: Increasingly, younger women (24–35 years) are diagnosed with cervical cancers who are interested in fertility preservation. Till recently, the standard treatment of early-stage cervical cancer was either abdominal radical hysterectomy or radiotherapy, both of which would deprive them of an opportunity of having babies. The radical trachelectomy is a new technique developed to preserve the reproductive function. This technique involves a laparoscopic pelvic lymphadenectomy followed by vaginal resection of a portion of the cervix, parametrium and upper one-third of the vagina, leaving the upper cervix and uterine corpus to allow for pregnancy. At the time of closure, a permanent prophylactic cerclage is placed for prevention of premature delivery following this procedure (Fig. 19.16) (Shepherd et al 2006; Hertel et al 2006).

Dargent from France first performed this procedure (1994). Many surgeons have reported their oncological and obstetrical experience since then. An abdominal approach for radical trachelectomy was also reported (Ungar et al 2005). The following

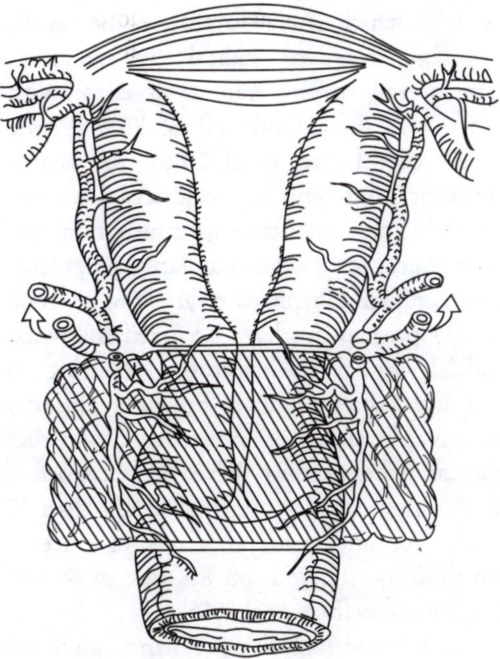

FIGURE 19.16: RADICAL TRACHELECTOMY

strict selection criteria are used to obtain optimal results.

1. Desire to preserve fertility
2. No clinical evidence of impaired fertility (relative contraindication)
3. FIGO stage IA1 with presence of vascular space invasion, IA2 and IB1
4. Lesion size less than 2.0 cm
5. Limited involvement of the upper endocervical canal determined by colposcopy or MRI
6. No evidence of pelvic node metastasis
7. Squamous-cell carcinoma or adenocarcinoma histologic subtypes

Outcome: Radical trachelectomy fulfils the needs of radicality along with the possibility of preserving childbearing capacity. Five hundred and thirty two cases of radical trachelectomy have been reported among seven centers worldwide till date. The cumulative data confirms an excellent oncological outcome with a recurrence rate of 4.3% and death rate of 1.5% which is comparable to the results following standard radical hysterectomy. The overall survival rate is excellent with a five-year disease survival of 95% (Plante et al 2004; Hertel et al 2006). As regards obstetrical outcome, the majority of women can anticipate spontaneous conception and deliver near term. The cumulative pregnancy rate is 52.8% (Shepherd et al 2006). A total of 211 pregnancies have occurred following radical vaginal trachelectomy resulting in 131 live babies till date. Frequent episodes of complications of pregnancy following radical trachelectomy have been reported. In 21 cases, delivery occurred in less than 32 weeks accounting for 16% risk of extreme prematurity. There is an 8% risk of second trimester loss (Boss et al 2005).

Established high-risk pregnancy units are required to manage pregnancies following radical trachelectomy. Successful pregnancies must be delivered by a classical cesarean section. Adequate neonatal intensive care must be available to take care of what will almost invariably be a premature baby after radical trachelectomy. There is a need for appropriate training to perform this procedure.

Table 19.15: Cervical cancer posttreatment surveillance

Post cone biopsy
- Pap and ECC every 3-4 months for 2 years
- Pap every 6 months for 3 years
- Annual thereafter

Post TAH or TVH
- Pap every 6 months for 2 years
- Annual thereafter

Post radical surgery or radiation therapy

First year
- Exam every three months, Pap and chest x-ray annually

Second year
- Exam every three months, chest x-ray biannually, Pap annually

Third and fourth year
- Exam every six months, chest x-ray biannually, Pap annually

Fifth year
- Exam every six months, chest x-ray and Pap annually

Nerve sparing radical hysterectomy:

The most common complication of radical hysterectomy is functional impairment of the bladder and anorectum resulting from damage to the autonomic nerve bundles. Various techniques have been described for preserving the autonomic nerve systematically without sacrificing the radicality of the radical hysterectomy procedure to preserve urinary function (Kuwabara et al 2000; Sakuragi et al 2005). It needs to be noted that the length of the vaginal cuff and the length of resected rectovaginal ligament correlated with bladder function and not the lateral parametrial resection (Zullo et al 2003; Benedetti-Panici et al 2004). Although attempts to spare the autonomic nerve fibres thus appear feasible and safe, it is limited to small volume disease without compromising radicality.

Role of sentinel node biopsy in the management of cervical cancer: The lymphatic spread of epithelial malignancies starts with the involvement of a first regional lymph node called the sentinel lymph node which drains a primary tumour. The sentinel lymph node would, therefore, reflect the pathological status of the remaining lymph nodes in the lymphatic basin (Ramirez and Levenback 2001). The aim of the sentinel node biopsy is to avoid systematic lymph node dissection in a patient who is lymph node-negative. The obturator lymph nodes were the most frequently involved, with a rate of 19% and it is proposed as sentinel nodes for cervical cancers. Although sentinel node biopsy is promising, it remains investigational at present.

SUMMARY

- Screening methods and recommendations are different for developed and developing countries.
- Pap smear is still the gold standard for screening and diagnosis of cervical cancer.
- Colposcopic evaluation is required in women with abnormal Pap smear for further management.
- Accurate staging of cervical cancer is critical in planning appropriate treatment.
- Staging for cervical cancer is based on clinical examination (FIGO).
- Surgery and chemoradiation are equally effective for early-stage disease.
- Microinvasive cancers can be managed with conservative surgery (conisation or extrafascial hysterectomy).
- Radical abdominal hysterectomy with bilateral pelvic lymphadenectomy is the standard surgical procedure in early stage cervical cancer.
- Addition of concurrent cisplatin-containing chemotherapy to radiotherapy for patients whose cancers have a high risk of locoregional recurrence is promising.
- Radical trachelectomy is promising fertility sparing surgery for very few selected cases of early cervical cancers.

REFERENCES

Albores-Saavedra J, D Gersell, CB Gilks et al. 1997. Terminology of endocrine tumours of the uterine cervix: Results of a workshop sponsored by the College of American Pathologists and the National Cancer Institute. *Arch Pathol Lab Med* 121:34–39.

American College of Obstetricians and Gynecologists Practice Bulletin. 2003. Clinical management guidelines for obstetrician gynecologists, no. 45, Cervical cytology screening. *Obstet Gynecol* 102: 417–427.

American College of Obstetricians and Gynecologists Practice Bulletin. 2005 Clinical management guidelines for obstetrician-gynecologists, no. 61. Human papillomavirus. *Obstet Gynecol* 105:905–918.

Amit A, D Beck, L Lowenstein, O Lavie, RB Shalom, Z Kedar, O Israel. 2006. The role of hybrid PET/CT in the evaluation of patients with cervical cancer. *Gynecol Oncol* 100:65–69.

Andersen W, H Frierson, S Barber et al. 1988. Sensitivity and specificity of endocervical curettage and the endocervical brush for the evaluation of the endocervical canal. *Am J Obstet Gynecol* 159:702–707.

Benedet JL, H Bender, H Jones III, HYS Ngan, S Pecorelli. 2000. FIGO Staging classifications and clinical practice guidelines in the management of gynecologic cancers. *Int J Obstet Gynecol* 170:209–262 (www.figo.org/content/PDF/staging-boklet.pdf.)

Benedet JL, F Odicino, P Maisonneuve, U Beller, WT Creasman, AP Heintz et al. 2001. Carcinoma of the cervix uteri. *J Epidemiol Biostat* 6:7–43.

Benedetti-Panici P, MA Zullo, F Plotti et al. 2004. Long-term bladder function in patients with locally advanced cervical carcinoma treated with neoadjuvant chemotherapy and type 3–4 radical hysterectomy. *Cancer* 100:2110–2117.

Bipat S, AS Glas, J van der Velden et al. 2003. Computed tomography and magnetic resonance imaging in staging of uterine cervical carcinoma: A systematic review. *Gynecol Oncol* 91:59–66.

Boss EA, RJT van Golde, CCM Beerendonk, LFAG Massuger. 2005. Pregnancy after radical trachelectomy: A real option? *Gynecol Oncol* 99: S152–S156

Chidanand MS, K Satyamoorthy, L Rai, AP Manjunath, VB Kartha. 2006. Optical diagnosis of cervical cancer by fluorescence spectroscopy technique. *Int J Cancer* 119:139–145.

Creasman WT, BF Fetter, DL Clarke-Pearson, L Kaufmann, RT Parker. 1985. Management of stage IA carcinoma of the cervix. *Am J Obstet Gynecol* 153:164-172.

Cronjé HS, GP Parham, BF Cooreman, A de Beer, P Divall, RH Bam. 2003. A comparison of four screening methods for cervical neoplasia in a developing country. *Am J Obstet Gynecol* 188:395–400.

Dargent D. 1994. La trachelectomie elargie (TE), une alternative a l'hysterectomieradicale dans le traitement des cancers infiltrants developpes sur la face externe du col uterin. *J Ob Gyn* 2:285–292.

Davy ML, TJ Dodd, CG Luke, DM Roder. 2003. Cervical cancer: Effect of glandular cell type on prognosis, treatment and survival. *Obstet Gynecol* 101: 38–45.

Davey E, A Barratt, L Irwig, et al. 2006. Effect of study design and quality on unsatisfactory rates, cytology classifications, and accuracy in liquid based versus conventional cervical cytology: A systematic review. *Lancet* 367: 122–132.

De Souza NM, R Dina, G Angus McIndoe, WP Soutter. 2006. Cervical cancer: Value of an endovaginal coil magnetic resonance imaging technique in detecting small volume disease and assessing parametrial extension *Gynecologic Oncology* 102:80–85.

Duyn A, M Van Eijkeren, G Kenter, K Zwinderman, A Ansink. 2002. Recurrent cervical cancer: Detection and prognosis. *Acta Obstet Gynecol Scand* 81:759–763.

Estape R, R Angioli, F Wagman et al. 1998. Significance of intraperitoneal cytology in patients undergoing radical hysterectomy. *Gynecol Oncol.* 68:169–171.

Fahey MT, L Irwig, P Macaskill. 1995. Meta-analysis of Pap test accuracy. *Am J Epidemiol* 141: 680–689.

Franchi M, F Ghezzi, F Zanaboni, et al. 1997. Nonclosure of peritoneum at radical abdominal hysterectomy and pelvic node dissection: A randomized study. *Obstet Gynecol* 90:622–627.

Goldie SJ, L Kuhn, L Denny et al. 2001 Policy analysis of cervical cancer screening strategies in low resource settings: Clinical benefits and cost-effectiveness. *JAMA* 285: 3107–3115.

Green J, J Kirwan, J Tierney et al. 2005. Concomitant chemotherapy and radiation therapy for cancer of the uterine cervix. *Cochrane Database Syst Rev*

Greenlee RT, T Murray, S Bolden et al. 2000. Cancer statistics. *CA Cancer J Clin* 2000 50:7–33.

Grigsby PW, BA Siegel, F Dehdashti. 2001. Lymph node staging by positron emission tomography in patients with carcinoma of the cervix. *J Clin Oncol* 19:3745.

Hamberger AD, GH Fletcher, JT Wharton. 1978. Results of treatment of early stage 1 carcinoma of the uterine cervix with intracavitary radium alone. *Cancer* 41:980–985.

Hertel H, C Kohler, G Grund, P Hilemanns, M Passover, W Michels and A Schneider. 2006. A. Radical vaginal trachelectomy (RVT) combined with laparoscopic pelvic lymphadenectomy: Prospective multicenter study of 100 patients with early cervical cancer. *Gynecol Oncol* 103:506–511.

Keys HM, BN Bundy, FB Stehman, et al. 2003. Radiation therapy with and without extrafascial hysterectomy for bulky stage IB cervical carcinoma: A randomized trial of the Gynecologic Oncology Group. *Gynecol Oncol* 89:343–253.

Kuwabara Y, M Suzuki, M Hashimoto, Y Furugen, K Yoshida, N Mitsuhashi. 2000. New method to prevent bladder dysfunction after radical hysterectomy for uterine cervical cancer. *J Obstet Gynaecol Res* 26:1–8.

Landoni F, A Maneo, A Colombo et al. 1997. Randomized study of radical surgery versus radiotherapy for stage 1b-lla cervical cancer. *Lancet* 350: 535–540.

Nanda K, DC McCrory, ER Myers et al. 2000. Accuracy of the Papanicolaou test in screening for and follow-up of cervical cytologic abnormalities: a systematic review. *Ann Intern Med* 132:810–819.

Narayan K. 2005. Arguments for a magnetic resonance imaging–assisted FIGO staging system for cervical cancer. *Int J Gynecol Cancer* 15:573–582.

Papanicolaou GN and HF Traut. 1941. The diagnostic value of vaginal smears in carcinoma of the uterus. *Am J Obstet Gynecol* 42:193–206.

Parker MF. 2005. Emerging technology in cervical cancer screening: Spectroscopy. *Clin Obstet Gynecol* 48:209–217.

Parkin DM. 2001. Global cancer statistics in the year 2000. *Lancet Oncol* 2: 533–543.

Peppercorn PD, AR Jeyarajah, R Woolas, JH Shepherd, DH Oram, IJ Jacobs et al. 1999. Role of MR imaging in the selection of patients with early cervical carcinoma forfertility-preserving surgery: Initial experience. *Radiology* 212:395–399.

Piver MS, F Rutledge, JP Smith. 1974. Five classes of extended hysterectomy for women with cervical cancer. *Obstet Gynecol* 44:265–272.

Plante M, MC Renaud, F Harel, M Roy. 2004. Vaginal radical trachelectomy: An oncologically safe fertility-preserving surgery. An updated series of 72 cases and review of the literature. *Gynecol Oncol* 94:614–623.

Ramanujam N, MF Mitchell, A Mahadevan et al. 1994. In vivo diagnosis of cervical intraepithelial neoplasia using 337-nm-excited laser-induced fluorescence. *Proc Natl Acad Sci USA* 91:10193–10197.

Ramanujam N, MF Mitchell, A Mahadevan-Jansen et al. 1996. Cervical precancer detection using a multivariate statistical algorithm based on laser-induced fluorescence spectra at multiple excitation wavelengths. *Photochem Photobiol* 64:720–735.

Ramirez PT and C Levenback. 2001. Sentinel nodes in gynecologic malignancies. *Curr Opin Oncol* 13:403–407.

Renju R and L Rai. 2005. Role of magnetic resonance imaging in carcinoma of the cervix uteri. MS (OBG) diss, Manipal Academy of Higher Education, Manipal.

Rose PG, LP Adler, M Rodriguez et al. 1999. Positron emission tomography for evaluating para-aortic nodal metastasis in locally advanced cervical cancer before surgical staging: A surgicopathological study. *J Clin Oncol* 17:41–45.

Sakuragi N, Y Todo, M Kudo, R Yamamoto, T Sato. 2005 A systematic nerve-sparing radical hysterectomy technique in invasive cervical cancer for preserving postsurgical bladder function. *Int J Gynecol Cancer*15:389–397.

Sankaranarayanan R, R Wesley, Thara S, Dhakad N, Chandralekha B, Sebastian P et al. 2003. Test characteristics of visual inspection with 4% acetic acid (VIA) and Lugol's iodine (VILI) in cervical cancer screening in Kerala, India. *Int J Cancer* 105:404–408.

Sankaranarayanan R, P Basu, R Wesley, C Mahé, N Keita, CC Gombe Mbalwa et al. 2004. Accuracy of visual screening for cervical neoplasia: Results from an IARC multicentre study in India and Africa. *Int J Cancer* 110:907–913.

Sankaranarayanan R, R Chatterji, S Shastri, R Wesley, P Basu, C Mahé et al. 2004. Accuracy of human papillomavirus testing in the primary screening of cervical neoplasia: Results from a multicentre study in India. *Int J Cancer* 112:341–247.

Sankaranarayanan R, SS Shastri, P Basu, C Mahé, R Mandal, G Amin et al. 2004. The role of low-level magnification in visual inspection with acetic acid for the early detection of cervical neoplasia. *Cancer Detect Prev* 28:345–251.

Sedlis A, BN Bundy, MZ Rothman et al. 1999. A randomized trial of pelvic radiation therapy versus no further therapy in selected patients with stage lB carcinoma of the cervix after radical hysterectomy and pelvic lymphadenectomy: A Gynecologic Oncology Group study. *Gynecol Oncol* 73:177–183.

Shastri SS, K Dinshaw, G Amin et al. 2005. Concurrent evaluation of visual, cytological and HPV testing as screening methods for the early detection of cervical neoplasia in Mumbai, India. *Bull World Health Organ* 83:186–194.

Shepherd JH, C Spencer, J Herod, Ind TEJ. 2006. Radical vaginal trachelectomy as a fertility-sparing procedure in women with early-stage cervical cancer—cumulative pregnancy rate in a series of 123 women. *Br J Obstet Gynaecol* 113:719–724.

Shimada M, J Kigawa, R Nishimura et al. 2006. Ovarian metastasis in carcinoma of the uterine cervix. *Gynecol Oncol* 101:234–237.

Smith RA, V Cokkinides and HJ Eyre. 2006. American Cancer Society Guidelines for the Early Detection of Cancer. *CA Cancer J Clin* 56:11–25.

Steed H and A Covens. 2003. Radical vaginal trachelectomy and laparoscopic pelvic lymphadenectomy for preservation of fertility. *Postgrad Obstet Gynecol* 23:1–6.

Tavassoli FA and P Devilee (eds). 2003. *World Health Organization Classification of Tumours: Pathology and Genetics of Tumours of the Breast and Female Genital Organs*. Lyon: IARC Press.

Ungar L, L Palfalvi, R Hogg, P Siklos, DC Boyle, G Del Priore et al. 2005. Abdominal radical trachelectomy: A fertility-preserving option for women with early cervical cancer. *Br J Obstet Gynaecol* 112:366–369.

Ungar L and L Palfalvi. 2003. Surgical treatment of lymph node metastases in stage IB cervical cancer: The laterally extended parametrectomy (LEP) procedure. *Int J Gynecol Cancer* 13:647–651.

Webb JC, CR Key, CR Qualls, HO Smith. 2001. Population-based study of microinvasive adenocarcinoma of the uterine cervix. *Obstet Gynecol* 97:701–706.

WHO Meeting. 1986. Control of cancer of the cervix uteri. *Bull World Health Org* 64:607–618.

Zullo MA, N Manci, R Angioli et al. 2003. Vesical dysfunction after radical hysterectomy for cervical cancer: A critical review. *Crit Rev Oncol Hematol* 48:287–293.

20

Carcinoma of the Endometrium

GRV Prasad

Endometrial cancer is often considered as gynecological cancer with favourable prognosis. The assumption is because of early presentation with postmenopausal bleeding leading to diagnosis in early stage of disease. Stage for stage, endometrial cancer is as lethal as cervical and ovarian cancer. It is mainly a disease of postmenopausal woman, though 25% of cases occur in premenopausal women and 5% occur in those younger than 40 years. African-American women have 40% lower risk of developing endometrial cancer but nearly 54% greater risk of dying of the disease, mainly because of delayed diagnosis (Madiason et al 2000).

Epidemiology: Most of the risk factors identified relate to prolonged unopposed estrogen stimulation. Infertility, nulliparity, anovulatory cycles increase the risk of endometrial cancer. Menopause occurring beyond age 52 increases the risk for endometrial cancer 2.4 times. The risk of endometrial cancer is increased with excess weight and the risk is nearly 10 times in those more than 50 pounds overweight, because of increased peripheral conversion of androstenedione to estrone.

Diagnosis: Endometrial cancer occurs in the sixth and seventh decades of life. Patients usually present with postmenopausal bleeding and/or discharge. Pain is usually a late symptom, either because of endocervical spread leading to pyometra or because of advanced disease with neural involvement. Hematuria and bleeding per rectum may indicate local spread to bladder and rectum, respectively. The standard method of approach in all such patients for diagnosing endometrial cancer is by performing formal fractional curettage. It should be remembered that a substantial number of these patients have additional medical problems like hypertension and diabetes and it is therefore preferable that these procedures are performed under general anesthesia. Also, proper fractional curettage ensures representative specimens from all the walls of the uterus, especially if the procedure is unaided by prior hysteroscopic evaluation to avoid false-negative pathologic report. Endocervical specimen should be collected before an endometrial specimen, though the current FIGO staging depends on final surgico-pathologic evaluation of hysterectomy specimen for staging purposes to document endocervical involvement.

Transvaginal ultrasound can be used as a useful adjunct in evaluating women with abnormal uterine bleeding, especially in the postmenopausal group. Endometrial thickness, greater than 4 mm, endometrial polyp and collection of fluid in the endometrial cavity mandate additional evaluation in the form of fractional curettage or hysteroscopy. However, it is not clear at present whether ultrasound findings can be used to safely eliminate the need for further evaluation in a woman who is symptomatic.

CT scan and MRI may be required in cases with abdominal mass, palpable extrauterine pelvic disease and clinical ascites. However, CT scan may not be of much use in the assessment of myometrial extension and the presence of nodal disease (Conor et al 2000; Zerbe et al 2000). MRI was evaluated for its efficacy as a tool for preoperative staging of disease by a National Cancer Institute cooperative study with 88 patients from five participating hospitals (Hricak et al 1991). For evaluating the depth of myometrial invasion the accuracy was 66% and for detection of paraaortic nodes 8%. Hence at present, MRI does not appear to be a cost-effective method to stage the disease preoperatively

Surgical staging for endometrial cancer (FIGO 1988)

Stage IA G123 Tumour limited to endometrium

Stage IB G123 Invasion to less than half of myometrium

Stage IC G123 Invasion to more than half of myometrium

Stage IIA G123 Extension to endocervical glands only

Stage IIB G123 Cervical stromal invasion

Stage IIIA G123 Tumour invasion to serosa and/or adnexa and/or positive peritoneal cytology

Stage IIIB G123 Presence of vaginal metastases

Stage IIIC G123 Metastases to pelvic and/or paraaortic lymph nodes

Stage IVA G123 Tumour invasion to bladder and rectal mucosa

Stage IVB G123 Distant metastases including intraabdominal and/or inguinal lymph nodes

Histopathology: Degree of Differentiation

Cases of carcinoma of the corpus should be classified (or graded) according to the degree of histologic differentiation:

G1 – 5% or less of a non-squamous or non-morular solid growth pattern

G2 – 6% to 50% of a non-squamous or non-morular solid growth pattern

G3 – More than 50% of non-squamous or non-morular solid growth pattern

Notes on Pathological Grading

1. Notable nuclear atypia, inappropriate for the architectural grade, raises the grade of a grade 1 or grade 2 tumour by 1.
2. In serous, clear cell and squamous cell carcinomas nuclear grading takes precedence.
3. Adenocarcinomas with squamous differentiation are graded according to nuclear grade of the glandular component.

Rules Related to Staging:

- Because the corpus cancer is now staged surgically, procedures previously used for determination of stages are no longer applicable, such as findings from fractional dilatation and curettage to differentiate stages I and II
- There may be a small number of patients with corpus cancer who will be treated primarily with radiation therapy. In that case, the clinical staging adopted by FIGO in 1971 would still apply, but designation of that staging system should be noted.
- Ideally, the width of the myometrium should be measured along with width of tumour invasion

Pathology: There can be several histological variants of endometrial carcinoma

Endometrioid adenocarcinoma
Variants—villoglandular, secretory, with squamous differentiation

Mucinous carcinoma
Papillary serous carcinoma
Clear cell carcinoma
Squamous carcinoma
Undifferentiated carcinoma
Mixed carcinoma

Endometrial cancer spreads through

- Direct extension into adjacent structures
- Lymphatic spread
- Hematogenous spread
- Exfoliation and trans-tubal spread

The spread to the cervix can be both by contiguous and lymphatic spread. In spite of direct lymphatic connections of fundus to paraaortic nodes through the infundibulo-pelvic ligament, it is rare to find paraaortic node metastases in the absence of pelvic node metastases. The vaginal metastases also appear to be because of lymphovascular spread rather than because of contiguous spread as they commonly occur in the absence of cervical involvement (Mackillop and Pringle 1985).

Prognostic factors: The various prognostic variables that may affect the outcome in endometrial cancer are classified as follows.

Gynecologic Oncology Group (GOG) tried to examine the concept of surgical staging by establishing prognostic factors in early stage endometrial cancer (Creasman et al 1987). In 621 cases it was found that 22% had extrauterine disease in the form of lymph node metastases, adnexal or intraperitoneal spread or positive peritoneal cytology. Univariate analysis showed uterine size and tumour differentiation as significant in predicting pelvic and paraaortic nodal disease. In multivariate analysis tumour grade, depth of myometrial invasion and intraperitoneal metastases were identified as independently significant for pelvic and paraaortic nodal metastases. The GOG could identify patients at high and low risk for nodal metastases using this data.

There was no pelvic lymph node disease when the tumour was well differentiated and there was no myometrial extension—this was considered a low risk group. Moderate or poorly differentiated tumours with superficial or middle third myometrial extension constituted the medium-risk group. There is 6% frequency of nodal metastases in this group. Those with intraperitoneal disease and/or deep myometrial disease constituted the high-risk group. Those with deep myoinvasion had an 18% risk of pelvic node metastases and those with intraperitoneal disease had a 33% risk. The incidence of pelvic lymph node involvement went up to 61% when both factors were present. In addition, paraaortic node involvement was 30% in this high-risk group.

The other important prognostic factors are

a. Histological type: In a retrospective study from Mayo clinic, out of 388 patients, 52 patients had an unusual histological subtype (20 adenosquamous, 14 serous papillary, 11 clear cell, 7 undifferentiated). In this study, the survival rate was 92% for endometrioid tumours and 33% for unusual histological types. As many as 62% of these patients with unfavourable histological types had extrauterine disease at the time of surgical staging (Wilson et al 1990). Papillary serous carcinomas have poor prognosis even in the absence of myometrial invasion with special predilection for intraabdominal metastases (Jeffrey et al 1986; Sherman et al 1992). Clear cell carcinomas tend to spread by the vascular route (Christopherson et al 1982).

Uterine factors	*Extrauterine factors*
Histological type Histological grading Myometrial invasion Cervical extension Vascular space invasion DNA ploidy	Adnexal disease Positive peritoneal cytology Intraperitoneal metastases Pelvic lymph node metastases Aortic node metastases Age

b. Histological grade and myometrial invasion: Increasing tumour grade and myometrial invasion are associated with increased frequency of pelvic and paraaortic lymph node metastases and therefore worse prognosis, as shown in the GOG study (Creasman et al 1987).
c. Cervical extension: If only the fundus is involved, 8% may have pelvic node metastases, whereas the risk doubles if isthumus and cervix is involved. The incidence of paraaortic node metastases is 4% with fundal lesions and 14% if the lower segment is involved (Creasman et al 1987).
d. Vascular space invasion: Abeler from the Norwegian Radium Hospital reported 5-year survival of 83.5% for patients without vascular space invasion compared with 64.5% for those with vascular space invasion (Abeler et al 1992). The frequency of vascular space invasion increases with increasing degree of myometrial invasion. Hanson reported vascular space invasion of 5% of the inner third of the myometrium compared with 70% for the outer third of the myometrium (Hanson et al 1985).
e. Peritoneal cytology: Significance of peritoneal positive cytology is controversial. The GOG study by Morrow et al (1991) reported a recurrence rate of 29.1% in those with positive peritoneal cytology compared to 10.5% in those with negative peritoneal cytology. GOG estimated that the relative risk of death for patients with positive peritoneal cytology was 3. Takeshima et al (2001) concluded that positive peritoneal washings are not independent risk factors for prognosis and that in the absence of other adverse prognostic factors, did not need upstaging of disease status. It may be explained that in several such cases of positive peritoneal cytology it is because of 'contamination' from primary tumour, because of tumour handling rather than potential viable cell capable of independent growth at the site of their retrieval.
f. DNA Ploidy: Presence of aneuploid tumours indicate worse prognosis. GOG estimates that the relative risk of disease-

	Pelvic lymph nodes (%)	*Para-aortic lymph nodes (%)*
Low risk		
Grade 1: No myometrial invasion and no intra-peritoneal disease	0	0
Moderate risk		
Inner/middle myometrial invasion		
Grade 2/3 tumour: No intraperitoneal disease		
- Only one factor	1	2
- Both factors	6	2
High risk		
Deep myometrial invasion	18	15
Intraperitoneal disease	33	8
Both factors	61	30

related death is 4.1 with aneuploid tumours (Zaino et al 1998).

Management of Primary Endometrioid Adenocarcinoma

Preoperative assessment: Thorough pathological review should form part of the initial assessment. In case of any disagreements about dysplasias and well differentiated cancer, the slides and specimen may be referred to a gynecology-oncology pathologist. The tumour must be graded accurately, clearly distinguishing papillary serous from clear cell tumours. Many of these patients are elderly, obese and have other medical complications like hypertension, diabetes and obstructive and restrictive lung diseases; appropriate medical and anesthetic consultations should be taken and a reasonable preoperative fitness must be ensured. Epidural anesthesia, need for prophylactic heparin and need for postoperative intensive care should be considered. Preoperatively, surgical options such as route of surgery (abdominal/vaginal/laparoscopic), need and extent of lymph node dissection and operative risks involved in the same may be discussed with the patient and her family and consent taken for the same.

Surgical approach: A midline vertical incision gives adequate access in most cases. However, high transverse suprapubic incision or a Maylard incision may be judiciously used in certain patients to decrease the chances of morbidity in obese diabetics without compromising surgical goals, especially if paraaortic node dissection is omitted. Collection of peritoneal fluid for cytology followed by total hysterectomy, bilateral salpingo-oophorectomy along with sampling or excision of any obvious metastatic areas is the performed at the initial surgery. In papillary serous carcinomas and clear cell carcinomas, the surgery considered is the same as that for ovarian cancer along with lymphadenectomy and omentectomy.

Management of Lymph Nodes in Endometrioid Adenocarcinoma

The therapeutic benefit of pelvic lymphadenectomy in endometrial endometrioid cancer has not been established. Kilgore et al (1995) suggested a benefit of survival in patients with lymph node sampling compared with those with no sampling. But the decision to remove lymph nodes was determined by patient characteristics such as weight and age which themselves may determine prognosis. The pathologic information obtained at lymphadectomy is useful in deciding which patients might benefit by adjuvant therapy like radiotherapy. The need for lymphadenectomy is determined by evaluation of the pathological factors preoperatively (histology and grade) and at the time of preoperative surgery (cervical extension, myometrial invasion and intraperitoneal disease). Frozen section pathological examination may further confirm some of these factors.

However, it should be borne in mind that there may be discrepancies in the histological evaluation of the preoperative specimen and the postoperative hysterectomy specimen. Grade 1 histology on endometrial biopsy is upgraded on review of hysterectomy specimen in approximately 20% of cases—FIGO Stage IC lesion will be found in patients with Grade 1 lesions in 17% cases.

The recommendations for performing pelvic and paraaortic node dissection are

- Clear cell, serous and squamous carcinomas
- Grade 2, 3 endometrioid carcinoma

- Cervical and isthmic extension
- Myometrial invasion more than 50%
- Tumour size more than 2 cm
- Extrauterine disease

Tumour histology and depth of myometrial invasion are the most important determinants of lymph node metastases.

Postoperative adjuvant therapy

Treatment of Clinical Stage I: Decisions about postoperative follow-up and adjuvant therapy are based on prognostic factors determined at surgicopathologic staging.

Observation: Those with Grade 1 and 2 lesions without myometrial invasion (Stage Ia, grade 1 and 2 lesions) do not require any postoperative therapy and need be kept under observational follow-up. In the PORTEC study (Postoperative Radiation Therapy in Endometrial Cancer), patients with intermediate risk (IC grade 1, all grade 2, IA and IB grade 3) were randomised to 46 Gy postoperative external beam radiotherapy (ERBT) or no radiotherapy (Creutzberg et al 2000). It was found that there was no difference in survival in the two groups, but those in the ERBT group had more locoregional recurrences (4% vs 14%). Equally good results in the observation group were explained by early detection of recurrences and effective treatment. Most of these recurrences were in the vault and were treated efficiently by further therapy. However, these results were not applicable to high-risk patients. The suggested postoperative therapy following surgical staging is as follows.

Treatment of Stage II: Involvement of cervix places the patient under worse prognosis because of the higher frequency of involvement of lymph nodes, as high as in a third of cases. However, it needs to be reemphasised that endocervical curettage has a relatively high false-positive (50%–80%) and false-negative rate for diagnosing endocervical involvement. Post-hysterectomy histological evaluation is the only definite proof. Preoperative MRI and hysteroscopy can diagnose cervical involvement better.

Radical hysterectomy with lymphadenectomy for Stage II patients allows accurate surgicopathologic evaluation besides being therapeutic with no further adjuvant therapy Patients for adjuvant therapy can be chosen based on surgicopathologic evaluation. However, given the incidence of false-positive cases, these may constitute overtreatment in certain cases. Besides, some of these patients who are elderly, obese and with medical complications may tolerate such extensive surgery poorly.

Another alternative—exploratory laparotomy with extrafascial hysterectomy and resection/sampling of any obvious extra-uterine—is increasingly finding favour, especially in the presence of poor reliability of preoperative diagnosis of cervical involvement. Depending on gross and/or frozen section, histology of cervical extension pelvic and/or aortic lymphadenectomy are done. Depending on final histological evaluation, patients are chosen for external pelvic or extended field radiotherapy and vaginal brachytherapy. Surveillance, epidemiology, and end results (SEER) in an analysis of 555 patients comparing the results of simple hysterectomy and radical hysterectomy in the treatment of Stage II endometrial cancer concluded that radical hysterectomy is associated with better survival (Cornelison et al 1999).

Treatment Of Stage III: The treatment of Stage III should be individualised. Surgical staging with abdominal hysterectomy (with bilateral oophorectomy) is the minimal initial goal whenever surgically and medically

Stage IA, Stage IB Grade 1,2	No further treatment
Stage IA, Stage IB, Grade 3 Stage IC any Grade 3	Vaginal cuff radiation
1 or 2 microscopically positive pelvic nodes	External pelvic radiotherapy
Positive nodes above level of common iliac nodes 3 or more microscopic nodes positive Grossly positive nodes	External field irradiation
Peritoneal metastases after complete resection	Whole abdomen irradiation

feasible. At the time of surgical exploration, every attempt must be made to resect any gross disease without undue morbidity. Postoperative whole abdomen irradiation may be appropriate in the presence of peritoneal metastases, especially if they are limited and if they are thoroughly resected to take care of diffuse micrometastases.

Regardless of how parametrial involvement is diagnosed preoperatively, external pelvic radiotherapy may be undertaken initially followed by surgical exploration later. Isolated vaginal metastases (Stage IIIB) are rare. Usually they are associated with peritoneal metastases (IIIC). Survival of those with vaginal metastases thus may not be different from those with IIIC.

Treatment Of Stage IV: The treatment of Stage IV needs to be tailored to the presentation of the disease. It often involves a combination of surgery, radiotherapy and chemotherapy to control spread and to provide relief from symptoms such as bleeding, discharge and pain. In some cases, preoperative progestin therapy may be given followed by hysterectomy and salpingo-oophorectomy. In selected patients with bladder and rectal involvement, extenteration may be offered.

Recurrent Endometrial Cancer

Nearly a fourth of patients treated for endometrial cancer have recurrent cancer. In a report from Norwegian Radium Hospital, local recurrence was found in 50% of patients, distant metastases in 29%, simultaneous local and distant metastases in 21%. Thirty four percent of all recurrences were within 1 year and 76% within 3 years of primary treatment (Aalders et al 1984). Isolated vaginal recurrences are amenable to therapeutic interventions in the form of cuff irradiation or surgical excision of bulky lesions followed by radiotherapy and show satisfactory salvage rates. However, vaginal recurrences require thorough investigation in the form of CT scan, CA125 and X-ray chest and fine needle aspiration cytology from suspicious areas to exclude pelvic, peritoneal and distant metastases.

Progestational agents and chemotherapy are reserved for advanced and distant disease often with palliative intent rather than curative intent.

References

Aalders J, V Abeler, P Kolstad. 1984. Recurrent adenocarcinoma of the endometrium: A clinical and histopathological study of 379 patients. *Gynecol Oncol* 17:85–103.

Abeler VM, KE Kjorstad, E Berle. 1992. Carcinoma of the endometrium in Norway: A histopathologic and prognostic survey of a total population. *Int J Gynecol Cancer* 2:9–22.

Christopherson WM, RG Alberhasky, PJ Connelly. 1982. Carcinoma of the endometrium: A clinicopathologic study of clear cell carcinoma and secretory carcinoma. *Cancer* 49:1511–1516.

Connor JP, JI Andrews, B Anderson, RE Buller. 2000. Computed tomography in endometrial carcinoma. *Obstet Gynecol* 95:692–696.

Cornelison TL, EL Trimble, CL Kosary. 1999. SEER data, corpus uteri cancer: Treatment trends versus survival for FIGO stage II, 1988–1994. *Gynecol Oncol* 74:350–355.

Creasman WT, CP Morrow, BN Bundy, HD Homesley, JF Graham, PB Heller. 1987. Surgical pathologic spread patterns of endometrial cancer. *Cancer* 60:2035–2041.

Creutzberg CL, WLJ van Putten, PCM Koper, MLM Lybeert, JJ Jobsen, CC Warlam-Rodenhuis et al. for the PORTEC Study Group. 2000. Surgery and postoperative radiotherapy versus surgery alone for patients with stage-1 endometrial carcinoma: Multicentre randomised trial - PORTEC study group post operative Radiation therapy in endometrial carcinoma *Lancet* 355:1404–1411.

Hanson MB, JR Van Nagell, DE Powell, ES Donaldson, H Gallion, M Merhige et al. 1985. The prognostic significance of lympho-vascular space invasion in stage I endometrial cancer. *Cancer* 55:1753–1757.

Hricak H, LV Rubinstein, GM Gherman, N Karstaedt. 1991. MR imaging evaluation of endometrial carcinoma: results of an NCI cooperative study. *Radiology* 179:829–34.

Jeffrey JF, GV Krepart, RJ Lotocki. 1986. Papillary serous adenocarcinoma of the endometrium. *Obstet Gynecol* 67:670–674.

Kilgore LC, EE Patridge, RD Alvarez, JM Austin, HM Shingleton, F Noojin III, et al. 1995. Adenocarcinoma of the endometrium: Survival comparisons of patients with and without pelvic node sampling. *Gynecol Oncol* 56:29–33

Mackillop WJ, JF Pringle. 1985. Stage III endometrial carcinoma: A review of 90 cases. *Cancer* 56:2519–2523.

Madison T, D Schottenfeld, V Baker. 1998. Cancer of corpus uteri in white and black women in Michigan, 1985–1994. *Cancer* 83:1546–1554.

Morrow CP, BN Bundy, RJ Kurman, WT Creasman, P Heller, HD Homesley et al. 1991. Relationship between surgico-pathologic risk factors and outcome in clinical stage I and II carcinoma of the endometrium: A Gynecologic Oncology Group study. *Gynecol Oncol* 40:55–65.

Sherman ME, P Bitterman, NB Rosenshein, G Delgado, RJ Kurman. 1992. Uterine serous carcinoma. *Am J Surg Path* 16:600–610.

Takeshima N, H Nishida, T Tabata, Y Hirai, K Hasumi. 2001. Positive peritoneal cytology in endometrial cancer: Enhancement of other prognostic factors. *Gynecol Oncol* 82:470–473.

Wilson TD, KC Podratz, TA Gaffey, GD Malkasian, PC O'Brien, JM Naessens. 1990. Evaluation of unfavourable histologic subtypes in endometrial adenocarcinoma . *Am J Obstet Gynecol* 162:418–426.

Zaino RJ, ATL Davis, BM Ohlsson-Wilhelm, VL Brunetto. 1998. DNA content is an independent prognostic indicator in endometrial adenocarcinoma. *Int J Gynecol Pathol* 17:312–319.

Zerbe MJ, R Bristow, FC Grumbine, FJ Montz. 2000. Inability of preoperative computed tomography scans to accurately detect the extent of myometrial invasion and extracorporeal spread in endometrial cancer. *Gynecol Oncol* 78:67–70.

21

Premalignant and Malignant Lesions of the Vulva

Poonam Goel | PK Saha

Premalignant Disorders of the vulva: There has been a marginal increase in the incidence and in the mortality rate from vulval cancer. The incidence has appreciably increased in the younger age group. The prognosis and conservation of vulval structures are best if this condition is diagnosed early, with a survival rate of over 90% in the absence of nodal involvement (Homesley et al 1991). It becomes imperative that the premalignant state be identified, treated and followed-up to prevent its progression to the stage of invasive cancer.

Vulval intraepithelial neoplasia (VIN), Paget's disease and melanoma in situ are important premalignant lesions. The malignant potential of lichen sclerosus, squamous hyperplasia and lichen planus is controversial. With the widespread use of the human papillomavirus vaccine, one half to two-thirds of vulval cancer can be prevented (Duong and Flowers 2007).

CLASSIFICATION

The International Society for the Study of Vulvar Disease (ISSVD) has recommended (Ridley et al 1989) a change in the terminology for vulval dystrophy and a re-classification as non-neoplastic epithelial disorders of skin and mucosa (Table 21.1). In 1966, Jeffcoate suggested that terms such as lichen sclerosus et atrophicus, sclerotic dermatosis, atrophic and hyperplastic vulvitis, leukoplakia and Kraurosis vulvae be clubbed under the umbrella of chronic vulval dystrophy as they denoted a common disease (Jeffcoate 1966). In 1986, the ISSVD came up with the term vulval intraepithelial neoplasia. Earlier in

Table 21.1: Classification of epithelial vulval diseases (ISSVD Classification)

Non-neoplastic epithelial disorders of the skin and mucosa
- Lichen sclerosis (Lichen sclerosis et atrophicus)
- Squamous hyperplasia (formerly hyperplastic dystrophy)
- Other dermatoses

Mixed non-neoplastic and neoplastic epithelial disorders

Intraepithelial neoplasia
- Squamous intraepithelial neoplasia
  - VIN 1
  - VIN 2
  - VIN 3 (severe dysplasia or carcinoma in situ)
- Non-squamous intraepithelial neoplasia
  - Paget's disease
  - Tumours of melanocytes, noninvasive

Invasive tumours

1976, ISSVD combined three nomenclatures—erythroplasia of Queyarat, Bowens disease and carcinoma in situ simplex into squamous cell carcinoma in situ as these three are variants of the same disease process (Ridley et al 1989).

In 2004, ISSVD eliminated VIN 1, as the diagnosis of this condition was not reproducible. They also combined VIN 2 and VIN 3 as it was difficult to reliably separate these two entities, so now the term VIN is applicable to histologically high grade squamous lesions only (Heller 2007). The current 2004 ISSVD disease terminology for VIN is given in table 21.2.

Lichen sclerosus (LS): This condition is mostly seen in postmenopausal women, but on rare occasions it may occur in younger women and in children. It is a chronic lymphocyte-mediated inflammatory dermatosis and has been linked to several autoimmune diseases, including Graves' disease and vitiligo (Thomas et al 1988), although infections, genetic and sex hormone factors have also been implicated in the causation. The most common symptom is pruritis but it can present with dyspareunia, dysuria and genital bleeding. The typical lesion is in the form of a well-defined white plaque with an atrophic wrinkled surface. However, they can progress to form large blisters, hemorrhagic bullous and ulcerative lesions. Prolonged disease can lead to labial shrinking, narrowing of the clitoral hood and introitus leading to dyspareunia. The classical histological features of uncomplicated LS include a thinned epidermis with hyperkeratosis, a wide band of homogenised collagen below the dermoepidermal junction and a lymphocytic infiltrate beneath the homogenised area. Some patients may have a thickened epidermis and these patients tend to have complicated disease that is not so responsive to treatment and may have a higher risk in the long term of developing an associated squamous cell carcinoma. Diagnosis is confirmed by biopsy. The first line of treatment is topical potent corticosteroids (Clobetasol propionate 0.05%), but not more than 30 gm is to be used in three months. Topical testosterone which was used earlier is not as effective as clobetasol but is more effective than an emollient. Cryotherapy, photodynamic and laser therapy have also been tried in resistant cases but with little success. Similarly, ciclosporin, retnoids, potassium para-amino benzoates and psoralen plus UV treatment has also been tried in resistant cases with mixed results. Recently, topical macrolide immunosuppressants such as pimecrolimus and tacrolimus, have been shown to be safe and effective treatment in a small series of patients (Assmann et al 2003). Another new promising treatment is focussed ultrasound therapy (Li et al 2004). Surgical intervention is indicated only for the complications of scarring or the development of malignancy.

TABLE 21.2: SQUAMOUS VULVAR INTRA-EPITHELIAL NEOPLASIA (VIN) CLASSIFICATION (ISSVD 2004)

I. VIN, usual type
   a) VIN, warty type
   b) VIN, basaloid type
   c) VIN, mixed (warty/basaloid) type
II. VIN, differentiated type
III. VIN, unclassified

Some reports have suggested that the lifetime risk of squamous cell carcinoma is about 4% (Wallace 1971). The role of HPV as an etiological agent in the progression to malignancy has not been clearly defined; however, 20% of cases of LS may carry the oncogenic HPV 16 (Kiene et al 1991). Women with this condition need lifelong follow-up, more so in patients who have difficulty in symptom control.

Lichen Planus

This is an inflammatory autoimmune disorder. This condition can present in different clinical pictures such as erosions, white plaques and hyperkeratotic and papulosquamous lesions. Common symptoms are pruritis, dyspareunia, burning and even destruction of the vulval architecture later. Treatment is by topical or systemic steroids. However, hydroxychloroquin, oral retenoid, methotrexate, tacrolimus and cyclophosphamide have also been tried. Their malignancy potential is uncertain.

Squamous Cell Hyperplasia

Squamous cell hyperplasia (SCH) is characterised by epidermal hyperplasia without inflammation, atypia or evidence of a specific dermatosis (Ridley et al 1989). It can occur alone or in association with LS. This being a premalignant condition is controversial, although some studies have shown genetic changes in SCH adjacent to invasive lesions; however, others have failed to show such changes (Lin et al 1998).

Vulval Intraepithelial Neoplasia (VIN)

VIN (usual type) is the one which is associated with high risk HPV subtype 16 and is often multifocal and progresses to invasive carcinoma. Differentiated type VIN is not associated with HPV but shows aneuploidy and genetic changes similar to that seen in invasive carcinoma. VIN is associated with underlying carcinoma 15% to 22% of the time (Thuis et al 2000). Of the usual type of VIN, the Basloid variety has more potential to undergo a malignant change. Risk factors for progression of HPV-associated VIN are immunocompromised status, age above 40 years, associated radiotherapy, previous lower genital tract neoplasia and proximity to the anal verge and squamous-columnar junction (van Seters et al 2005).

Clinical features and pathology: VIN does not have a unique pattern and can be diagnosed incidentally or because of symptoms. Common symptoms include chronic itching, burning, pain, dyspareunia and bleeding. The posterior vulva or the periclitoral region is involved initially and then it extends to other areas of the vulva. VIN usual type presents as multifocal lesions which are usually elevated with a rough surface and sharp margins resembling flat warts. VIN differentiated type is often seen in areas of lichen sclerosus and lichen planus and they are often symptomatic with a longstanding history of itching and burning.

Diagnosis: Vulval biopsy is the gold standard modality for diagnosis. The role of vulvar cytology remains investigational. Toluidine blue staining to pick up suspicious areas for biopsy has not yielded good results because of high false positive and false negative rates (Collins et al 1996). Colposcopy directed biopsy after application with 5% acetic acid is helpful. Evaluation of the whole of the vulva is mandatory to rule out multifocal lesions.

Treatment: Treatment of VIN is necessary and it can be treated with surgery, laser ablation or topical agents. As these lesions are occurring in the younger age group, therapy has to be conservative and should not result in distorting the normal anatomy. Standard treatment of VIN remains surgery, as outcomes are similar or better to other modalities. Conservative surgery in the form of wide excision, superficial vulvectomy or skinning vulvectomy is done. Wide local excision with at least 5 mm normal margin should be done for a localised lesion (Disaia and Creaseman 1997). If the dissection is extensive, split thickness grafts may also be required. In skinning vulvectomy, the subcutaneous tissue is preserved which maintains function and gives good cosmetic results. More extensive lesions require a simple vulvectomy. Laser treatment is becoming popular because it is as effective as surgery and gives good cosmetic results, especially in multifocal disease. The disadvantage with laser ablation is that it does not give a pathology specimen, it is painful, expensive and expertise is required. Topical agents that have been tried are 5–flurouracil, bleomycin and dinitrochlorobenzene, but the experience with these is limited and these are not ideal for the treatment of VIN. Recently, a new drug, imiquimod, has been tried in a small trial with promising results (van Seters et al 2008). All these agents cause severe inflammation.

Paget's Disease Of The Vulva

This condition is rare, apocrine in origin and occurs in the seventh decade of life in women but can occur in the younger age group as well. The most common presenting feature is pruritis. Vulval lesions are typically hyperemic, sharply demarcated with areas of excoriation and induration. This disease is usually intraepithelial, although underlying adenocarcinomas may be associated with it. The lesion is mostly localised to one labium but the entire vulva may also be involved. Other areas of involvement are the perineum, buttocks, inguinal area and mons. Diagnosis is by biopsy which should be deep, to rule out associated adenocarcinoma. Histopathology reveals large cells of clear cytoplasm in a heavy lymphocytic infiltration in the dermis. These findings can sometimes be confused with melanoma. It can be associated with carcinomas of the cervix, colon, bladder, gall bladder in 4% of cases and associated with vulvar cancer in 15% to 25% of cases (Duong and Flowers 2007). Treatment consists of wide local excision as recurrences are common because it is usually present beyond the gross lesion. If it is associated with invasive carcinoma, the management adopted will be that of squamous cell carcinoma of the vulva.

Malignant Lesions Of The Vulva

Epidemiology and pathology: Vulval cancer is relatively uncommon and accounts for approximately 5% of all female genital malignancies. It occurs in 2 per 100,000 women per year in developed countries but is 2–3 times more common in developing nations (Platz and Benda 1995). This cancer occurs more frequently in elderly women aged 65–75 years (Landis et al 1998); however, 15% of all vulval cancers occur in women, younger than 40 years of age (Creasman et al 1997) and they correlate to human papillomavirus infection. The overall incidence over the years has increased marginally but one study has shown that in women younger than 50 years of age, the incidence has increased from 2% to 21% over the past 20 years (Jones et al 1997). Incidence is higher in women who smoke, are immunosuppressed, have multiple sexual partners and have other diseases that are HPV related.

Nearly 90% of vulval cancers are squamous cell carcinomas. Other less common malignant lesions are melanoma, verrucous carcinoma, basal cell carcinoma, adenocarcinoma, Bartholin gland tumours and sarcomas. Lymphoma, endodermal sinus tumour, Merkeles cell carcinoma, dermatofibrosarcoma protuberans and malignant schwannoma are some of the other rare tumours of the vulva (Hacker 2000). Eight per cent of vulval tumours are metastatic. Vulval cancer exists as two separate diseases; one involves the human papilloma virus (HPV) infection which progress to VIN and cancer. The second type involves non-neoplastic epithelial disorders progressing to cellular atypia and cancer seen in the elderly.

Staging: The International Federation of Gynecology and Obstetrics (FIGO) introduced a new surgical/pathological staging system in 1988, replacing the clinical staging system of vulval carcinoma because the results of clinical assessment of lymph node status were inaccurate. This was again modified in 1995, where Stage I was subdivided into the two stages (Tables 21.3) (Beller et al 2003).

Spread: Vulval cancer spreads by direct extension into adjacent structures, by embolisation to the regional lymph nodes (inguinal and femoral) nodes, with little or no opportunity for metastatic sites to develop along the pathway (the intervening skin bridge) and by hematogenous spread to distant sites (bone, liver and lungs) (Disaia and Creaseman 1997). Metastasis to lymph nodes is earlier. Vulval cancer spreads to the lymph nodes in a very systematic way and skipping of the nodes is very rare. Initially it spreads to the inguinal lymph nodes followed by femoral nodes. However, rarely, femoral nodes can be involved without the involvement of the inguinal nodes from the clitoris and the Bartholin glands to these nodes. Contralateral lymph nodes, in the absence of involvement of ipsilateral lymph nodes, are very rarely seen in lateral tumours. However, lymphatic

Table 21.3: Revised FIGO surgical staging for vulvar cancer

FIGO stage	*Clinical / Pathologic findings*
Stage 0	Carcinoma in situ, intraepithelial carcinoma
Stage I	Tumour confined to vulva and/or perineum, ≤2 cm in greatest dimension, nodes are negative
Stage I a	Stromal invasion ≤1 mm (from epi)
Stage I b	Stromal invasion >1 mm
Stage II	Tumour confined to vulva and/or perineum, >2 cm in greatest dimension, nodes are negative
Stage III	Tumour of any size with 1. Adjacent spread to lower urethra, vagina or anus or 2. Unilateral regional lymph node metastasis
Stage IV a	Tumour of any size with 1. Adjacent spread to upper urethra, bladder mucosa, rectal mucosa, pelvic bone or 2. Bilateral regional lymph node metastasis
Stage IV b	Any distant metastasis, including pelvic lymph nodes

drainage from the midline structures like the clitoris, perineum and the anterior labia minora is bilateral (Hacker and Van der Velden 1993).

Diagnosis: The most common symptom of vulval cancer is a long history of pruritis. Other less common symptoms include pain, dyspareunia, discharge, vulval bleeding, a mass, a lump in the groin and dysuria. Patients can even be asymptomatic at the time of diagnosis. In such cases, diagnosis of this condition is often delayed significantly. A high index of suspicion and biopsy of any vulval abnormality can help in early detection.

On clinical examination, vulval carcinoma is usually raised and may be fleshy, ulcerated, leukoplakic or warty in appearance (Hacker 2000). Most of the lesions occur on the labia majora (50%) and are unifocal. Other sites of involvement are the labia minora (15%–20%), clitoris, perineum and 5% are multifocal.

Biopsy is required for diagnosis which can be done in the outpatient department under local anesthesia but before that a through clinical examination to know the extent of lesion, whether unifocal or multifocal, should be performed. Pelvic examination, colposcopy of the cervix and the vagina is necessary to rule out other associated premalignant and malignant lesions. If the lesion is smaller than 1 cm, excision biopsy should be done. The biopsy specimen should incorporate the underlying dermis and some normal-looking surrounding tissue for better evaluation by a pathologist.

Cystoscopy, proctoscopy, x-ray examination of the lungs and intravenous urography as needed can be used for staging. CT scan and MRI can be used for evaluating the lymphatic spread; however, the sensitivity is poor. PET to diagnose small nodal metastasis is promising but still investigational in vulvar carcinoma.

Prognosis: Lymph node metastasis is the single most important prognostic factor in vulval cancer. Gynecological oncology group trials have shown that five-year survival rate with negative inguinal lymph nodes is 91% and five-year survival rate fell to 75%, 36%, 24% and 0% in patients with one or two, three or four, five or six or seven or more positive lymph nodes respectively (Homesley et al 1991). Tumour thickness, depth of invasion, presence of lymph-vascular invasion, tumour grade are other factors which are not independent prognostic factors but are predictive of lymph node metastasis. Patients with aneuploid tumours have a poorer five year survival rate than patients with diploid tumours (Kaern 1992). The five-year survival rate in stage I is 98%, stage II is 85%, stage III is 74% and stage IV is 31% (Homesley et al 1991). The presence of extra-capsular tumour cells in the node and size of node more than 15 mm of size is also associated with poor prognosis.

Management of sqamous cell carcinoma (major changes over the years): There is no other gynecological cancer that has undergone so much change in the management as vulval cancer. En bloc radical vulvectomy and bilateral dissection of the groin and pelvic nodes was the standard treatment for operable vulvar cancer (Taussing 1940; Way 1960). Such radical surgery was associated with much morbidity although the cure rates were good. It was viewed that if en block dissection is not performed and separate incisions are given for lymph node removal, the intervening tissue left between the primary tumour and the regional lymph nodes may have microscopic tumour foci and act as a site of recurrence.

The current approach to vulval cancer now

involves individualisation and conservation; and this has been possible because of better understanding of the lymphatic pathways, the finding that local radical excision with a good margin was as equally effective as radical vulvectomy in terms of local recurrence rate in early stage carcinoma (Hoffman et al 1989; Hacker and Van der Velden 1993; Ansink 1999) and that separate incisions rarely result in the metastases in skin bridges (Hacker et al 1981). Conservation of the non-involved skin of the vulva and thigh by the 'triple incision' technique has considerably reduced wound breakdown and prolonged hospitalisation. Reports of chemoradiation being successful in vulval carcinoma has resulted in decreasing the complications and disfigurement because of exenterative procedures in advanced stages. Now, the clitoris and periclitoral lesions in younger women can be treated with chemoradiation, avoiding serious psychosexual morbidity.

Role of sentinel lymph node: Sentinel node implies the first node in the lymphatic system that receives the lymphatic flow from the primary tumour. Sentinel lymph node mapping is done by technetium 99m labelled noncolloid or isosulfun blue dye injected into the peritumoral area intraoperatively. It is a new technology in which the selective removal of the first node draining a tumour is possible thus allowing deletion of the full lymphadenectomy procedure. In a review, some studies have shown that with Technetium labelled nonocolloid, sentinel node detection rate sensitivity and specificity has been almost 100% for vulval carcinoma (Ayhan et al 2008). This method is still being investigated and until we know the rate of recurrence in uninvolved sentinel nodes (lymph node dissection omitted), the standard treatment of inguinofemoral lymphadenectomy in early stage cancer should continue. Recent studies have shown that in early stage vulval cancer, patients with a negative sentinel node and omitting the lymphadenectomy, the groin recurrence rate is low, survival is excellent and treatment related morbidity is minimal (Van der Zee et al. 2008).

Stage 1 Vulval cancer: Therapy is still not standardised. The procedure to be undertaken should be one which minimises physical and psychosocial morbidity and gives a good cure rate. Microvasive lesions (<1 mm invasion) are treated with wide excision and groin dissection is omitted. For other Stage I lesions, if well lateralised, with 5 mm or less of the invasion, a radical local excision (with at least 1 cm normal margin) with unilateral lymphadenectomy should be performed, and other sided lympadenectomy to be performed if the contralateral lymph nodes are positive. Lateral tumours of the vulva spread to the ipsilateral inguinal lymph nodes and can even be treated effectively with radical hemivulvectomy; and ipsilateral superficial lymph node dissection and deep inguinal lymphadenectomy is to be done only when the superficial inguinal lymph nodes are positive (DeSimone 2007). Studies have shown that the recurrence after radical local excision with margins negative is not higher than after radical vulvectomy (Hoffman et al 1989; Ansink 1999). Recent studies have shown that > or =8 mm pathologic margin clearance leads to a high rate of loco-regional control (Chan et al 2007). Patients with bulky, midline lesions involving clitoris, posterior fourchette and anterior labia minora should undergo radical vulvectomy with bilateral inguino femoral lymphadenectomy using separate incisions (triple incision technique) (Iversen and Aas 1983). If more extensive dissection has been done at the vulva, the defect can be repaired by full thickness skin flaps, gracilis or tensor fascia lata myocutaneous flaps. Radiotherapy as the primary modality to treat the ingunofemoral lymph nodes as compared to surgery to decrease the morbidity was reviewed and it showed that although radiotherapy was associated with less morbidity, there was higher incidence of groin recurrence (van der Velden and Ansink 2001). Only patients not fit for surgery should be treated with primary radiotherapy. Young patients with small clitoral or periclitoral tumours can be treated by chemoradiation to prevent any psychosexual problem developing later.

Stage II Vulval cancer: Standard treatment is radical vulvectomy with bilateral inguinal and femoral node dissection by using separate groin incision. The margin of the surgical resection should clear the tumour by 10 mm. But in early stage II disease in young patients, and involving the posterior half of the vulva radical local excision will preserve the clitoris, mons pubis and seems to have the same recurrence rate as radical vulvectomy, as long as surgical margins of 1 cm are achieved (Farias-Eisner et al 1994). Adjuvant local radiation therapy may be indicated if surgical margins are less than 8 mm, invasion greater than 5 mm, lymphovascular invasion and positive nodes (Thomas et al 1991; Faul et al 1997). Pelvic and groin radiation is indicated with three or more micrometastasis in the inguinal nodes, bilateral groin metastasis and with node size more than 10 mm. Primary radiation therapy to the groin is an alternative to groin dissection and should only be undertaken (as in stage I) in patients who refuse or who are unfit for surgery.

Advanced vulval cancer (stage III and stage IV): Management of advanced cancer vulva is difficult and requires a multidisciplinary approach.

Patients in this group require radical vulvectomy with inguinofemoral lymphadenectomy and pelvic exenteration. This type of surgery is associated with increased morbidity (physical and psychological) and mortality. Chemoradiation preoperatively in selected patients has been shown to be effective in some small trials to improve operability and this is becoming the first line of treatment in the management of this advanced disease (Thomas et al 1989; Berek et al 1991). Study by Landrum et al (2008) showed that patients treated with primary surgery or primary chemoradiation in advanced cancer have no differences in overall survival, progression free survival or recurrence rates.

Recurrent vulval cancer: More than 80% of the recurrences occur in the first two years of therapy. The vulva is the most common site of recurrence (69.5%), followed by groin nodes (24.3%), pelvis (15.6%) and distant metastasis (18.5%) (Piura et al 1993). Prognosis is poor as treatment is difficult. Local recurrence is treated by radical excision, alternatively, radiation therapy with or without chemotherapy may be used in patients with small local recurrences. Resection of a groin recurrence is not recommended and should be managed by radiotherapy. Distant metastases are treated with chemotherapy.

Radiotherapy: This has an important role in the treatment of vulval cancer. Recently its use with concomitant chemotherapy is gaining popularity in the treatment of this condition. It is mostly used as an adjuvant in postoperative treatment for positive lymph nodes or with positive margins of the resected tumour. Radiotherapy, with or without chemotherapy, is being increasingly used preoperatively in the management of advanced inoperable vulval cancer. Preoperative radiotherapy in such patients allows a less radical surgery. Primary radiotherapy is also used in women who are not fit enough to withstand surgery but primary radiotherapy to avoid groin dissection in early stage carcinoma is not recommended as highlighted earlier. Intensity-modulated radiation therapy (IMRT) is a new technology that allows delivery of radiation dose in a more conformal manner by varying the radiation beams spatially or temporally. Locally advanced vulval cancers were treated using preoperative chemotherapy with IMRT and it was seen that they were well tolerated with good clinical response and early clinical outcome; however, more studies are required (Beriwal et al 2008).

Chemotherapy: It has been used in vulval carcinoma for the treatment of recurrent disease for a number of years. Recently, its effective use with radiotherapy in advanced disease has made the role of chemotherapy in treating vulval cancer more important. This modality of treatment is becoming popular as in carcinoma cervix and a number of trials are going on. Chemotherapy has been used in the following situations—preoperatively (radiation dose of 55Gy with 5-fluorouracil) with radiotherapy in patients with inoperable disease to make it suitable for surgery later, postoperatively as an adjuvant with radiotherapy for node positive disease and for recurrent and metastatic disease. The most common agents used for concomitant use with radiotherapy are 5-fluorouracil and cisplatinum.

Complications of treatment and follow-up: The most important morbidity as related to surgery is the breakdown of the vulval and groin wound, but with radical local excision and groin dissection by separate incision, this complication has decreased appreciably. The incidence of major breakdown occurs in 14% of patients (Hopkins et al 1993). Other complications include seromas in femoral triangle, urinary tract infection, deep vein thrombosis, pulmonary embolism, inguinal lymphocysts and psychosexual problems. Chronic lymphoedema and introital stenosis are important late complications. Rarely urinary stress incontinence, pubic osteomyelites, rectovaginal fistula, genital prolapse, femoral hernia and recurrent leg lymphnagitis may occur. Preservation of the long saphenous vein may reduce both the groin wound and subsequent lower limb problems.

There is no well-defined protocol for follow-up of these patients after treatment. Patients after completing treatment can be followed-up every 3 to 4 weeks for 2 years and then every 6 months for the next 3 years and then annually.

Vulval melanoma: Melanoma is the second most common malignancy of the vulva with an incidence of 0.1 to 0.19 per 100,000 women (Ragnarsson-Olding et al 1993; Weinstock 1994). It accounts for approximately 10% of vulval cancers and mainly occurs in white women. Some patients may have itching or bleeding, but most of them may not have any symptoms except for a pigmented lesion which keeps enlarging. The common sites of involvement are the labia minora and the clitoris. Three histopathologic types of vulval melanoma have been described. These are mucosal lentiginous melanoma, superficial spreading melanoma and nodular melanoma. Prognosis depends on the depth of the tumour rather than on the diameter of the lesion, so FIGO staging used for squamous lesion is not applicable to this condition (Podratz et al

1983).

The main treatment modality for vulval melanoma is surgical. It is advisable that if the lesion shows less than 1 mm of invasion it should be treated by radical local excision alone with 2 cm margins. For intermediate invasion (1–4 mm), lymph node dissection gives better results. Patients with deeper invasion (more than 4 mm) would not benefit from lymph node dissection because of the high incidence of systemic metastasis (Chung et al 1975; Phillips et al 1982).

Melanomas have an overall poor prognosis with a five-year survival rate of about 50% (Suwandinata et al 2007).

Bartholin's gland carcinoma: Primary carcinoma of the Bartholin's gland accounts for about 5% of vulval malignancies. It generally occurs in older women and is rare in patients under 50 years of age. Patients usually present with an enlargement in the gland that may be mistaken for a cyst.

Bartholin's gland carcinoma is usually treated by radical vulvectomy with bilateral groin and pelvic node dissection (Barclay et al 1964). As these tumours are deep, more radical surgery is usually needed followed by radiotherapy. Lesions that are less deep without the involvement of lymph nodes can be managed by hemivulvectomy or radical local excision (Copeland et al 1986). However, a recent study has shown primary radiation or chemoradiation therapy to be an effective alternative to surgery in the treatment of Bartholin gland carcinoma with preservation of genital function and low morbidity (Lopez-Varela et al 2007).

Basal cell carcinoma and verrucous carcinoma: These squamous variants are very rare tumours.They are rarely associated with lymph node metastases, so these lesions can be managed by wide local excision. Basal cell carcinomas can also be managed by radiotherapy if resection would compromise function of the sphincter. The local recurrence rate is about 20% (Palladino et al 1969; Breen et al 1975; Hoffman et al 1988).

Vulval sarcomas: Leiomyosarcoma is the most common vulval sarcoma and accounts for 1.5% of vulval malignancies. Aggressive resection of primary tumour followed by radiation therapy helps decease recurrences. However, the natural history of vulval leiomyosarcoma is characterised by a protracted course of frequent local recurrence followed by distant fatal metastases. Chemotherapy is used chiefly for palliation rather than for cure (Ulutin et al 2003). Other sarcomas which can involve the vulva are epitheloid sarcoma, fibrosarcoma, liposarcoma, rhabdomyosarcoma and neurofibrosarcoma.

Other rare malignancies: The vulva may be involved primarily by lymphoma or as a part of the systemic disease. Treatment is by surgical excision followed by chemotherapy and radiation or both (Harris and Scully 1984). The vulva can be involved as a metastatic site from other primaries such as the cervix, endometrium, kidney and urethra.

Summary: Cancer of the vulva is a relatively rare neoplasm, accounting for approximately 5% of all gynecologic malignancies and less than 1% of all cancers in women. There are definite premalignant conditions, and if these are diagnosed early and treated, can decrease the incidence of vulvar cancer appreciably. Squamous cell carcinoma is the most common and represents approximately 90% of all vulval cancers. Most women present with vulval pruritis and a recognisable lesion in the vulva. A high index of suspicion and early biopsy of any abnormal vulval lesion will also help in the diagnosis of premalignant and malignant conditions of the vulva early.

Management of vulval cancer has evolved over the past two decades. Each case has to be individualised. This individualisation includes careful consideration of less radical surgery for early-stage disease and the incorporation of radiation and chemotherapy into the treatment regimen of locoregionally advanced disease. A more conservative approach to treatment has significantly decreased the associated physical and psychological morbidity without compromising overall survival in vulval cancer.

References

Ansink A. 1999. Surgical interventions for early squamous cell carcinoma of the vulva. *Cochrane Database Syst Rev* (4):CD002036.

Assmann T, P Becker-Wegerich, M Grewe, M Megahed and T Ruzicka. 2003. Tacrolimus ointment for the treatment of vulvar lichen sclerosus. *J Am Acad Dermatol* 48 (6):935–937.

Ayhan A, H Celik and P Dursun. 2008. Lymphatic mapping and sentinel node biopsy in gynecological cancers: A critical review of the literature. *World J Surg Oncol* 6:53.

Beller U, P Maisonneuve, JL Benedet, AP Heintz, HY Ngan, S Pecorelli, F Odicino, WT Creasman. 2003. Carcinoma of the vulva. *Int J Gynaecol Obstet* 83 Suppl 1:7–26.

Berek JS, JM Heaps, YS Fu, GJ Juillard, NF Hacker. 1991. Concurrent cisplatin and 5-fluorouracil chemotherapy and radiation therapy for advanced-stage squamous carcinoma of the vulva. *Gynecol Oncol* 42 (3):197–201.

Boreal S, D Coon, DE Heron, JL Kelley, RP Edwards et al. 2008. Preoperative intensity-modulated radiotherapy and chemotherapy for locally advanced vulvar carcinoma. *Gynecol Oncol* 109(2):291–295.

Breen JL, RD Neubecker, E Greenwald, CA Gregori. 1975. Basal cell carcinoma of the vulva. *Obstet Gynecol* 46 (2):122–129.

Canavan TP and D Cohen. 2002. Vulvar cancer. *Am Fam Physician* 66 (7):1269-1274.

Chan JK, V Sugiyama, H Pham, M Gu et al. 2007. Margin distance and other clinico-pathologic prognostic factors in vulvar carcinoma: A multivariate analysis. *Gynecol Oncol* 104 (3):636–641.

Chu J, HK Tamimi, DC Figge. 1981. Femoral node metastases with negative superficial inguinal nodes in early vulvar cancer. *Am J Obstet Gynecol* 140 (3):337–339.

Chung AF, JM Woodruff and JL Lewis, Jr. 1975. Malignant melanoma of the vulva: A report of 44 cases. *Obstet Gynecol* 45 (6):638–646.

Copeland LJ, N Sneige, DM Gershenson, VB McGuffee et al. 1986. Bartholin gland carcinoma. *Obstet Gynecol* 67 (6):794-801.

Creasman WT, JL Phillips, HR Menck. 1997. The National Cancer Data Base report on early stage invasive vulvar carcinoma. The American College of Surgeons Commission on Cancer and the American Cancer Society. *Cancer* 80 (3):505–513.

DeSimone CP, JS Van Ness, AL Cooper, SC Modesitt et al. 2007. The treatment of lateral T1 and T2 squamous cell carcinomas of the vulva confined to the labium majus or minus. *Gynecol Oncol* 104(2): 390–395.

Disaia PJ and WT Creaseman. 1997. Invasive cancer of the vulva. In *Clinical Gynecologic Oncology*, edited by PJ Disaia and WT Creaseman. St Louis: Mosby-Year Book, 202–232.

Duong TH and LC Flowers. 2007. Vulvo-vaginal cancers: Risks, evaluation, prevention and early detection. *Obstet Gynecol Clin North Am* 34(4):783–802.

Farias-Eisner R, FD Cirisano, D Grouse, RS Leuchter et al. 1994. Conservative and individualized surgery for early squamous carcinoma of the vulva: The treatment of choice for stage I and II (T1-2N0-1M0) disease. *Gynecol Oncol* 53 (1):55–58.

Faul CM., D Mirmow, Q Huang, K Gerszten et al. 1997. Adjuvant radiation for vulvar carcinoma: Improved local control. *Int J Radiat Oncol Biol Phys* 38 (2):381–389.

Hacker NF. 2000. Vulvar cancer. In *Practical Gynecologic Oncology,* 3rd ed. Philadelphia: Williams & Wilkins, 553–596.

Hacker NF, RS Leuchter, JS Berek, TW Castaldo, LD Lagasse. 1981. Radical vulvectomy and bilateral inguinal lymphadenectomy through separate groin incisions. *Obstet Gynecol* 58 (5):574–579.

Hacker NF and J Van der Velden. 1993. Conservative management of early vulvar cancer. *Cancer* 71 (4 Suppl):1673–1677.

Harris NL and RE Scully. 1984. Malignant lymphoma and granulocytic sarcoma of the uterus and vagina. A clinicopathologic analysis of 27 cases. *Cancer* 53 (11):2530–2545.

Heller DS. 2007. Report of a new ISSVD classification of VIN. *J Low Genit Tract Dis* 11 (1):46–47.

Hoffman MS, WS Roberts, JP Lapolla, D Cavanagh. 1989. Recent modifications in the treatment of invasive squamous cell carcinoma of the vulva. *Obstet Gynecol Surv* 44 (4):227–233.

Hoffman MS, WS Roberts, EH Ruffolo. 1988. Basal cell carcinoma of the vulva with inguinal lymph node metastases. *Gynecol Oncol* 29 (1):113–119.

Homesley HD, BN Bundy, A Sedlis, E Yordan et al. 1991. Assessment of Current International Federation of Gynecology and Obstetrics staging of vulvar carcinoma relative to prognostic factors for survival (a Gynecologic Oncology Group study). *Am J Obstet Gynecol* 164 (4):997-1003; discussion 1003–1004.

Hopkins MP, GC Reid and GW Morley. 1993. Radical vulvectomy. The decision for the incision. *Cancer* 72 (3):799–803.

Iversen T and M Aas. 1983. Lymph drainage from the vulva. *Gynecol Oncol* 16 (2):179–189.

Jeffcoate TN. 1966. Chronic vulval dystrophies. *Am J Obstet Gynecol* 95 (1):61–74.

Jones RW, J Baranyai and S Stables. 1997. Trends in squamous cell carcinoma of the vulva: The influence of vulvar intraepithelial neoplasia. *Obstet Gynecol* 90 (3):448–452.

Kaern J. 1992. Flow cytometric DNA measurements in squamous cell carcinoma of the vulva an important prognostic method. *Int J Gynecol Cancer* 2:169–175.

Kiene P, K Milde-Langosch and T Loning. 1991. Human papillomavirus infection in vulvar lesions of lichen sclerosus et atrophicus. *Arch Dermatol Res* 283 (7):445–448.

Landis SH, T Murray, S Bolden and PA Wingo. 1998. Cancer statistics, 1998. *CA Cancer J Clin* 48 (1):6–29.

Landrum LM, Skaggs V, Gould N, Walker JL, McMeekin DS. 2008. Comparison of outcome measures in patients with advanced squamous cell carcinoma of the vulva treated with surgery or primary chemoradiation. *Gynecol Oncol* 108(3):584–590

Li C, D Bian W Chen, C Zhao, N Yin and Z Wang. 2004. Focused ultrasound therapy of vulvar dystrophies: a feasibility study. *Obstet Gynecol* 104 (5 Pt 1):915–921.

Lin MC, GL Mutter, P Trivijisilp, KA Boynton et al. 1998. Patterns of allelic loss (LOH) in vulvar squamous carcinomas and adjacent noninvasive epithelia. *Am J Pathol* 152 (5):1313–1318.

López-Varela E, Oliva E, McIntyre JF, Fuller AF Jr. 2007. Primary treatment of Bartholin's gland carcinoma with radiation and chemoradiation: A report on ten consecutive cases. *Int J Gynecol Cancer* 17(3):661–667.

Meyrick Thomas RH, CM Ridley, DH McGibbon, and MM Black. 1988. Lichen sclerosus et atrophicus and autoimmunity: A study of 350 women. *Br J Dermatol* 118 (1):41–46.

Palladino VS, JL Duffy and GJ Bures. 1969. Basal cell carcinoma of the vulva. *Cancer* 24 (3):460–470.

Phillips GL, LB Twiggs and T Okagaki. 1982. Vulvar melanoma: A microstaging study. *Gynecol Oncol* 14 (1):80–88.

Piura B, A Masotina, J Murdoch, A Lopes et al. 1993. Recurrent squamous cell carcinoma of the vulva: A study of 73 cases. *Gynecol Oncol* 48 (2):189–195.

Platz CE and JA Benda. 1995. Female genital tract cancer. *Cancer* 75 (1 Suppl): 270–294.

Podratz KC, TA Gaffey, RE Symmonds, KL Johansen and PC O'Brien. 1983. Melanoma of the vulva: An update. *Gynecol Oncol* 16 (2):153–168.

Ragnarsson-Olding B, H. Johansson, LE Rutqvist and U Ringborg. 1993. Malignant melanoma of the vulva and vagina. Trends in incidence, age distribution, and long-term survival among 245 consecutive cases in Sweden 1960-1984. *Cancer* 71 (5):1893–1897.

Ridley CM, O Frankman, IS Jones, SH Pincus et al. 1989. New nomenclature for vulvar disease: International Society for the Study of Vulvar Disease. *Hum Pathol* 20 (5):495–496.

Suwandinata FS, RM Bohle, CA Omwandho, HR Tinneberg and SE Gruessner. 2007. Management of vulvar melanoma and review of the literature. *Eur J Gynaecol Oncol* 28 (3):220–224.

Taussing FJ. 1940. Cancer of the vulva: An analysis of 155 cases. *Am J Obstet Gynecol* 40:764–777.

Thomas G, A Dembo, A DePetrillo, J Pringle et al. 1989. Concurrent radiation and chemotherapy in vulvar carcinoma. *Gynecol Oncol* 34 (3):263–267.

Thomas GM, AJ Dembo, SC Bryson, R Osborne, AD DePetrillo. 1991. Changing concepts in the management of vulvar cancer. *Gynecol Oncol* 42 (1):9–21.

Thuis YN, M Campion, H Fox and NF Hacker. 2000. Contemporary experience with the management of vulvar intraepithelial neoplasia. *Int J Gynecol Cancer* 10 (3):223–227.

Ulutin HC, RC Zellars and D Frassica. 2003. Soft tissue sarcoma of the vulva: A clinical study. *Int J Gynecol Cancer* 13 (4):528–531.

van der Velden K and A Ansink. 2001. Primary groin irradiation vs primary groin surgery for early vulvar cancer. *Cochrane Database Syst Rev* (4):CD002224.

Van der Zee AG, MH Oonk, JA De Hullu, AC Ansink et al. 2008. Sentinel node dissection is safe in the treatment of early-stage vulvar cancer. *J Clin Oncol* 26 (6):884–889.

van Seters M, M. van Beurden, AJ de Craen. 2005. Is the assumed natural history of vulvar intraepithelial neoplasia III based on enough evidence? A systematic review of 3322 published patients. *Gynecol Oncol* 97 (2):645–651.

van Seters M, M van Beurden, FJ ten Kate, I Beckmann et al. 2008. Treatment of vulvar intraepithelial neoplasia with topical imiquimod. *N Engl J Med* 358 (14):1465–1473.

Wallace HJ. 1971. Lichen sclerosus et atrophicus. Trans St Johns Hosp Dermatol Soc 57 (1):9–30.

Way S. 1960. Carcinoma of the vulva. *Am J Obstet Gynecol* 79:692–697.

Weinstock MA 1994. Malignant melanoma of the vulva and vagina in the United States: Patterns of incidence and population-based estimates of survival. *Am J Obstet Gynecol* 171 (5):1225–1230.

22

Malignant Epithelial Ovarian Tumours

Pralhad Kushtagi

Ovarian cancer continues to have the highest mortality of all gynecological malignancies and is the least able to be diagnosed at an early stage. It is the fourth most common cause of cancer death in women, and the leading cause of gynecologic cancer death in the developed world (Boring et al 1994). Approximately 90% are epithelial carcinomas, and nearly 75% will have spread beyond the ovaries at the time of diagnosis (Young et al 1993). Since only a minority of women present with surgically curable localised disease, systemic chemotherapy has become the mainstay of treatment. Although much progress has been made in this regard over the last 20 years, the high response rates observed with chemotherapy have not readily translated into major long-term survival gains, and the overall 5-year survival is still less than 30% (Neijt et al 1991). The need for new therapeutic strategies is therefore paramount.

Etiopathology: The risk for developing ovarian cancer increases after 40 years of age, with the peak incidence between the ages of 50 and 55, and a median age of 59. General trends of higher incidence in the upper middle class especially in industrialised countries suggest environmental, dietary or pregnancy practices as possible etiologic factors in ovarian cancer. Environmental factors such as industrial pollutants, talc and asbestos have been implicated. So are a high-fat diet, hormonal, genetic and hereditary factors, number of pregnancies and, to a lesser degree, specific blood group factors and viruses have all been believed to contribute to the cause. In an attempt to unite several theories of the development of ovarian carcinoma, a theory of pathogenesis has been suggested (Cramer and Welch 1983).

Epithelial ovarian tumours arise from surface epithelium of the ovary which develops from the celomic epithelium (mesothelium) of the embryonic gonad. The latter epithelium is continuous with the celomic epithelium that penetrates the underlying mesenchyme to form the müllerian duct. This proximity is reflected in the various directions of müllerian differentiation pursued by the surface epithelium when it undergoes neoplasia in the postnatal ovary, that is fallopian tube epithelium, in cases of serous neoplasia, endometrial epithelium in case of endometroid tumours, and endocervical epithelium in cases of mucinous neoplasia. Although common epithelial tumours (Table 22.1) may arise directly from the surface epithelium and grow exophytically, more commonly, they appear to originate from its

TABLE 22.1: COMMON EPITHELIAL TUMOURS—HISTOLOGICAL WHO CLASSIFICATION OF OVARIAN TUMOURS

	Type	*Borderline*	*Malignant*
A	Serous tumours	serous cystadenoma, papillary serous cystadenoma, surface papilloma adenofibroma cystadenofibroma	cystadenocarcinoma, papillary serous cystadenocarcinomama, papillary adenocarcinoma; malignant adenofibroma,cystadenofibroma
B	Mucinous	mucinous cystadenoma, adenofibroma cystadenifibroma	cystadenocarcinoma, cystadenocarcinoma; malignant adenofibroma,cystadenofibroma
C	Endometroid	adenoma, cystadenoma adenofibroma, cystadenofibroma	adenocarcinoma, adenoacanthoma, malignant adenofibroma and cystadeno fibroma; endometrial stromal sarcoma; mixed mesodermal tumours-homologous and heterologous
D	Clear cell (Mesonephroid)	clear cell adenoma	carcinoma, adenocarcinoma
E	Brenner	proliferating tumour	malignant tumour
F	Undifferentiated	-	carcinoma
G	Mixed	borderline tumour	malignant tumour
H	Unclassified	-	-

(Source: Serov et al, 1973)

inclusion glands, accounting for the basically cystic or endophytic nature of most of these tumours. Initially, inclusion cysts containing surface epithelium are formed by entrapment of ovarian surface epithelium in the ovarian stroma. This is followed by abnormal proliferation and malignant transformation of the epithelial lining of the inclusion cyst. They become solid when they contain a large component of ovarian stromal origin or when malignant neoplastic cells proliferate to form masses containing varying amounts of tumour cells and stroma. The abnormal proliferation of epithelial lining of inclusion cysts and to some extent, their malignant transformation, may occur by stimulation of high levels of gonadotrophins or estrogens. Both oral contraceptive use and pregnancy decrease the pituitary gonadotrophin excretion, and are associated with significantly lower incidence of ovarian cancer. These may exert their protective effects by inhibiting incessant ovulation, a proposed cause of inclusion cyst formation. High gonadotrophins increase with age, and reach their peak at the age when the incidence of ovarian cancer is highest. Premature ovarian failure, such as depletion of oocytes from mumps virus or chemicals such as talc or asbestos, would also be associated with high levels of gonadotrophin early in life. High levels of gonadotrophins could reflect estrogen degradation in the liver caused by exogenous toxic chemicals or drugs. High estrogen sources could be exogenous, non-contraceptive estrogens, or endogenous in diseases that cause high estrogen levels from extra-glandular sources secondary to increased estrogen stores in adipose tissue in obese individuals.

Compiling the family cancer history through second degree relatives could, in certain circumstances, show at a glance that one may be dealing with a cancer aggregation consonant with hereditary cancer.

Screening: Screening for epithelial ovarian tumours remains one of medicine's greatest challenges after enormous advances in tumour marker and ultrasound technology, combined with sophisticated statistical analysis. A premalignant precursor lesion for ovarian cancer has not been identified, limiting the focus of screening at present to detection of asymptomatic, early stage disease. The relationship between stage at presentation and survival in ovarian cancer has long provided a rationale for efforts to improve outcome by detection of early stage disease. An attempt has been made to apply WHO screening criteria to ovarian cancer to assess the potential for early detection of the disease (Rosenthal and Jacobs 1998).

Specificity is a major consideration in ovarian cancer screening because the majority of women who test positive will require exploratory surgery. A variety of different modalities have been used to detect ovarian cancer in asymptomatic women. Although vaginal examination remains important in the assessment of women presenting with gynecological symptoms, it cannot be recommended as a first line screening tool in asymptomatic women (MacFarlane et al 1955; Andolf et al 1986; Jacob and Oram 1990).

A variety of ovarian tumour markers have been studied. The most extensively investigated of these is measurement of the tumour marker cancer antigen 125 (CA125) in serum. The use of combination of markers to increase the sensitivity and specificity has been widely investigated. The marker that appeared to exhibit complementarity to CA125 was OVX1 (Xu et al 1993; Woolas et al 1993), a monoclonal antibody developed using sequential immunisation with three different ovarian cancer cell lines. It is unstable unless serum is rapidly separated: a viable humoral marker has not yet been found. Ovarian Cancer Activating Factor, a species of lysophosphatidic acids capable of stimulating cancer cell proliferation which correlates with surgical stage did promise, but the procedure is quite involved for a screening test (Xu et al 1998). Serum analysed by an iterative searching algorithm that identified a proteomic pattern, could completely distinguish patients with cancer from those without with 100% sensitivity (95% CI 93–100) and 95% specificity (Petricoin III et al 2002; Singh et al 2006). Prostacin, a potential serum marker for ovarian cancer identified through microarray technology, demonstrates utility of expression arrays in identifying genes that may lead to the discovery of novel tumour markers (Mok et al 2001). Digital analysis of single nucleotide polymorphism (SNP) appears to detect ovarian cancer very well and is far more precise than other available tests. It is claimed to detect "allelic imbalance" in 87% of early disease, 95% of late disease and none in healthy controls (Chang et al 2002). However, as of now it is expensive and labour intensive.

Current screening methods include transvaginal ultrasound scanning of the ovaries and measurement of CA125 in serum. Although several other tumour markers have been associated with ovarian cancer, they have not been widely tested for screening purposes. When used for screening, CA125 measurement is usually followed by ultrasound scanning in women with abnormal levels. The definition of abnormal level varies with menopausal status. The presence of rising CA125 levels obtained by serial measurements has also been used to indicate possible tumour activity. A sophisticated approach to interpretation of CA125 using an algorithm incorporating age and rate of change of CA125 as well as absolute levels has been made. The algorithm uses an individual's sequential CA125 results, from which the slope and intercept are calculated. The higher the slope or intercept, the greater is the risk of ovarian cancer (Skates et al 1995).

Transvaginal ultrasound scanning which offers greater resolution by virtue of closer proximity of the probe to the ovaries would be a sensitive tool. There are no universally-accepted criteria for distinguishing between benign and malignant conditions on the basis of ultrasound findings. Several systems for classifying and scoring abnormalities in the form of a morphological index (Sassone et al 1991; Learner et al 1994; Bourne et al 1993; Ferrazzi et al 1997) have been described. At the moment, no test has been proved reliable enough to screen for ovarian cancer in the general population. Two distinct screening strategies have emerged, one ultrasound based and the other based on measurement of the serum tumour marker CA125, with ultrasound as the secondary test (multimodal screening). Overall, the interim data from large prospective studies of screening for ovarian cancer in the general population (UKCTOCS; US Preventive Services Task Force 2004) suggest that sequential multimodal screening has superior specificity and positive predictive value compared with strategies based on transvaginal ultrasound alone. However, ultrasound as a first-line test may offer greater sensitivity for early stage disease. Other high modalities, such as radioimmunoscintigraphy, may yet have a role as second- or third-line tests, but will never be practical for mass screening.

To help determine preoperatively the patients with adnexal mass(es) as benign or likely to be malignant, various scoring systems to calculate risk of malignancy index using menopausal status, CA125 value and ovarian morphological scores have been proposed (Jacobs et al 1990; Tingulstad et al 1996; Tingulstad et al 1999). The value of detection of normal ovarian tissue (ovarian crescent sign) in the differential diagnosis of adnexal masses is suggested (Hillaby et al 2004) and appears simple, immediate and comparable to the scorings of malignancy indices (Kalghatgi 2006).

Staging: In order to manage patients with ovarian cancer properly, surgical exploration of abdomen cavity is necessary at the outset of therapy, and surgical staging has become mandatory, by convention, to document the precise extent of disease prior to the recommendation of adjuvant therapy, because occult dissemination may have occurred in patients whose disease is apparently confined to the ovaries. It has been seen that in many patients who were not subjected to rigorous staging, the overall 5-year survival rates for patients with apparent early stages (stage I and II) was lesser, with relatively significant relapse in these patients (Buchsbaumm and Lifshitz 1984; Fisher and Young 1977). Transcelomic spread by exfoliation of cells is the most common mode, but the malignant cells can also metastasise via the lymphatic or blood vessels.

The staging according to the Federation of Obstetrics and Gynecology (FIGO) is listed in Table 22.2 (Benedet et al 2000).

While in some patients the diagnosis of a malignant ovarian neoplasm is strongly suspected preoperatively, the actual diagnosis is frequently not confirmed until after laparotomy. Often the diagnosis is an incidental or completely unexpected finding.

In older patients, particularly those who are postmenopausal, an adnexal mass must be presumed to be a malignancy until proved otherwise. For preoperative assessment, in addition to a complete blood count, renal and liver function tests should be obtained. Serum levels of CA125 and Carcinoembryo Antigen be obtained, and if the levels are found to be elevated they prove useful in following the progress of the disease during subsequent

TABLE 22.2: FIGO STAGING OF CARCINOMA OF THE OVARY

Staging is based on findings at clinical examination and surgical exploration. The final histologic findings (cytologic, when required) after surgery are to be considered in the staging			***TNM***
Stage I	Growth limited to ovaries		T1
	A	Growth limited to one ovary, no ascites containing malignant cells; no tumour on the external surface, capsule intact.	T1a
	B	Growth limited to both ovaries, no ascites containing malignant cells; no tumour on the external surface, capsule intact.	T1b
	C	Tumour either stage IA or IB, with any of the following: tumour on external surface of one or both ovaries, capsule ruptured or with ascites containing malignant cells or with positive peritoneal washings.	T1c
Stage II	Growth involving one or both ovaries with pelvic extension		T2
	A	Extension and/or metastasis to the uterus and/or fallopian tubes; no malignant cells in ascites or peritoneal washings	T2a
	B	Extension to other pelvic tissues; no malignant cells in ascites or peritoneal washings	T2b
	C	Tumour either stage IIA or IIB; malignant cells in ascites or peritoneal washings	T2c
Stage III	Growth involving one or both ovaries with microscopically confirmed peritoneal metastases outside the pelvis and/or regional lymph node metastases		T3 &/or N1
	A	Microscopic peritoneal metastases beyond pelvis	T3a
	B	Macroscopic peritoneal metastases beyond pelvis, 2 cm or less in greatest dimension	T3b
	C	Macroscopic peritoneal metastases beyond pelvis, more than 2 cm in greatest dimension and/or regional lymph node metastases	T3c and/or N1
Stage IV	Distant metastases beyond peritoneal cavity.		M

Note: Liver capsule metastases is Stage III; Liver parenchymal metastases is Stage IV; Pleural effusion must have positive cytology

Source: FIGO Committee on Gynecologic Oncology, 2000

chemotherapy. Radiographic studies should include a chest x-ray which may reveal pleural effusion or may suggest lung parenchymal metastatic disease that might alter the extent of attempted tumour resection in the peritoneal cavity. Pelvic and abdominal ultrasound is useful and necessary. CT or MRI scan are not mandatory, since surgical exploration and intravenous urogram are necessary. An upper gastrointestinal series and intestinal evaluation should be performed, if symptoms and signs suggest this or if stools are positive for occult blood. The technique of surgical staging (Table 22.3) is described very well in most textbooks.

If the gastrocolic ligament is palpably normal, it does not routinely require resection, since occult metastases are more often located in the infracolic omentum. The retroperitoneal spaces should be explored to document lymph node metastases. A particularly thorough dissection is warranted in lesions apparently confined to the ovary, because the discovery of disease in this situation will require adjuvant therapy.

Reports from literature document occult metastasis in over 25% of cytologic specimens, about 7% of diaphragm and periaortic lymph node biopsies, and 6% of pelvic lymph node and 8% of omental biopsies in apparent stages I and II epithelial ovarian malignancies (Berek and Hacker 1987).

Management

Despite advances, novel approaches and the wide variety of different therapies, surgery has been the cornerstone in all treatment modalities for ovarian cancers. The optimal surgical approach to a malignant tumour is resection of the tumour with wide margins of normal tissue. In many patients with ovarian cancer, it is not attainable because of the existence of early metastases. Hence, the concept of cyto (tumour) reductive surgery or debulking surgery is applied for these patients where tumour is partially removed without curative intent, in the hope of making subsequent therapy more effective (Silberman 1982). The rationale is mainly based on three theoretical considerations: first, tumour mass excision provides physiological benefit by restoring gastric function, improving nutritional status, and thereby improving the general condition of the patient, temporarily interrupting the natural course of the disease (Fuller and Griffiths 1979). Second, the cell kinetic and tumour perfusion considerations: cytoreductive surgery will remove poorly diffused masses that have tenuous vascularisation and oxygenation and decreased growth fraction rendering the tissue sensitive to carcinochemotherapeutic agents or radiotherapy. The possible role of the immune system in the defence against cancer is formulated. The surveillance hypothesis is based on the assumption that cancer cells have surface antigens and immune system producing antibodies which destroy these malignant cells as long as only a small number of such cells are present. Once the tumour has begun to grow, it starts to interfere with the host's immune mechanisms to facilitate its own growth. The role of the surgeon could be to lower the level of immune suppression by resecting the bulk of tumour.

The main goal of cytoreductive surgery is to resect all visible tumours. The benefit of reducing burden to an optimal status, if only incomplete resection is possible, is described by several authors. The considered optimal status of tumour reduction has varied from a maximum tumour diameter of as small than 5 mm (Griffiths 1975) to less than 15 mm (Hacker et al 1983).

Table 22.3: Staging laparotomy

Preoperative preparation	1. Mechanical and antibiotic bowel preparation 2. Systemic prophylactic antimicrobials
Incision	1. Midline or paramedian - preferred 2. Low transverse (inadvertent) - divide/detach rectus muscles from symphysis; may extend the incision upward on the right side
Exploration	Careful inspection and palpation of all intraabdominal surfaces and viscera proceeding in a clockwise fashion: cecum, pericolic gutter, right kidney, liver, gall bladder, right diaphragm, entrance to lesser sac at periaortic area, left side of falciform ligament, spleen, left kidney; entire length of small intestine from ligament of Trietz to cecum, including peritoneal surfaces of intestinal mesentery; ascending, transverse and sigmoid colon
Sampling	1. Malignancy confined to pelvic viscera or ovaries a. Sample all sites in upper abdomen b. Retrieve ascetic fluid if present c. Obtain peritoneal washings after instilling 50–100 ml normal saline in five sites i. Pelvic cul-de-sac ii. Each pericolic gutter iii. Under each half of diaphragm* 2. If no macroscopic evidence of disease a. Multiple intraperitoneal biopsies including pelvic cul de sac, pericolic gutters, peritoneum over bladder and rectum, small intestinal mesentery, under surfaces of diaphragm† b. Biopsy from adhesions, irregularities c. 'Pap' smear of diaphragm surface 3. All cases—exploration of retroperitoneal spaces: resection of enlarged nodes; if not enlarged, representative nodal tissue from a. Periaortic area b. Iliac area—along external, internal and common iliac vessels 4. Young patient, disease apparently confined to one ovary (stage 1A) where fertility preservation is planned—arrange for frozen section evaluation a. Biopsy from other ovary b. Plus as in (b) and (c) above
Procedures	Bilateral salpingoovariectomy, total hysterectomy, infracolic omentectomy, maximum tumour resection (in fertility-preserving surgery, only removal of affected ovary and infracolic omentectomy; other ovary, tube and uterus are preserved)

** Collection can be facilitated by the use of rubber catheters attached to bulb syringe*
† laparoscope facilitated biopsy

Early stage (Stage I or Stage II disease): Although the preliminary radiological findings may seem to corroborate with clinical findings of early disease, it is imperative that these patients still undergo a thorough surgical staging. The prognosis of adequately staged patients with Stage IA and Stage IB Grade I cystadenocarcinoma is extremely good:

adjuvant chemotherapy would not provide further benefits. For higher grade tumours and for patients with Stage IC, adjuvant platinum based chemotherapy should be considered, although this practice remains controversial. All patients with Stage II disease should receive adjuvant chemotherapy. The number of cycles of chemotherapy has also not been clarified but are usually 3–6 (Dembo et al 1990; Young et al 1990; DiSaia and Creasman 2002; Bell et al 2003). Although it is axiomatic that pelvic radiation therapy has no role in the treatment of early staged ovarian cancer, the role of whole-abdomen irradiation, either open field or moving strip, remains unclear.

Fertility sparing surgery: Conservative surgery for invasive epithelial ovarian cancer is controversial. However, epithelial ovarian cancer does arise in young women who have yet to complete childbearing, and conservation of the uterus and opposite ovary in stage IA cancer may be considered for these patients. The situation and surgical possibilities should be discussed preoperatively. First, frozen sections should be obtained from the involved ovary, followed by staging exploration as outlined in Table 22.3. Because of the problems associated with frozen section reporting, efforts are on to find an alternative method and evaluation of the tissues through optical diagnosis by Raman microspectroscopy and this has shown encouraging results (Muralikrishna et al 2005). If there are no high-risk features (Table 22.4) and contralateral ovary appears to be normal, then fertility sparing surgery may be an option. If high-risk features are discovered on the final histopathology, or completion of childbearing, consideration should be given to a completion hysterectomy and unilateral salpingo-ovariectomy.

Borderline tumours: Borderline tumours or those of low malignant potential tend to remain confined to the ovary for long periods and are associated with good prognosis. Although uncommon, metastatic implants may occur and these may be invasive or non-invasive. The diagnosis is based on histopathological features that is characterised by the absence of stromal invasion (Bell 1991). The principal treatment of borderline ovarian tumours is surgical resection of the primary tumour. There is no evidence that either subsequent chemotherapy or radiation therapy improve survival. For patients in whom an ovariectomy or cystectomy has been performed and a border tumour is later documented, no additional immediate surgery is necessary.

Advanced Stage (Stage III and IV): The patients in advanced disease are usually quite symptomatic from the intra-abdominal disease. This may affect performance status and fitness for surgery. However, as mentioned above, one of the most critical prognostic indicators in patients with advanced stage ovarian cancer is the volume of residual disease. Therefore, all patients whose medical condition and fitness for surgery permits should undergo primary laparotomy, with maximal attempt at optimal cytoreduction (Omura 1991; DiSaia and Creasman 2002).

It should be remembered that even large epithelial ovarian cancers tend not to infiltrate deeply in the peritoneum of the pelvic wall, or invade the lumina of the colon or bladder. Hence, retroperitoneal approach for pelvic tumour dissection, entering the retroperitoneum laterally along the surface of the psoas makes surgery easier and helps to avoid the iliac vessels and the ureter. The technique of reverse hysterectomy, which uses

TABLE 22.4: RISK VARIABLES IN EARLY STAGE EPITHELIAL OVARIAN CANCER

Variable	*Low risk*	*High risk*
Grade	Low	High
Histologic type	Non clear cell	Clear cell
Capsule	Intact	Tumour growth through capsule
Surface excrescenses	No	Present
Ascites	No	Present
Peritoneal cytological findings	Negative	Positive
Rupture	Unruptured or intraoperative	Preoperative
Dense adherence	Absent	Absent
Ploidy	Diploid	Aneuploid

(Source : Berek and Hacker, 2000)

a transvaginal entry to the rectovaginal space, is particularly helpful in situations in which the posterior cul-de-sac is obliterated with tumour. The disease may involve focal areas of the small or large intestine, and resection should be performed if it would permit the removal of all or most of the abdominal metastases. Apart from the rectosigmoid colon, the most frequent sites of intestinal metastases are the terminal ileum, the cecum and the transverse colon. The resection of one or more of these segments of the bowel may be necessary. It is rarely necessary to resect portions of the lower urinary tract. Resection of portion of the bladder may be required which can be accomplished through cystotomy (Heintz 1986). If possible, all metastases larger than 15 mm in diameter are removed from parietal the peritoneum. If larger metastases are located on the liver serosa or diaphragm, removal is not advised because it is technically difficult and is associated with high morbidity. Large pelvic and para-aortic nodes are only removed if removal contributes to the optimal status.

Induction chemotherapy: Optimal cytoreduction at primary laparotomy is considered to be impossible in certain patients if there are localisations where tumour masses of more than 15 mm cannot be removed. This is usually the case if masses of this size are located near the base of the small bowel mesentery, close to the origin of the superior mesenteric artery, in paraaortic nodes above the renal artery, in the porta hepatis, in the liver parenchyma or in the lungs, and if there is extensive involvement of the peritoneum with tumour plaques of more than 15 mm in diameter (Griffiths and Fuller 1978). In such cases, interval debulking may be considered after three cycles of systemic chemotherapy (van der Burg 1995; DiSaia and Creasman 2002). This also applies to patients who could not, in lieu of physical fitness, undergo primary cytoreduction prior to chemotherapy. Such an approach is termed neoadjuvant or upfront cytoreductive chemotherapy. This does render operability to the presumed inoperable cases. In addition, it provides information about in vivo tumour sensitivity to the used carcinotherapeutic agents. The chemotherapy may dry up the effusions, improve the patient's performance status, and decrease postoperative morbidity. Survival of these patients treated with cytoreductive chemotherapy was found comparable to patients historically treated conventionally (Griffiths and Fuller 1978; Schwartz et al 1999). For adopting upfront chemotherapy, it is necessary that there is cytological or histopathological evidence of adenocarcinoma, at least sonographic information that it could be ovarian with extra-pelvic metastasis, and that serum CA125 levels are high.

Adjuvant chemotherapy: Patients who have had cytoreduction should receive adjuvant chemotherapy (Aabo et al 1998; DiSaia and Creasman 2002). Several combinations have been studied. Median and overall survival has improved, but the long-term survival rates have been disappointing. Thus, the priority is a more effective first-line therapy. For systemic chemotherapy, a combination of a Paclitaxel or Docetaxel with Carboplatin is the first choice. Docetaxel is considered because of its favourable neurotoxicity profile (Vasey 2002). It is hoped that gemicitabine, topotecan, doxorubicin, and prolonged use of etoposide will provide effective disease-free status.

Secondary cytoreduction: The term secondary cytoreductive surgery could be applied to cytoreductive operations performed on patients who have a recurrence after adequate initial surgery followed by complete first line chemotherapy. The term is also used by some authors to describe cytoreductive after-induction chemotherapy in patients in whom optimal cytoreductive surgery was not performed initially. Others use the name to describe tumour resections in patients who were partial responders on first-line therapy. It is preferable to restrict the use of term secondary cytoreductive surgery to those patients who undergo tumour debulking at the completion of the prescribed course of primary chemotherapy. In patients with residual lesions of more than 10 mm after primary cytoreductive surgery, secondary debulking significantly increases the progression-free and overall survival.

Second-look operation: The 'second-look' operation remains a technique for documenting response to therapy in those patients with ovarian cancer who are clinically free of disease at the time that reassessment is deemed necessary. A negative second-look operation is one that documents no pathologic evidence of persistent cancer, including all cytologic and histologic specimens. The achievement of a negative second-look is, unfortunately, no guarantee that the lesion will not recur. Indeed, the reported recurrence rates after negative second-look range from 12% to 30% over 1 to 2 years. There have been many trials studying the benefits of second-look operations. Patients who had residual disease at the end of chemotherapy treatment seem to benefit from second-look surgery while patients who were optimally debulked at initial diagnosis did not benefit. This strategy in the management of advanced ovarian cancer is therefore not considered standard (Nicoletto et al 1997; Hoskins et al 1989; Bertelsen 1990; Potter 1993). The principal value of the performance of second-look operation appears to determine when to discontinue therapy. However, if no subsequent therapy is planned, a case can be made for omission of the second-look surgery.

Laparoscopy in ovarian cancer: The role of the laparoscope in the management of patients with ovarian cancer is somewhat limited as of now. Possible uses for the procedure are for second-look in patients who either refuse a laparotomy or are considered medically unfit to undergo a laparotomy, for the follow-up of patients with neoplasms of low malignant potential, for the evaluation of patients with low-grade stage I tumours who have received no adjuvant therapy, and for certain patients on treatment protocols which require some operative documentation of response, particularly to second line therapies (Berek and Hacker 1983). Laparoscopy has been used immediately before a planned laparotomy. If gross disease is detected and secondary dissection of the tumour is not possible, a laparotomy can be omitted. Analysing the series which report the findings of laparotomy performed immediately following a laparoscopy, it is projected that laparoscopy was able to detect disease in only two-thirds of the patients with persistent disease (Lele and Piver 1986).

Maintenance chemotherapy: At the end of six cycles of chemotherapy, maintenance chemotherapy with Paclitaxel has been shown to improve disease-free interval but not overall survival (Markman et al 2003). However, this treatment must only be offered if a patient achieves complete response to treatment, and understands the aim of treatment and its potential toxicities. There is no consensus in prolonging the treatment after complete response. Systemic chemotherapy, external radiation, intraperitoneal chemotherapy, use of radioisotopes and use of novel approaches such as biological agents and radioimmunotherapy are all suggested as measures to consolidate the disease free status after the initial treatment. The role of intraperitoneal chemotherapy remains controversial.

MONITORING AFTER TREATMENT

There is no evidence to show that intensive clinical monitoring in asymptomatic women has any positive impact on overall survival or on the quality of life. Nonetheless, early diagnosis of recurrence after a prolonged progression free interval is thought to offer the best results. The objectives of follow-up could be to determine patient's immediate response to the treatment employed, early recognition and prompt management of any treatment-related complications, including any psychological sequelae and early detection of persistent or recurrent disease. In general, during the first year following treatment, patients should be seen every three months with a gradual increase in intervals to every four to six months and annually after the fifth year. At each follow-up, the patient should have her history retaken; complete physical examination (including breast, pelvic and rectal examination) performed to exclude any clinical signs of recurrence. The CA125 may also be checked at regular intervals. It is unclear as to the utility of such a practice on survival impact (Bast et al 1998). Radiological tests such as ultrasonography of the pelvis, CT scans or MRI scans should only be performed when the clinical findings or the tumour markers suggest possible recurrences. All patients with intact cervix should receive a regular pap smear. All patients above the age of 40 should undergo an yearly routine mammogram, as should younger patients with a strong family history of breast cancer.

The treatment of an asymptomatic patient with recurrent disease based on tumour marker alone is difficult. When CA125 rises to twice the upper limit of normal, close observation or hormonal therapy with agents such as tamoxifen can be considered (Hatch et al 1991). In the former situation, their treatment is deferred until clinical relapse. It is important that the patient understands that chemotherapy responses do not necessarily translate into meaningful survival prolongation. Often, improvement in quality of life and optimisation of functionality become the goals of treatment.

Management of recurrences: The majority of patients treated for advanced epithelial ovarian tumours will unfortunately relapse. Patients who had a disease-free interval of at least 6 months can be considered platinum sensitive and those patients whose disease-free interval is less than 6 months can be considered platinum refractory. Trials have also shown that the longer the platinum-free interval, the higher the response rate to further platinum, as well as non platinum treatment (Markman et al 1991; DiSaia and Creasman 2002). For patients who are platinum sensitive, Carboplatin or Cisplatin can be offered. Combination with other cytotoxic or non-cytotoxic agents may be preferable. But there are no randomised studies to suggest that combination therapy is superior to single agent platinum in terms of overall survival. Patients with localised recurrences after a long disease-free interval may benefit from a secondary cytoreduction. Repeat cytoreduction for this group of patients has hitherto been controversial.

The patients who are considered platinum refractory may be provided the option of further non-platinum chemotherapy. There are a number of choices for chemotherapy: liposomal doxorubicin, topotecan (Gordon et al 2001), etoposide (Hoskins and Swenerton 1994; Rose et al 1998) and gemcitabine (Shapiro et al 1996; Friedlander et al 1998) have all shown a response ranging between 10% and 15%, either as a single agent or in combination. There is a pressing need to evaluate the many biological or molecular-targeted agents such as inhibitors of angiogenesis (for example, the monoclonal antibody Bevacizimab), epidermal growth factor receptor tyrosine kinase inhibitors (for example, gefitinib, erlotinib, cetuximab) which are emerging rapidly from the pharmaceutical industry's drug development programmes.

Refractory ovarian cancer: The optimal management of a patient with refractory ovarian cancer requires careful assessment of the patient's physical, mental and spiritual condition. It is pertinent to identify any physical condition that may immediately affect a patient's survival or quality of life, so that adequate appropriate treatment can be given. Such physical conditions include systemic infections, intestinal obstruction, ascites, pleural effusion, and unusual metastases to organs such as the brain, liver or bone. The hitherto lack of quality of life and palliative index measurements in salvage chemotherapy treatment of these patients makes it difficult to recommend the best option. It is important to bear in mind the function of the bone marrow in the dosing of chemotherapy in patients who have had many lines of chemotherapy.

The prognosis for patients with epithelial ovarian cancer relates to several clinical variables such as the patient's age, tumour stage and tumour grade at the start of the chemotherapy, residual disease, status at second-look, patient performance status and above all, the tumour behaviour. One should remember that the patients in any particular stage do not behave as a homogenous group. They have different molecular biological characteristics. In the same vein, patients from different stages may have homogenous characteristics. To understand and manage malignant epithelial tumours, we need to know these molecular determinants.

Conclusions

- An attempt has been made to apply WHO screening criteria to ovarian cancer to assess the potential for early detection of the disease.
- Sequential multimodal screening (CA125 estimation and transvaginal sonography) has superior specificity and positive predictive value.
- Presence of normal ovarian tissue ('Ovarian Crescent Sign') and low score from any of the risk of malignancy indices will help to differentiate adnexal masses.
- Surgery is the cornerstone in all treatment modalities employed for ovarian cancers.
- The concept of cytoreductive surgery or debulking surgery is applicable in the management of ovarian cancer.
- In adequately staged patients with Stage IA and Stage IB Grade I disease, adjuvant chemotherapy would not provide further benefits.
- In the absence of high risk features, fertility sparing surgery may be an option for stage IA disease.
- Surgical resection of the primary tumour is the principal treatment of borderline tumours and there is no evidence that either subsequent chemotherapy or radiation therapy would improve survival.
- Epithelial ovarian tumours do not infiltrate the peritoneum or lumina of intestine and bladder deeply.
- Primary debulking surgery remains the cornerstone of treatment of epithelial ovarian carcinoma, survival of patients with an optimal primary cytoreductive surgery (taken as $<$ 5 to 15 mm of residual disease) being superior.
- All cases of advanced ovarian carcinoma should receive adjuvant chemotherapy which has a platinum-based combination.
- Induction chemotherapy can be considered in patients in whom optimal cytoreduction at primary laparotomy is considered to be impossible.
- Interval debulking in advanced ovarian cancer significantly increases the survival and progression free interval.
- The 'second-look' operation helps in documenting response to therapy in those patients with ovarian cancer who are clinically free of disease. But a negative second-look is, unfortunately, no guarantee that the lesion will not recur.
- The role of laparoscopy in the management of patients with ovarian cancer is somewhat limited to either for second-look or in advanced cases where surgery is not feasible, to avoid laparotomy.
- The treatment of an asymptomatic patient with recurrent disease based on tumour marker alone is difficult.
- Patients with relapse are managed based on disease free interval after primary platinum based chemotherapy.

References

Aabo K, M Adams, P Adnitt, DS Alberts, A Athanazziou, V Barley, DR Bell, U Bianchi et al. 1998. Chemotherapy in advanced ovarian cancer: Four systematic meta-analyses of individual patient data from 37 randomized trials. Advanced Ovarian Cancer Trialists' Group. *Br J Cancer* 78:1479–1487.

Andolf E, E Svalenius, B Astedt. 1986. Ultrasonography for early detection of ovarian cancer. *Br J Obstet Gynecol* 93:1286–1289

Bast RC Jr, FJ Xu, YH Yu, S Barnhill, Z Zhang, GB Mills. 1998. CA 125: The past and the future. *Int J Biol Markers* 13:179–187.

Bell DA. 1991. Ovarian surface epithelial stromal tumours. *Hum Pathol* 22:750–762.

Bell J, M Brady, J Lage, KY Look, N Spirtos, J Walker, GS Rose, RC Young. 2003. A Randomized Phase III Trial of Three versus Six Cycles of Carboplatin and Paclitaxel as Adjuvant Treatment in Early Stage Ovarian Epithelial Carcinoma: A Gynecologic Oncology Group Study. *Proceedings of 34th Annual Meeting of the Society of Gynecologic Oncologists*:Abstract 1:70.

Benedet JL, H Bender, H Jones III, HYS Ngan, S Pecorelli. 2000. Staging classifications and clinical practice guidelines of gynecologic cancers. *Int J Gynecol Obstet* 70:207–312.

Berek JS and NF Hacker 1983. Laparoscopy in the management of patients with ovarian carcinoma. In *Ovarian Cancer* ed. Alberts DS, Surwit EA:69, Boston: Martinus Nijhoff Publishers. ch. 5.

Berek JS and NF Hacker. 1987. Staging and second-look operations in ovarian cancer. In *Ovarian Malignancies–Diagnostic and Therapeutic Advances.* ed. Piver MS, 112. New York: Churchill Livingstone.

Berek JS and NF Hacker (eds). 2000. *Practical Gynecologic Oncology*, 3rd ed. Philadelphia: Lippincott Williams & Wilkins, 3–38.

Bertelsen K. 1990. Tumour reduction surgery and long-term survival in advanced ovarian cancer: A DACOVA study. *Gynecol Oncol* 38:203–209.

Boring CC, TS Squires, T Tong. 1994. Cancer statistics. *CA Cancer J Clin.* 44:7–26.

Bourne TH, S Campbell, KM Reynolds, MI Whitehead, J Hampson, P Royston, TJB Crayford, WP Collins. 1993. Screening for early familial ovarian cancer with transvaginal ultrasonography and colour blood flow imaging. *Br Med J* 306:1025–1029.

Buchsbaumm HJ and S Lifshitz. 1984. Staging and surgical evaluation of ovarian cancer. *Semin Oncol* 11:227.

Chang HW, SM Lee, SN Goodman, G Singer, SK Cho, LJ Sokoll, FJ Montz, R Roden et al. 2002. Assessment of plasma DNA levels, allelic imbalance, and CA 125 as diagnostic tests for cancer. *J Natl Cancer Inst* 94:1697–1703.

Cramer DW and WR Welch. 1983 Determinants of ovarian cancer risk. II. Inferences regarding pathogenesis. *J Natl Cancer Inst* 71:717.

Dembo AJ, M Davy, AE Stenwig, EJ Berle, RS Bush, K Kjorstad. 1990. Prognostic factors in patients with stage I epithelial ovarian cancer *Obstet Gynecol* 75:263–273.

DiSaia P and W Creasman. 2002. Epithelial Ovarian Cancer. In *Clinical Gynecologic Oncology,* ed P DiSaia, W Creasman, 6th Ed, New York: Mosby, 289–350.

Ferrazzi E, G Zanetta, D Dordoni, N Berlanda, R Mezzopane, G Lissoni. 1997. Transvaginal ultrasonographic characterization of ovarian masses: Comparison of five scoring systems in a multicenter study. *Ultrasound Obstet Gynecol* 10:192–197.

Friedlander M, MJ Millward, D Bell, R Bugat, P Harnett, JA Moreno, L Campbell, C Varette, V Ripoche, L Kayitalire. 1998. A phase II study of gemcitabine in platinum pre-treated patients with advanced epithelial ovarian cancer. *Ann Oncol* 9:1343–1345.

Fisher R and R Young. 1977 Advances in the staging and treatment of ovarian cancer. *Cancer* 39:967.

Fuller AF and CT Griffiths. 1979. Ovarian cancer cachexia, surgical interactions. *Gynecologic Oncology* 9:301–310.

Gordon AN, JT Fleagle, D Guthrie, DE Parkin, ME Gore, AJ Lacave. 2001. Recurrent epithelial ovarian carcinoma: A randomized phase III study of pegylated liposomal doxorubicin versus topotecan. *J Clin Oncol* 19:3312–3322

Griffiths CT. 1975. Surgical resection of tumour bulk in the primary treatment of ovarian carcinoma. *National Cancer Institute Monograph* 42:101–104.

Griffiths CT and AF Fuller. 1978. Intensive surgical and chemotherapeutic management of advanced ovarian cancer. *Surg Clin North Am* 58:131–142.

Hacker NF, JS Berek, ID Lagasse, RK Nieberg, RM Elashoff. 1983. Primary cytoreductive surgery for epithelial ovarian cancer. *Obstet Gynecol* 61:413–420.

Hatch KD, JB Beecham, JA Blessing, WT Creasman. 1991. Responsiveness of patients with advanced ovarian carcinoma to tamoxifen. A Gynecologic Oncology Group study of second-line therapy in 105 patients. *Cancer* 68:269–271.

Heintz AM, NF Hacker, JS Berek, TP Rose, AK Munoz, LD Lagasse. 1986. Cytoreductive surgery in ovarian carcinoma: Feasibility and morbidity. *Obstet Gynecol* 67:783–788.

Hillaby K, N Aslam, R Salim, A Lawrence, KS Raju, D Jurkovic. 2004. The value of detection of normal ovarian tissue (ovarian crescent sign) in the differential diagnosis of adnexal masses. *Ultrasound Obstet Gynecol* 23:63–67.

Hoskins PJ and KD Swenerton. 1994. Oral etoposide is active against platinum-resistant epithelial ovarian cancer. *J Clin Oncol* 12:60–63.

Hoskins WJ, SC Rubin, E Dulaney, D Chapman, L Almadrones, P Saigo, M Markman, T Hakes, B Reichman, WB Jones et al. 1989. Influence of secondary cytoreduction at the time of second-look laparotomy on the survival of patients with epithelial ovarian carcinoma. *Gynecol Oncol* 34:365–371.

Jacobs IJ and DH Oram.1990. Potential screening tests for ovarian cancer. In *Ovarian Cancer* ed. Sharp F, Mason WP, Leake RE London: Chapman and Hall Medical. 197–205.

Jacobs I, D Oram, J Fairbanks, J Turner, C Frost, JG Grudzinskas. 1990. A risk of malignancy index incorporating CA125, ultrasound and menopausal status for the accurate preoperative diagnosis of ovarian cancer. *Br J Obstet Gynecol* 97:922–929.

Kalghatgi K. 2006. Ovarian crescent sign: A sonological marker for ovarian malignancy. Dissertaion submitted to Manipal Academy of Higher Education.

Learner JP, IE Timor-Tritsch, A Federman, G Abramovich. 1994. Transvaginal ultrasonographic characterization of ovarian masses with an improved, weighted scoring system. *Am J Obstet Gynecol* 170:81–85.

Lele SB and MS Piver 1986. Interval laparoscopy prior to second look laparotomy in ovarian cancer *Obstet Gynecol* 68:345–347.

Markman M, R Rothman, T Hakes, B Reichman, W Hoskins, S Rubin, W Jones, L Almadrones, JL Lewis Jr. 1991. Second-line platinum therapy in patients with ovarian cancer previously treated with cisplatin. *J Clin Oncol* 9:389–393.

Markman M, PY Liu, S Wilczynski, B Monk, LJ Copeland, RD Alvarez, C Jiang, D Alberts. 2003. Phase III Randomized Trial of 12 versus 3 Months of maintenance after Paclitaxel in Patients with Advanced Ovarian Cancer Complete Response to Platinum and Paclitaxel-Based Chemotherapy: A Southwest Oncology Group and Gynecologic Oncology Group Trial. *J Clin Oncol* 21:2460–2465.

McFarlane C, MC Sturgis, FS Fetterman. 1955. Results of an experiment in the control of cancer of the female pelvic organs and report of fifteen year research. *Am J Obstet Gynecol* 69:294–299.

Mok SC, J Chao, S Skates, KK Wong, GK Yiu, MG Muto, RS Berkowitz, DW Crame. 2001. Prostacin: A potential serum marker for ovarian cancer. Identification through microarray technology. *J Natl Cancer Inst* 93:1458–1464.

Muralikrishna C, GD Sockalingam, L Venteo, P Kushtagi, RA Bhat, M Pluot, M Manfait. 2005. Evaluation of the suitability of ex vivo handled ovarian tissues for optical diagnosis by Raman Microspectroscopy. *Biopolymers* 79:269–276.

Neijt JP, WW ten Bokkel Huinink, ME van der Burg, AT van Oosterom, PH Willemse, JB Vermorken, AC van Lindert, AP Heintz, E Aartsen, M van Lent et al. 1991. Long-term survival in ovarian cancer. Mature data from The Netherlands Joint Study Group for Ovarian Cancer. *Eur J Cancer* 27:1367–1372.

Nicoletto MO, S Tumolo, R Talamini, L Salvagno, S Franceschi, E Visona, G Marin, Angelini et al. 1997. Surgical second look in ovarian cancer: A randomized study in patients with laparoscopic complete remission: A Northeastern Oncology Cooperative Group–Ovarian Cancer Cooperative Group Study. *J Clin Oncol* 15:994–999.

Omura GA, MF Brady, HD Homesley, E Yordan, FJ Major, HJ Buchsbaum, RC Park. 1991. Long-term follow-up and prognostic factor analysis in advanced ovarian carcinoma: The Gynecologic Oncology Group experience. *J Clin Oncol* 9:1138–1150.

Potter ME. 1993. Secondary cytoreduction in ovarian cancer: Pro or con? *Gynecol Oncol* 51:131–135.

Rose PG, JA Blessing, AR Mayer, HD Homesley. 1998. Prolonged oral etoposide as secondline therapy for platinum-resistant and platinum-sensitive ovarian carcinoma: A Gynecologic Oncology Group study. *J Clin Oncol* 16:405–410.

Petricoin III EF, AM Ardekani, BA Hitt, PJ Levine, VA Fusaro, SM Steinberg, GB Mills, C Simone, DA Fishman, EC Kohn, LA Liotta. 2002. Use of proteomic patterns in serum to identify ovarian cancer. *Lancet* 359:572–577.

Rosenthal A and I Jacobs. 1998. Ovarian cancer screening. *Semin Oncol* 25:315–325.

Sassone AM, IE Timor-Tritsch, A Artner, C Westhoff, WB Warren. 1991. Transvaginal sonographic characterization of ovarian disease: Evaluation of new scoring system to predict ovarian malignancy. *Obstet Gynecol* 78:70–76.

Schwartz PE, TJ Rutherford, JT Chambers, EI Kohorn, RP Thiel. 1999. Neoadjuvant chemotherapy for advanced ovarian cancer: Long-term survival. *Gynecol Oncol* 72:93–99.

Serov F, RE Scully, LH Sobin. 1973. Histological typing of ovarian tumours. International Classification of Tumours No 9. Geneva: World Health Organization.

Shapiro JD, MJ Millward, D Rischin, M Michael, V Walcher, PA Francis, GC Toner. 1996. Activity of gemcitabine in patients with advanced ovarian cancer: Responses seen following platinum and paclitaxel. *Gynecol Oncol* 63:89–93.

Silberman AW. 1982. Surgical debulking of tumours. *Surg Gynecol Obstet* 155:577–585.

Singh SK, RI Martis, Sujatha, RA Bhat, P Kushtagi, L Rai, VB Kartha, C Santhosh. 2006. Protein profile study of clinical samples of ovarian cancer using high-performance liquid chromatography-laser induced fluorescence (HPLC–LIF). In *Ultrasensitive and Single–Molecule Detection Technologies* eds. Jörg Enderlein, Zygmunt K. Gryczynski Proc. SPIE 6092, 149–157.

Skates SJ, FJ Xu, YH Yu, K Sjovall, N Einhorn, Y Chang, RC Bast Jr, Knapp RC. 1995. Toward an optimal algorithm for ovarian cancer screening with longitudinal tumour markers. *Cancer* 76: 2004–2010.

Tingulstad S, B Hagen, FE Skjeldestad, M Onsrud, T Kiserud, T Halvorsen and K Nustad 1996. Evaluation of a risk of malignancy index based on serum CA125, ultrasound findings and menopausal status in the pre-operative diagnosis of pelvic masses. *Br J Obstet Gynecol* 103:826–831.

Tingulstad S, B Hagen, FE Skjeldestad, T Halvorsen, K Nustad, M Onsrud. 1999. The risk of malignancy index to evaluate potential ovarian cancers in local hospitals. *Obstet Gynecol* 93:448–452.

UK Collaborative Trial of Ovarian Cancer Screening www.ukctocs.org.uk

US Preventive Services Task Force. *Screening for Ovarian Cancer: Brief Evidence Update.* May 2004. Agency for Healthcare Research and Quality, Rockville, MD. http://www.ahrq.gov/clinic/3rduspstf/ovariancan/ovcanup.htm

van der Burg ME, M van Lent, M Buyse, A Kobierska, N Colombo et al. 1995. The effect of debulking surgery after induction chemotherapy on the prognosis in advanced epithelial ovarian cancer. Gynecological Cancer Cooperative Group of the European Organization for Research and Treatment of Cancer. *N Engl J Med* 332:629–34.

Vasey PA. 2002. On behalf of the Scottish Gynecological Cancer Trials Group, CRC Trials Unit Glasgow, UK. Survival and longer-term toxicity results of the SCOTROC study: Docetaxel-carboplatin (DC) vs. paclitaxel-carboplatin(PC) in epithelial ovarian cancer (EOC). *ASCO Proceedings of the American Society of Clinical Oncology* Abstract 804.

Woolas RP, FJ Xu, IJ Jacobs, YH Yu, L Daly et al. 1993. Elevation of multiple serum markers in patients with stage I ovarian cancer. *J Natl Cancer Inst* 85:1748–751.

Xu FJ, YA Yu, L Daly, K DeSombre et al. 1993. OVX1 radioimmunoassay compliments CA125 for predicting the presence of residual ovarian carcinoma at second look surgical surveillance procedures. *J Clin Oncol* 11:1506–1510.

Xu Y, Z Shen, DW Wiper, M Wu et al. 1998. Lysophosphatidic acid as a potential biomarker for ovarian and other gynecologic cancers. *JAMA* 280:719–723.

Young RC, LA Walton, SS Ellenberg, HD Homesley et al. 1990. Adjuvant therapy in stage I and stage II epithelial ovarian cancer: Results of two prospective randomized trials. *N Engl J Med* 322:1021–1027.

Young RC, CA Perez, WJ Hoskins. 1993. Cancer of the ovary In *Cancer: Principles and Practice of Oncology,* ed. VT DeVita, S Hellman, SA Rosenberg, 4th ed. Philadelphia: JB Lippincott Co.

23

Role of Chemotherapy in Epithelial Ovarian Cancers

Rakesh Kapoor

Ovarian cancer is the leading cause of death among all gynecological cancers and is the fifth most common cancer among women in the United States. Despite the advances in surgical and chemotherapeutic management of this disease, the five-year survival rate for woman with Stage III/IV epithelial ovarian cancer has remained as low as 12% over the past thirty years.

Even though aggressive surgery remains the cornerstone in the management of ovarian cancers, the chances of relapse following surgery alone are high. Thus, further management includes adjuvant therapy in all but a small proportion of patients. In recent years, the role of chemotherapy has been more firmly established in this neoplasm. Anticancer medication can eradicate primary disease and possibly sterilise micrometastasis.

Therationalebehindtheuseofchemotherapy is to treat gross or micrometastasis within or outside the peritoneal cavity. Chemotherapy can be used as single agent/multidrug therapy. There has been a significant amount of research on epithelial ovarian cancer in the recent past, probably as a result of factors such as the following:

- Its occurrence in a population that is at the peak of productivity (age 40–60 years)
- Its general responsiveness to therapy suggests curability and
- The standard treatment for advanced ovarian cancer is still suboptimal in terms of long-term survival.

A minority of patients with ovarian cancer present with early disease (Stage I and II). Most of these patients are offered some form of adjunctive therapy postoperatively, because there will be a recurrence of approximately 40%, after surgery alone.

The majority of patients, however, present with advanced disease (Stage III and IV). These patients usually succumb after an initial encouraging response, followed by the emergence of resistance clones and clinical progression. A small subgroup of patients fail primary therapy and these patients with primary drug resistance present an even greater challenge. The current chemotherapy approach to primary treatment of epithelial ovarian tumour of all stages is discussed in detail. Chemotherapy options commonly used in epithelial ovarian tumour could be as single agents or in combination with chemotherapy

Useful single agents for ovarian cancer

- Cisplatin

- Carboplatin
- Paclitaxel
- Docetaxel
- Cyclophosphamide
- Doxorubicin
- Epirubicin
- Ifosfamide
- Chlorambucil
- Melphalan
- Treosulfan
- Altretamine (Hexamethylmelamine)

Combination chemotherapy

- Cisplatin with cyclophosphamide (CC)
- Cisplatin with cyclophosphamide with Doxorubicin (CAP)
- Paclitaxel with cisplatin/carboplatin
- Ifosfamide with cisplatin/carboplatin

Alkylating Agents

The alklylating agents were the first drugs used as chemotherapy for ovarian malignancy. They act by forming a highly reactive ammonium ion binding to the 7-nitrogen group of the nucleic acid guanine. This causes a miscoded base pair resulting in intrastrand and interstrand DNA cross-linking between guanine pairs and the breakage of DNA strands. Early studies showed the use of single agent alkylating agents usually given orally (melphalan, altretamine) or their use in combination therapy. In untreated patients, the response rate was 40% with a median survival of 12 to 14 months. Overall survival was 50% at five years (Neijt et al 1984). European clinicians still consider them to be appropriate agents, particularly if given by mouth, for those elderly or frail patients who cannot easily travel to the cancer centre for intravenous chemotherapy or tolerate the toxicity of more aggressive therapy. The most commonly prescribed drugs are melphalan, chlorambial, altretamine and treosulphan (Masding 1988). They are given orally, their main toxicity being myelosuppression which can be cumulative and prolonged. Currently, intravenous alkalating agents are more widely used with cyclophosphamide or ifosfamide (Sultton et al 1989), the preferred agent, usually in combination with a platinum analogue (Gallghar et al 1989).

Cyclophosphamide: This is a chemical derivative of mechlorethamine synthesised in Germany in 1958. It was developed as a highly alkylating agent that could be activated preferentially by tumour-associated intracellular enzymes. Cyclophosphamide acts as a classic alkylating agent resulting in apoptosis (Meyn et al 1994; Naruse et al 1994). Myelosuppression and hemorrhagic cystitis are the usual forms of dose limiting toxicity with standard doses. Cyclophosphamide is available as oral tablets as 25 or 50 mg, or as lyophilised or non-lyophilised powder for intravenous administration (100, 200, 500 mg and 1 and 2 g). Oral dose: Continuous therapy with single agent cyclophosphamide is 1 to 2.5 mg/kg/day in divided doses.

Intravenous dose: 40 to 50 mg/kg divided over a point of 2 to 5 days with concomitant intravenous hydration (500–1000 ml of normal saline).

Ifosfamide was synthesised in the mid-1960s in West Germany as an isomer of cyclophosphamide in which one chloroethyl group is present on each of the nitrogen atoms. Initial preclinical studies of the drug demonstrated severe dose-limiting unothelial toxicity. However, the use of ifosfamide with the radical scavenger, mesna, has led to a renaissance of interest in the drug (Zulpoln and Balker 1988).

The mechanism of action of ifosfamide is presumed to be identical to that of cyclophosphide. Mesna decreases the urotoxicity of ifosfamide, prior or concurrent use of cisplatin may increase the neurotoxicity or nephrotoxicity of the drug (Pratt et al 1990; Rossi et al 1994). Sedation, such as lorazepam and opiates, may potentiate the neurotoxicity of ifosfamide. Methylene blue may be an antidote for cerebral toxicity due to ifosfamide (Kupfer et al 1994). Ifosfamide is available in 1 and 3 g vials package with 200 mg and 400 mg ampoules of Mesna. Dose is 1.2 g/m^2 slow intravenous infusion over at least 30 minutes daily for four days. Ifosfamide is given with 2L of hydration per day plus Mesna.

Melphalan: A phenylalamine derivative of mechlorelteamine, was synthesised by Bergel and Stock in 1955. It is available for oral or intravenous administration.

Oral: Absorption of melphalan is erratic with bioavailability varying from 32% to 100%. The time of peak plasma levels is about six hours, 2 mg tablets are available for oral use prescribed with a dose of 0.25 mg/kg/day for four to five days repeated, four-weekly intervals.

For intravenous use: Dose is 16 mg/m^2 over 15–20 minutes, four weekly, for 4–6 doses.

Toxicity: The major dose-limiting toxicity of melphalan is reversible myelosuppression, GI toxicity, and other rare reactions such as hypersensitivity, mucositis skin ulceration in the area of intravenous drug extravasation, vasculitis, pulmonary fibrosis, hyperuricemia, cataract, infertility and carcinogenicity.

Chlorambucil, an aromatic derivative of mechlorethamine, was developed at the Chester Beauty Research Institute in England. It is the slowest acting, and generally, least toxic of the alkylating agents in common use. The mechanism of action and side effects are similar to mechlorethanamine. The dose is 2 mg orally. The desired effect is usually achieved in 3–6 weeks; thereafter, maintenance therapy with 2–4 mg/day is continued.

Altratamine was originally synthesised as a derivative of melamine. It is a synthetic S-triazime derivative that functions as a non-classic alkylating agent but the precise mechanism of action is unknown.

It is also known as hexamethylmelamine. Altretamine has a wide spectrum of antitumour activity in humans (Foster et al 1986). The drug is non-toxic in itself and requires conversion to the active metabolites of pentamethyl melamine and tetramethyl melamine. Absorption is variable after oral administration. It is used as a single agent for the palliative treatment of recurrent or persistent ovarian cancer failing front line therapy with alkylating agents.

Side effects are mild to moderate neutropenia, nausea with or without emesis, anorexia, peripheral neuropathy and CNS reactions. The dose consisting of 50 mg capsules (260 mg/m^2/day in four divided oral doses) is given for two weeks in a 28-day cycle.

Platinum Compounds

In the late 1970s, platinum drugs were found to have high activity in ovarian disease. Cisplatin was the first to be used, followed by its analogue, carboplatin. Cisplatin was found to produce a 60% objective response rate. Complete response was seen in 20%–40% of patients (Wiltshaw et al 1986). The importance of cisplatin was summarised in a meta-analysis of 45 randomised trials that compared primary treatment with regimens containing this agent, with a regimen that did not include cisplatin (Stewart 1991).

Cisplatin (Cis-diamine dichloroplatinum II): Cisplatin is an inorganic complex formed by an atom of platinum-II surrounded by chlorine and ammonia atoms in the cis position of the horizontal plane. In plasma, the cisplatin complex is thought to be un-ionised, thus allowing passage of drug into cells. Inside the cell, chloride concentration is low; water displaces the chloride ligands of the complex, forming positively charged platinum complexes that are highly reactive. These complexes inhibit DNA synthesis to a much greater extent than RNA synthesis or protein synthesis.

Toxicity: Vomiting, renal dysfunction, and mild to moderate peripheral neuropathy are the predominant form of toxicity at standard doses. Patients receiving high doses of cisplatin have myelosuppression and severe neuropathy.

The lower dose is 50 mg/m^2 infusion in two hours, the high dose 100–120 mg/m^2 infused over 2–6 hours with large volumes of fluid repeated every three to four weeks.

Carboplatin: This was developed at the Michigan State University to develop cisplatin analogues that might retain efficacy but will have reduced toxicity. Carboplatin appears to have the same spectrum of anti-tumour activity as cisplatin, but with a very different spectrum of toxicity. The choice of platinum analogue is usually based on the type of tumour, the intent of treatment and the pharmacologic characteristics of other drugs used in the treatment regimen (Lokich and Anderson 1998). Carboplatin and cisplatin are considered to share the same mechanism of cytotoxicity.

Toxic effects are similar to those of cisplatinum, but are much less severe. Dose-related cumulative myelosuppression, anaphylaxis and vomiting can occur; a high dose of carboplatin may, in rare cases, cause multi-organ failure.

Iproplatin is a platinum analogue that reportedly lacked cross-resistance with other platinum compounds, used in treatment of refractory ovarian cancers. Administration of iproplatin was limited by hematological toxicity. Response rates for iproplatin in untreated patients were similar for cisplatin and carboplatin.

Taxanes: In the 1980s, the taxanes were shown to possess significant activity against platinum resistant ovarian cancers. Based on their experience, two Phase-III randomised trials assigned patients with suboptimally resected Stage III and IV ovarian cancer, to one of two combined chemotherapy combinations and showed that there was statistically significant high objective response rate and improved progression free and overall survival with paclitaxel plus cisplatin combination (McGuirexel et al 1996; Piccart et al 2000).

Paclitaxel is a complex plant alkaloid derived from the bark of the Pacific yew tree (*Taxus brevifolia*). It was discovered in late 1960s by the National Cancer Institute, USA. The drug is highly lipophilic and is insoluble in water; it is therefore provided in solution with polyoxyethylated castor oil. The drug is the first among a new class of agents, the taxanes (Rowinsky et al 1990). Paclitaxel is also known as taxol and NSC-125973.

Paclitaxel is a microtubule inhibitor that works by stabilising intracellular microtubules in susceptible cells (Rowinsky et al 1990; Matsuoka et al 1994; Amos and Lowe 1999). This stabilisation of microtubules leads ultimately to apoptosis.

Toxicities include myelosuppression, hypersensitivity reactions and neuropathy. The hypersensitivity reactions require pretreatment proplylaxis with corticosteroids, diphenhydramine and a H_2-receptor antagonist. The dose is 135 mg/m² or 175 mg/m² for three or four hours, every 21 days.

MANAGEMENT OF EARLY STAGE DISEASE (I AND II)

Only 20%–25% of women with ovarian cancer present with early stage disease, so clinical research in this area has been limited by low patient number.

A study initiated by the Gynecological Oncology Group (GOG) in the early 1970s, for Stage I disease compared to postoperative therapy, postoperative pelvic radiation therapy and 18 months of phenyl alamine mustard (0.2 mg/kg once a day for five days every 28 days). The total number of patients was 100 and was not staged by present standards. Survival comparisons between any of two groups were not statistically significant—the group that received radiation therapy had the poorest outcome and the group that received chemotherapy did significantly better than the other two groups combined.

The important information generated by this study was a better understanding of differences in prognosis for the subgroup of patients with early stage disease. Patients with high-grade tumour and extension of tumour through the capsule that caused adherence to peritoneal structure were found to have a high relapse rate (20%–35%), while patients with low-grade tumour and tumour confined to the ovary displayed greater than 90% disease-free survival at five years. Although this study did not help define optimal therapy for early stage disease, it did help to delineate two groups of patients with early disease that have been handled separately in many subsequent treatment protocols.

The studies conducted in the 1980s included detailed staging, which made the groups relatively homogenous and easier to compare.

Two national trials were initiated (Young et al 1990). The first, which included 81 patients, evaluated no postoperative therapy versus chronic oral phenylalamine mustard (0.2 mg/kg/day to 5 mg every four to six weeks for 12 months) in patients with stage IA or IB tumours, Grades 1 and 2. With a median follow-up of more than seven years, no significant differences were seen in the outcome. Disease-free survival and survival were predicted to be in excess of 90% in both groups. Because of the risks of alkylating agent induced leukemia in the treated group and the excellent survival demonstrated in both groups, this study suggests no postoperative therapy for low-grade Stage I disease.

In the second-trial, 141 patients with poorly differentiated stage IA, IB, IC or II tumours of all grades were randomised to phenylalamine mustard, as above, versus a single dose of intreperitoneal ^{32}P (15 mCi). Again, no significant differences were observed between the two groups for five-year DFS or overall survival, both being about 80%.

About 30%–45% of patients from this study are expected to have recurrence; review of prognostic factors does not allow the selection of favourable and non-favourable groups for study. As ^{32}P is less toxic and easier to administer than melphalan, the standard of care for patients with early stage is held by many to be ^{32}P, although the authors made no recommendation for one therapy over the other.

In these two trials, a significant number of patients with borderline ovarian tumours were included. These tumours have an indolent natural history and may show favourable prognosis for survival (Massad et al 1991). Additionally, no prospective trials have compared ^{32}P to no therapy in high-risk, low-grade patients, and the acceptance of ^{32}P as the standard is thus based on comparisons to historical controls in which 30%–45% of such patients failed after surgery alone. These historical control patients, however, often were not staged according to modern standards. Many have been understaged, and they may have had significantly different pretreatment prognostic factors that make these comparisons less than optimal.

Current protocol: Trials performed in the past fifteen years by the gynecologic oncology group identified the platinum/taxane combination as optimal and the backbone to treat chemonaive ovarian cancer (These are patients who have a recurrence after initial complete surgical resection of low-risk stage I disease, about 10%, who have undergone surgical resection only and will have received no prior systemic therapy; hence, they are classified as chemonaive).

In early ovarian cancer, the similarity in efficacy of the treatment employed (7601, 7602), the lack of control arms (7602, 95, 157), and the less than anticipated effect of platinum-based therapy must call into question the value of any therapy in this population. Nevertheless, the GOG has assumed that the therapy is beneficial and will continue to pursue therapy in all patients considered at high risk for recurrence (stage IC and high grade stage IA or IB patient). Only those patients with low-risk disease are recommended to have no postoperative therapy. Future studies in high-risk disease will likely use a platinum/Ttxane backbone and explore angiogenesis inhibitors.

Ongoing trials in Europe are addressing the relative value of therapy versus observation—results are awaited. Finally, when one compares all studies in early ovarian cancer, it becomes clear that our ability to separate patients into different risk groups is far from adequate as best evidenced by the recent Italian study in which disease-free survival (DFS) was similar in the intermediate- and high-risk groups. A better staging system is needed and could incorporate molecular markers and ploidy, which is prognostic and more reproducible than current descriptive staging and grading systems.

Disease of low stage confined to one or both ovaries with no evidence of capsular invasion (Ia/Ib, G, G_2) should be treated with surgery alone—the five-year survival rates are in excess of 85%.

In a study by GOG in 81 patients, no adjuvant treatment was compared to oral intermittent melpharlan for a total course of 12. The GOG trial (n = 81) observation is:

Oral melphalan showed a five-year DFS of 91%–98% and a five-year overall survival of 94%–98% at a median follow-up of six years. Only six deaths have been reported in 81 patients, four in the observation group and two in the group receiving melphalan.

Patients with preoperative cyst rupture, penetration of the capsule or poorly differentiated histology might benefit from adjuvant chemotherapy (Young et al 1990).

Clinicopathologic factors currently used by GOG to define unfavourable prognosis in the early stage include FIGO stage II, IcG3, clear cell histology disease and tumour adhesions. In a study by Bolus et al (1995) with 85 patients, observation versus cisplatin for six cycles showed five-year DFS of 65% and 82% in both the groups, whereas the five-year overall survival was 83% and 88% respectively with a p value of 0.021 and 0.773. There has been an improvement in the five-year DFS (65% vs 82%), but there is no difference in overall survival.

The author's study by EORTC–ACTION (2003 trial) included 448 patients of early stage disease (IA, IB G2 G3, IC, IIA).

These patients were either kept on observation or received platinum-based chemotherapy. The five-year DFS was 68% versus 75%, whereas overall five-year survival was 76% versus 85%, respectively, in both the groups. It is apparent that the optimum postoperative treatment for patients with early stage ovarian cancer with unfavourable prognostic factors remains to be established.

MANAGEMENT OF ADVANCED-STAGE DISEASE (STAGE III AND IV)

In the majority of patients present with advanced disease (Stage III and IV), systemic chemotherapy forms the cornerstone of successful management of advanced disease.

In advanced ovarian cancer, Stage III patients are sub-classified based on the amount of postoperative residual disease, because this factor has been shown to be prognostic for outcome in multiple studies and multivariate analyses performed on large populations (Hoskins and Rubin 1991). Additional factors found to be prognostic indicators for a positive outcome include low tumour grade (Neijt et al 1991), young age, good performances status, absence of ascitis, cell type other than mucinous or clear cell and treatment with cisplatinum (van Houwelingen et al 1989; Marsoni et al 1990; Omura et al 1991; Neijt et al 1991).

Contemporary studies use 1 cm residual mass size as the breakpoint between optimally and sub-optimally cytoreduced patient within Stage III, while studies performed prior to 1995 usually used 2 to 3 cm as the breakpoint. Its effect on outcome must be considered when studies from different time periods are compared.

Patients with optimally debulked Stage III disease rarely have measurable tumour at the completion of staging laboratory. With the exception of few patients whose disease progresses during therapy, determination of response usually depends on findings at second-look laparotomy.

As with most tumours, the attainment of a complete pathologic response may result in 'cure' of advanced ovarian cancer. Patients with persistent disease after primary therapy are rarely alive three years later. Progression-free survival or overall survival has been used to measure the effectiveness of primary therapy. Cisplatin-based combination therapy is more effective in the initial treatment of ovarian cancer than single agent alkylating agents (Williams et al 1995) or combination without cisplatin (Neijt et al 1984; Omura et al 1986).

This improvement in efficacy, applies only to response rates and possibly to DFS. No significant impact on long-term survival has been noted, perhaps because of the frequent use of platinum compounds as salvage therapy in patients who fail non-platinum regimens. About 30%–40% of patients with disease that is refractory to standard alkylating agents will respond to cisplatin for long periods and with prolongation of survival. In the era of primary therapy with cisplatin combinations, response rates have risen to 70%–80% (20%–50% complete pathological response). The greatest activity is noted in patients who are optimally cytoreduced. Combination chemotherapy has replaced single drug therapy. The first study that showed significant benefit of the multiagent chemotherapy as compared to single agent was the Gynecology Oncology group trial.

In patients with bulky advanced disease, the GOG protocol compared melphalan alone to melphalan plus haxanethylmelamine or to doxorubicin plus cyclophosphamide. The only statistically significant difference observed was a greater complete response rate in those treated with doxorubicin plus cyclophosphamide as compared to melphalan alone (32% versus 20%) (Omura et al 1983).

Subsequently, studies have addressed the issue of adjuvant chemotherapy in patients with minimal residual disease and also aggressive chemotherapy in advanced disease. The three-drug regimen cyclophosphamide, adriamycin and cisplatin has been compared to the two-drug regimen (adriamycin plus cyclophosphamide [CAP vs AC]). Cisplatin-based chemotherapy (cisplatin plus cyclophosphamide or standard three-drug CAP regimen) is now considered the ideal schedule in ovarian cancer. Evidence suggests that cisplatin may have improved the five-year survival in epithelial ovarian cancers by 10% (Neijt et al 1991).

Conclusion: Chemotherapeutic management of epithialial ovarian tumours has evolved with better understanding of surgical staging, identification of optimal debulking and molecular genetics. Though it may appear difficult to lay down standard guidelines for individual patients, certain conclusions have been formulated from trials on different group of patients.

FIRST-LINE CHEMOTHERAPY

The benefit of adjuvant chemotherapy in Stage IA or IB with a well- or moderately differentiated tumour is controversial, since the five-year survival rates following surgery are in the range of 91%–98% (Kumar et al 1996).

Patients with poorly differentiated Stage IA or IB, IC and any Stage II, high risk early stage ovarian carcinoma, are considered for postoperative adjuvant therapy (Gerhenson and McGuire 1998).

Cisplatin-based chemotherapy is the preferred treatment choice. Six cycles of cisplatin and cyclophosphosphamide are given at three-weekly intervals. Chiara et al, observed 61% relapse-free survival and 76% overall survival rate at seven years (Redman et al 1993).

Radiation therapy has also been compared with cisplatin-based chemotherapy in early ovarian cancer patients. In a randomised study, patients received either five cycles of cisplatin or whole abdomen radiotherapy (WAR) by 'moving strip technique'. There was no difference in the five-year survival between both arms, 62% versus 58% (Cannistra 1993). Presently, all high-risk patients in the early stage of ovarian carcinoma are treated by cisplatin-based adjuvant chemotherapy. In some institutes, paclitaxel is combined with cisplatin for stage IIB and IIC (Gerhenson and McGuire 1998).

The greatest number of studies, related to chemotherapy in ovarian cancer, has been carried out in Stage III and IV disease. The overall survival of these patients depends upon the stage and amount of residual disease after surgery. Improvement in surgical therapy has resulted in more patients without measurable tumour. Patients with Stage III disease who have less than 1–2 cm residuum have a four-year survival rate of 30%. Patients with Stage IV or those suboptimally debulked Stage III ovarian cancer have a long-term survival rate of approximately 10% (Cannistra 1993).

Indiana University evaluated the three-drug combination of cisplatin, adriamycin and cyclophosphamide as first-line chemotherapy in Stage III and IV cancer. They reported a complete remission (CR) rate of 37% in 35 evaluable patients with an overall response rate of 68.5%. This series was updated in 1983 and the overall response rate was reported to be 82% (Ehrlich et al 1983).

A meta-analysis of 1194 patients has demonstrated a survival benefit of 7% at six years for the PAC (cisplatin-doxorubicin-cyclophosphamide) regimen as compared to PC (AOCTG 1991).

During the last fifteen years or more, advanced ovarian cancer has been treated with platinum-based regimens. Several trials have shown that extending treatment with cisplatin-based combination chemotherapy from six to twelve cycles has only increased toxicity with no improvement in progression-free survival (PFS) or overall survival (Hakes et al 1992).

Other studies have examined the role of cisplatin dose intensity in ovarian cancer. Retrospective reviews of 33 trials suggested that greater dose intensity may be associated with superior outcome. But prospective phase III trials failed to reveal an advantage for increasing cisplatin dose intensity beyond 75 mg/m^2 (McGuire et al 1995).

Since the mid-1990s, paclitaxel has been introduced into the chemotherapy schedule GOG of USA randomised trial of 386 patients of Stages III and IV to paclitaxel and cisplatin versus cisplatin and cyclophosphamide. The paclitaxel group showed better response rate (73% versus 60%) ($P = 0.01$) and improved median survival (38 months versus 24 months) (McGuire et al 1999). However, it has been opined that survival data from the paclitaxel study is still not mature and it may take another decade of comparison with cisplatin (Gerhenson and McGuire 1998). Epithelial ovarian cancers are highly drug sensitive and approximately 60% to 80% of patients will achieve an objective response to a cisplatin-based chemotherapy regimen. Unfortunately, complete clinical remission is not tantamount to a cure and approximately 50% of advanced ovarian cancer will relapse within 1–2 years after treatment. Though, second-line treatment may show clinical response, survival for these patients is usually less than 12 months (after relapse).

A multiplicity of biologic, pharamacologic and biochemical factors are likely to interact to limit the effectiveness of chemotherapeutic agents in ovarian cancer, thus opening the door to second-line drugs.

SECOND-LINE CHEMOTHERAPY

Despite the good response to first-line treatment, patients still have a 40%–50% chance of disease relapse within two years. Two distinct groups of patients are identified. The first group consists of those who originally responded to platinum and had PFS (progression-free survival) of at least six months, these patients can be successfully retreated with platinum compounds—their response rate will depend on the initial disease-free interval (Markman et al 1991).

The second group are the patients who show earlier relapse from platinum based combination chemotherapy at less than six months or have true platinum refractory disease. The only effective cytotoxic agents available for these patients are ifosfamide and paclitaxel which show RR > 15%. Ifosfamide has limited activity of 12% in platinum resistant patients and 20% in patients who showed a response to first-line therapy. This includes patients who received cyclophosphamide as first-line treatment (Markman et al 1992a). Long-term low-dose etoposide has shown some activity in platinum resistant ovarian cancer and may be useful palliative therapy (Markman et al 1992b).

Newer Drugs

A number of new drugs are undergoing evaluation in advanced ovarian cancer.

These are docetaxel, camptothecane and gemcitabine.

Docetaxel: In trials involving hundreds of patients, docetaxel has shown similar activity to paclitaxel but with greater toxicity that is, peripheral edema, pleural effusion, skin and nail toxicity and lethargy (Francis et al 1994).

Comptothecans (Kundella et al 1993): Topotecan is a new topoisomerase I inhibitior. Various studies indicate that it is active in refractory ovarian cancer with an RR of 14%. Dose limiting toxicity in myelo-suppressive neutropenia and thrombocytopenia; other side effects are mild; the drug is well tolerated, and similar response rates are seen with irinotecan.

Gemcitabine: A pyrimidine analogue showed an objective response rate of 23% in 45 treated patients of ovarian cancer with an average duration of five months.

In this study, there seemed to be a lack of cross resistance with platinum (Lund et al 1993).

INTRAPERITONEAL CHEMOTHERAPY IN OVARIAN CANCER

One of the main routes of dissemination of ovarian cancer is via the transcelomic route; it is therefore logical that attempts have been made to target drugs in relatively high concentrations via the intraperitoneal route.

Large volumes are required for homogeneous drug distribution and even this gives a tumour penetration of 1 to 2 mm only. Drugs which are ideally suited for intraperitoneal use are those with large molecules which will not be readily cleared, and are less likely to diffuse into the tumour deposits. In addition, the recognition of significant intraperitoneal disease in the pelvic and para-arotic lymph nodes has dampened initial enthusiasm to this approach (Lorigan et al 1996).

Markman reviewed the role of intraperitoneal therapy in ovarian cancer—there have been numerous Phase I and II trials of intraperitoneal therapy using drugs such as methotrexate, 5 FU; doxorubicin, cisplatin, carboplatin and paclitaxel. The widest experience is with intraperitoneal cisplatin and from these trials, two conclusions have been reached:

1. Intraperitoneal chemotherapy is unlikely to be beneficial to patients who have other than small amounts of disease, since drug penetration into larger tumour nodules is limited (Ozols et al 1999). In Sloan Kettering, there was complete response rate to intraperitoneal chemotherapy in patients with microscopic disease in 4%, compared to 5% complete response rate in patients who had tumour nodules greater than 1 cm (Markman et al 1991).
2. The patients who are resistant to intravenous cisplatin could not be successfully treated by intraperitoneal platinum. There was a 33% surgically documented complete response rate to salvage intraperitoneal cisplatin in patients who had shown prior response to intravenous cisplatin, in those who had failed to respond to prior systemic therapy, there was only a 3% response to intraperitoneal drug delivery (Markman et al 1991).

Current trials: GOG/SWOG study initiated in 1985 studied the role of IP chemotherapy as initial therapy in optimal Stage III disease patients. These 600 patients were treated with intraperitoneal or intravenous cisplatin; all patients also received intravenous cyclophosphamide.

Surgically defined complete response rate

for intraperitoneal patients was 47% compared to 36% for those receiving intravenous cisplatin. The median survival was 49 months compared to 41 months.

There was no obvious advantage for intraperitoneal therapy in patients with microscopic disease. This study did not alter general practice as the control arm consisted of patients taking intravenous cyclophosphamide and cisplatin which is no longer considered standard therapy (Alberts et al 1996).

Standard CCT (concomitant chemotherapy) for previously untreated patients is paclitaxel with a platinum compound (McGuire and Ozols 1998).

Another GOG trial (protocol 114) studied 523 patients. The study was randomised to treatment with six courses of intravenous cisplatin (75 mg/m^2) plus paclitaxel (135 mg/m^2) or to an experimental arm which consisted of two courses of carboplatin followed by six cycles of intraperitoneal cisplatin with intravenous paclitaxel (135 mg/m^2). Patients in the experimental arm had statistically significant improvement in recurrence-free survival (27.6 months vs 22.5 months), but no significant improvement in overall survival. The intraperitoneal arm was associated with myelotoxicity, without any improvement in overall survival. Modest improvement seen could be due to two cycles of high dose carboplatin (Markman and Bundy 1998).

Another trial of intraperitoneal therapy was in patients with <1 cm stage III disease; the control arm consisted of six cycles of intravenous cisplatin with paclitaxel; the experimental arm consisted of intravenous paclitaxel on day 1 and intraperitoneal platinum on day 2 and intraperitoneal paclitaxel on day 8.

In Phase II trials, patients were treated with intraperitoneal paclitaxel 60 mg/m^2 weekly for 16 weeks. It was well tolerated—of 28 patients, 17 (61%) achieved a surgically confirmed complete response, only 3% achieved complete response (Markman et al 1992).

Thus, intraperitoneal therapy has no established role in the treatment of patients with advanced ovarian cancer. It does play two major roles—as part of consolidation treatment and as part of initial therapy. Until such trials are completed, its role should be considered investigational.

References

Advanced Ovarian Cancer Trialists Group (AOCTG). 1991. Chemotherapy in advanced ovarian cancer. An overview of randomized clinical trials. *Br Med J* 303:884–893.

Alberts DS, PY Lui, EV Hannigan et al. 1996. Intraperitoneal cisplatin plus intravenous cyclophosphamide versus intravenous cisplatin plus intravenous cyclophosphamide for stage III ovarian cancer. *N Engl J Med* 335:1950–1955.

Amos LA and J Lowe. 1999. How Taxol stabilizes microtubule structure. *Chem Biol* 6:R65–69.

Cannistra SA. 1993. Cancer of the ovary. *New Engl J Med* 329:1550–1559.

Ehrlich GE, L Einhorn, F Stehman et al. 1983. Treatment of advanced epithelial ovarian cancer using cisplatin, adriamycin and cytoxan. The Indiana University experience. *Clin Obstet Gynecol* 10:325.

Foster BJ, BJ Harding, B Leyland-Jones, D Hoth. 1986. Hexamethylmelamine: A critical review of an active drug. *Cancer Treat Rev* 13:187–217.

Francis P, J Shneides, L Hann et al. 1994. Phase-II trial of docetaxel in platinum refractory advanced ovarian cancer. *J Clin Oncol* 12:2301–2308.

Gallaghar CJ, E Witshaw, RE Coleman et al. 1989. A dose escalation study of Carboplatin and Ifosfamide in advanced ovarian cancer. *Cancer Chemother Pharmacol* 24:54–57.

Gerhenson DM and WP McGuire (eds). 1998. *Ovarian cancer: Controversies in Management.* New York: Churchill Livingstone.

Hakes T, E Chalas, WJ Hoskins et al. 1992. Randomized prospective trial of 5 versus 10 cycles of cyclophosphamide, doxorubicin, and cisplatin in ovarian cancer. *Gynecol Oncol* 42–284.

Hoskins WJ and SC Rubin. 1991. Surgery in treatment of patients with advanced ovarian cancer. *Sem Oncol* 18:213–221.

Hreshchyshyn MM, RC Park, JA Blessing et al. 1980. The role of adjuvant therapy in stage I ovarian cancer. *Am J Obstet Gynecol* 138:139–145.

Kumar L, L Chandy, A Kriplani, S Kumar et al. 1996. Chemotherapy in epithelial ovarian cancer. *Asian J Obstet Gynecol* 1:35–39.

Kundella A, C Edwards, R Freedmans et al. 1993. An open phase-II study to evaluate the efficacy and toxicity of topotecan administered intraveneonsly as 5 daily infusions every 21 days to women with advanced epithelial ovarian cancer. *Proc Am Soc Clin Oncol* 12:821.

Kupfer A, C Aeschliomann, B Wermuth, T Corney. 1994. Prophylaxis and removal of Ifosfamide encephalopathy with methylene blue. *Lancet* 343:763–764.

Lokich J and N Anderson. 1998. Carboplatin versus cisplatin in solid tumors: An analysis of the literature (erratum published in Ann Oncol). *Ann Oncol* 9:13–21.

Lorigan P, T Crospy, RE Coleman. 1996. Current drug treatment guideline for epithelial ovarian cancer *Drugs* 51(4):571–584.

Lund B, OP Hansen, K Therlade et al. 1993. Phase II study of gemcitabine in previously platinum treated ovarian cancer patients. *J Natl Cancer Inst* 15:30.

Markman M and B Bundy. 1998. Randomized phase III study of i/v cisplatin, paclctaxel varsus moderately high dose i/v carboplatin followed by i/v PAC and IP cisplatin in optimal reduced ovarian cancer. An inter group trial (GOG, SCO OG, ECOB). *Proc Am Soc Clin Oncol* 17:361(a) Abstr.

Markman M, B Reichman, T Hakes et al. 1991. Responses to second-line cisplatin based intraperitoneal therapy in ovarian cancer: Influence of a prior response to intravenous cisplatin. *J Clin Oncol* 9: 1801–1805.

Markman M, Hakes T, Rothman P et al. 1991. Second line platinum therapy in patients with ovarian cancer previously treated with platinum. *J Clin Oncol* 9:389–393.

Markman M, T Hakes, B Reichman et al. 1992a. Ifosfamide and Mesna in previously treated advanced epithtial ovarian cancer, activity in platinum resistant disease. *J Clin Oncol* 10:2438.

Markman M, E Rowinsky, T Hakes et al. 1992. Phase I trial of intraperitoneal taxol: A gynecologic oncology group study. *J Clin Oncol* 10:1485–1491.

Markman M, T Hakes, B Reichman, et al. 1992b. Phase II trial of chronic low close oral etoposide as salvage therapy or platinum refractory ovarian cancer. *J Cancer Res Clin Oncol* 119:55–57.

Marsoni S, V Torri, MG Valsecchi et al. 1990. Prognostic factors in advanced epithelial ovarian cancer. *Br J Cancer* 62:444–450.

Masding JE. 1988. Treosulfan Zur Behand lung Fortgeschrittur ovarialkarzinoma. *Aktuel Onkol* 45:57–74.

Massad LS, VJ Hunter, CA Szpak et al. 1991. Epithelial ovarian tumor of low malignant potential. *Obstet Gynaecol* 78:1027.

Matsuoka H, M Furusawa, H Tomoda, Y Sew. 1994. Difference in cytotoxicity of paclitaxol against neoplastic and normal cells. *Anticancer Res* 14:163–167.

McGuire WP, WJ Hoskins, MF Brady et al. 1995. Assessment of dose intensive therapy in suboptimally debulked ovarian cancer: A gynecologic oncology group study. *J Clin Oncol* 13:1589.

McGuire WP, WJ Hoskin, MF Brady et al. 1996. Cyclophosphamide and cisplatin compared with paclitaxel and cisplatin in patients with stage III and IV ovarian cancer. *N Engl J Med* 334:1.

McGuire WP and RF Ozols. 1998. Chemotherapy of advanced ovarian cancer. *Semin Oncol* 25:3408.

McGuire WP, WJ Hoskins, MF Brady et al. 1999. The Gynaecological Oncology Group experience in ovarian cancer. *Ann Oncol* 10 (Suppl1):29–34.

Meyn RE, LC Stephens, NR Hunter, L Miles. 1994. Introduction of apoptosis in murine tumors by cyclophosphamide. *Cancer Chemother Pharmacol* 33:410–414.

Naruse I, H Keino, Y Kawarada. 1994. Antibody against single-stranded DNA detects both programmed cell death and drug induced apoptosis. *Histochemistry* 101:73–78.

Neijt JP and WW ten Bokkel-Huinink. 1984. Randomized trial comparing two combination chemotherapy regimens (HEXA-CAF VS CHAP-S) in advanced ovarian cancer. *Lancet* 2:594–600.

Neijt JP, WW ten Bokkel Huinink, MEL van der Burg et al. 1984. Current status of systemic chemotherapy in the treatment of advanced ovarian cancer with emphasis on CHAP-5 *Radiother Oncol* 2:19–29.

Neijt JP, WW ten Bokkel-Huinink, ME van der Burg et al. 1991. Long-term survival in ovarian cancer. Mature data from the Netherlands Joint Study Group for Ovarian Cancer. *Eur J Cancer* 27:1367–1372.

Omura G, P Marrow, J Blessing et al. 1983. A randomized comparison of melphalan versus melphalan plus hexamethylmine versus adriamycin plus cyclophosphamide in ovarian carcinoma. *Cancer* 51: 783–789.

Omura GA, JA Blessing, CE Ehrlich et al. 1986. A randomized trial of cyclophosphamide and doxorubicin with or without cisplatin in advanced ovarian cancer. *Cancer* 57:1725–1730.

Omura GA, MF Brady, HD Homesley et al. 1991. Long term follow-up and prognostic factor analysis in advanced ovarian carcinoma: The Gynecological Oncology Group experience. *J Clin Oncol* 9: 1138–1150.

Ozols RF, M Gore, C Trope, S Grenman. 1999. Intraperitoneal treatment and dose intensity therapy in ovarian Cancer. *Ann Oncol* 19(Suppl 1):559–564.

Piccart MJ, K Bertelsen, K James et al. 2000. Randomised metagroup trial of cisplatin–paclitaxel verse cisplatin–cyclophosphamide in women with advanced epithelial ovarian cancer: Three years results. *J Natl Cancer Inst* 92:699.

Pratt CB, MP Goven, WH Meyer et al. 1990. Ifosfamide nephrotoxicity is related to previous cisplatin treatment for paediatric solid tumors. *J Clin Oncol* 8:1399–1401.

Redman CWE, J Mould, J Warwick et al. 1993. The West Midlands epithelial ovarian cancer adjuvant therapy trial. *Clin Oncol* 5:1.

Rossi R, A Godde, A Kleimebrend, et al. 1994. Unilateral nephrectomy and cisplatin as risk factors of Ifosfamide induced nephrotoxicity. Analysis of 120 patients. *J Clin Oncol* 12:159–165.

Rowinsky EK, LA Cazenave, RC Donchowar. 1990. Taxol: A novel investigational anti microtubule agent. *J Natl Cancer Inst* 82:1247–1259.

Rowinsky EK. 1997. The development and clinical utility of the taxane class of microtubule chemotherapy agents. *Ann Rev Med* 48:353–374.

Stewart LA, for the advanced ovarian cancer trialists group (AOCTG). 1991. Chemotherapy in advanced ovarian cancer: An overview of randomized clinical trials. *Br Med J* 303–887.

Sutton GP, JA Blessing, HD Homesley, et al. 1989. Phase II trial of Ifosfamide and mesna in advanced ovarian carcinoma: A Gynaecological Oncology Group study. *J Clin Oncol* 7:172–176.

Thigpen JT et al. 1989. Chemotherapy in ovarian carcinoma: Present role and future prospects. *Sem Oncol* **16:58–65.**

van Houwelingen JC, WW ten Bokkel Huinink, ME van der Burg et al. 1989. Predictability of the survival of patients with advanced ovarian cancer. *J Clin Oncol* Jun; 7(6):796–773.

Williams CJ, GM Mead, FR Macbeth et al. 1995. Cisplatin combination chemotherapy versus chlorambucil in advanced ovarian carcinoma: Mature results of a randomized trial. *J Clin Oncol* 3: 1455–1462.

Wiltshaw E, B Evans, C Rustin et al. 1986. A prospective rendomised trial compring high dose cisplatin with low dose cisplatin and chlorambucil in advanced ovarian cancer. *J Clin Oncol* 4:722–729.

Young RC, LA Walton, SS Ellenberg et al. 1990. Adjuvant therapy in stage I and stage II epithelial ovarian cancer. *N Engl J Med* 322:1021–1027.

Young RC, LA Walton, SS Ellenberg et al. 1990. Adjuvant therapy in stage I and stage II epithelial ovarian cancer. Results of two prospective randomized trials. *N Engl J Med* 322:1021.

Zulupoln M and LH Balker. 1988. Ifosfamide. *J Natl Cancer Inst* 80:566.

24

Radiotherapy in Gynecology

MS Vidyasagar

Introduction to radiation oncology: Radiation oncology is a subject which deals with ionising radiation in the treatment of benign and malignant tumours. Radiation was used to treat malignant disorders within a few years of its discovery by Roentgen in November 1895. The last four decades have seen a major revolution in this field with the advent of mega-voltage therapy—better imaging techniques, modern planning systems, remote after-loading brachytherapy and computerised dosimetry systems.

Biological effects of radiation: Ionizing radiation causes damage to the DNA and other sub-cellular components of the cell. It has either a direct effect or an indirect effect. A direct effect causes either single-strand or double-strand breaks in the DNA, while the indirect effect involves interaction with water-generating free radicals (for example, hydroxyl ions).

The damaged cell undergoes changes in its structure and function, and further attempts at division causes cell death. Those cells, which are not lethally damaged, can undergo repair. This repair can be either potentially lethal damage repair (PLR) (Little et al 1973), which designates the increase in cell survival as a result of post-irradiation environmental conditions or sublethal damage repair (SLR) (Elkind and Sutton 1959) which denotes increase in cell survival due to rejoining and repair of double-strand breaks in DNA. The repair of normal cells is better than malignant cells. This differential repair mechanism is utilised in fractionated radiotherapy, so that malignant cells are killed and normal cells recover and repair themselves.

Radiation response modifiers

Response to radiation depends on various factors:

1. Oxygen: Cellular oxygen plays a very significant role in response to radiation. The radiation dose required to kill a hypoxic cell is much more than to kill well-oxygenated cells. Studies with hypoxic cell sensitisers, like misonidazole or metronidazole, did not show any significant advantage and hence these methods are not being used except under clinical trials.

A promising Phase I study of tirapazamine and cisplatin in recurrent cervical carcinoma (Aghajanian et al 1997) and also its combination with radiotherapy for the primary treatment of cervical cancer have demonstrated safety and feasibility (Craighead et al 2000).

2. Hemoglobin: Anemia contributes to an inadequate response to radiation. Studies on the addition of erythropoietin during radiotherapy are in progress, especially in carcinoma cervix, however, there is currently no proof that the use of erythropoietin is in any way superior to transfusions with respect to impact on clinical outcome.

3. Cell cycle: Response to radiation depends on cells in different phases of the cell cycle. A cell is most sensitive to radiation in the M and late G2 phases of the cell cycle and least sensitive in the S and G1 phase.

4. Chemotherapy: Cisplatin, 5 FU, hydroxyurea and other drugs are used along with radiation to enhance the response. Recent results of chemo-radiation in cancer cervix suggest that chemotherapy delivered along with radiation enhances the response to radiation and yields better results.

5. Hyperthermia: As an adjuvant to external radiotherapy hyperthermia acts synergistically. Hyperthermia acts on S-phase of cells, which is resistant to radiation. Clinical Phase II and Phase III studies showed a clear and significant benefit with the addition of hyperthermia to standard radiotherapy, especially in superficial tumours and head and neck cancers.

Types of radiation treatment: Radiation, for treatment purposes, is delivered by three modalities—teletherapy, brachytherapy and systemic therapy.

In teletherapy, the source of radiation is at a distance from the body and treatment is delivered by a Telecobalt or Linear accelerator. In brachytherapy, the radiation source is implanted directly into the tumour tissue or placed in the adjacent region. Sources used are Co60, Cs137 or Ir192. In systemic therapy, radiation is delivered through the oral route or by intravenous injection, for example, I131 for thyroid ablation or strontium 90 for bone metastases.

Megavoltage therapy units: External beam radiation is delivered by megavoltage therapy units. These units produce either high energy gamma rays or photon beams. The advantages of megavoltage therapy are:

1. Skin sparing effect which leads to better cosmesis.
2. Deep seated tumours can be treated effectively.
3. Improved dose distribution.
4. Bone sparing effect

Telecobalt therapy unit: The Telecobalt unit used to be the backbone of most departments till linear accelerators came into existence. The source of radiation is Co60 which emits gamma rays. Its average energy is 1.25 Mev, with a half-life of around 5.2 years.

Linear accelerators: Most modern radiotherapy centers are equipped with linear accelerators which generate both electrons and photons. The advantages of a linear accelerator over cobalt are that the beams are much sharper, treatment is shorter and the depth of penetration is higher and both electrons and photons can be generated by linear accelerators. Photon energy varies from 4 to 18 MV and electrons between 3 to 24 Mev.

Brachytherapy: This involves the placement of radiation sources within an existing cavity, like the vagina or the uterus (intracavitary treatment), or within the tumour (interstitial therapy) or by surface applicators. The advantage of brachytherapy over external beam radiotherapy is that a maximum dose can be delivered to the tumour with minimal normal tissue damage. There is a rapid fall-off of the dose due to the inverse square law which states that the dose of radiation varies inversely with the square of the distance.

Techniques: Brachytherapy techniques are broadly classified in terms of surgical approach to the target volume (interstitial, intracavitary, intraluminal or mould technique), and the means of controlling the dose delivered (temporary or permanent implants). Another classification would be in terms of source-loading technology (preloaded, manually after-loaded or remotely after-loaded) and the dose rate used (low, medium or high).

Based on the dose rate delivered, there are two types of techniques—low dose rate (LDR) 40–200 cGy/hr and high dose rate (HDR) >200 cGy/minute. In the LDR technique, the treatment lasts for 24 to 72 hours and the patient has to remain in protected areas for a longer time. In the HDR technique, the treatment time varies from 5 to 30 minutes and therefore, it can be performed as an outpatient procedure. The isotopes usually used are Ir192, Co60 or Cs137. Pulsed dose brachytherapy (PDR) simulates a continuous LDR interstitial treatment lasting several days with a series of short (about 10 minutes) HDR radiations, usually delivered every hour.

Special applicators are available for intracavitary brachytherapy like the Fletcher-Suit applicator. Earlier, the physician used to directly handle the radiation sources and hence this was known as a preloaded technique. Presently, empty catheters or applicators are placed and after verifying the position of the applicators, the radiation source is introduced and its movement is computer controlled. Hence, this technique is referred to as a remote after-loading technique. With this technology, radiation exposure to the treating personnel is minimal. Since the physician is not directly handling the radioisotope, he can place the applicators accurately, check the same with the simulator and allow the physicist/dosimetrists to calculate the time for a prescribed treatment. Recent brachytherapy equipment are well connected to computers and it is possible to manipulate the dose in such a way that the dose to the tumour is maximised, sparing normal tissue.

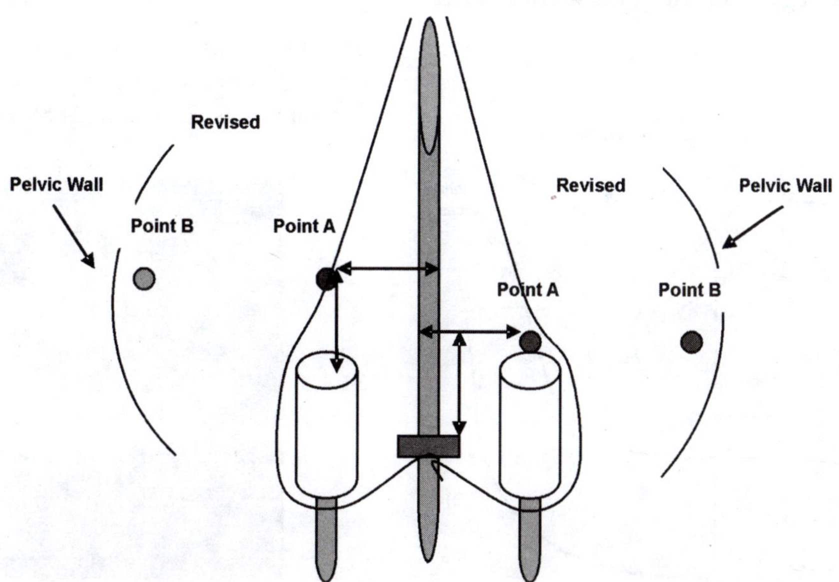

FIGURE 24.1: REFERENCE POINTS FOR BRACHYTHERAPY IN CARCINOMA CERVIX

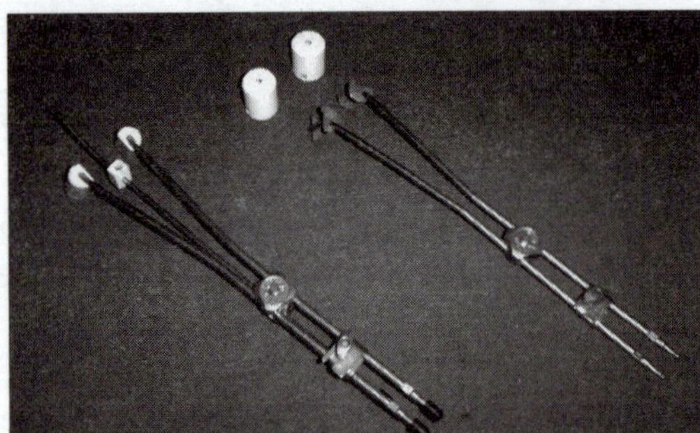

FIGURE 24.2: INTRACAVITARY RADIOTHERAPY APPLICATOR

Initially, three systems for intracavitary brachytherapy were developed—the Paris, the Stockholm and the Manchester systems. The systems differed in the type of applicator used, the strength of the source and time of administration. Today, most systems are derivations of the Manchester technique. Point A is 'classically' defined as being 2 cm above the mucous membrane of the lateral vaginal fornix and 2 cm lateral to the center of the uterine canal, which corresponds to the paracervical triangle, in the medial edge of the broad ligament, where the uterine vessels cross the ureters. Point B which is 5 cm from the midline, at the same level as Point A, was intended to quantify the dose delivered to the obturator nodes.

In current practice, Point A dose is used to approximate the average or minimum dose to the tumour. A later definition 'revised' Point A as being 2 cm above the distal end of the lowest source in the cervical canal and 2 cm lateral to the tandem. This is currently accepted as the standard. In practice, the os is radiographically demarcated by the tandem collar, whereas the lateral fornix is indicated by the colpostat surface.

Various applicators have been designed based on the Manchester system with minor modifications, for example, Williamson-Fletcher, Howard, Delclos Suit etc

Ideally, the tandem should be in the midline, as equidistant as possible from the lateral pelvic wall, crossing the mid-long axis of the ovoids, and the vaginal colpostats should be symmetrically positioned against the cervix in relation to the tandem.

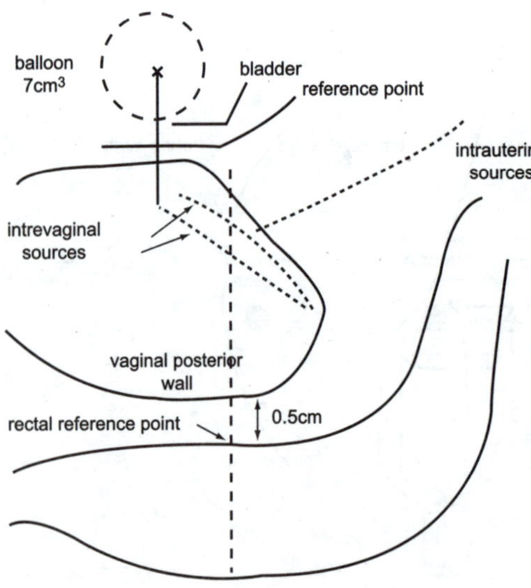

FIGURE 24.3: ICRU REFERENCE POINTS

Brachytherapy planning for carcinoma cervix: After orthogonal x-rays (AP and Lateral) (Figs 24.4 and 24.5) are obtained,

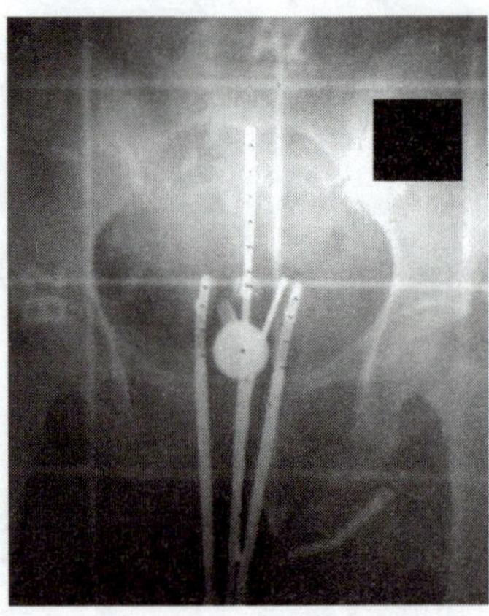

FIGURE 24.4: INTRACAVITARY RADIOTHERAPY—AP

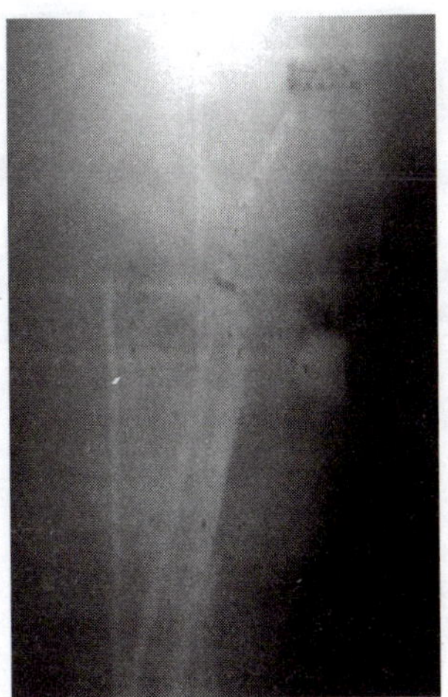

FIGURE 24.5: INTRACAVITARY RADIOTHERAPY—LATERAL

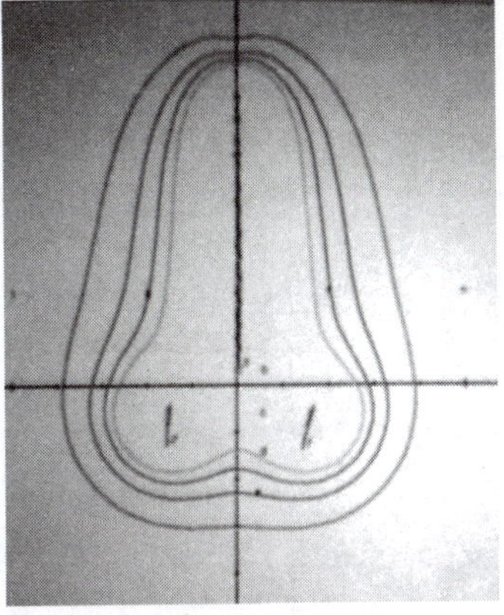

FIGURE 24.6: AP INTRACAVITARY RADIOTHERAPY—DOSE DISTRIBUTION

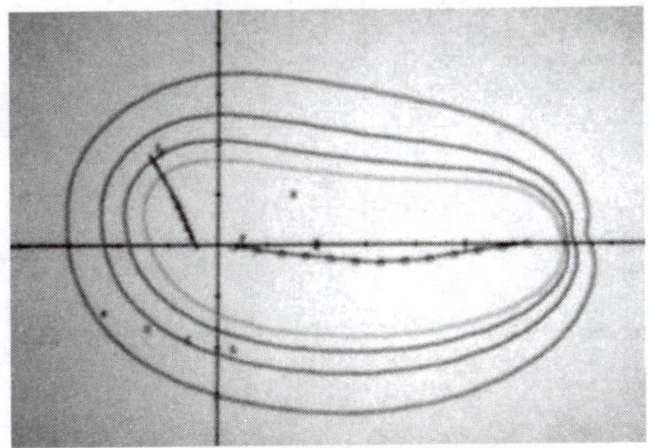

FIGURE 24.7: LATERAL INTRACAVITARY RADIOTHERAPY—LATERAL DISTRIBUTION

Point A , Point B, the bladder and the rectum reference points are marked on the films. Dose distribution is calculated after the films are digitised (Figs. 24.6 and 24.7)

Complications due to radiation

RADIATION EFFECTS ON COLON AND RECTUM: The tolerance of the colon and rectum depends upon the volume of tissue radiated and the total dose. Small portions of the colon and rectum can tolerate up to 70 Grays in 1.8–2 Gy per fraction or 1 Gy/hr in LDR brachytherapy (Fajardo et al 2001). The greater the dose per fraction, the lesser the total dose required to produce severe effects. It causes damage of rapidly proliferating mucosal cells. Radiation also causes mast cell hyperplasia, which induces both inflammatory and fibrotic changes.

Radiation causes a dose dependent decrease in water absorption and sodium and chloride and a twofold increase in the secretion of potassium (Dublineau et al 2000). The dose of 50 Gy in 25 fractions or above, causes fibrosis of the intestine after two years.

Clinically, patients develop diarrhea during the second to third weeks of radiotherapy. It may appear earlier when chemoradiation is given. The diarrhea can be controlled by oral medications like loperamide, low residue diet and plenty of oral fluids with salt.

The risks of developing hematochezia and GI fistula at five years are 0.7% and 1.7%, respectively. Bowel fistulas are more common than urinary fistulas, and these fistulas rarely close spontaneously and frequently require diversion of the fecal stream.

RADIATION EFFECT ON BLADDER AND URETHRA: Complications due to radiotherapy on the bladder and urethra usually occur much later than GI complications, typically after two to three years. Acute effects arise from injury to the rapidly dividing basal cells (Benedetti-Panici et al 1993). Marks et al (1995) in a

TABLE 24.1: ACUTE RADIATION MORBIDITY SCORING CRITERIA (RTOG)

Grade → Site ↓	[0]	[1]	[2]	[3]	[4]
SKIN	No change over base-line	Follicular, faint or dull erythema/ epilation/dry desquamation/ decreased sweating	Tender or bright erythema, patchy moist desquamation/ moderate edema	Confluent, moist desquamation other than skinfolds, pitting edema	Ulceration, hemorrhage, necrosis
MUCOUS MEMBRANE	No change over base-line	Injection/may experience mild pain not requiring analgesic	Patchy mucositis which may produce an inflammatory serosanguinitis discharge/ may experience moderate pain requiring analgesia	Confluent fibrinous mucositis/may include severe pain requiring narcotic	Ulceration, hemorrhage or necrosis
LOWER GI INCLUDING PELVIS	No change	Increased frequency or change in quality of bowel habits not requiring medication/rectal discomfort not requiring analgesics	Diarrhea requiring parasympatholytic drugs (for example, Lomotil)/ mucous discharge not necessitating sanitary pads/ rectal or abdominal pain requiring analgesics	Diarrhea requiring parenteral support/ severe mucous or blood discharge necessitating sanitary pags/ abdominal distention (flat plate radiograph demonstrates distended bowel loops)	Acute or subacute obstruction, fistula or perforation/GI bleeding requiring transfusion/ abdominal pain or tenesmus requiring tube decompression or bowel diversion
GENITOURI-NARY	No change	Frequency of urination or nocturia twice pretreatment habit/dysuria, urgency not requiring medication	Frequency of urination or nocturia which is less frequent than every hour. Dysuria, urgency, bladder spasm requiring local anesthetic (for example, Pyridium)	Frequency with urgency and nocturia hourly or more frequently/dysuria, pelvis pain or bladder spasm requiring regular, frequent narcotic/gross hematuria with/ without clot passage	Hematuria requiring transfusion/acute bladder obstruction not secondary to clot passage, ulceration or necrosis

review of clinical literature estimated the whole bladder tolerance dose for late effects at 45 Gy with conventional fractionation. A dose of 67 Gy to less than 30% of the bladder volume and 75 Gy to less than 10% was seen to be tolerable. The risk of hematuria and developing fistula at five years are 2.6% and 1.6% respectively.

The patients have hematuria due to chronic cystitis, increased frequency due to bladder fibrosis or ureteric stricture. Increased fluid intake, antibiotics and antispasmodics may be useful. Patients may complain of bladder or urethral irritation. The symptoms can be treated with pyridium or antispasmodics. If a patient has flank pain or fever, she should be evaluated for pyelonephritis, especially in advanced stages of the disease.

Radiation effect on vagina: Mild to moderate vaginal ulceration or necrosis seen in 5%–10% of patients usually occurs within 12 months of treatment. Maximum tolerable dose to the proximal vagina is 150 Gy and to the distal vagina, it is 90 to 100 Gy. Treatment includes vaginal estrogen cream application or 50% hydrogen peroxide douches. Vaginal shortening is also seen mostly in postmenopausal women and in those women who are sexually inactive. Dilatation, starting during and after radiation, is recommended for patients who are sexually inactive.

Small bowel complications: Small bowel obstruction is usually seen in patients who underwent surgery (especially transperitoneal lymphadenectomy), followed by external radiotherapy. Occasionally, HDR brachytherapy can deliver a high dose of radiation to a loop of the small bowel causing fibrosis, obstruction or fistula, if the patient had undergone prior surgery. It is also seen in patients who are thin and those with pelvic infection and those who receive more than 50 Gy to the central pelvis.

Intracavitary brachytherapy can, occasionally, cause thromboembolic events (0.3%). The risk is more in patients who had extensive disease that may have obstructed flow in pelvic vessels. Less serious complications include uterine perforation (2.8%) and vaginal laceration (0.3%) (Jhingran and Eifel 2000).

Late complications: Most late complications involve the rectum, bladder and small bowel. Rectal complications usually occur within the first three years of treatment, serious side effects can occur several years after treatment. The most common side effects are stricture, fistula and fibrosis. The treatment of bleeding includes stool softeners, steroid enemas and cauterisation.

Carcinoma of the cervix: Incidence of carcinoma of the cervix varies in different regions of the world. It is more in India, Latin America, Southern and Eastern Africa and South East Asian countries. In the USA, around 12,000 new cases of cervical cancer were expected to be diagnosed in 2003 and 4100 patients were expected to die of cervical cancer (American Cancer Society 2001). With effective screening methods adopted in developed western countries, the incidence as well as deaths due to cancer cervix has reduced considerably. But it still remains the leading cause of cancer death among women in developing countries.

Behaviour of carcinoma cervix: Cervical carcinoma usually originates at the junction between the pre-columnar epithelium of the endocervix and the squamous epithelium of the ectocervix. It takes nearly 15 years for a woman to develop frank malignancy from the stage of CIN. (Walton 1976; Kivlahan and Ingram 1986)

Local spread: Once the malignant process breaks through the basement membrane of the epithelium, it invades the stroma. The tumour spreads endocervically, equally in all directions. It can spread superiorly to the uterus in 10% to 30% of cases, inferiorly to the vagina or laterally to the right and left parametrial tissue in 28% and 34% of cases, respectively. It can also spread anteriorly through the vesicocervical ligament (anterior parametrium) to the bladder in 23% of cases or posteriorly through the rectovaginal septum to the rectum in 15% of cases (Landoni et al 1995).

LYMPHATIC SPREAD: The uterine lymphatics drain primarily through the paracervical nodes to the parametrial nodes, and thence to the external iliac nodes (of which the obturator nodes are the most medial) and the hypogastric nodes. The pelvic lymphatics drain into the common iliac and the para-aortic nodes. Regional lymphatic dissemination need not usually follow an orderly sequence; however, there is a close correlation between the involvement of the parametrial lymph nodes and the pelvic lymph nodes. Most commonly involved nodes are the medial group of external iliac and obturator nodes.

The incidence of positive pelvic nodes in Stage 1A1 is 1%, 1A2 5.8%, 1B 12%, 2B 21% and between 30% to 40% in Stage 3B. The incidence of positive para-aortic nodes is 3.3% in Stage 1B and 2B, less than 4 cm in Stage 2B and more than 13% in Stage 3B (Benedetti-Panici et al 1996).

METASTASIS: The most frequently observed metastasis were in the lungs (21%), followed by the abdominal cavity, liver and the gastrointestinal tract (GIT). The incidence of clinically apparent lymph node involvement was 22%, predominantly to the para-aortic, supraclavicular and inguinal nodes. Bone metastases occurred in 16%, most commonly to the lumbar and thoracic spine (Fagundes et al 1992).

Recurrence: When recurrence occurs after therapy, the majority of patients will be symptomatic. The median interval to recurrence is 17 months, although a small percentage may be detected after five years.

Diagnostic work up: Every patient should be jointly evaluated by a radiation and a gynecologic oncologist. After a general exam, paying special attention to the supraclavicular areas, abdomen and liver, a careful pelvic exam including inspection of the external genitalia, vagina and the uterine cervix, rectal examination and bimanual palpation of the pelvis should be done. Cystoscopy or proctosigmoidoscopy should be performed in all patients with Stage IIB, III and IVA or those with early stages who have a history of urinary or lower GI tract disturbances. Other standard investigations to be done are chest x-ray, intravenous pyelography, complete blood count, renal function tests and urinalysis.

Clinical classification system is commonly followed. The FIGO staging is based predominantly on clinical EUA, ultrasonography, intravenous urography, cystoscopy, proctoscopy and chest radiography. Significant inaccuracies occur in this staging because of possible errors in gynecologic examination (24%–39%) (Subak et al 1995; Lai et al 1999, Won Park et al 2005).

The various imaging modalities have a complementary role in the accurate staging and complete evaluation of the cancer and have important therapeutic implications. These include CT, MRI or PET scans. Although results from these investigations cannot be used for staging, they can be used for treatment planning and evaluating response to treatment. CT is valuable in the evaluation of para-aortic nodes and MRI is useful to detect

Table 24.2: Staging 1997: FIGO

TNM	FIGO	
TX		Primary tumour cannot be assessed
T0		No evidence of primary tumour
TIS	0	Carcinoma in situ (preinvasive carcinoma)
T1	I	Cervical carcinoma confined to the uterus (extension to corpus should be disregarded)
T1a	IA	Invasive cancer identified only microscopically. All gross lesions, even with superficial invasion, are stage T1b/IB cancers.
T1a1	IA1	Stromal invasion no greater than 3.0 mm in depth and no wider than 7.0 mm
T1a2	IA2	Measured invasion of stroma, greater than 3.0 mm and no greater than 5.0 mm with horizontal spread 7.0 mm or less
Note: The depth of invasion should not be more than 5 mm taken from the base of the epithelium, either surface or glandular, from which it originates. Vascular space involvement, either venous or lymphatic, should not alter the staging, but should be specifically recorded so as to determine whether it should affect treatment decisions in the future.		
T1b	IB	Clinical lesions confined to the cervix or microscopic lesion greater than T1a2/IA2
T1b1	IB1	Clinical lesions not greater than 4.0 cm in size
T1b2	IB2	Clinical lesions greater than 4.0 cm in size
T2	II	Tumour invades beyond the uterus but not to the pelvic wall or to the lower third of the vagina
T2a	IIA	Without parametrial invasion
T2b	IIB	With parametrial invasion
T3	III	Tumour extends to the pelvic wall and/or involves the lower third of the vagina and/or causes hydronephrosis or a non-functioning kidney
T3a	IIIA	Tumour involves the lower third of the vagina, no extension to the pelvic wall
T3b	IIIB	Tumour extends to the pelvic wall and/or causes hydronephrosis or a non-functioning kidney
T4	IVA	Tumour invades the mucosa of the bladder or rectum and/or extends beyond the true pelvis Note: the presence of bullous edema is not sufficient to classify a tumour as T4
M1	IVB	Distant metastasis

extrauterine extension. The hybrid CT-PET scanner is likely to prove superior in spatial resolution and anatomic localisation.

Treatment: Treatment of carcinoma of the cervix depends on the stage of the disease. Other factors, which can influence the treatment, include age, size of the tumour, histological features, lymph node involvement and contraindications for particular type of treatment like chemotherapy, chemo-radiotherapy, radiotherapy or surgery.

General consensus on the treatment strategy depends upon the stage of the disease.

Stage 0 There is no significant role of radiotherapy.

Stage IA, IB, IIA Is managed either with radical surgery or radical radiotherapy.

Stage IIB-IVA Is managed with radiotherapy or with the addition of chemotherapy to radiation.

Recent results with randomised clinical trials of chemo-radiation with cisplatin have shown a significant improvement in survival rates.

Stage IA: Radiotherapy also gives as good results as surgery. Radiotherapy is preferred in patients who have medical problems that contraindicate surgery. Progression-free 10-year survival rate for these patients, treated with radiation, is around 100%. Hamberger et al (1978) reported 89%–96% survival in Stages IA and IB disease with intracavitary radiation alone.

Stage IB and IIA disease: The choice of treatment for early carcinoma of the cervix, that is, Stages IB and IIA disease, is either radical hysterectomy or radical radiotherapy.

Radical hysterectomy: This includes removal of the uterus, cervix and paracervical, parametrial and paravaginal tissues up to the lateral pelvic wall. Removal of the ovaries may be deferred in a woman below 40 years; however, preservation of ovarian function is seen in only 50%–60% of surgically treated patients, not receiving irradiation (Feeney et al 1995). Radical surgery has only a 1% risk of operative mortality, yet this exceeds that of radiation.

Radiotherapy: Radical radiotherapy gives the same results as radical surgery. The patients are treated with a combination of external beam radiotherapy and intracavitary treatment. The total dose to point A will be 80–85 Gy. With combined EBRT and brachytherapy, the usual five-year survival for stage IB is 86%–92% and for stage IIA, it is approximately 75%. The overall pelvic failure rate in Stage IB is 5%–8% and in Stage IIA, it is 15%–20% (Perez et al 1986).

Combined treatment with surgery and radiotherapy: Postoperative radiotherapy decreases the risk of pelvic recurrence in patients, who have lymph node metastases, deep stromal invasion, incomplete resection, positive margins and parametrial involvement. In a prospective Gynecologic Oncology Group (GOG) trial in women who had deep stromal invasion, lymphovascular space invasion or large tumour diameter, >4–5 cm, the patients were assigned to either postoperative radiotherapy or there was no further therapy. Local recurrence was not observed in 84.7% as compared to 72% in patients who had no postoperative radiation (Sedlis et al 1999).

In another study by Peters et al (2000), where patients received postoperative radiotherapy and cisplatin, those who had positive nodes, parametrial involvement or positive surgical margins demonstrated a significant improvement in survival with chemotherapy and radiotherapy.

Post irradiation hysterectomy: Many studies done recently suggest that there is no advantage of combining surgery following radical radiation therapy. Although, it was thought to be the choice of treatment for large tumours of size 4 cm or more, Keys et al (1997) reported no improvement in survival among patients who had hysterectomy after radical radiotherapy. Adjuvant surgery may be indicated for these patients where brachytherapy is not feasible following external beam radiotherapy. It is also indicated in patients with uterine fibroids or narrow vagina, where it is not possible to deliver an adequate dose with brachytherapy.

Combination of surgery, radiotherapy and chemotherapy: There are very few studies in early carcinoma of cervix, where neoadjuvant chemotherapy followed by surgery and radiotherapy has been used. Andi et al in their study reported improved survival in patients who had tumours larger than 4 cm in diameter. Most of the studies, including GOG, have not shown any significant differences in survival between combination therapies versus radiotherapy alone.

Stage IIB, III, IVA disease: Radiotherapy is

the treatment of choice in locally advanced cervical carcinoma. Radiotherapy is usually delivered by combining external beam therapy with intracavitary radiotherapy. External radiotherapy usually shrinks the tumour enabling appropriate placement of intracavitary sources. As a result, the primary tumour receives a very high dose of radiation. The unusually high radiation tolerance of cervix, vagina and uterus is exploited in the treatment of this disease. The cervix can usually tolerate up to a dose of 150 Gy. The dose limiting organs are the bladder and the rectum. The survival rates for IIB and IIIB range between 35% and 70%.

External beam radiotherapy: The dose administered is usually 45–50 Gy in 4–5 weeks and five days per week.

Tumour volume for external beam radiotherapy includes the primary tumour, surrounding lymph nodes, obturator nodes and external iliac nodes up to the junction of the L4–L5 region.

Prophylactic extended field radiotherapy to the para-aortic nodes was tried in two randomised trials. The five-year disease-free survival rate was not statistically significant although an absolute five-year survival was significantly better. In patients with para-aortic node involvement, external field radiotherapy may be advocated which increases the survival rate by 25%–50%.

Para-aortic nodal Irradiation: The incidence of para-aortic node involvement in cancer of the cervix depends upon the stage of the disease. The higher the FIGO stage, the higher the incidence of para-aortic node involvement. It can be as high as 30%–50% in Stage III and Stage IV disease. A European Organisation for Research and Treatment of Cancer (EORTC) study compared pelvic radiotherapy alone to pelvic radiotherapy with para-aortic node irradiation to a total dose of 45 Gy. This study did not show any significant difference in survival, regional disease control or metastatic rate. A Radiation Therapy Oncology Group (RTOG) study, 1990–2001, also showed no significant difference in long-term survival, although early analysis suggested an improvement in survival rates, from 55% to 65% in favour of para-aortic node irradiation. But these studies demonstrated more morbidity in the para-aortic node group. Para-aortic node irradiation could improve the survival in poor prognosis Stage IB and II B disease.

In the presence of enlarged para-aortic nodes at the time of diagnosis, it is reasonable to treat these patients with extended field radiation fields that will irradiate both the pelvis and the para-aortic nodes. The dose recommended to para-aortic nodes is 45 Gy in 25 fractions. The five-year survival of these patients is around 24%, with a median survival of around 18 months.

Chemoradiation in locally advanced carcinoma cervix: Recent studies, including five randomised clinical trials (Table 24.1) and two meta-analyses (Green et al 2001; Lukka et al 2002), on the role of concurrent chemotherapy with cisplatin and radiation showed statistically significant survival benefit. These results have prompted the National Institute of Health to alert the clinicians to adopt chemo-radiation as a standard of care for patients with locally advanced cancer.

The chemo-radiation administered concurrently, has given better results with the advent of platinum-based chemotherapy like cisplatin and carboplatin (Table 24.1). It is shown to act synergistically with radiotherapy. It inhibits the potentially lethal damage or sublethal damage repair of tumour cells and increases the radiosensitivity of hypoxic cells.

Trials of chemoradiation using a cisplatin-based regimen have demonstrated consistent improvements in survival. Three trials, including the one from the RTOG and two from the GOG, all evaluated the use of cisplatin-based chemoradiation in patients with Stages IIB–IVA disease (RTOG 90-01 also included some patients with bulky Stage IB or IIA disease). All the trials showed an improvement in local control, overall survival and disease-specific survival. A recent update of this trial presented at the annual American Society for Therapeutic Radiology and Oncology meeting, pointed

TABLE 24.3: RESULTS OF CHEMORADIOTHERAPY IN CARCINOMA CERVIX

Reference	*Eligibility*	*Patient (no.)*	*CT: Investigational Arm*	*CT: Control Arm (no.)*	*Relative risk of Recurrence*	*p Values*
Rose et al 1999	FIGO IIB-IVA	526	Cisplatin 40 mg/m²/week (up to 6 cycles)	HU 3 g/m² (2×/week)	0.57 (0.42-0.78)	<0.001
			Cisplatin 50 mg/m²;HU 2 g/m² (two times per week) (2 cycles)	HU 3 g/m² (2×/week)	0.55 (0.40-0.75)	<0.001
Morris et al 1999	FIGO IB-IIA (≥5 cm); IIB-IVA or pelvic nodes involved	403	Cisplatin 75 mg/m²; 5-FU 4 g/m²/96 h (3 cycles)	None	0.48 (0.35-0.66)	<0.001
Keys et al 1999	FIGO IB (≥4 cm)	369	Cisplatin 40 mg/m²/week (up to 6 cycles)	None	0.51 (0.34-0.75)	0.001
Whitney et al 1999	FIGO IIB-IVA	368	Cisplatin 50 mg/m²;5-FU 4 g/m²/96 h (2 cycles)	HU 3 g/m² (2×/wk)	0.79 (0.62-0.99)	0.03
Peters et al 2000	FIGO I-IIA after radical hysterectomy with nodes, margins, or parametrium positive	268	Cisplatin 50 mg/m²;5-FU 4 g/m²/96 h (2 cycles)	None	0.50 (0.29-0.84)	0.01
Pearcey et al 2002	FIGO IB-IIA (≥5 cm), IIB-IVA or pelvic nodes involved	259	Cisplatin 40 mg/m²/wk (up to 6 cycles)	None	0.91 (0.62–1.35)	0.43

CI = confidence, interval; FU = 5-Flurouracil; HU = hydroxyurea; PA = para-aortic; RT = radiotherapy to a trend towards better overall survival in patients with Stage IIIB–IVA disease, treated with chemoradiation (59% vs 45%, p = 0.07). The cause-specific survival rate, however, was significantly higher in patients treated with chemoradiation (62% vs 51%, *p* = .05) (Eifel et al 2004).

Cisplatin, the present standard, is administrated as a single agent with 40 mg/m^2 once a week along with external radiation. The RTOG and the Southwest Oncology Group (SWOG) trials of cisplatin plus 5-FU and the GOG trials of weekly cisplatin, all showed reductions in the risk of progression and a death rate of 40% to 50%. Although the body of evidence supporting the combination of cisplatin and 5-FU is arguably somewhat stronger than that for weekly cisplatin, both regimens are considered highly effective, and the two regimens are considered approximately equally effective.

In women with doubtful compliance or tolerance to combined modality treatment, radical radiotherapy alone, without compromising the doses and duration, can still be considered as the gold standard treatment approach (EBM 2005).

INDICATIONS OF CHEMORADIATION THERAPY

1. Loco-regionally advanced cervical cancer (that is, Stage IB2 or greater or with positive pelvic lymph nodes) that is confined to the pelvis are candidates for chemoradiotherapy.
2. Patients who require post-hysterectomy radiotherapy due to high-risk disease (positive lymph nodes, parametrium or margins).
3. Patients with high intermediate-risk factors, particularly close margins or high-grade adenocarcinoma.
4. Localised recurrences of cervical cancer.

Stage IV B disease: The objective of treatment of Stage IVB disease is palliation. They should be managed in an individualised manner with treatment directed to the region of distress. A hemostatic dose of radiation to reduce uterine bleeding can be delivered using external beam radiotherapy. The bleeding can also be controlled by intracavitary radiotherapy. Skeletal metastases can be treated with external radiation of a single fraction of 800 Gy or 30 Gy in 10 fractions over two weeks. Palliative treatment can also be given to relieve obstructive symptoms like ureteric obstruction due to growth or lymph nodes, spinal cord compression or obstruction to the bronchus due to metastases.

External RT techniques: About 45–50 Gy of EBRT is required for microscopic disease in the regional lymph nodes. Higher doses up to 60 Gy are needed for heavy microscopic infestation (for example, sites of close or positive margins; extracapsular lymph node extension).

EBRT is delivered before intracavitary radiation with sedation using cylinders (ICR) in patients with:

1. Bulky cervical lesions in order to improve the geometry of ICR application,
2. Exophytic, easily bleeding tumours,
3. Tumours with necrosis or infection
4. Parametrial involvement.

Pelvic field: Superior border is kept at the L4–L5 interspace. Lateral margins are kept at a 2 cm margin, lateral to the bony pelvis. If there is no vaginal extension, the lower margin is at the mid portion of the obturator foramen and in case of vaginal extension, the field should extend distally beyond the tumour with a margin of 4 cm.

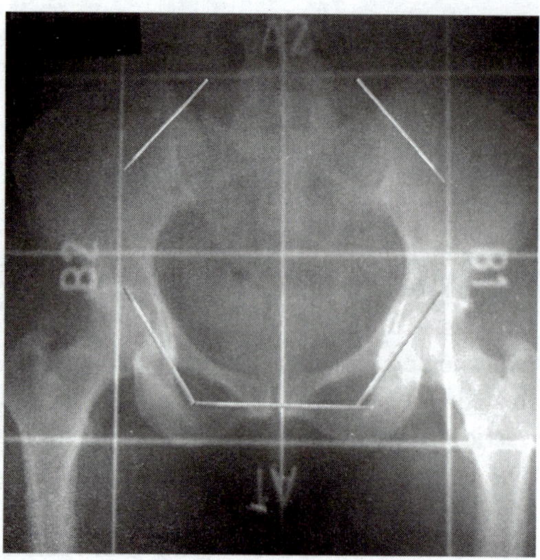

FIGURE 24.8: AP SIMULATION FILM OF THE PELVIS ILLUSTRATING PORTALS USED FOR EXTERNAL RADIATION

Carcinoma of the endometrium: Carcinoma of the endometrium is the most common malignancy of the female genital tract in developed countries and peak incidence occurs in those between 50 to 70 years of age, with 75% of all cases occurring in postmenopausal women.

ROLE OF RADIOTHERAPY

Adjuvant radiation therapy: Radiotherapy can be given either preoperatively or postoperatively as adjuvant treatment for inoperable carcinoma or for recurrent disease. The mainstay of treatment for adenocarcinoma of the endometrium is surgery. Preoperative radiotherapy has not shown any benefit over postoperative radiotherapy. It is also possible to assess the extent of the growth and pathological grade after surgery. Hence, postoperative radiotherapy is the more preferred choice of treatment.

Preoperative radiotherapy: Preoperative radiation is generally used to reduce the tumour burden before surgery. A few studies have showed the benefit of preoperative radiotherapy, especially for local control rate and also survival benefit in grade 3 disease, when compared to primary surgery alone (76% vs 53%) (Lewis et al 1977; Eifel et al 1983). Preoperative radiotherapy can be delivered by both intracavitary treatment or by external radiation or a combination of both.

Postoperative radiotherapy: The role of postoperative radiotherapy depends upon the stage of the disease, grade and the extent of myometrial invasion and lymph node involvement.

Stage I and II disease: Numerous studies have focused on early stage patients treated with postoperative radiotherapy. It is clearly observed that the rate of local recurrence has decreased considerably with postoperative radiotherapy.

Vaginal brachytherapy may be used in stage IA and IB with Grade 2 patients (Chadha et al 1999, Anderson et al 2000). All other stages, like stage IB Grade 3 and Stage II patients may receive both external pelvic radiotherapy and intravaginal brachytherapy (Calvin et al 1999).

Radical radiotherapy (RT) should be considered for women with endometrial cancer who suffer a localised relapse following surgery. RT can be curative in a select group of previously nonirradiated women with small vaginal recurrences.

The influence of prior RT on survival after relapse of endometrial cancer can be illustrated by results from the PORTEC trial, in which women with Stage I endometrial cancer were randomly assigned to surgery alone or followed by adjuvant pelvic RT (Creutzberg et al 2000, 2003). Actuarial three-year survival rates after any first relapse in the control and RT groups were 51% and 19%, respectively, as were five-year survival rates after an isolated vaginal relapse (65% versus 43% for surgery alone and adjuvant RT, respectively) (Creutzberg et al 2000).

Long-term survival rates in women, who undergo irradiation after relapse, range from 18% to 71% (Kuten et al 1989; Pai et al 1997, Curran et al 1998; Jhingran et al 2003). As illustrated by the PORTEC trial discussed above, the best outcomes are seen in patients with an isolated vaginal recurrence (Creutzberg et al 2003, Jhingran et al 2003). Besides location and no prior RT, other factors associated with improved survival in these patients include a long relapse-free interval, low-grade histology and endometrioid adenocarcinoma as compared to other histologies (Morgan et al 1993; Hart et al 1998).

Local control can be achieved in approximately 40% to 75% of patients treated with salvage RT, and like survival, is highest in those with an isolated vaginal relapse (75% in one series of 91 patients (Jhingran et al 2000; 2003). A major determinant of local control is tumour size at relapse (Hoekstra et al 1993; Curran et al 1998, Wylie et al 2000). Five-year local control rates were significantly higher for tumours ≤2 cm compared to larger ones (80 vs 54%, p = 0.02) (Wylie et al 2000).

Stage III and Stage IV disease: For high-risk extrauterine disease, adjuvant RT plays an important role, although no prospective randomised trial has been performed to evaluate the benefit of adjuvant RT in these patients. Indirect evidence is derived from nonrandomised reports (Morrow et al 1991; Rose et al 1992; Schorge et al 1996). In GOG Trial 33, there was an improvement in loco-regional control for irradiated women with adverse pathologic features (that is, positive nodes, adnexal involvement, capillary lymphatic space invasion, isthmus/cervical involvement, positive cytology and/or gross extrapelvic disease) (Morrow et al 1991).

Patients whose disease is limited to the pelvis typically undergo pelvic RT vaginal brachytherapy. Women with extrauterine disease extension undergo more comprehensive treatment, including extended field RT (EFRT) or whole abdominal RT (WART) (Greven et al 1993; Dusenbery et al 2005). Intraperitoneal administration of radioactive phosphorus (32P) has also been used in the past (Soper et al 1985; Heath et al 1988).

Considerable attention has been focused on the use of adjuvant RT in patients with node-positive (stage IIIC) endometrial cancer. Long-term RFS has been reported in women with positive para-aortic nodes who receive extended field RT (Rose et al 1992). Patients with isolated pelvic nodal involvement represent a favorable group (Nelson et al 1999).

Combined adjuvant chemotherapy and RT is also being explored (Reisinger et al 1996; Onda et al 1997; Frigerio et al 2001; Greven et al 2004). Promising results have been reported in a small series of patients with stage IIIC disease using this approach (Onda et al 1997).

The Radiation Therapy Oncology Group (RTOG) conducted a study of postoperative whole pelvis RT (45 Gy) with cisplatin (50 mg/m^2 on days 1 and 28) in 46 women with high-risk endometrial cancer (grade 2 or 3 with >50% myometrial invasion, extrauterine extension or stromal invasion) (Greven et al 2004). In a preliminary analysis with 29 month median follow-up, rates of pelvic, regional and distant metastasis were 2%, 3% and 17%, while disease-free survival and overall survival rates were 83% and 90%, respectively.

GOG recently completed a clinical trial comparing cisplatin plus doxorubicin *versus* cisplatin plus doxorubicin and paclitaxel in optimally debulked women with Stage III or IV disease (GOG 184). All patients received adjuvant RT (either pelvic or extended field RT) tailored to their specific pathologic features.

In more recent years, interest is shifting away from RT and towards adjuvant chemotherapy in high-risk patients with extrauterine involvement.

Uterine papillary serous carcinoma: Uterine papillary serous carcinoma (UPSC) is a distinct morphological type of endometrial cancer associated with a significantly worse prognosis. In the 1980s and 1990s, adjuvant treatment for resected Stage I and II UPSC or clear cell endometrial cancers generally involved RT, which was also recommended following debulking surgery for Stage III or IV disease (Craighead et al 2000b; Mehta et al 2003, NCCN 2005). The benefit of WART is particularly unclear for stage I–II tumours. In women with surgical Stage I UPSC, who are treated with WART, reported five-year survival rates are 70% to 80%, results which do not seem significantly different from that achieved with pelvic irradiation or observation alone (Huh et al 2003; Mehta et al 2003; Fleming 2004; Goff 2005). Various GOG trials have been conducted testing the role of whole abdominal radiotherapy (WART) in stage II and stage IV (Randall et al 2003). Chemotherapy proved to be superior to WART in terms of two-year overall survival and progression-free survival (PFS).

Uterine sarcoma: The role of radiotherapy in the treatment of early stage uterine sarcoma (I and II) is less well established than for endometrial carcinoma. Randomised trial that has completed accrual, from EORTC, randomly assigned 222 women with resected surgical Stage I or II uterine sarcomas (103 leiomyosarcomas, 91 carcinosarcomas, 28 endometrial stromal sarcomas) to pelvic external beam RT or observation (Reed et al 2003). The study ended in 2001, and a preliminary report in 2003 suggested a lower rate of local recurrence in the radiated group, but no improvement in survival. Retrospective series suggest the possibility of a survival benefit in addition to improvement in local control (Moskovic et al 1993; Knocke et al 1998; Molpus et al 1998; Ferrer et al 1999; Weitmann et al 2001).

Stage III uterine sarcomas are usually referred for postoperative radiotherapy as well as chemotherapy in view of the high risk of local-regional and systemic relapse. Radiotherapy is again an effective treatment modality for control of symptoms such as bleeding and pain in the palliative setting for patients with stage IV uterine sarcoma.

Carcinoma vulva: Invasive carcinoma of the vulva is a very rare neoplasm affecting around 4% of women with gynecological malignancies (Jemal et al 2005). They usually tend to occur in the older age group, with a median age group of occurrence between 65 to 70 years. These tumours are usually associated with HPV infection.

Prognostic factors: Tumour size, depth of invasion, tumour thickness, presence or absence of lympho-vascular space invasion and extra capsular extension of tumour strongly correlates with the prognosis.

Treatment Decisions

Stage IA: Radical local excision without lymph node dissection is the treatment of choice in patients with less than 1 mm of stromal invasion (stage IA) since inguinofemoral lymph node metastases are rare (< 1%) (Farias-Eisner et al 1994)

Stage IB: For lesions with ≥1 mm of stromal

invasion (stage IB), the risk of inguinofemoral lymph node metastases is at least 8%. Thus, all patients with stage IB disease should undergo ipsilateral inguinofemoral lymph node dissection for lateralised lesions, and bilateral lymph node dissections for central lesions (Hacker et al 1984). In a randomised trial, groin dissection was more effective in reducing the frequency of groin relapse than primary groin radiation without resection (Stehman et al 1992).

Modified radical vulvectomy and inguinofemoral lymphadenectomy are the mainstays of treatment for stage II disease.

Adjuvant radiotherapy: Indications for postoperative radiotherapy are grossly positive inguinal node, more than one positive inguinal node, extracapsular extension of nodal disease, medical contraindication for inguinofemoral dissection, vulvar resection margin of less than 8 mm or positive margins, the depth of tumour invasion more than 5 mm. In a retrospective series study of women with resected vulvar cancer with bilateral groin lymphadenectomy, adjuvant radiation therapy (RT) appeared to benefit those with either positive inguinal lymph nodes or positive/close surgical margins (Homesley et al 1986). The two-year survival rate was significantly better in the irradiated group (68% vs 54%). Patients with close or positive surgical margins may also benefit from postoperative RT. In one nonrandomised series of 62 such patients with invasive vulvar cancer at high risk of recurrence because of positive or close margins, 31 patients received postoperative RT and 31 did not (Faul et al 1997). Compared with the unirradiated patients, local recurrence rates were lower (16% vs 58%) and survival was significantly improved in those who received radiation. GOG (145) trial demonstrated five-year survival rates in patients who underwent surgery alone with no postoperative radiotherapy, even for positive inguinal nodes—91% for patients with negative nodes, 75% for those with one or two positive nodes, 36% for those with three to four positive nodes, 24% for those with five to six positive nodes.

Stage III and IV: Advanced vulvar squamous cell carcinoma involving the anus, rectum, rectovaginal septum or proximal urethra can be resected by radical vulvectomy combined with pelvic exenteration. Preoperative RT may downstage the tumour, allowing a more conservative surgical resection (Hacker et al 1984). Chemoradiotherapy is another alternative therapeutic approach to upfront exenterative surgery for locally advanced vulvar cancer. Squamous cell cancers are chemotherapy-sensitive tumours. This has been seen with cisplatin and 5-fluorouracil (5-FU) given during the first and last weeks of radiotherapy to women with advanced vulvar cancer (Berek et al 1991; Eifel et al 1995; Cunningham et al 1997; Moore et al 1998).

Verrucous carcinoma of vulva: Radical local excision is usually adequate. Suspicious lymph nodes should be biopsied; if positive, then inguinofemoral lymphadenectomy is indicated. RT is contraindicated because it can induce anaplastic transformation and increase the likelihood of metastases (Demian et al 1973).

Sarcomas: Wide local excision is the standard approach to treatment of most vulvar sarcomas. Rhabdomyosarcomas in children are treated with primary chemotherapy followed by surgery (Martelli et al 1999).

Melanoma: of the vulva and vagina are uncommon and are treated by wide local excision or radical vulvectomy for large tumours.

Vulval Paget's disease: Treatment consists of wide local excision or vulvectomy

RT Dose: After gross total resection, a dose of 50 Gy is adequate. In the presence of extra capsular extension of nodal disease, the dose is increased up to 60 Gy to the groins. In the presence of gross residual disease at the primary site, a dose of 65 Gy to 70 Gy is required.

Management of acute radiotherapy reactions: Confluent desquamation of the skin sets in by the fourth to fifth week of radiotherapy causing significant discomfort to the patient. Therefore, the patient requires reassurance before starting the treatment. The following measures can help alleviate the discomfort and minimise the chances of treatment interruptions.

- The patient should be encouraged to wear loose fitting garments
- Trauma to the skin should be avoided
- A Sitz bath with lukewarm water may be used for perineal hygiene
- The patient may be started on a regular dose of analgesics
- Systemic therapy for candidal infection should be started at the earliest possible

Acute hematological toxicity due to pelvic irradiation may warrant the use of colony-stimulating factor or blood transfusion. Treatment interruption or modification may be required.

Vaginal Cancer

Primary cancer of the vagina comprises approximately 3% of all malignant neoplasms of the female genital tract (Jemal et al 2005).

Treatment: Stage I lesions in the upper vagina that are less than 2 cm in diameter may be treated with either surgery or intracavitary radiation therapy. Lesions in the mid-to lower vagina are typically treated with radiation therapy. Surgical treatment, with or without adjuvant radiotherapy, the mean five-year survival for stage I, II, III and IV disease was 77%, 52%, 44% and 14%, respectively (Tewari et al 2001).

Radiation: Although more superficial lesions may be treated with brachytherapy alone, the treatment, of stage I lesions that are greater than 2 cm in diameter and all patients with stage II to IV disease, is external beam radiation with or without intracavitary or interstitial brachytherapy (Prempree and Amornmarn 1985; Spirtos et al 1989; Reddy et al 1991; Perez et al 1999, Grigsby 2000).

A total external radiation dose of 40–50 Gy is usually necessary for adequate treatment of the primary tumour and the regional lymphatics. In addition, inguinofemoral lymph node irradiation is indicated when the primary tumour involves the mid or distal third of the vagina.

Pelvic external beam radiation may be followed by intracavitary or interstitial radiation to a total tumour dose of approximately 75 Gy. Chemotherapy with 5-fluorouracil (5-FU) and/or cisplatin, is used along with radiotherapy in locoregionally advanced disease (Rubin et al 1985).

Treatment-related complications: Of the patients treated for vaginal cancer, 10%–15% will develop treatment related complications (Kirkbride et al 1995). These include rectovaginal or vesicovaginal fistulas, radiation cystitis or proctitis, rectal and vaginal strictures.

Prognosis: The most important variable affecting prognosis is the stage at the time of presentation, reflecting the size and depth of tumour penetration (Nori et al 1983;

Prempree and Amornmarn 1985; Brady et al 1986; Grigsby 2002).

Ovarian cancer

Epithelial ovarian cancer constitutes around 80% of all ovarian tumours. Others include germ cell and stromal tumours which are around 20%. The five-year survival rate for carcinoma of the ovary has improved from 37% in the 1970s to 44% in 2000 due to advances in treatment (Jemal et al 2005). In the early stages of the disease, the survival rate is around 95% and in stage IV disease, the survival rate is around 37%.

Treatment: Surgery is the treatment of choice in the management of ovarian cancer (Morton and Thomas 1994). Patients with stage I disease with unfavorable prognostic factors, such as grade II or III, and patients with stage II and III disease are often recommended to have surgery, followed by intravenous (IV) carboplatin and paclitaxel chemotherapy, since there is often at least a 30% risk of recurrence (Marsden et al 2000). Recent trials have shown that platinum-based adjuvant chemotherapy improved survival and recurrence-free survival in early-stage ovarian cancer (ICON 1 2003).

The role of radiation: With the advent of chemotherapy, the role of radiation in the management of carcinoma of the ovaries has diminished. Although radiation therapy has been proven in several trials to be effective adjuvant therapy in certain stages and to a certain extent (Morton and Thomas 1994), there are no randomised clinical trials comparing platinum-based chemotherapy to whole abdomen therapy. However, radiotherapy does have a role in both curative and palliative treatment of carcinoma of the ovary.

At Princess Margaret Hospital, randomised trial of 147 patients compared radiotherapy alone or with chlorambucil chemotherapy to whole abdomen radiotherapy in patients with stage I–III disease. After a seven-year follow-up, the 10 year difference in survival was significantly higher in the 76 patients treated with whole abdomen radiation compared to the 71 patients treated with pelvic irradiation and chlorambucil. The survival benefit was seen in patients who had residual tumour, less than 2 cm or no tumour at all, postoperatively. In patients who had gross residual tumour, there was no difference seen in either arm of treatment (Dembo et al 1979).

These trials have validated that radiation therapy is an effective adjuvant therapy in patients with minimal residual disease or no residual disease.

Salvage with radiation: Although very high incidence of clinical response is seen initially, the rate of recurrence after cisplatin/paclitaxel based chemotherapy is around 40%–50% (Gonzalez-Martin et al 2003). Ovarian cancer patients who had recurrent or persistent disease after surgery and chemotherapy were next treated with whole abdomen radiotherapy as salvage therapy with curative intent. Survival rates from one through five years was 66%, 48%, 26%, 15% and 15% respectively. The study found that patients who had only microscopic residual disease or disease confined to the pelvis had significantly longer recurrence-free survival (Sedlacek et al 1997).

Consolidative radiotherapy: Carboplatin/paclitaxel chemotherapy is an established standard treatment for ovarian carcinoma. Though initial response rates are good, there is a very high incidence of residual disease and failure rates after initial chemotherapy. Consolidated radiotherapy following chemotherapy with carboplatin/paclitaxel may offer improved tumour control in selected patients (Dinniwell et al 2005).

Sorbe et al (2002) conducted a trial with 98 patients with stage III ovarian cancer who had initial cytoreductive surgery followed by chemotherapy with complete pathologic response. They were randomly assigned whole abdomen radiotherapy, chemotherapy or no further treatment. The patients who had whole abdomen radiotherapy had better survival rates (56%) compared to chemotherapy (36%) and no further treatment (33%).

Palliative radiation therapy: The role of radiotherapy as a palliation is useful especially in reducing pain due to skeletal metastases, pelvic pain, large bowel obstruction, pulmonary compromise. There is a good response in patients with pain and bleeding.

Conclusion: Currently, chemotherapy is the standard of care after surgery due to the lack of large prospective randomised trials involving postoperative radiotherapy. Radiation may be utilised as salvage therapy in patients who have failed surgery followed by chemotherapy. Optimal results have been found in patients who have microscopic residual disease or disease confined to the pelvis. Radiotherapy can also be considered as consolidative therapy following optimal cytoreductive surgery and platinum-based chemotherapy for select individuals with intermediate or high risk of relapse.

Treatment dose: The prescribed dose is 22–30 Gy with 1–1.2 Gy per fraction to whole abdomen with a pelvic boost to a total dose of 45–50 Gy.

Dysgerminoma: This mainly occurs in younger patients (89% of patients, younger than 29 years of age). It is highly sensitive to radiation therapy. Usually, the tumour is confined to one ovary only at the time of diagnosis. Because dysgerminoma has been shown to be curable with chemotherapy, radiotherapy management has changed appreciably over the time. Bleomycin, etoposide and cisplatin combination chemotherapy is highly effective. Radiation is considered for stage IA only. The dose administered is 25 Gy in 20–25 fractions to whole abdomen with possible boosts of 10 Gy to sites of bulky disease (Gonzalez-Martin et al 2003). In uncontrolled disease, where chemotherapy has failed, radiation may provide excellent palliation.

Granulosa cell tumour: The majority of granuloma cell tumours are at stage I at diagnosis and do not need any further therapy, except surgery. However, recurrences many years after primary surgery can occur. Such recurrences can be treated with chemotherapy and radiation. Abdominopelvic radiation may be offered to patients with bilateral, metastatic, high risk non-metastatic, or recurrent granuloma cell tumour, provided the residual bulk is not large.

References

American Cancer Society. 2001. *Cancer Facts and Figures*. Atlanta: American Cancer Society.

Anderson JM, B Stea, AV Hallum et al. 2000. High-dose-rate postoperative vaginal cuff irradiation alone for stage IB and IC endometrial cancer. *Int J Radiat Oncol Biol Phys* 46:417.

Averette HE, HN Nguyen, DM Donato. et al.1993. Radical hysterectomy for invasive cervical cancer. A 25-year prospective experience with the Miami technique. *Cancer* 1422–1437.

Aghajanian, C, C Brown, C O'Flaherty, A Fleischauer, J Curtin, R Roemeling, DR Spriggs. 1997.

Phase I study of tirapazamine and cisplatin in patients with recurrent cervical cancer. *Gynecologic Oncology*, 67: 127–130

Beller U, M Sideri, P Maisonneuve et al. 2001. Carcinoma of the vulva. *J Epidemiol Biostat*; 6:155.

Benedetti-Panici P, S Greggi, G Scambia, et al. 1993. Cisplatin (P), bleomycin (B), and methotrexate (M) preoperative chemotherapy in locally advanced vulvar carcinoma. *Gynecol Oncol* 50:49.

Benedetti-Panici P, Maneschi F, Scambia G et al. 1996. Lymphatic spread of cervical cancer: An anatomical and pathological study based on radical hysterectomies and pelvic and aortic lymphadenectomy. *Gynaecol Oncol* 62:19–24.

Berek JS, JM Heaps, YS Fu et al. 1991. Concurrent cisplatin and 5-fluorouracil chemotherapy and radiation therapy for advanced-stage squamous carcinoma of the vulva. *Gynecol Oncol* 42:197.

Bethesda MD. 1985. International Commission of Radiation Units and Measurements Dose and Volume specifications for reporting intracavitary therapy in gynecology. ICRU38.

Bolis G, G Scarfone, G Giardina, A Villa. 2001. Carboplatin alone vs carboplatin plus epidoxorubicin as second-line therapy for cisplatin- or carboplatin-sensitive ovarian cancer. *Gynecol Oncol* 81:3.

Boyce J, R Fruchter, A Nicastri et al. 1981. Prognostic factors in stage I carcinoma of the cervix. *Gynecol Oncol* 12: 154

Brady LW, CA Perez, JM Bedwinek. 1986. Failure patterns in gynecologic cancer. *Int J Radiat Oncol Biol Phys* 12:549.

Calvin DP, PP Connell, J Rotmensch et al. 1999. Surgery and postoperative radiation therapy in stage II endometrial carcinoma. *Am J Clin Oncol* 22:338.

Chadha M, PJ Nanavati, P Liu et al. 1999. Patterns of failure in endometrial carcinoma stage IB grade 3 and IC patients treated with postoperative vaginal vault brachytherapy. *Gynecol Oncol* 75:103.

Craighead PS, K Sait, GC Stuart et al. 2000a. Management of aggressive histologic variants of endometrial carcinoma at the Tom Baker Cancer Centre between 1984 and 1994. *Gynecol Oncol* 77:248.

Craighead PS, R Pearcey, G Stuart. 2000. A phase I/II evaluation of tirapazamine administered intravenously concurrent with cisplatin and radiotherapy in women with locally advanced cervical cancer. *International Journal of Radiation Oncology, Biology, Physics,* 48: 791–795.

Creutzberg CL, WL Van Putten, PC Koper et al. 2000. Surgery and postoperative radiotherapy versus surgery alone for patients with stage-1 endometrial carcinoma: Multicentre randomised trial. PORTEC Study Group. Post Operative Radiation Therapy in Endometrial Carcinoma. *Lancet* 355:1404.

Creutzberg CL, WL van Putten, PC Koper et al. 2003. Survival after relapse in patients with endometrial cancer: Results from a randomized trial small star, filled. *Gynecol Oncol* 89:201.

Cunningham MJ, RP Goyer, SK Gibbons et al. 1997. Primary radiation, cisplatin and 5-fluorouracil for advanced squamous carcinoma of the vulva. *Gynecol Oncol* 66:258.

Curran WJ Jr, R Whittington, AJ Peters, J Fanning. 1988. Vaginal recurrences of endometrial carcinoma: The prognostic value of staging by a primary vaginal carcinoma system. *Int J Radiat Oncol Biol Phys* 15:803.

Delgado G, BN Bundy, WC Fowler et al. 1989. A prospective sugical pathological study of stage I squamous carcinoma of the cervix: A Gynecologic Oncology Group study. *Gynecol Oncol* 36: 314–320

Dembo A 1992. 'Epithelial Ovarian Cancer: The Role of Radiotherapy.' *Int J Radiation Oncology Biol Phys* 22:835–845.

Dembo AJ, RS Bush, FA Beale, HA Bean, JF Pringle, J Sturgeon, JG Reid. 1979. Improved survival following abdominopelvic irradiation in patients with a completed pelvic operation. *Am J Obstet Gynecol* 134: 793800.

Demian SD, FL Bushkin, RA Echevarria. 1973. Perineural invasion and anaplastic transformation of verrucous carcinoma. *Cancer* 32:395.

Dinniwell R, M Lock, M Pintilie, A Fyles, S Laframboise, D Depetrillo, W Levin, L Manchul, J Murphy, A Oxa, B Rosen, J Sturgeon, M Milosevic. 2005. Consolidative abdominopelvic radiotherapy after surgery and carboplatin/paclitaxel chemotherapy for epithelial ovarian cancer. *Int J. Radiation Oncology Biol Phys* 62:104–110.

Dublineau I, B Ksas, NM Griffiths. 2000. Functional changes in the distal colon after whole body irradiation: Dose-response and temporal relationships. *Radiat Res* 154:187–195.

Dusenbery KE, RA Potish, DG Gold, MP Boente. 2005. Utility and limitations of abdominal radiotherapy in the management of endometrial carcinomas. *Gynecol Oncol* 96:635.

EBM. 2005. Evidence based management guidelines: Challenges in the practice of practices of evidence based oncology in developing countries—Cervical cancers. Tata Memorial Hospital vol. IV 97–146

Eifel PJ, J Ross, M Hendrickson et al. 1983. Adenocarcinoma of the endometrium. Analysis of 256 cases with disease limited to the uterine corpus: treatment options. *Cancer* 52:1026–1031.

Eifel PJ, M Morris, TW Burke et al. 1995. Prolonged continuous infusion cisplatin and 5-fluorouracil with radiation for locally advanced carcinoma of the vulva. *Gynecol Oncol* 59:51.

Eifel PJ, K Winter, M Morris, et al. 2004. Pelvic radiation with concurrent chemotherapy versus pelvic and para-aortic radiation for high-risk cervical cancer: An update of radiation therapy oncology group trial (RTOG) 90-01. *J Clin Oncol* 22:872.

Elkind MM and HF Sutton. 1959. X Ray damage and recovery in mammalian cells in culture. *Nature* 184: 1293.

Fagundes H, CA Perez, PW Grigsby et al. 1992. Distant metastasis after irradiation alone in carcinoma of cervix. *Int J Radiat Oncol Biol Phys* 24:197–204.

Fajardo LF, M Berthrong, RE Anderson. 2001. Large intestine and anal canal In *Radiation Pathology.* New York: Oxford University Press 239–247.

Farias-Eisner R, FD Cirisano, D Grouse et al. 1994. Conservative and individualized surgery for early squamous carcinoma of the vulva: The treatment of choice for stage I and II (T1-2N0-1M0) disease. *Gynecol Oncol* 53:55.

Faul CM, D Mirmow, Q Huang, et al. 1997. Adjuvant radiation for vulvar carcinoma: Improved local control. *Int J Radiat Oncol Biol Phys* 38:381.

Feeney DD, DH Moore, KY Look et al. 1995. The fate of the ovaries after radical hysterectomy and ovarian transposition. *Gynaecol Oncol* 56:3.

Fernandes DJ, T Joseph. MS Vidyasagar, et al 1995 . Synchronous chemotherapy 5 FU + Mitomycin C and Radiotherapy in the treatment of locally advanced carcinoma of the uterine cervix. (eds). M Krishnan Nair, Proceedings of the 16th AROI Congress. Regional Cancer Center, Trivandrum. PP:97–102.(Cochrane reviewed)

Ferrer F, S Sabater, B Farrus et al. 1999. Impact of radiotherapy on local control and survival in uterine sarcomas: A retrospective study from the Group Oncologic Catala-Occita. *Int J Radiat Oncol Biol Phys* 44:47.

Fleming G. 2004. *Systemic management of endometrial cancers with unusual histology.* American Society of Clinical Oncology Educational Book, 40th Annual Meeting. p 293.

Frank SJ, A Jhingran, C Levenback, PJ Eifel. 2005. Definitive radiation therapy for squamous cell carcinoma of the vagina. *Int J Radiat Oncol Biol Phys* 62:138.

Frigerio L, G Mangili, G Aletti et al. 2001. Concomitant radiotherapy and paclitaxel for high-risk endometrial cancer: First feasibility study. *Gynecol Oncol* 81:53.

Goff BA. 2005. Uterine papillary serous carcinoma: What have we learned over the past quarter century? *Gynecol Oncol* 98:341.

Gonzalez-Martin AA, E Calvo, I Bover et al. 2003. Randomised phase II study of carboplatin versus paclitaxel-carboplatin in platinum-sensitive recurrent advanced ovarian carcinoma with assessment of quality of life: a GEICO study (Spanish Group for Investigation on Ovarian Carcinoma) (abstract). *Proc Am Soc Clin Oncol* 22:451a.

Green J, J Kirwan, Tierney et al. 2001. Concomitatnt chemotherapy and Radiation therapy for cancer of the uterine cervix. *Cochrane Database Systamatic Review* (4) : CDO 02225.

Green JA, JM Kinwan, Tierney et al. 2001. Survival and recurrence after concomitant chemotherapy and radiotherapy for cancer of the cervix. Metanalysis. *Lancet* 358:781

Greven KM, RM Lanciano, B Corn et al. 1993 . Pathologic stage III endometrial carcinoma. Prognostic factors and patterns of recurrence. *Cancer* 71:3697.

Greven K, K Winter, K Underhill et al. 2004. Preliminary analysis of RTOG 9708: Adjuvant postoperative radiotherapy combined with cisplatin/paclitaxel chemotherapy after surgery for patients with high-risk endometrial cancer. *Int J Radiat Oncol Biol Phys* 59:168.

Grigsby PW. 2002. Vaginal cancer. *Curr Treat Options Oncol* 3:125.

Hacker NF, JS Berek, GJ Juillard, LD Lagasse. 1984. Preoperative radiation therapy for locally advanced vulvar cancer. *Cancer* 54:2056.

Hacker NF, JS Berek, LD Lagasse et al. 1984. Individualization of treatment for stage I squamous cell vulvar carcinoma. *Obstet Gynecol* 63:155.

Hamberger AD, GH Fletcher, JT Wharton. 1978. Results of treatment of early stage I carcinoma cervix with intracavitary radium alone. *Cancer* 41: 980–985.

Hart KB, I Han, F Shamsa et al. 1998. Radiation therapy for endometrial cancer in patients treated for postoperative recurrence. *Int J Radiat Oncol Biol Phys* 41:7.

Heath R, J Rosenman, M Varia, L Walton. 1988. Peritoneal fluid cytology in endometrial cancer: Its significance and the role of chromic phosphate (32P) therapy. *Int J Radiat Oncol Biol Phys* 15:815.

Hoekstra CJ, PC Koper, WL van Putten. 1993. Recurrent endometrial adenocarcinoma after surgery alone: prognostic factors and treatment. *Radiother Oncol* 27:164.

Homesley HD, BN Bundy, A Sedlis, L Adcock. 1986. Radiation therapy versus pelvic node resection for carcinoma of the vulva with positive groin nodes. *Obstet Gynecol* 68:733.

Huh WK, M Powell, CA Leath III, et al. 2003. Uterine papillary serous carcinoma: Comparisons of outcomes in surgical Stage I patients with and without adjuvant therapy. *Gynecol Oncol* 91:470.

ICON 1 - International Collaborative Ovarian Neoplasm 1 Collaborators; European Organisation for Research and Treatment of Cancer Collaborators—Adjuvant Chemotherapy in Ovarian Neoplasm. 2003. "International Collaborative Ovarian Neoplasm Trial 1 and Adjuvant Chemotherapy in Ovarian Neoplasm trial: Two parallel randomized phase III trials of adjuvant chemotherapy in patients with early-stage ovarian carcinoma." *J Natl Cancer Inst* 95:105–112.

Jemal A, T Murray, W Ward, et al. 2005. Cancer Statistics, 2005. *CA Cancer J Clin* 55:10.

Jereczek-Fossa B, A Badzio, J Jassem. 2000. Recurrent endometrial cancer after surgery alone: Results of salvage radiotherapy. *Int J Radiat Oncol Biol Phys* 48:405.

Jhingran A, TW Burke, PJ Eifel. 2003. Definitive radiotherapy for patients with isolated vaginal recurrence of endometrial carcinoma after hysterectomy. *Int J Radiat Oncol Biol Phys* 56:1366.

Jhingran A and PJ Eifel. 2000. Perioperative and post operative complications of intracavitary radiation for FIGO stage I-III carcinoma of the cervix. *Int J Radiat Oncol Biol Phys* 46:1177–1183

Keys H, B Bundy, F Stehman et al. 1997. Adjuvant hysterectomy after radiation therapy reduces detection of local recurrences in 'bulky' stage IB cervical carcinoma without improving the survival: Results of a prospective randomized GOG trial. *Cancer J Sci Am* 3:117 (abstr).

Keys HM, BN Bundy, FB Stehman et al. 1999. Cisplatin, radiation and adjuvant hysterectomy for bulky stage IB cervical carcinoma. *N Engl J Med* 340:1154.

Kirkbride P, A Fyles, GA Rawlings, et al. 1995. Carcinoma of the vagina: Experience at the Princess Margaret Hospital (1974-1989). *Gynecol Oncol* 56:435.

Kivlahan C and E Ingram. 1986. Papanicolaou smears without endocerviccal cells. Are they inadequate? *Acta Cytol* 20: 258–260

Knocke TH, H Kucera, D Dorfler et al. 1998 . Results of postoperative radiotherapy in the treatment of sarcoma of the corpus uteri. *Cancer* 83:1972.

Kurtz JE, G Deplanque, B Duclos, F Eichler. 1998. Paclitaxel-anthracycline combination chemotherapy in relapsing advanced ovarian cancer after platinum-based chemotherapy: A pilot study. *Gynecol Oncol* 70:414.

Kuten A, PW Grigsby, CA Perez, et al. 1989. Results of radiotherapy in recurrent endometrial carcinoma: A retrospective analysis of 51 patients. *Int J Radiat Oncol Biol Phys* 17:29.

Lai CH, JH Hong, S Hsueh, KK Ng, TC Chang, CJ Tseng et al.1999. Preoperative prognostic variables and the impact of postoperative adjuvant therapy on the outcome of stage IB and II cervical carcinoma patients with or without pelvic lymph-node metatases: An analysis of 891 cases. *Cancer* 85:1537–1546.

Landoni F, L Boccilone, P Perego et al. 1995. Cancer of cervix, FIGO stages Ib and IIa: Patterns of local growth and paracervical extension. *Int J Gynaecol Cancer* 5:329–334.

Landoni F, A Maneo, A Colombo et al. 1997. Randomised study of radical surgery versus radiotherapy for stage Ib–IIa cervical cancer. *Lancet* 350:535–40

Landoni F, A Maneo, G Zanetta et al. 1996. Concurrent preoperative chemotherapy with 5-fluorouracil and mitomycin C and radiotherapy (FUMIR) followed by limited surgery in locally advanced and recurrent vulvar carcinoma. *Gynecol Oncol* 61:321.

Lewis GC, R Mortel, NH Slack. 1977. Adenocarcinoma of the body of uterus. *J Obestet Gynaecol Br Commw* 77:342–348

Little JB, GM Hahn, E Frinfel, M Tubiana. 1973. Repair of potentially lethal radiation damage in vitro and in vivo. *Radiology* 106:689–694.

Lukka H, H Hirtle, G Thomas et al. 2002. Concurrent cisplatin based chemotherapy plus radiotherapy for cervical cancer–A Meta-analysis. *Clinical Oncology* (3) 203–212

Lupi G, F Raspagliesi, R Zucali et al. 1996. Combined preoperative chemoradiotherapy followed by radical surgery in locally advanced vulvar carcinoma. A pilot study. *Cancer* 77:1472.

Marks LB, PR Carroll, TC Dugan et al. 1995. The response of the urinary bladder, urethra and ureter to radiation and chemotherapy. *Int J Radiat Oncol Biol Phys* 31: 1257–1280.

Marsden DE, M Friedlander, NF Hacker. 2000. Current Management of Epithelial Ovarian Carcinoma: A Review. *Semin Surg Oncol* 19:11–19.

Martelli H, O Oberlin, A Rey et al. 1999. Conservative treatment for girls with nonmetastatic rhabdomyosarcoma of the genital tract: A report from the Study Committee of the International Society of Pediatric Oncology. *J Clin Oncol* 17:2117.

Mehta N, SD Yamada, J Rotmensch, AJ Mundt. 2003. Outcome and pattern of failure in pathologic stage I-II papillary serous carcinoma of the endometrium: Implications for adjuvant radiation therapy. *Int J Radiat Oncol Biol Phys* 57:1004.

Molpus KL, S Redlin-Frazier, G Reed et al. 1998. Postoperative pelvic irradiation in early stage uterine mixed mullerian tumors. *Eur J Gynaecol Oncol* 19:541.

Moore DH, GM Thomas, GS Montana et al. 1998. Preoperative chemoradiation for advanced vulvar cancer: a phase II study of the Gynecologic Oncology Group. *Int J Radiat Oncol Biol Phys* 42:79.

Morgan JD III, S Reddy, P Sarin et al. 1993. Isolated vaginal recurrences of endometrial carcinoma. *Radiology*. 189:609.

Morris M, PJ Eifel, J Lu et al. 1999. Pelvic radiation with concurrent chemotherapy compared with pelvic and paraaortic radiation for high-risk cervical cancer. *N Engl J Med* 340: 1137.

Morrow CP, BN Bundy, RJ Kurman et al. 1991. Relationship between surgical-pathological risk factors and outcome in clinical stage I and II carcinoma of the endometrium: A Gynecologic Oncology Group study. *Gynecol Oncol* 40:55.

Morton G and GM Thomas. 1994. Role of Radiotherapy in the Treatment of Cancer of the Ovary. *Semin Surg Onc* 10:305–312 .

Moskovic E, E MacSweeney, M Law, A Price. 1993. Survival, patterns of spread and prognostic factors in uterine sarcoma: A study of 76 patients. *Br J Radiol* 66:1009.

Mulayim N, D Foster Silver, PE Schwartz, S Higgins. 2004. Chemoradiation with 5-fluorouracil and mitomycin C in the treatment of vulvar squamous cell carcinoma. *Gynecol Oncol* 93:659.

NCCN. 2005. National Comprehensive Cancer Network guidlines available online at www.nccn.org/professionals/physician_gls/default.asp (Accessed 3/8/05).

Nelson G M Rabdall, G Sutton, D Moore, J Hurtean, K Look. 1999. FIGO stage IIIC endometrial carcinoma with metastases confined to pelvic lymph nodes: Analysis of treatment outcomes, prognostic variables and failure patterns following adjuvant radiation therapy. *Gynecol Oncol* 75:211.

Nori D, BS Hilaris, G Stanimir, JL Lewis Jr. 1983. Radiation therapy of primary vaginal carcinoma. *Int J Radiat Oncol Biol Phys* 9:1471.

Onda T, H Yoshikawa, K Mizutani et al. 1997. Treatment of node-positive endometrial cancer with complete node dissection, chemotherapy and radiation therapy. *Br J Cancer* 75:1836.

Pai HH, L Souhami, BG Clark, T Roman. 1997. Isolated vaginal recurrences in endometrial carcinoma: treatment results using high-dose-rate intracavitary brachytherapy and external beam radiotherapy. *Gynecol Oncol* 66:300.

Patricia J. Eifel, 2006. Chemoradiotherapy in the treatment of cervical cancer. *Emin Radiat Oncol* 16:177–185.

Pearcey R, M Brundage, P Drouin et al. 2002. Phase III Trial comparing radical radiotherapy with and without cisplatin hemotherapy in patients with advanced squamous cell cancer of the cervix. *JCO* 20:966–972

Perez CA, PW Grigsby, HM Camel et al. 1986. Randomized study of preoperative radiation and surgery or irradiation alone in the treatment of Stage IB and IIA carcinoma cervix: final report. *Gynaecol Oncol* 23:127–140.

Perez CA, PW Grigsby, M Garipagaoglu et al. 1999. Factors affecting long-term outcome of irradiation in carcinoma of the vagina. *Int J Radiat Oncol Biol Phys* 44:37.

Peters WA III, PY Liu, RJ Barrett II et al. 2000. Concurrent chemotherapy and pelvic radiation therapy compared with pelvic radiation therapy alone as adjuvant therapy after radical surgery in high-risk early-stage cancer of the cervix. *J Clin Oncol* 18:1606–1613.

Prempree T and R Amornmarn 1985. Radiation treatment of primary carcinoma of the vagina. Patterns of failures after definitive therapy. *Acta Radiol Oncol* 24:51.

Randall ME, G Brunetto, H Muss, et al. 2003. Whole abdominal radiotherapy versus combination doxorubicin-cisplatin chemotherapy in advanced endometrial carcinoma: A randomized trial of the Gynecologic Oncology Group (abstract). *Proc Am Soc Clin Oncol* 22:2.

Reddy S, VS Saxena, S Reddy et al. 1991. Results of radiotherapeutic management of primary carcinoma of the vagina. *Int J Radiat Oncol Biol Phys* 21:1041.

Reed NS, C Mangioni, H Malmstrom et al. 2003. First results of a randomized trial comparing radiotherapy versus observation postoperatively in patients with uterine sarcomas. An EORTC-GCG Study (abstract). *Int J Gynecol Cancer* 13(suppl 1);4.

Reisinger SA, R Asbury, SY Liao, HD Homesley. 1996. A phase I study of weekly cisplatin and whole abdominal radiation for the treatment of stage III and IV endometrial carcinoma: A Gynecologic Oncology Group pilot study. *Gynecol Oncol* 63:299.

Roberts WS, MS Hoffman, JJ Kavanagh et al. 1991. Further experience with radiation therapy and concomitant intravenous chemotherapy in advanced carcinoma of the lower female genital tract. *Gynecol Oncol* 43:233.

Rose PG, SD Cha, WK Tak et al. 1992. Radiation therapy for surgically proven para-aortic node metastasis in endometrial carcinoma. *Int J Radiat Oncol Biol Phys* 24:229.

Rose PG, BN Bundy, J Watkins et al. 1999. Concurrent cisplatin-based chemotherapy and radiotherapy for locally advanced cervical cancer. *N Engl J Med* 340:1144.

Rubin P and GW Cassarett. 1968. *Clinical Radiation Pathology*, Philadelphia: WB Saunders.

Rubin SC, J Young, JJ Mikuta. 1985. Squamous carcinoma of the vagina: Treatment, complications and long-term follow-up. *Gynecol Oncol* 20:346.

Schorge JO, Kh Molpus, A Goodman, N Nikrui, AF Fuller Jr. 1996. The effect of post-surgical therapy on stage III endometrial carcinoma. *Gynecol Oncol* 63:34–39.

Sedlacek TV, P Syropoulus, R Cifaldi, J Glassburn, S Fisher. 1997. Whole-abdomen radiation therapy as salvage treatment for epithelial ovarian carcinoma. *Cancer J Sci Am* 3:358–363.

Sedlis A, BN Bundy, MZ Rotman et al. 1999. A randomized trial of pelvic radiation therapy versus no further therapy in selected patients with stage IB carcinoma of the cervix after radical hysterectomy and pelvic lymphadenectomy. GOG Study. *Gynaecol Oncol* May. 73(2):177–183.

Soper JT, WT Creasman, DL Clarke-Pearson, et al. 1985. Intraperitoneal chromic phosphate P 32 suspension therapy of malignant peritoneal cytology in endometrial carcinoma. *Am J Obstet Gynecol* 153:191.

Sorbe B. 2002. Consolidated treatment of advanced (PIGO Stage III) ovarian carcinoma in complete surgical remission after induction chemotherapy: A randomized, controlled, clinical trial comparing whole-abdominal radiotherapy, chemotherapy and no further treatment. Swedish-Norwegian Ovarian Cancer Study Group. *Int J Gynecol Cancer.* 12:250.

Spirtos NM, BP Doshi, DS Kapp, N Teng. 1989. Radiation therapy for primary squamous cell carcinoma of the vagina: Stanford University experience. *Gynecol Oncol* 35:20.

Stehman FB, BN Bundy, G Thomas et al. 1992. Groin dissection versus groin radiation in carcinoma of the vulva: A Gynecologic Oncology Group study. *Int J Radiat Oncol Biol Phys* 24:389.

Subak LL, H Hricak, CB Powell, L Azizi, JL Stern. 1995. Cervical carcinoma: Computed tomography and magnetic resonance imaging for preoperative staging. *Obstet Gynecol* 86:43–50

Sutton G, JH Axelrod, BN Bundy et al. 2005. Whole abdominal radiotherapy in the adjuvant treatment of patients with stage III and IV endometrial cancer: A gynecologic oncology group study. *Gynecol Oncol* 97:755.

Tewari KS, F Cappuccini, AA Puthawala et al. 2001. Primary invasive carcinoma of the vagina: Treatment with interstitial brachytherapy. *Cancer* 91:758.

Walton RJ. 1976. Editorial: The task force on cervical cancer screening programs. *Can Med Assoc J* 114:981

Weitmann HD, TH Knocke, H Kucera, R Potter. 2001. Radiation therapy in the treatment of endometrial stromal sarcoma. *Int J Radiat Oncol Biol Phys* 49:739.

Whitney CW, W Sause, BN Bundy et al. 1999. A randomized comparison of fluorouracil plus cisplatin versus hydroxyurea as an adjunct to radiation therapy in stages IIB–IVA carcinoma of the cervix with negative para-aortic lymph nodes: A Gynecologic Oncology Group and Southwest Oncology Group study. *J Clin Oncol* 17:1339.

Won Park, Young Je Park, Seung Jae Huh et al. 2005 .The Usefulness of MRI and PET Imaging for the detection of parametrial involvement and lymph node metastasis in patients with cervical cancer. *Japanese Journal of Clinical Oncology* 35(5):260–264

Wylie J, C Irwin, M Pintilie, et al. 2000. Results of radical radiotherapy for recurrent endometrial cancer. *Gynecol Oncol* 77:66.

25

Screening for Gynecological Cancers

Suresh Kumarasamy

Screening is defined as a procedure to help identify, in an organised way, a specified disease or condition among asymptomatic individuals. Population screening programmes are applied to a general population to detect disease early, in order to facilitate effective treatment. Screening may also be applied for the purpose of separating apparently healthy individuals into groups with high and low probabilities for a given disorder, so that further health resources can be targeted more efficiently on those who have a high probability for the identified disorder. The objectives of population screening programmes are to reduce morbidity and mortality, and improve quality of life.

For a screening programme to be successful, the following criteria should be fulfilled (Wildschut et al 1996):

1. The condition being screened should be an important health problem
2. The screening test and its consequences (in terms of further diagnostic tests and subsequent treatment) should be acceptable to the population screened.
3. The target conditions should have a recognisable latent or early symptomatic phase and the natural history of the target condition should be well understood.
4. The screening test should be reliable and valid.
5. There should be adequate facilities to confirm the diagnosis and provide adequate treatment.
6. The screening process should be a continuing process and not a 'once and for all' project
7. Early treatment of the target condition should be effective
8. The objectives of the screening programme should justify the cost.

OVARIAN CANCER

Ovarian cancer is the most common gynecological malignancy and the fourth most common cause of death from cancer in the developed world. Ovarian cancer carries the worst prognosis among the gynecological cancers, with an overall five-year survival rate of only 30%, as the diagnosis is often made when the disease has reached an advanced stage. This is because the disease is often asymptomatic in the early stages. Seventy percent of women are diagnosed with stage III or IV disease, with five-year survival rates of 15% to 20% and less than 5%, respectively (Teneriello and Park 1995).

The prognosis in women where the cancer

is diagnosed at an early stage is good, with survival rates of 80% for stage I disease and more than 90% for those with stage Ia disease (Nguyen et al 1993). This fact has generated interest in screening for ovarian cancer with the aim of detecting the disease at an early stage resulting in an improvement of prognosis.

Ovarian cancer fulfills some of the criteria for a successful screening programme. Elevated CA 125 levels have been detected years before the diagnosis of ovarian cancer by retrospective serum analysis. However, there is no known pre-malignant precursor lesion, limiting the focus of screening at present to the detection of asymptomatic, early stage disease. There is also no data on how long ovarian cancer takes to progress from early to advanced disease. Both transvaginal ultrasound and CA 125 blood tests have been found to be acceptable tests by patients in large prospective trials. CA 125 and ultrasound as well as facilities for treatment of ovarian cancer, both surgical and medical, are widely available.

CA 125: Serum CA 125 was initially proposed as a screening test following the work of Bast and colleagues. This group first demonstrated that elevations of CA 125 were seen more frequently in women with ovarian cancer (82%) than in women in the general population (1%) (Bast et al 1983). Elevated CA 125 levels were found in 50% of patients with stage I disease and more than 90% of women with more advanced disease (Jacobs and Bast 1989). Further studies showed that CA 125 could be elevated in the preclinical asymptomatic phase of the disease, as raised levels were found in 25% of 59 stored serum samples collected five to twelve years prior to the diagnosis of ovarian cancer (Zurawski et al 1988).

Unfortunately, CA 125 was also found to be elevated in a number of conditions other than ovarian cancer. It was found to be elevated in 6% of women with benign disease, as well as in 28.5% of women with non-gynecologic cancers. Table 25.1 shows a list of conditions other than ovarian cancer associated with raised CA 125.

Prospective studies that followed did not show that CA 125 when used alone was useful as a screening test to detect ovarian cancer. Einhorn et al (1992) conducted a longitudinal study on a cohort of women, selected from a population of healthy women who were found to have CA 125 greater than 30 U/ml. Serial CA 125 measurements, pelvic examinations, and transabdominal ultrasound scans were performed at regular intervals. Six ovarian cancers (two each in stages Ia, IIb

Table 25.1: Some conditions in which CA 125 may be elevated

Gynecological Conditions
Ovarian cancer
Endometriosis
Fibroids
Hemorrhagic ovarian cycsts
Menstrualtion
Acute pelvic inflammatory disease
Endometrial cancer
Non-gynecological Conditions
Acute pancreatitis
Colitis
Chronic active hepatitis
Cirrhosis
Diverticulitis
Pericarditis
Renal disease
Systemic lupus erythematosis
Non-gynecological Malignancies
Bladder cancer
Breast cancer
Lung cancer
Liver cancer
Pancreas cancer
Non-Hodgkin's lymphoma

and IIIc) were diagnosed during the period of follow up. Three patients in the group with normal CA 125 developed cancer. The number of positive screens per cancer detected was 29. Helzlsouer et al (1993) analysing CA 125 levels in over 11,000 women over a 12-year period showed that the sensitivity of CA 125 for ovarian cancer within three years of diagnosis was 57%.

Analysis of CA 125 levels has revealed that CA 125 levels in women without ovarian cancer were static or decreased with time, while pre-clinical levels associated with malignancy tended to rise. This has resulted in attempts to develop a more sophisticated approach to interpretation of CA 125 results than a fixed absolute cut-off level. A computer based mathematical model has been developed by Skates, Pauler and Jacobs (2001) using the absolute level of CA 125 as well as the rate of rise over time, together with the individual's age specific risk of ovarian cancer. The algorithm is called the Risk of Ovarian Cancer Algorithm (ROCA). The algorithm has a specificity of 99.7%, with a sensitivity of 83% and a positive predictive value of 16%. This is being tested in the ongoing United Kingdom Trial of Ovarian Cancer Screening trial (UKCTOCS).

Ultrasound: Vaginal ultrasound has been assessed in the early detection of ovarian cancer. Van Nagell et al (1995) studied transvaginal ultrasonography as a screening method for the detection of early ovarian cancer in 8500 asymptomatic women. Of them 121 women had a persisting abnormality on TVS and underwent surgery. Eight patients had ovarian cancer and 57 patients had serous cystadenomas. Six of the patients with ovarian cancer had stage I disease, one patient had stage IIc disease and one patient had stage III cancer. Only one of these patients had a palpable ovarian enlargement on clinical examination, and only one had an elevated serum CA 125. There were 8379 women with normal screens. One patient with a family history of ovarian cancer was noted to have ovarian cancer at prophylactic oophorectomy 11 months after a normal screen.

The authors concluded that while TVS could detect ovarian cancer, there was a low positive predictive value (7%). The low specificity of ultrasonography for malignant ovarian lesions, combined with recent findings of a high prevalence of benign ovarian lesions in older asymptomatic women results in many women requiring further investigations and undergoing potentially unnecessary surgery when ultrasonography alone is used for screening (Menon 2004).

Multimodal screening: Jacobs and colleagues have reported on a randomised controlled trial using sequential CA 125 determinations and ultrasonography (1999): 22,000 women who were older than 45 years or postmenopausal were randomised to screening and a control group.

The screening strategy involved initial screening with a CA 125 measurement and ultrasonography for all women with CA 125 levels above 30 U/ml. Women with abnormal ultrasound findings were referred for surgical investigations. Of 29 patients referred for surgical intervention, 6 index cancers (of the ovary or fallopian tube) were detected. There were 23 patients with false positive results (14 with benign tumours, 4 with fibroids, 2 with adenocarcinoma of unknown origin and 3 with no abnormality). The positive predictive value of screening was 20.7%

When these women were followed up for eight years from randomisation, interesting results were observed. Another 10 women developed cancer in the screened group and 20 women developed cancer in the control group. Survival time was significantly longer in the screened group than in the control group ($p = 0.0112$). The median survival time of women with index cancers in the screened group was 72.9 months compared to 41.8 months in the control group.

The promising results of this trial have formed the basis of the United Kingdom Trial of Ovarian Cancer Screening (UKCTOCS). This study aims to recruit 200,000 women and randomise them to a 1:1:2 ratio, into ultrasound screening, multimodality screening and control group. The results of this trial are due in 2014.

In the United States, a similar trial, the Prostate, Lung, Colorectal and Ovarian Cancer Screening Trial (PLCO) has just completed enrollment (74,000 women). The screening strategy involves CA 125 and vaginal scans for 3 years followed by CA 125 for another 2 years. The follow-up is planned for 13 years with the results expected in 2012.

Until at least one of the trials described is completed and the impact on disease-specific mortality is assessed along with other outcome measures, CA 125 screening for ovarian cancer should be performed only in the context of clinical research,

Screening in high-risk women: Hereditary syndromes account for approximately 5% to 10% of ovarian cancers. Women who are of high risk of ovarian cancer have been identified by virtue of family history, genetic predisposition or both (Menon and Jacobs 2002). There is a lack of data from optimally conducted trials on the value of screening in these populations.

Jacobs (2005) in a recent editorial has suggested a number of points that high risk women considering screening should be informed about. First, there is no definitive evidence that screening will reduce mortality from ovarian cancer. He pointed out that the benefits (or lack of benefits) of screening will only be known when the large randomised trials currently in progress are complete. As these trials are in the general population, there is likely to be debate on the applicability of using this general population data when available to the high risk group. This is due to the possibility of differences in the tumour biology of cancers in the high risk group. Another important point to note was that neither CA 125 nor ultrasounds will detect all occurrences of cancer; therefore, women should be told that screening will miss some occurrences of ovarian cancer as well as most occurrences of primary peritoneal cancer. Women considering screening should therefore be counselled about the false positive rate (which is higher in premenopausal women, for both ultrasound and CA 125) as this may lead to anxiety and sometimes even unnecessary surgery.

Up to eight women will undergo surgery for each woman with a screening-detected ovarian cancer, and a small proportion will be exposed to the risk of complications as a result of surgery. Some women may, however, value the short term reassurance when they are screen negative.

ENDOMETRIAL CANCER

The majority of patients with endometrial cancer have symptoms, with more than 90% presenting with postmenopausal bleeding. In addition, the majority of patients who have endometrial cancer have early disease at first presentation, as symptoms often occur when the disease is at an early stage (Hawwa et al 1970).

Screening: There is no indication for universal screening in endometrial cancer as there is no data confirming the efficacy of screening in the general population. In a study of 801 asymptomatic perimenopausal and premenopausal women who underwent endometrial biopsies, only one well differentiated endometrial cancer was detected (Archer et al 1991).

Our efforts on detecting endometrial cancer should focus on detecting it in women with symptoms. Assessment of all women who have post menopausal bleeding should include an endometrial biopsy as between 4% to 24% of them will have endometrial cancer. An endometrial biopsy, should also be performed in perimenopausal and premenopausal women with irregular bleeding, prolonged menorrhagia or metorrhagia.

Screening in high-risk women: There are certain groups of women who are at high risk for developing endometrial cancer. These include women who are taking tamoxifen, women who have a genetic predisposition to endometrial cancer and obese women.

Women on tamoxifen: Tamoxifen is often used as adjuvant treatment in patients with breast cancer. It has been shown to be associated with a 2.2- to 7.5-fold increased risk of endometrial cancer (Fornnander et al 1989). Two screening strategies have been suggested to evaluate these women, transvaginal ultrasonography and endometrial biopsy.

Tamoxifen causes the endometrium as visualised by transvaginal ultrasound to appear thickened. There is however, poor correlation between the endometrial thickness and endometrial hyperplasia and cancer. Gerber et al (2000) screened 247 postmenopausal women taking adjuvant tamoxifen and 98 controls in a prospective trial using transvaginal ultrasonography. Of these, 52 asymptomatic women had a thickened endometrium on scan. Of these women, four had endometrial hyperplasia and one had endometrial cancer; 20 of the women in the trial developed abnormal bleeding. When the women with abnormal bleeding were evaluated, four had hyperplasia and two had cancer. The authors concluded that transvaginal sonography is not indicated for routine screening in asymptomatic women taking tamoxifen, but all women with abnormal bleeding should be evaluated.

Barakat et al (2000) evaluated an alternative strategy performing serial endometrial biopsies at baseline, every six months for two years and then yearly for a further three years to evaluate 159 tamoxifen treated women. One case of complex hyperplasia and no cases of endometrial cancer were detected in this cohort.

The current evidence indicates that screening, both by transvaginal ultrasound and endometrial biopsy, are not useful for women on tamoxifen. Women on tamoxifen should have a baseline pelvic assessment prior to starting tamoxifen and be advised to report abnormal bleeding which should then be evaluated.

Women with heriditary non-polyposis colorectal cancer: Women with hereditary non-polyposis colorectal cancer (HNPCC), have a 40%–60% lifetime risk of endometrial cancer, a 60%–80% lifetime risk of colon cancer and a 13% risk of ovarian cancer (Watson et al 1994; Dunlop et al 1997)

Annual screening with colonoscopy has been shown to improve survival in these women. There have, however, been few studies evaluating the benefit of endometrial cancer screening in women with HNPCC.

Women with HNPCC-related endometrial cancer are usually diagnosed with the cancer at a younger age than that of the general population. The mean age at diagnosis in these women is 48 to 51 years (Watson et al 1994; Dunlop et al 1997). There have been recommendations to carry out screening from the age of 25 to 35 years (Burke et al 1997).

Two methods of screening have been evaluated in this group of women—transvaginal ultrasonography and office endometrial biopsy. In a study of 269 women from HNPCC families, no cases of endometrial cancer were detected by abnormal findings during sonography alone. Two patients in this series were diagnosed with stage I endometrial cancer. They presented with postmenopausal bleeding, and continuous vaginal bleeding respectively (Dove-Edwin et al 2002). This highlights the importance of counselling this group of patients to report symptoms of abnormal menstrual bleeding and postmenopausal bleeding.

Some authors have recommended annual office endometrial biopsies in these women (Ramondetta and Lu 2004). However, further research is needed to address the efficacy of office endometrial biopsy as a screening tool in this situation. It is also important to assess the tolerability of the procedure, particularly in postmenopausal women. The role of prophylactic hysterectomy and bilateral salpingo-oophorectomy should be discussed with these women.

Obese women: Women who are obese have an increased risk of endometrial cancer. An increased risk of up to ninefold in women who are 50 pounds heavier than their ideal weight has been described (Ramondetta and Lu 2004). However, there has been no study that has shown a benefit of endometrial cancer screening in these women. These women should also be counselled on the importance of reporting symptoms of abnormal menstrual bleeding and postmenopausal bleeding.

CERVICAL CANCER

Cervical cancer is the most common cancer affecting females in the developing world. In 2000, it was estimated that there were 470,600 new cases diagnosed and 233,400 deaths from cervical cancer worldwide, with 83% of these cases occurring in developing countries (Ferlay et al 2001). Cervical cancer is both preventable and curable, provided it is detected at an early stage.

The aim of cervical screening is to reduce the morbidity and mortality from cervical cancer which is unique in that there is a well defined precancerous stage as well as a method to detect this stage.

The fact that CIN develops into cervical cancer is proven by situations where CIN has been observed without treatment. In New Zealand, a group of 131 women who had proven CIN 3 by cervical biopsies were followed up untreated. In most cases, the diagnosis had been made by cone biopsy which probably removed most of the lesion. After 20 years, 36% had developed cervical cancer (McIndole et al 1984)

The cell changes associated with pre-malignant disease was first described by Babes of Bacharest in 1927. Cytologic evaluation of cells obtained from the cervix (and vagina) was first proposed by George Papanicolaou in 1943. Since then, cervical cytology has proven to be an efficient and effective method for cervical cancer screening.

There have been no randomised controlled trials to evaluate the impact of cervical cancer screening on cervical cancer incidence and mortality. There has, however, been a marked decrease in the incidence and mortality of cervical cancer observed in a number of countries following the introduction of cervical cancer screening programmes.

British Columbia, Canada, was one of the first places to have an organised cervical cancer screening programme. As a result of the screening programme, the incidence of cervical cancer dropped from 25 cases per 100,000 women in 1954 to 8 cases per 100,000 women in 1884, and the death rate dropped from 13 cases per 100,000 in 1962 to 3 cases per 100,000 in 1983 (Boyes 1980).

Similar results were obtained in the Scandinavian countries. A comparison of trends in the mortality from cervical cancer showed that the rate fell steeply in Iceland, Finland and Sweden after the introduction of organised screening programmes, but fell very little in Norway, where only 5% of the population was screened (Laara et al 1987).

Following an analysis of several of the largest screening programmes in the world, the International Agency for Research on Cancer (IARC) (1986) concluded that the factors that determined the success of screening programme, were the extent of the coverage of the population, the target age of the women screened and the reliability of cytology services.

For a cervical cancer screening programme to reduce the incidence and mortality from cervical cancer, it is important that a wide coverage of the target population is obtained. This was demonstrated by the rapid decline in mortality in England and Wales after changes were implemented in the screening programme in 1988 (Quinn et al 1999). Organised programmes have resulted in a larger reduction in the disease than opportunistic screening because a higher compliance of the target population is reached.

Recommendations for optimal screening schedules vary. The First Canadian Task Force recommended that a woman should enter a screening programme when she becomes sexually active or at the age of 18, whichever is later, should have a repeat smear a year later, smears three-yearly to the age of 35 and smears five-yearly to the age of 60, provided these smears were satisfactory and without atypia. The Second Task Force subsequently recommended annual screening to the age of 35.

In the United States, the American Cancer Society recommended three-yearly screening from the onset of sexual activity, based on a mathematical model. The American Cancer Society and the American College of Obstetricians and Gynecologists' latest recommendation is that all women have annual Papanicolaou smears and pelvic examinations from the age of 18 or onset of sexual activity. After three or more consecutive normal examinations, the Papanicolaou test may be performed less frequently at the discretion of her physician.

The World Health Organization recommends screening according to the resources of the relevant country, pointing out that even a single smear in a lifetime, if appropriately timed, will produce some benefit. It makes more sense in healthcare economic terms to use resources to increase the number of women being screened for the first time than to increase the frequency of screening in women previously screened (Chan and Luesley 2004)

After a negative smear, the protection remains high for two years and subsequently decreases with time. A working group from the International Agency for Research on Cancer concluded that screening of women aged 20 to 64 years, every five years, would protect 84% of them, whereas smears taken every 3 years would protect 91% and annual smears would protect 93% (Ponten et al 1995).

There is debate on the appropriate age to stop screening. Some series suggest that the screening of women older than 65 is of benefit with a 63% improvement in five-year mortality (Fletcher 1990), whereas other data on well screened populations suggest that a woman who has had regular normal smears up to the age of 50 is at a very low risk of cervical cancer and can stop being screened (Fahs et al 1992).

The Bethesda System

The United States, National Institutes of Health constituted a consensus panel to develop a uniform terminology for reporting cervical cytology results. This was called the Bethesda System. The Bethesda system was modified in 1991. The Bethesda system attempts to separate epithelial changes secondary to inflammation or repair from pre-malignant lesions. The terms, low-grade and high-grade squamous intraepithelial lesions (SIL), are used to designate cytologic changes that correlate with low and high grade SIL obtained by histology. The main features of the system is that it requires an estimate of the adequacy of the specimen, a general categorisation of the specimen (within normal limits, benign cellular changes related to inflammation or having an epithelial abnormality) and a descriptive diagnosis that includes evidence of infection, inflammation and reactive changes, as well as a descriptive diagnosis (Wright 2000). The 1991 Bethesda System is described in Table 25.2 (Solomon et al 2001).

False negative as well as false positive reports arise with cervical cytology. False negative reports can result in delays in diagnosis and in obtaining the appropriate medical care. False negative results may also be a medicolegal challenge.

A study comparing the results of two smears taken simultaneously, but examined independently, estimated a false negative rate of 18.5% (Beilby et al 1982). The actual false negative rate could possibly have been higher as lesions may have been missed by both smears. In another study, where asymtomatic women were examined, both cytologically and colposcopically, a false negative rate of 48% was reported (Kesic et al 1993). A recent meta-analysis suggested that a single conventional cervical smear misses between 40% and 50% of biopsy confirmed high-grade SIL (Nanda et al 2000). Sampling the endocervical canal can reduce the false positive rate. Studies have reported a higher CIN detection rate when the cytobrush is used (Boon et al 1986).

In spite of the relatively high false negative rate, cervical cytology is effective in preventing cervical cancer because of the natural history of cervical cancer, with slow progression of CIN to invasive cancer in the majority of cases. Also, because smears are repeated at intervals as part of a cervical screening programme, a lesion missed at an earlier screen may be detected at a subsequent screen.

A number of factors can decrease the false negative rate. They include using a proper technique to sample the smears, rapidly fixing the slides to prevent air drying and subsequent artifacts in the slides, as well as ensuring good quality control in the cytology laboratory.

The false positive rate of cervical cytology can vary from 5% to 70%. This can result in anxiety. Also, many women who do not have an abnormality end up being needlessly investigated by colposcopy.

Liquid based cytology: This is a recent development to reduce the false negative rate of conventional smears. With this method, the clinician obtains a specimen from the cervix in the conventional manner. A number of

TABLE 25.2: THE 2001 BETHESDA SYSTEM FOR REPORTING RESULTS OF CERVICAL CYTOLOGY

Specimen Adequacy
Satisfactory for evaluation (note presence/absence of endocervical/transformation zone component)
Unsatisfactory for evaluation (specify reason)
Specimen rejected/not processed (specify reason)
Specimen processed and examined, but unsatisfactory for evaluation of epithelial abnormality because (specify reason)

General Categorisation (Optional)
Negative for intraepithelial lesion or malignancy
Epithelial cell abnormality
Other

Interpretation/Result
Negative for intraepithelial lesion of malignancy
Organisms
Trichomonas vaginalis
Fungal organisms morphologically consistent with *Candida* species
Shift in flora suggestive of bacterial vaginosis
Bacteria morphologically consistent with *Actinomyces* species
Cellular changes consistent with herpes simplex virus
Other non-neoplastic findings (optional to report; list not comprehensive)
Reactive cellular changes associated with
- Inflammation (includes typical repair)
- Radiation
- Intrauterine contraceptive device
- Glandular cells status post hysterectomy
- Atrophy

Epithelial cell abnormalities
Squamous cell
Atypical squamous cell (ASC)
Of undetermined significance (ASC-US)
Cannot exclude HSIL (ASC-H)
Low grade squamous intraepithelial lesion (LSIL)
Encompassing: human papillomavirus/mild dysplasia/cervical intraepithelial neoplasia (CIN 1)
High-grade squamous intraepithelial lesion (HSIL)
Encompasing moderate and severe dysplasia, carcinoma in situ; CIN 2 and CIN 3
Squamous cell carcinoma
Glandular cell
Atypical glandular cells (AGC) (specify endocervical, endometrial or not otherwise specified)
Atypical glandular cells, favour neoplastic (specify endocervical or not otherwise specified,
Endocervical adenocarcinoma in situ (AIS)
Adenocarcinoma
Other (list not comprehensive)
Endometrial cells in women ≥40 years of age

collection devices can be used, including the conventional Ayers spatula and cytobrush or one of the newer collecting devices. The collection device is rinsed in a vial of buffered alcohol preservative fluid.

The cells in the fluid are made into a slide with a thin well distributed layer of cells. The slides are of better quality and less likely to be compromised by blood, mucous or inflammatory debris. A number of trials have demonstrated increased detection of SIL with liquid cytology (Austin and Ramzy 1998). Another advantage of liquid based cytology is that the remaining fluid can be used for human papillomavirus (HPV) testing. This may be useful in management decisions when the result has been reported as ASCUS.

HPV testing: It is an established fact that infection with HPV causes cervical cancer. High-risk types of HPV have been identified. Persistent infection with these high risk types of HPV lead to the development of high grades of CIN and cervical cancer (Rozendaal et al 1996). Patients infected with low-risk types of HPV rarely progress to CIN and cervical cancer.

HPV can be detected by a number of techniques including Hybrid Capture II (HC II) and polymerase chain reaction (PCR). Studies using HC II have demonstrated a sensitivity of over 90% in predicting high grade CIN or cervical cancer (Manos et al 1999).

HPV testing can be used to help in the triaging and subsequent management of patients with abnormal smears. Patients with abnormal smears who are HPV positive have a higher risk of having or developing high-grade lesions and are advised immediate colposcopy. Conversely, patients with abnormal smears who are HPV negative have a lower risk of developing high grade lesions and can be managed more conservatively

Another benefit of HPV testing is to detect women who are of low risk of developing high-grade lesions. A combination of normal cytology and a negative HPV test carries a negative predictive value of 97% –100%. The screening interval of such women could be increased or screening can be stopped in older women with safety as they have a low risk of developing high grade lesions and cancer.

Low technology screening tests: Though cervical cytology programmes have significantly reduced the incidence and mortality of cervical cancer, these are not feasible in many developing countries due to costs and technical constraints. Low technology approaches based on visual inspection has been proposed as an alternative approach.

The performance of unaided visual inspection has been unsatisfactory; 10%–70% of women were found to have an abnormal cervix, depending on the criteria used by the investigators to define an abnormal cervix. The sensitivity varied from 50% to 93.8% and the specificity varied from 30.5% to 55.2% to detect invasive cervical cancer. For preinvasive lesions, the sensitivity and specificity was low (50% and 30% respectively) (Sujathan et al 1995). Any attempt to improve the specificity by restricting the criteria used to define an abnormal cervix resulted in an unacceptable low sensitivity (31%–60%) (Wesley et al 1997).

Visualisation of the cervix to detect subjects with intense aceto-white areas after the application of 3%–5% acetic acid is termed as direct visual inspection (DVI) or visual inspection with acetic acid (VIA). Results from pooled analysis of data from two studies indicated an approximate sensitivity of 93.4%

and specificity of 85.1% for VIA to detect CIN 2 or worse lesions; the corresponding figures for cytology were 72.1% and 91.6% (Sankaranarayanan et al 2003).

Other studies to evaluate the safety, acceptability and impact of VIA on cancer incidence are underway. There are a number of randomised trials underway evaluating 'screen and treat' approaches using both VIA and HPV testing. The results of these trials will contribute valuable information to guide the development of public health policies on cervical cancer prevention in countries with poor resources.

Conclusion: There is insufficient evidence to date to support screening for ovarian cancer. A number of large randomised trials are underway to assess the value of screening for ovarian cancer. Until the results of these trials are available, ovarian cancer screening should only be carried out in the context of clinical trials. The issue of screening in high-risk populations is more contentious. Unfortunately, there is a lack of good data from optimally conducted trials on the value of screening in these populations

There is no indication for universal screening in endometrial cancer. Our efforts on detecting should focus on detecting endometrial cancer in women with symptoms of abnormal bleeding. There is also no good evidence to support screening in women who are at higher risk of endometrial cancer.

Cervical cancer screening with the Papanicolou smear is an effective method to decrease the incidence and mortality from cervical cancer. Successful screening programmes are well organised and managed, cover a large segment of the population, screen women of the appropriate age and must be backed by reliable cytology services. Low technology screening tests like aided visual inspection (VIA) need to be further evaluated. They may have a role in developing countries with insufficient resources to institute well run cervical smear based screening programmes.

Prophylactic HPV vaccines, recently developed, have been shown to be effective in preventing high risk HPV infection in randomised trials (Koutsky et al 2002; Harper et al 2004). They may be the ultimate solution to the prevention of cervical cancer. There are however, still unanswered questions regarding the duration of protection and long term safety. The vaccines developed to date also do not protect against all the subtypes of HPV that may cause cervical cancer.

References

A WHO Meeting. 1986. Control of cancer of the cervix uteri. *Bull Wld Hlth Org* 64:107

American Cancer Society. 1980 Guidelines for the cancer related check up. Recommendations and rationale *CA* 30:193

American College of Obstetricians and Gynecologists. 1995. ACOG committee opinion: Recommendations on frequency of Pap test screening. *Int J Gynecol Obstet* 49:210.

Archer DF, K McIntyre-Seltman, WW Wilborn et al. 1991. Endometrial morphology in asymptomatic postmenopausal women. *Am J Obstet Gynecol* 165:317–322.

Austin RM and I Ramzy. 1998. Increased detection of epithelial cell abnormalities by liquid based cytology preparations. A review of accumulated data. *Acta Cytol* 42:178.

Barakat RR, TA Gilweski, L Almadrones et al. 2000. Effect of adjuvant tamoxifen on the endometrium in women with breast cancer: A prospective study using office endometrial biopsy *J Clin Oncol* 18: 3459–3463.

Bast RC, TL Klug, E St John et al. 1983.A radioimmununoassay using a monoclonal antibody to monitor the course of epithelial ovarian cancer. *N Eng J Med* 309:883–887.

Bast RC, F Seigal, C Runowicz et al. 1985. Elevation of serum CA 125 prior to diagnosis of an epithelial ovarian carcinoma. *Gynecol Oncol* 22:115–120.

Beilby JOW, R Bourne, J Guillebaud, ST Steele. 1982. Paired cervical smears: A method of reducing the false negative rate in population screening. *Obstet Gynecol* 60:46–48.

Boon ME, JJM Alons-van Kordelaar, PEM Rietveld-Scheffers. 1986. Consequences of the introduction of combined spatula and cytobrush sampling for cervical cytology: Improvements in smear quality and detection rates. *Act Cytol* 30:264.

Boyes DA. 1980. The value of a Pap smear programm and suggestions for its implementation. *Cancer* 48:613.

Burke W, G Petersen, P Lynch et al. 1997. Recommendations for follow-up care of individuals with an inherited predisposition to cancer. *JAMA* 277:915–919 .

Chan YM and Luesley. 2004. Screening, diagnosis and staging of cervical cancer *Gynecologic Cancer: Controversies in Mangement* eds Gershenson DM, McGuire WP, Gore M, Quinn MA, Thomas G. New York: Elsevier Churchill Livingstone.

Dove-Edwin I, D Boks, S Goff et al. 2002. The outcome of endometrial carcinoma surveillance by ultrasound in women at risk of hereditary non polyposis colorectal carcinoma and familial colorectal carcinoma *Cancer* 94:1708–1712.

Dunlop MG, SM Farrington, AD Carrothers et al. 1997. Cancer risk associated with germline DNA mismatch repair gene mutations. *Hum Mol Genet* 6:105–110.

Einhorn N, K Sjovall, RC Knapp et al. 1992. Prospective evaluation of serum CA 125 levels for early detection of ovarian cancer. *Obstet Gynecol* 80(1):14–18.

Fahs MC, J Mandelblatt, C Schechter et al. 1992. Cost effectiveness of cervical cancer screening for the elderly. *Ann Intern Med.* 117:520–527.

Ferlay J, F Bray, P Pisawi, DM Parkin. 2001. GLOBOCAN 2000 Cancer Incidence, Mortality and Prevalence Worlwide. Version 1.0 IARC Cancer Base No.5. Lyon: IARC Press.

Fink DJ. 1988. Change in American Cancer Society checkup guidelines for detection of cervical cancer. *CA* 38:127

Fletcher A. 1990. Screening for cancer of the cervix in elderly women. *Lancet* 335:97–99

Fornnander T, LE Rutquist, B Cedernark et al. 1989. Adjuvant tamoxifen in early breast cancer: Occurrence of new primary cancers. *Lancet* 1:117–120.

Gerber B, A Krause, H Muller et al. 2001. Ultrasonic detection of asymptomatic endometrial cancer in postmenopausal patients offers no prognostic advance over symptomatic disease discovered by uterine bleeding. *Eur J Cancer* 37:67–71.

Harper DM, EL Franco, C Wheeler et al. 2004. Efficacy of a bivalent L1 virus-like particle vaccine in prevention of infection with human papilloma virus types 16 and 18 in young women: A randomized controlled trial. *Lancet* 364:1757–1764.

Hawwa ZM, WA Nahhas, EH Copenhaver. 1970. Postmenopausal bleeding, *Br J Obstet Gynecol* 102: 133–136.

Helzlsouer KJ, TL Bush, AJ Alberg et al. 1993. Retrospective study of serum CA 125 levels as markers of ovarian cancer. *JAMA* 269:1123–1126.

IARC Working Group on Evaluation of Cervical Cancer Screening Programmes. 1986. Screening for squamous cervical cancer: The duration of low risk after negative result of cervical cytology and its implication for screening policies.1986. *BMJ* 293:659–64.

Jacobs I and RC Bast. 1989. The CA 125 tumour associated antigen: A review of the literature. *Hum Reprod* 4(1):1–12.

Jacobs I. 2005. Screening for Familial Ovarian Cancer: The need for well designed prospective studies. *J Clin Oncol* 23(24):5443–5445.

Jacobs IJ, SJ Skates, N MacDonald et al. 1999. Screening for ovarian cancer: A pilot randomized controlled trial. *Lancet* 353:1207–1210.

Kesic VI, WP Soutter, V Sulovic, N Juznic, M Aleksic, A Ljubic. 1993. A comparatison cytology and cervicography in cervical screening. *Int J Gynecol Oncol* 3:395–398.

Koutsky LA, KA Ault, CM Wheeler et al. 2002. A controlled trial of a human papilloma virus type 16 vaccine. *N Eng J Med* 347:1645–1647.

Laara E, NE Day, M Hakama. 1987. Trends in the mortality from cervical cancer in the Nordic countries associated with organized screening programmes *Lancet* ii:247–249.

Manos MM, WK Kinney, LB Hurley et al. 1999. Identifying women with cervical neoplasia: Using human papillomavirus DNA testing forquivocal Papanicolaou results *JAMA* 281:1605–1610.

McIndole WA, MR McLean, RW Jones, PR Mullins. 1984. The invasive potential of carcinoma in situ of the cervix. *Obstet Gynecol* 64:451–458.

Menon U and IJ Jacobs. 2002. The current status of screening for ovarian cancer In *Ovarian Cancer* ed CN Hudson. London: Oxford University Press.

Menon U. 2004. Ovarian cancer screening. *CMAJ* 171(4):323.

Nanda K, DC McCrory, ER Myers et al. 2000. Accuracy of the Papanicolaou test in screening for and follow-up of cervical cytologic abnormalities: A systemic review. *Ann Intern Med*: 132:810–819.

Nguyen HN, HE Averette, W Hoskins et al. 1993. National survey of ovarian carcinoma.VI. Critical assessment of International Federation of Gynecology and Obstetrics staging system. *Cancer* 72: 3007–3011.

Ponten J, HO Adami, R Bergstrom et al. 1995. Strategies for global control of cervical cancer. *Int J Cancer* 60:1–26

Quinn M, P Babb, J Jones et al. 1999. Effect of screening on incidence of and mortality from cancer of cervix in England: Evaluation based on routinely collected statistics. *BMJ* 318:904–908.

Ramondetta L and KH Lu. 2004. Controversies in Endometrial Cancer Screening and Diagnosis. *Gynecologic Cancer: Controversies in Mangement* ed DM Gershenson, WP McGuire, M Gore, MA Quinn, G Thomas, New York: Elsevier Churchill Livingstone.

Rozendaal L, JM Walboomers, JC van der Linden et al. 1996. PCR-based high risk HPV test in cervical cancer screening gives objective risk assessment of women with cytomorphologically normal cervical smears *Int J Cancer* 68:766–769

Sankaranarayanan R, BM Nene, K Dinshaw, R Rajkumar, S Shastri, R Wesley et al. 2003. Early detection of cervical cancer with visual inspection methods: a summary of completed and on-going studies in India. *Salud Publica Mex* 45(Suppl 3):S399–407.

Skates SJ, DK Pauler, I Jacobs. 2001. Screening based on the risk of ovarian cancer calculation from Bayesian hierarchical change point and mixture models of longitudinal markers. *J Am Stat Assoc* 96: 429–439.

Solomon D, D Davey, R Kurman et al. 2002. The 2001 Bethesda System: Terminology for reporting results of cervical cytology. *JAMA* 287:2116.

Sujathan K, S Kannan, KR Pillai, A Mathew, M Joseph, B Syamalkumari, MK Nair. 1995. Implications of gynecological abnormalities in pre-selction criteria for cervical cancer screening: Preliminary evaluation of 36022 subjects in South India *Cytopathology* 6:75–87.

Task Force. 1976. Cervical Cancer Screening Programme. The Walton Report. *Can Med Ass J* 114:1003.

Task Force. 1982. Cervical Cancer Screening Programme: Summary of the 1982 Canadian task force report. *Can Med Ass J* 127:581

Teneriello MG and RC Park. 1995. Early detection of ovarian cancer. *CA Cancer J Clin* 45:71–87.

Van Nagell JR, HH Gallion, EJ Pavlik et al. 1995. Ovarian cancer screening. *Cancer* 76: 2086–2091.

Watson P, HF Vasen, JP Mecklin et al. 1994. The risk of endometrial cancer in hereditary non polyposis colorectal cancer. *Am J Med* 96:516–520.

Wesley R, R Sankaranarayanan, B Mathew, B Chandralekha, A Aysha Beegum, NS Amma, MK Nair. 1997. Evaluation of visual inspection as a screening test for cervical cancer *Br J Cancer* 75(3):436–440.

Wildschut HIJ, CP Weiner, TJ Peters, ed. 1996. *When to screen in Obstetrics and Gynecology*. London: WB Saunders Company Ltd.

Wright TC. 2000. Pathogenesis and diagnosis of preinvasive lesions of the lower genital tract. *Principles and Practice of Gynecologic Oncology* ed JW Hoskins, CA Perez and RC Young, 3rd edition. Philadelphia: Lippincott Williams & Wilkins.

Zurawski VR, H Orjaster Jr, A Andersen, E Jellum. 1988. Elevated serum CA 125 levels prior to diagnosis of ovarian neoplasia: Relevance for early detection of ovarian cancer. *Int J Cancer* 42(5): 677–680.

26

Palliative Care for Patients with Gynecological Cancers

Firuza D Patel | Lee Hsueh Ni | Suresh C Sharma

Palliative care for the terminally ill patient with gynecological cancer has to be an effort involving the family caregivers and a dedicated medical team, which should include the palliative care physician, oncologists, experienced staff nurses, a psychologist and others. Communication involving the patient and her family and relatives is of paramount importance to assure effective end of life care. Despite the advances in modern medicine and its related disciplines, the dying are the most neglected, and of them, women are the worst affected. A dying woman in a developing country often tries to spare her loved ones the anguish of her pain and also the financial burden, by making light of her suffering. The challenge is exacerbated at the end of life due to accumulating debility, distressful symptomatology and increasing dependence upon limited family carers. The changing demographic profile and social structure, together with the emergence of the nuclear family norm, challenges health care providers to deliver quality care to this vulnerable group.

Goals of care at the end of life: The ability to make the passage from life to death with dignity, and the ability to create a positive meaning for those who are leaving as well as those who remain (professional and family alike), all fall under the broad category of goals of care at the end of life.

The four principle needs identified as important to provide care of the terminally ill are social support, psycho-spiritual support, nursing care and medical clinical management (Uys and Cameron 2003). The main aim of all medical caregivers should be to provide relief for the patient from all unnecessary suffering, whatever its cause. Various physical and psychological symptoms, in particular anxiety, grief and depression, need to be addressed by the physician. Care of the terminally ill is an important part of palliative care and usually refers to the management of patients during their last few days or weeks of life. From the point at which it becomes clear that the patient is in a progressive state of decline, the therapeutic focus shifts from cure to comfort. The focus of care also needs to shift from the patient alone to the family as a whole, and bereavement support for the family is an integral part of palliative care.

The World Health Organization defines palliative medicine as: 'the active total care of patients whose disease is not responsive to curative treatment. Control of pain, of other symptoms, and of psychological, social and spiritual problems is paramount. The goal of palliative care is achievement of the best quality of life for patients and their families. Many aspects of palliative care are also applicable earlier in the course of their illness in conjunction with anticancer treatment' (MacDonald 1997).

Palliative Care (Neighbourhood Network in Palliative Care 2006)

- Affirms life and regards dying as a normal process
- It neither hastens nor postpones death
- It provides relief from pain and other distressing symptoms
- It integrates the psychological and spiritual aspects of patient care
- It offers a support system to help patients live as actively as possible until death
- It offers a support system to help the family cope during the patient's illness and in their own bereavement.

Pain and its management: The International Association for the Study of Pain defines pain 'as an unpleasant sensory and emotional experience associated with actual or potential tissue damage or described in terms of such damage'. The rider that pain is always subjective and the inclusion of the term, emotional experience, is very important and also that, pain is a somatopsychic experience. It emphasises the fact that a variety of different factors may cause or aggravate pain, all of which need to be considered in assessment and treatment.

A more practical clinical definition is 'pain is what the patient says hurts'—it is what the patient describes and not what others think it ought to be—it is subjective, and achieving pain relief is a major clinical challenge for caregivers.

The number of cancer patients experiencing pain increases with progression of the disease. Nearly 74% of patients with metastatic disease and up to 87% patients at the end of life experience pain (Seal and Cartwright 1994; Neighbourhood Network in Palliative Care 2006). However, in a majority of oncological situations, nearly 40%–50% patients fail to achieve adequate pain relief (Bonica et al 1990; Brescia et al 1990; Cleeland 1991; Portenoy et al 1992, Von Roenn et al 1993). Pain is inevitable in cancer, but suffering is not. There needs to be an adequate concept and a logical way to achieve pain relief in an individual patient (Lickiss 2001). Thus, pain evaluation is necessary. To treat pain, one must know its origin. Pain in a cancer patient is not due to a single cause, there may be a multitude of causes interacting at one point of time (Twycross and Fairfields 1982). The pain experience of the cancer patient is the result of nociceptive sources, specific pain syndromes and behavioural contributions (Ashburn and Lipman 1993) resulting in fatigue, pain and distress (Curtis et al 1991; Portenoy et al 1994). The attending physician must be aware that not all pain is related to malignancy, and its cause may be altered with progression of the underlying disease (Banning et al 1991).

Causes of chronic pain syndromes in gynecological malignancy:

1. Cancer-related pain:

a. Tumour-related pain syndromes

- Pain due to primary tumour—soft tissue extension
- Back pain
- Pain syndromes of the bony pelvis and hip
- Multiple or generalised bone pain due to bone metastases

b. Tumour—involvement of peripheral nervous system

- Malignant lumbosacral plexopathy
- Tumour-related mononeuropathy

C. Pain syndromes of the viscera

- Peritoneal carcinomatosis
- Midline retroperitoneal syndrome
- Hepatic distension syndrome
- Paraortic lymphadenopathy
- Chronic intestinal obstruction
- Malignant perineal pain
- Ureteric obstruction

2. Treatment-related pain:

a. Chronic postradiation pain syndromes

- Plexopathies
- Chronic radiation enteritis and proctitis
- Burning perineum syndrome

b. Chronic postsurgical pain syndromes

- Postoperative scars
- Postoperative adhesions

c. Chronic postchemotherapy pain syndromes

- Neuropathy

3. Associated factors unrelated to cancer:

a. Constipation
b. Pressure sores
c. Bladder spasm
d. Arthritis
e. Post-herpatic neuralgia

Development of an effective and successful strategy requires a broad-spectrum approach. Goals of treatment need to be defined. Besides drug management, necessary interventions like surgery, radiation or palliative chemotherapy should be kept in mind. In this way, chronic cancer pain can be successfully alleviated in nearly 70% of patients (Ventafridda et al 1987; Walker et al 1988; Schug et al 1990; Vainio and Auvinen 1996).

A proper evaluation of pain is essential for proper treatment. The body chart is a useful tool in pain evaluation. The different sites of pain should be marked, along with the nature of each at the time of evaluation, so that it is available at the time of subsequent review. To assess the success of treatment, some form of quantification of pain is necessary. The Visual Analogue Scale (VAS), which is a 100 mm scale with no pain at one end and the worst imaginable pain at the other, is the one most commonly used. It is also important to assess the other factors which may influence pain—physical, psychological, social, cultural and spiritual factors. Table 26.1 illustrates factors affecting the pain threshold.

Factors affecting pain threshold:

Therapeutic approaches: Pain caused by cancer will require drugs which will give adequate relief, provided the right drug is administered at the right dose at the right time intervals. Cancer patients require a fixed dose scheduling to control the constant nature of pain. As and when required, a rescue dose needs to be incorporated for breakthrough pain. There is no paucity of data regarding pain management. The WHO has recommended the 3-step 'analgesic ladder', a classical approach in selecting drugs for managing pain (WHO 1996).

The WHO Ladder

A simple, well-validated and effective method for assuring the rational titration of therapy for cancer pain was devised by WHO in 1996. It has been shown to be effective in relieving pain in approximately 90% of patients with cancer and in over 75% of cancer patients who are terminally ill. This approach is based on the concept of an analgesic ladder.

The five essential concepts in the WHO approach to drug therapy of cancer pain are:

- By the mouth
- By the clock

- By the ladder
- For the individual
- With attention to detail

The use of analgesics for the treatment of acute pain in patients with cancer is the same for those not suffering from cancer. It is the treatment of chronic pain which is often poorly managed and requires a different approach.

The selection of a drug or drugs to use involves:

- Selecting a drug appropriate for the type of pain
- Selecting a drug appropriate to the severity of pain
- Using combinations of drugs, not combined preparations
- Using adjuvant analgesics
- Never using a placebo

Drug selection depends upon the type and severity of the pain. Different types of pain respond to different analgesics (Table 26.2). It is important that pain be brought under control as quickly as possible, so start with a stronger analgesic and subsequently wean the patient on to a weaker drug.

TYPE OF PAIN AND IMPLICATIONS FOR TREATMENT

When prescribing for patients with chronic pain, it is commonplace to use more than one drug. Different drugs should be given independently and compound preparations avoided because, if it is necessary to escalate the dose of one of the drugs, the dose of the second will also be increased and may cause unwanted toxicity.

If the prescribed analgesia is insufficient, or if the patent's disease progresses, analgesia is escalated in an orderly manner from non-opioid to weak opioid to strong opioid, as illustrated in the World Health Organization's analgesic ladder (Table 26.3). Non-opioid analgesics should be continued when opioid drugs are commenced, as their action can be complementary and allow lesser doses of opioids to be used. Adjuvant analgesics should be used whenever indicated.

Table 26.1: Factors affecting pain threshold

Threshold lowered	*Threshold raised*
Discomfort	Relief of symptoms
Anger	Relaxation
Insomnia	Sleep
Fatigue	Understanding
Anxiety	Companionship
Sadness	Anxiety reduction
Depression	Mood elevation
Boredom	Anxiety reduction
Mental isolation	Analgesics
Social abandonment	Antidepressants
Fear	Activity

The WHO Analgesic Ladder For Cancer Pain Management

The scheduling of drugs is according to the pharmacological properties and duration of clinical action. It is important that drugs are given according to a strict schedule, determined by the duration of clinical action, in order to prevent the recurrence of pain. Patients given doses that are too small or too infrequent may behave in a manner suggestive of psychological dependence, badgering the staff for extra doses of medication; this has been termed 'iatrogenic pseudoaddiction' and is resolved by the prescription of doses adequate in amount or frequency to provide continuous pain relief.

There is no place in the treatment of chronic cancer-related pain for giving analgesics on an 'as required' basis or pro re nata (PRN). As required or PRN orders invite inadequate treatment—staff may not enquire about pain and patients may not realise they have to ask for analgesics; staff or patients may minimise the number of doses for fear of addiction; or staff may be too busy to attend to requests, all of which result in unrelieved or recurrent pain.

Nonsteroidal anti-inflammatory drugs: Non-opioid analgesics, acetaminophen and the NSAIDS are the recommended first line drugs for cancer pain treatment (Lomen et al 1986; Ventafridda 1989; Mercadante 2001; Wallenstein and Portenoy 2002). They are highly effective in inflammatory conditions and bone pains with minimal effects on neuropathic pain (Mercadante et al 1997). NSAIDS inhibits the enzyme cyclooxygenase (COX), which has 2 forms—COX-1 and COX-2 that reduce the production of prostaglandins, compounds that sensitise nociceptive primary afferent neurons (Vane et al 1998). COX-2 inhibitors like rofecoxib, valdecoxib and celecoxib have the least risk of inducing gastrointestinal side effects, as compared to indomethacin (COX-1) (Mercadante 2001). NSAIDS must be administered with great care in patients with peptic ulcer disease, bleeding tendency, renal insufficiency (Mercadante 2001), advanced age or when used with steroids (Hernandez Diaz and Roderiguez 2000). Proton pump inhibitors, thus, have to be given in conjunction with NSAIDS (Hawkey et al 1998; Hawkey 1998; Yoemans et al 1998) to reduce the risks of gastrointestinal damage.

Opioids: The word 'weak' is a misnomer as none of these drugs incorporate a ceiling effect limiting its use. The initial WHO recommended subclassification, into a 'weak' or 'strong' opioid, is more functional than pharmacologic (WHO 1996). On the basis of receptor interactions, opioids may be divided into pure agonists and agonist–antagonists. Pure agonists, that is, morphine, binds directly at the 'μ' receptor subtype. The latter group which plays a limited role in chronic cancer pain management comprises mixed agonist–antagonist subtypes, which may be weak agonists at the 'μ' receptor (buprenorphine) and antagonists at other receptor subtype or vice versa (pentazocine, nalbuphine and

Table 26.2: Response to analgesics

Nociceptive		
Bone, soft tissue	Mild, moderate	Non-opioid (opioids if required)
	Severe	Opioids + non-opioid
	Visceral	Mild non-opioid (optional if required)
	Moderate, severe	Opioids ± non-opioid
Neuropathic		
	Nerve compression	Opioids + corticosteroid
	Nerve infiltration, damage	Tricyclic antidepressant or anti-convulsant or oral local anesthetic drug
	Sympathetic-type pain	(sympathetic nerve block)
Other		
	Raised intracranial pressure	Corticosteroid
	Muscle spasm	Muscle relaxant

TABLE 26.3: ANALGESICS FOR PAIN CONTROL

		Analgesics	*Drug of choice*	*Alternative*
Step 1	pain	non-opioid±adjuvant	aspirin/NSAID	paracetamol
Step 2	pain persists or increases	weak opioid drug± non-opioid±adjuvant	codeine	oxycodone tramadol
Step 3	pain persists or increases	strong opioid± non-opioid±adjuvant	morphine	methadone hydromorphone

butorphanol) (Hoskins and Hanks 1991). They have a threshold dose for pain, with a propensity to cause an abstinence syndrome, in patients already physically dependent on an agonist drug. The following principles should be observed:

- A weak opioid should be added to a non-opioid, not substituted for one
- If a weak opioid is inadequate when given regularly, switch to morphine

Weak opioids: Commonly used 'weak' opioids for managing pain of moderate intensity are codeine, dihydrocodeine, hydrocodone, propoxyphene and oxycodone, which is available in combination with acetaminophen. Codeine has about a tenth of the potency of morphine, in terms of pain relief. It is more constipating than other weak opioids and not generally recommended. The dose of an opioid combined with a coanalgesic, like aspirin or acetaminophen, can only be escalated until the dose of the adjuvant drug reaches its toxicity level. The dose may be increased to maximal safe limits of the coanalgesic, that is, 4 g per day of acetaminophen. Patients not benefiting from this combination need to be stepped up to the next level.

Tramadol: It has a dual mechanism of action, partly via opioid receptors and partly by blocking the presynaptic re-uptake of serotonin and noradrenaline. The dual analgesic action is synergistic. Undesirable opioid effects are significantly less than with codeine and morphine (Vickers et al 1992). It is less constipating (Wilder-Smith and Bettiga 1997) and relatively more effective in neuropathic pain (Sindrup and Jensen 1999).

Strong opioids: Morphine, oxymorphone, hydromorphone, fentanyl and methadone are examples of 'strong' opioids used for managing pain of severe intensity. For continuous chronic pain, opioids need to be administered around-the-clock, and several long-acting formulations are available, that require administration only once or twice daily like, levorphanol and methadone (half life 12–190 hrs). In the case of morphine, specific counselling concerning 'myths' like fears of tolerance, addiction or dying must be done. In the Indian context, successful palliation of agonising pain has been possible with the use of intravenous morphine (Rajagopal 1998; Sureshkumar et al 2000; Harris et al 2003). Adverse effects include constipation, nausea, vomiting and sedation (Nicholson 2003). It is irresponsible to use an opioid, without prescribing a laxative (Lickiss 2001). Morphine must be cautiously prescribed in patients with renal insufficiency as it has a high potential to accumulate the metabolites (morphine-3-glucuronide and morphine-6-glucuronide), resulting in toxicity. These patients must be managed, preferably with alternative compounds like fentanyl or hydromorphone. Thus, before prescribing an opioid, the clinician must be well armed in advance to deal with all its side effects.

General comments and cautions regarding the use of opioid analgesics:

- Drugs of choice for severe cancer-related pain. Opioids do not have an analgesic ceiling effect, and therefore, dose can be titrated to achieve maximum pain relief.
- Constipation is a universal complication of opioid use, so all patients should receive prophylactic stimulant laxative therapy unless otherwise contraindicated (e.g. chronic diarrhea).
- Sedation is a frequent side effect of initial opioid use; however, tolerance develops soon in most of the patients.
- Respiratory depression rarely occurs except in opioid-naiive patients and those with significant pulmonary disease.
- True sensitivity reactions to opioids are rare. If patients experience such reactions, it is often possible to administer an opioid from another subclass. The subclasses are: phenanthrene derivatives—morphine, codeine, hydromorphone, oxycodone; phenypiperidine derivatives—meperidine, fentanyl; diphenylheptane derivatives—methadone.
- The use of opioid antagonists such as naloxone can immediately reverse all opioid effects including analgesia. Such reversal results in acute withdrawal, which may be complicated by excruciating pain and seizures. Therefore, opioid antagonists are never recommended to reverse non life-threatening effects such as confusion or sedation. If used to reverse life-threatening respiratory depression or hypotension, they should be titrated cautiously.

Adjuvant drugs: These drugs enhance the efficacy of analgesics and are used to treat co-existing symptoms (Mercadante and Portenoy 2001). They are generally 'add on' drugs supplementing the impact of an NSAID and an opioid. Nearly 60% of patients with gynecological neoplasm suffer from neuropathic pain which may be opioid-refractory. Hence, these cases will require co-administration of antidepressants, anticonvulsants or steroids (Portenoy 1998; Portenoy and Frager 1999; Lickiss 2001). Excellent analgesic efficacy of amitryptyline, a tricyclic antidepressant (Rowbotham 1998; Caraceni et al 1999; Watson 2000; Bosnjack et al 2002) and gabapentin, an anticonvulsant (Backonja et al 1998; Rowbotham et al 1998) are reported. Newer antidepressants with lower adverse effects that are available include bupropion, paroxetine and citalopram. The newer gabapentin analogues marketed are lamotrigine, topiramate, oxcarbazepine and zonisamide. Nearly 90% of patients with pain from nerve injury respond well to the systematic use of non-opioids, opioids and adjuvant analgesics (Twycross and Wilcock 2001). The remainder require spinal analgesia (for example, morphine + bupivacaine ± clonidine) or a neurolytic procedure to attain pain relief. Some patients derive benefit from other non-drug measures, like transcutaneous electrical nerve stimulation (TENS). Corticosteroids have found a wide acceptance with proven efficacy in the management of cancer pain with added advantages of improving appetite, nausea and malaise. They are indicated as adjuvant drugs in visceral, neuropathic and bone pains. Recommended initial doses range from as low as 1–2 mg, to as high as 10 mg of dexamethasone or 10 mg prednisolone, administered once or twice daily (Watanabe and Bruera 1994). Gradual tapering off of the higher doses will be required weekly, so as to reach the minimally effective dose (Wooldridge et al 2001). For the management of severe debilitating pain, an intravenous administration of a single bolus of dexamethasone 100 mg, followed by lower doses with subsequent tapering, is given 3–4 times a day (McDonnell et al 2001).

NMDA (n-methyl-d-aspartate) receptor antagonists: For neuropathic pain, which is refractory to standard treatment measures, a trial with NMDA inhibitors, which includes dextromethorphan, amantadine and ketamine, may be given. Ketamine when given in subanesthetic doses and administered orally, has a more favourable side effect profile than the parenteral route. Doses ranging from 0.2 mg/kg to 0.5 mg/kg Q6-8H are used. Benzodiazepine or a neuroleptic is co-administered, so as to prevent the exemplification of the psychomimetic syndromes commonly encountered with this drug (Bells et al 2003).

Ziconotide (PRIALT) is a newer N-type calcium channel blocker non-opioid drug, with a promising role in refractory cancer pain. It results in the selective blockade of neuronal N-type voltage-sensitive calcium channels. It has shown good efficacy in cases, which are not amenable to systemic analgesics or intrathecal morphine (Prommer 2005).

Nausea and vomiting: Nausea and vomiting may affect nearly 40%–70% of patients (Fainsinger et al 1981; Doyle 1983; Regnard and Tempest 1992). Nausea and vomiting is a common accompaniment of malignancies, as well as an adverse effect of its treatment. A careful understanding of its underlying mechanism along with a sympathetic attitude is helpful in managing this condition. Nausea causes more misery than vomiting, many patients can tolerate one or two vomits a day but prolonged nausea is profoundly debilitating. Dehydration, electrolyte imbalance, neutropenia, renal sufficiency resulting in uremia are the main causative factors for nausea (Coates et al 1983; Bliss et al 1992; Cooper and Georgior 1992).

When considering drug treatment for emesis,. the clinician must have an understanding of the underlying reflex pathways causing these symptoms. Emesis in malignancy is more of a physiologic process, in which the body attempts to rid itself of noxious substances. This reflex arc consists of various afferent limbs, a vomiting centre (VC) and efferent pathways which activate muscle groups to cause a response. The afferent pathways are

a. the chemoreceptor trigger zone (CTZ) which is rich in dopaminergic (D_2), mucarinic cholinergic (Ach), histamine type 1 (H1) and serotonin type 3($5HT_3$) receptors;
b. the peripheral pathway, where receptors in the gut wall send signals via the vagus nerve;
c. the cerebrocortical pathway; and
d. the vestibular limb, activated by positional change (Borison and Wang 1953; Soukop and Cunningham 1987; Kris et al 1993).

The CTZ is sensitive to chemotherapeutic agents, uremia and ketosis. As it is rich in serotonin receptors, drugs containing specific serotonin inhibitors like ondansetron or granisetron are the gold standard in managing chemotherapy-induced vomiting (Kris et al 1993; Lichter 1993). Table 26.4 illustrates the various causative factors of vomiting and its management. Haloperidol, when used at low doses of 1.5–3 mg, is one of the most potent dopaminergic (D_2) antagonists, acting at the CTZ and is an effective agent for controlling symptoms of nausea and vomiting (Petouka and Synder 1982). Metochlopromide and domperidone, preferentially act upon the gut to antagonize D_2 receptors and stimulate the $5HT_4$ receptors. The local cholinergic response mediated by the stimulation of $5HT_4$ receptors, results in normal peristalsis in the upper gastrointestinal tract, by reversing gastroparesis (Cassileth et al 1983; Linnik et al 1991). Cisapride, a prokinetic drug increases peristalsis from the esophagus to the rectum

CAUSES OF VOMITING AND ITS MANAGEMENT

Other families of antiemetic agents include corticosteroids, benzodiazepines and cannabinoids. Corticosteroids, like dexamethasone and prednisolone are moderately effective antiemetic agents when used alone, and are known to possess additive effects, when used along with other classes of antiemetic drugs (Cassileth et al 1983; Aapro 1991; Diehl and Marty 1994). Benzodiazepines (diazepam, lorazepam, alprazolam) are anxiolytic and sedative agents with little intrinsic antiemetic properties; they are helpful in blunting the effect of psychogenic, anticipatory vomiting (Greenberg et al 1987). Cannabinoids (nabilone, dronabinol) are potent antiemetics with a relatively severe toxicity profile that includes hallucination, disorientation, sedation, dizziness and dysphoria (Tyson et al 1985). They are used only when all other agents have failed to achieve a response.

Bowel Obstruction

Intestinal obstruction is due to occlusion of the lumen, or a lack of normal propulsion which prevents or delays the passage of bowel contents along the gastrointestinal tract. This may be the presenting symptom of a malignancy or it may occur during the course of the disease (Baines 1997). In gynecological malignancies, it is most commonly seen in carcinoma ovary at all stages, Tunca et al (1981) found an incidence of 25%, while Beattie et al (1989) found a 42% incidence of bowel obstruction. The attending clinician must be aware of the various factors that may predispose to bowel obstruction. In gynecological malignancies, the obstruction is generally extraluminal due to surrounding peritoneal disease and is often at multiple sites. Malignant abdominal or pelvic adhesions are commonly encountered in ovarian cancers. Other causes of obstruction may be mesenteric or omental masses causing direct compression. Motility disorders without any mechanical obstruction are also common in these patients (Yuhasz et al 1985). Electrolyte imbalances, drugs, for example, opioids, antihistamines, tricyclic antidepressants and neuroleptics may be other causative factors.

Patients may present with a typical vomiting pattern ranging from several times daily to once every few days. Vomitus may be large volume, feculent, associated with colicky pain. Patients may say that vomiting helps to relieve their nausea.

Management of bowel obstruction includes an erect and a supine radiography of the abdomen to look for multiple air-fluid levels, fecolith impaction and signs of imminent bowel rupture. A gastrograffin enema will help in distinguishing between large and small bowel obstruction. A CT scan of the abdomen will reveal the tumour masses, but not the site of obstruction and will seldom enlighten us upon the necessity of a surgical intervention. Prior to any form of surgical approach, if there are no signs of imminent rupture, a wait and watch policy may be adopted.

Symptomatic measures using medication are the mainstay of treatment avoiding the standard 'drip and suck' approach, which may be distressing and is ineffective in 80% of patients. Hence, the following measures should be tried.

Bowel wall edema reduction: Corticosteroids have found a definite role in the management of bowel obstruction in advanced malignancy. It is hypothesised that steroids decrease edema of the bowel wall, subsequently improving luminal patency. Dexamethasone, administered parenterally at a dose of 4–8 mg, given daily for 3–5 days, has been shown to relieve obstruction in various clinical settings (Twycross 1992; Philip et al 1994). If this is helpful and vomiting subsides, many physicians continue with oral steroids for example, prednisolone, 60–100 mg/day.

Gut motility stimulation: Metochlopromide 30–20 mg/24 hr may be given subcutaneously. This remedy must be stopped if obstruction does not resolve and care must be taken in case of increase in gut colic.

Other measures for management of intestinal obstruction: If obstruction is not relieved with the above measures within 24–48 hours, the focus must be shifted to treating symptoms rather than the underlying cause:

- Relieve nausea and vomiting—haloperidol 3–5 mg/24h rs sc
- Relieve colic—hyoscine butylbromide (buscopan) 40–100 mg/24hrs sc
- Ensure constant pain relief–morphine sc when required
- Relieve constipation by prescribing docusate, 200 mg tds, if obstruction is partial

To reduce or to encourage reabsorption of gut secretions and to reduce intestinal motility use hyoscine butylbromide, 40–100 mg/24 h sc; alternatively, octreotide 300–600 µg/24 h may be infused. If vomiting does not subside, or becomes distressing and/or feculent, it may be necessary to use a nasogastric tube after a thorough discussion with the patient and caregivers.

Role of surgery in relieving intestinal obstruction: Surgery should only be undertaken after an in-depth consideration of the etiology, after ruling out all medically correctable causes, with due consideration for the general status of the patient. The potential mortality and morbidity associated with surgery should be weighed against the quality of life in a patient in whom prognosis is poor. Clarke et al (1987), in their data on surgery for bowel obstruction in ovarian malignancy found that 30 (61.2%) patients had small bowel, 16 (32.6%) had large bowel and three (6%) had concurrent small and

Table 26.4: Drugs to deal with vomitting

Cause of vomiting	*Drug of choice*
Drug or toxin-induced	Haloperidol 1.5-2 mg bd or hs
Radiation therapy	Ondansetron 8 mg stat, 4 mg tds, granisetron1mg bd
Metabolic e.g. uremia	Haloperidol 1.5 mg hs or bd
Cytotoxic drugs	Ondansetron 4 mg tds; granisetron 1mg bd; dexamethasone 4-8 mg od prior to chemotherapy;metochlopromide 20 mg qid
Raised intracranial tension	Olanzapine 2.5 mg hs; dexamethasone 8-32 mg od
Intestinal obstruction	Hyoscine butylbromide 40-100 mg sc; olanzapine 2.5 mg hs
Delayed gastric emptying	Metochlopromide 10-20 qid; domperidone 10-20 mg qid
Gastritis	Omeprazole 20 od; lansoprazole 40 mg od; metochlopromide 10 mg qid

large bowel involvement. Progression of the malignancy was the main cause of obstruction in 86% of the patients. Major postoperative complications were encountered in 49% of patients in the form of wound infections, sepsis and enterocutaneous fistulas. They emphasised the need for judicious preoperative selection of patients who would likely benefit from this procedure. Krebs and Goplerud (1983), performed surgery in 98 patients in advanced ovarian neoplasms. They found an inoperability rate of 12% and a postoperative mortality rate of 12%. Thirty-five per cent of the patients died within 8 weeks of surgery, thus, no benefit was achieved in these cases. They proposed six prognostic factors index—

- Patient's age
- Nutritional status
- Tumour spread
- Presence of ascites and the type and amount of prior chemotherapy and/or radiation therapy
- All of which correlated well with the patients' outcome in their series

Intestinal obstruction encountered in advanced gynecological malignancies needs to be managed prudently. Utmost care needs to be taken when opting for surgery after conservative management failure. In end stage patients, it is always best to offer conservative management.

CONSTIPATION

Any factor that causes a decrease in motility, secretions or an increase in absorption will lead to constipation. In addition, the local functions, rectal tone, capacity, sensation and anal sphincter reflexes are important determinants of normal bowel function (Richter 1991). In advanced cases of gynecological malignancies, patients may become bedridden, resulting in decreased activity, diminished fluid intake, dehydration, hypercalcemia and low stool bulk. Neurologic and mechanical changes from presence of mass may also lead to a progressive loss of normal tone and sensation in the anorectal region with resultant constipation (Wald 1995).

Many medications used in the terminal phase are known to cause constipation. Opioids are the most notorious causative agents; the attributes that are so therapeutic for diarrhea become pathologic in this setting. The effects of this class of agents on the bowel include inhibition in the contraction of longitudinal muscles and in the secretion of intestinal secretagogues. They increase colonic circular muscle tone, and decrease overall intestinal transit time. There is subsequent increased intestinal absorption of fluid and electrolytes. Further, opioids cause impairment of normal anorectal tone and sensation, leading to frank bowel dysfunction (Bouvier et al 1987). Various other drugs commonly prescribed are also implicated to cause constipation. These include tricyclic antidepressants, anticonvulsants, diuretics, calcium and aluminium compound antacids (De Luca and Coupar 1996).

Management of constipation: Initial preventive strategy must include an attempt at increasing fibre intake so as to increase the stool bulk and subsequently prevent constipation, though most researchers have found that attempting to increase fibre intake is ineffective in managing constipation in the setting of advanced cancer (Bruera et al 1994; Rowinski and Donehower 1998). An important supportive care is that a bowel regimen must always accompany the use of opioids and steroids (Seynaeve et al 1991). Hydration in the form of increasing intake of oral fluids and fruit juices is accepted, and is somewhat beneficial, both as a preventive and also therapeutically, but it is often difficult to achieve orally (Glare and Lickiss 1992).

For treatment, initial assessment of the patient must include a rectal examination. Information obtained will include rectal tone, presence or absence of a mass, quantity and consistency of stools in the rectal vault (Glare and Lickiss 1992). We must try and keep the patient ambulatory for as long as possible. If hard stools are present, the initial intervention must be disimpaction. Table 26.7 illustrates the various drugs and their mechanism of action. Bisacodyl suppositories are stimulants and are an appropriate first measure if stool is adequately soft. Glycerine suppositories are useful in hard stools because they soften and lubricate the rectal contents, promoting less painful defecation. Two of the most potent laxatives for long term use are the non-absorbable sugars, lactulose and sorbitol. Lactulose is a synthetic disaccharide that is poorly absorbed in the digestive tract. There is no enzymatic degradation in the small intestine, so it reaches the colon intact, where it is metabolised to lactic acid and causes an increase in osmotic pressure, thus softening the stools. Its initial effect is delayed by 24–48 hours. Dose is to be titrated from 15 ml/day to 30 ml bd. A randomised study by Lederle et al (1990), in cancer patients comparing lactulose to sorbitol found the two equally effective and well tolerated. In a study by Wirz et al (2005), a combination of polyethylene glycol (PEG) 3350/electrolyte solution, sodium picosulphate and liquid paraffin was found to be highly effective in cases of opioid-related constipation, though further investigations are warranted.

Anorexia and cachexia: Anorexia and cachexia are commonly encountered in patients with advanced gynecological malignancies. Eating and drinking is essential not only for living, but is also an essential component of maintaining a healthy, social, interpersonal relationship. An insight into these sensitive issues must be kept in mind when caring for these patients.

In a cancer patient, high levels of circulating cytokines like interleukin-1, interleukin-6, cachectin, tumour necrosis factor are produced from macrophages in the body, resulting in a mobilisation of resources both from the fat and skeletal muscles (Backwich et al 1986; Bodnar et al 1989; Body 1992; Mantovani et al 1998). Thus, it is important to educate the patient and the caregivers, about the futility of forced feeding due to its unique underlying mechanism. Listed below are some of the common causes of cachexia and anorexia in advanced cancer:

- Paraneoplastic-cytokine production by host cells for example, tumour necrosis factor (TNF), Interleukin (IL-6), IL-1. Proteolysis producing factors result in abnormal protein, carbohydrate metabolism and altered fat metabolism
- Increased metabolic rate leading to increased energy expenditure
- Deficient food intake due to vomiting, diarrhea, malabsorption, bowel obstruction
- Debilitating effect of surgery, radiotherapy or chemotherapy

Patients present with marked weight loss, weakness, anorexia and fatigue. Associated physical features include pallor, edema due to hypoalbuminemia and altered taste sensation.

Treatment of associated symptoms like nausea, constipation, gastric stasis is paramount. Both medroxyprogesterone acetate and megestrol acetate have shown activity in improving appetite in patients suffering from cancer-related cachexia (Mantovani et al 1998). Various randomised, double blind, placebo-controlled trials evaluating megestrol acetate have been reported (Bruera et al 1990; Loprinzi et al 1990; Tchekmedyian et al 1990; Vadell et al 1998). Loprinzi et al (1990) used 800 mg/day of megestrol acetate or placebo in 133 patients. They found the drug was capable of stimulating appetite and weight gain of up to 6.75 kg in 11 of the 67 (16%) patients receiving megestrol acetate as compared with 1 of 66 (2%) patients receiving the placebo (P = 0.003). In patients on high doses, minimal side effects like hypercalcemia, edema and Cushingoid distribution of fat was noted. De Conno et al (1998), in a randomised trial found that using 320 mg per day of megestrol acetate, resulted in stimulation of appetite in 88% of patients, suffering from end stage malignancy, within 7 days of use, versus only 25% in the placebo group. Vadell et al (1998), in a double blind controlled trial, compared different dosages of megestrol acetate, 160 mg and 480 mg per day. They concluded that the latter dose resulted in a significant improvement in weight and tricep skinfold thickness, compared to the control group or the group receiving the lower dose.

Use of corticosteroids, in the form of low dose dexamethasone or intravenous methyl prednisolone, has been shown to improve appetite, food intake and performance status (Schell 1972; Bruera et al 1985).

Cyproheptadine, an antihistamine with antiserotonergic activities, has demonstrated similar activities in cancer-related anorexia (Pawlowski 1975; Editorial Lancet 1978; Nobel 1989). In a randomised, double blind clinical trial, oral cyproheptadine, 8 mg tds, administered in 295 patients, was found to improve appetite, but it did not prevent the progressive weight loss seen in these patients (Kardinal et al 1990). Gogos et al (1998) reported on the benefits of using omega-3 polyunsaturated fatty acids, at a dose of 18 mg of fish oil capsules along with vitamin E supplements, for end stage malignant disease. In a review of 55 randomised controlled studies (Yavuzsen et al 2005), only progestins and corticosteroids were found to be useful agents in stimulating appetite. They found no benefit with the use of hydrazine sulphate.

MALIGNANT ASCITIES

The healthy peritoneal cavity constitutes about 50 ml of fluid. The formation and drainage rates are about 4–5 ml/min (Hirabayashi and Graham 1970). Circulation of fluid from the peritoneal cavity is directly related to the increase in intraabdominal pressure and a ten-fold increase may be seen in the setting of malignancy. Lymphatic obstruction may also cause ascitis (Coates et al 1973). Locally mediated immune modulators, IL-1β-triggers vascular endothelial growth factor (VEGF), matrix metalloproteinases, kallikrien-4 and vascular permeability factor production by neoplastic cells increases permeability of new vessels as a result of tumour angiogenesis, and is an important mechanism of generation of ascitis (Aslam and Marino 2001; Davidson et al 2005; Stadlmann et al 2005). Another mechanism is the elevated renin activity resulting in sodium and water retention via the renin-angiotensin-aldosterone pathway. Beta-glucuronidase, β-galactosidase and α-mannosidase activity is increased in peritoneal fluid from patients with gynecological cancer, thus it is a useful diagnostic tool (Beratis et al 2005). Newer therapies in the form of immunomodulators offer an opportunity for the development of

TABLE 26.5: MANAGEMENT OF CONSTIPATION

Class	Drugs	Mechanism	Onset	Contraindication
Stool softener	Docusate sodium	Increases mixing of fat and water, easy stool penetration		
Hydrophilic	Dietary bran, fibre, psyllium	Retain water in colon, bulk forming	12–72 hrs	In cases of fecal impaction and the patient is bedridden
Osmotic agents	Epsom salts, milk of magnesia, lactulose, sorbitol, PEG-S	Water content in intestine increases peristalsis	0.5–3 hrs	Fecal impaction may cause renal failure in rare cases
Lubricants	Glycerine suppositories, mineral oil	Prevents water retention	6–8 hrs	Avoid mineral oil in elderly patients
Enemas/ suppositories	Proctoclysis	Distends colon and reflex evacuation	2–60 min	Interferes with fat soluble vitamin absorption

newer, targeted therapies for the management of ascites (Aslam and Marino 2001).

Patients present with abdominal discomfort, pain, inability to sit upright, nausea, vomiting, dyspepsia, early satiety, sour eructation and anorexia. Associated symptoms include weight gain with manifestation of muscle wasting. Due to elevation of diaphragm, tachypnea, dyspnea or orthopnea may occur. On physical examination, there is distension of abdomen with eversion of the umbilicus and bulging of the flanks. Free fluid can be elicited by shifting dullness.

Radiography will demonstrate abdominal haziness. Ultrasonography can detect quantities of fluid, even as little as 100 ml (Goldberg et al 1970; Michaud 1995). Diagnostic paracentesis is an important investigation done from a flank or a low midline site. Fluid aspirated must be examined for its physical appearance, colour, cell count, protein, sugar content, presence of microorganisms and malignant cells. Cytological examination detects malignant cells in 40%–70% effusions attributed to neoplasm (Sears and Hajdu 1987; Runyon 1988; Runyon 1994; Parsons et al 1996; Davidson 2004). The specificity of cytological examinations is nearly 100%.

The management of ascitis is done based on the knowledge of its formation. The diagnosis of a malignant effusion signifies disease progression and is associated with a worse prognosis regardless of the site of tumour. It includes the following.

Paracentesis: The mainstay of management of symptomatic ascitis is repeated large volume paracentesis which results in rapid symptom control. It should be the treatment of choice in patients with limited life expectancy, of less than 4–6 weeks. Up to 5–7 litres may be removed without colloidal support (Kao et al 1985; Pinto et al 1988;). In ovarian carcinomas, the principle followed is tap till dry. In this way, paracentesis provides relief in up to 90% of patients (Fevery et al 1996; Smith and Jayson 2003). Various studies have shown that removal of 2.4–11 litres within 30 min did not cause any significant changes in hemodynamics, serum electrolyte concentrations or hematocrit values within 24–48 hours post procedure (Kao et al 1985; Pinto et al 1988). Gines et al (1988) reported a lower incidence of asymptomatic abnormalities of electrolytes, creatinine and plasma renin in patients who received albumin after large-volume paracentesis. Cost of the expensive albumin must be considered. Infusion of dextran, a volume expander which is a much cheaper option has helped in preventing the asymptomatic abnormalities in laboratory values that may occur after paracentesis (Planas et al 1990).

Diuretics: These must be considered when the expected life prolongation is more than 4 weeks. As secondary hyperaldosteronism and increased plasma rennin activity are an important etiopathogenesis of ascitis, an aldosterone antagonist, spironolactone, used alone or in combination with proximal-segment diuretics like furosemide has been found to be effective in controlling ascitis (Fogel et al 1981; Greenway et al 1982; Arroyo et al 1989; Pockros et al 1992). Furosemide alone is less effective and results in more hypokalemia than spironolactone, thus the latter drug is preferred (Fogel et al 1981; Perez-Ayusho et al 1983). A normal renal profile and electrolyte value is mandatory, before starting diuretics. A daily dose started at 100 mg of spironolactone given once in the morning improves compliance with no resultant pharmacokinetic aberrations. Doses may be doubled to 200–400 mg, in cases where there is no decrease in body weight. Furosemide may be added for achieving a rapid response. The patient should be closely monitored for dehydration and serial monitoring of electrolytes; both sodium and potassium and the renal profile help to determine the optimal diuretic dose. A negative sodium balance with a weight loss of 0.5 kg per day should be the target (Shear et al 1970; Pockros and Reynolds 1986). In combination with dietary sodium restriction, this medical approach is effective in over 90% of patients (Fogel et al 1981; Perez-Ayusho et al 1983; Arroyo et al 1989; Stanley et al 1989) and as long as it continues to be effective, no other treatment for ascites is needed.

Peritoneovenous shunts: If diuretics are unsuccessful in managing ascitis, shunting may be considered. In the 1980s, peritoneovenous (for example, LeVeen or Denver shunts) shunting became very popular for the treatment of ascites. Complications like infections and shunt malfunctions decreased enthusiasm for this approach. The Veterans Administration Cooperative Study which screened 3860 patients was a controlled trial of treatment of diuretic-resistant ascites (Stanley et al 1989). This study could not document improved survival in patients treated with shunts, as compared with patients treated medically. Another recent controlled trial comparing shunting with therapeutic paracentesis, demonstrated approximately 50% survival at one year with either approach (Zanon et al 2002). Although survival is not prolonged, shunting may improve patients' comfort by reducing the volume of ascitic fluid. Use of shunts prevents the need for repeated paracentesis, while maintaining normal serum albumin concentrations. Blockage occurs in 25% of shunts, thus it is contraindicated in the presence of heavily bloodstained ascites because of the risk of occlusion (Smith and Jayson 2003). In a study by Zanon et al (2002), use of Denver shunts resulted in relief of symptomatic ascites in 87.5% of cases, with reduction of dyspnea, and subsequent improvement in appetite and ambulation. They concluded that careful patient selection, a close follow-up and appropriate device modifications may improve shunt performance, allowing a wider application of the Denver peritoneovenous shunt.

Chemotherapy: In the majority of cases in a palliative setting, therapy is aimed at symptom control. In an occasional patient, chemotherapy, either systemic or intraperitoneal, may be tried if the prognosis of the patient warrants it.

OBSTRUCTIVE UROPATHY

Advanced cancer cervix predisposes to the development of ureteric obstruction in nearly two-thirds of patients (Watkinson et al 1993). The patient may present with anorexia, anuria/oliguria, confusion, nausea, edema, hypertension and increased susceptibility to infections. Both blood urea and creatinine levels will be high, potassium levels may also be raised. Ultrasound will confirm obstruction to the renal outflow tract and, in a majority of cases it will be able to demonstrate the cause of the obstruction. If left untreated, progressive disease will lead to acute or chronic renal failure. However, a careful consideration of the stage of the patient's disease and prognosis is required before embarking on therapy. Patients suffering from advanced, disseminated disease, with no effective anticancer treatment available, that allow the patient to die with progressive uremia, without submitting them to painful, invasive procedures, may be the least distressing course.

If appropriate, the obstruction needs to be promptly relieved before irreversible damage to the kidneys occurs. Acute management of the associated hyperkalemia, metabolic acidosis and fluid overload may be necessary if renal deterioration is rapid. Symptomatic measures include hydration so as to replace losses and prevent thirst while avoiding fluid overload and pulmonary edema. All drugs should be used with caution in renal failure. Haloperidol, 1.5–5 mg od to tds orally or 5–20 mg/24 h by subcutaneous infusion, will help control nausea, myoclonic jerks, confusion and agitation. Pain from hydronephrosis and other aspects of the malignant disease may require strong opioids. Morphine and other opioids accumulate in renal failure and should be used with longer dosing intervals. Fentanyl has little excretion and accumulates less in renal failure than in other opioids (Faull and Barton 2001).

Relief of the ureteric obstruction by percutaneous nephrostomy (PCN), which has a very low complication rate, is a relatively simple procedure, and it may precede some form of permanent diversion so as to restore the renal function. One major contraindication of this procedure is progression of the disease during therapy. In a study by Lau et al (1995), PCN in patients with advanced carcinoma with obstructive uropathy without any further treatment resulted in a median survival of only 6.5 weeks (Lau et al 1995). Chan et al (1980) reported that the value of PCN in recurrent and advanced disease is very limited. Thus, an important question arises—is relief of the obstruction, and subsequent prolongation of life, in the patient's best interests? A careful selection of patients is required. At times, diversion may prolong life but at the cost of denying a terminally-ill patient with cancer, a painless death due to uremia.

Fistulas: The development of a vesicovaginal (VVF) or a rectovaginal fistula (RVF) may complicate recurrent or advanced gynecological neoplasms. It results in intense irritation and ulceration of the skin around the fistula. On occasions, a three way fistula may develop in the form of a 'cloaca'. Primary management measures include scrupulous management of perineal hygiene, use of adult diapers or tampons and use of creams like 1% silver sulphadiazine as local barriers. Occasionally, in cases of a low fistula, an indwelling catheter may relieve the incontinence due to a VVF, or a ureteric stent may be helpful in bypassing a ureteric fistula. The ideal management is excision of the fistula with primary repair but, this is seldom practical. Small fistulas may be dealt with in this way, using healthy tissue from the omentum or a labial fat pad as in a Martius rotational graft. Usually, a urinary diversion will be needed, either in the form of an ileal conduit or a nephrostomy, although in very ill or dying patients bilateral nephrostomy drainage may be adequate. RVF results in the passage of flatus, liquid or formed stools in varying amounts. A diversion or end colostomy is the most practical approach in such cases. If needed, a separate mucous fistula can be developed at the inferior margin of the abdominal incision (Ball et al 2003). If this is not possible, then barrier creams and douching with saline and betadine may be done.

Malodorous discharge: Infections with the vaginal and cervical flora are a major cause of morbidity and mortality, in women with advanced cases of carcinoma cervix, vagina, vulva or endometrium. Malodour, discharge, disfigurement leads to a loss of self esteem and social withdrawal.

In a healthy patient, the flora consists of anerobes like clostridium species, anerobic streptococci, bacteroids, Prevotella species (*B. fragilis* and *P. bivius*) along with aerobes, like *Escherichia coli,* Klebsiella, Enterobacter and gram positive cocci—enterococci and streptococci (Swenson 1973; Bartlett et al 1977). Any of the above organisms may become pathogenic and cause disease if the protective integument of the vagina, cervix, uterus and tubes are compromised in the setting of a malignancy, previous radiation therapy and prior antibiotic use, with resultant malodorous discharge, leading to increased exudate formation, pain and pyrexia (Gilstrap et al 1986; Gordon et al 1989; Thomas 1990). Other predisposing factors include the use of an indwelling urinary catheter and proximity of the gynecologic organs to the urinary and gastrointestinal tract, thus allowing easy access to the bloodstream. The malodour associated with the discharge can cause great distress as the individual feels permanently unclean, and may isolate her, minimising social interaction for fear of offending others. The odour is commonly caused by anerobic bacteria that inhabit hypoxic and necrotic tissues. Regular change of perineal pads is necessary. In a resource-poor setting, where diapers are unaffordable, pads made of folds of newspaper wrapped in layers of cotton has been shown to be an inexpensive and effective alternative. It is often helpful to provide an air-conditioning facility for individuals with discharge, or consider the use of air fresheners or aromatherapy oils—whichever is found to be effective (Casilda and Krishnaswamy 2005).

Successful treatment involves the use of metronidazole. However, the incidence of nausea associated with this drug may reduce its compliance. It has been reported that clindamycin 300 mg qid may be more effective than metronidazole (Grocott 1995). Some centres have found honey and activated charcoal useful for combating malodour (Williams 1999). Regular douching with warm water or dilute betadine solution is necessary for all patients with vaginal discharge. This can be followed by metronidazole irrigation. Some centres use vaginal douche pumps with an attached catheter. The irrigation catheter is gently introduced as far back into the vagina as possible. Wounds around the perineum or anus may benefit from a sitz bath, twice daily (Casilda and Krishnaswamy 2005).

Bleeding: Bleeding from a patient with gynecological cancers may occur due to:

- Bleeding directly from the tumour for example, cervix, vagina, vulva or it may occur from penetrating ulcerated inguinal lymph nodes, major vessel bleed due to direct nodal invasion
- Bleeding secondary to thrombocytopenia sometimes as a result of cancer treatment; uremia; disseminated intravascular coagulation (DIC); or the use of anticoagulants

Management: (Robert 2004) includes pressure dressings or vaginal packing with subsequent hospitalisation and bed rest which may be successful in most of the patients. Supportive measures in the form of intravascular replacement are recommended for a hemoglobin level of 7 g/dl or less and in patients with hypotension. An antibiotic cover is essential to lower the chances of mixed flora infections which are commonly encountered. Drugs which decrease the tendency to bleed may be helpful. For example, tranexamic acid 500 mg to 1 gram qid or ethamsylate 500 mg qid. Topical adrenaline 1:1000 may be used when dressings are changed, and is found to be useful in capillary bleeding. In rare cases of cancer cervix where re-irradiation is not possible, bleeding is intractable and facilities are available, arteriography can demonstrate the bleeding site and show whether a unilateral or bilateral internal iliac embolisation is needed. Sometimes, only selective injection of the small branches can identify the bleeding site. Cessation of hemorrhage after selective embolisation can be seen at fluoroscopy. In rare cases, hypogastric ligation may be done if embolisation fails.

Bleeding can be a very debilitating symptom for the patient, both physically as well as psychologically, confining her to bed and at times it may get very difficult to control. Rebleeding within two months is common; often patients die soon after from the underlying malignancy.

Lymphedema: This is a progressive condition which results from insufficiency or failure of the lymphatic system, with or without coexisting venous insufficiency (Farncombe et al 1994). It results in the accumulation of protein-rich fluid in the subcutaneous tissues. It is a considerably distressing condition, and if left untreated, can become a crippling handicap to patients who are already weakened by advanced malignancy. A heavy, edematous limb has debilitating physical and psychological effects and may impair mobility, independence and quality of life. Physical disabilities include pain, heaviness, skin fragility and sensory disturbances in the affected limb (Granda 1994).

Lymphedema occurs when there is a disturbance of the equilibrium between the transport capacity of the lymphatic system and the load of the lymph to be cleared. This may be due to:

- Impaired lymphatic drainage: Lymph node irradiation or lymph node dissection obstructs lymphatic drainage routes, and may result in the remaining vessels becoming overloaded. At particular risk are the patients with genital or pelvic tumours who have undergone surgery and/or irradiation to a major group of lymph nodes (Farncombe 2003)

- Increased lymphatic load: This is due to venous insufficiency or acute tissue inflammation. Initially, the lymphatic system will respond by increasing lymph flow, but if the load keeps on increasing, drainage fails as the vessels become overloaded
- Gravitational effect: Dependent edema occurs due to a lack of propulsion of blood and lymph in a limb, mostly seen in bedridden patients
- Pressure effect: A large lymph nodal mass or the primary tumour itself may impede lymphatic clearance

In initial cases, lymphedema is soft, pitting and responsive to limb elevation. As chronicity sets in, typical changes of hyperkeratosis, lymphangiomatosis and papillomatosis are seen (Veitch 1993).

Symptoms includes tightness, heaviness, a bursting feeling if there is acute exacerbation, impaired function, pain due to lumbosacral plexopathy and psychosocial distress due to altered body image.

Aims of management include prevention of further development, reduction of the swelling, alleviating the symptoms and maximising control. There are two major phases of management:

Intensive phase: In this phase, the skin is prone to infections, so great care has to be taken. This is achieved by keeping the skin supple and intact. Instructions for skin care (Twycross et al 2000) should be given and the patient should be advised to avoid injury to the affected limb. Normal movements or gentle active or passive movements must be encouraged. Exercise is important as it stimulates the muscle pump, improves joint mobility and improves posture and functional activities, thus promoting lymph drainage. External compression is achieved by the daily application of multilayer, graduated compression bandages. Manual lymphatic drainage (MLD) is also important when done by an expert physiotherapist and should be taught to the patient or the attendant. The procedure commences with massage from the toes upwards to the legs, the inner aspect of the upper thigh, the procedure is then repeated for the top of the thigh followed by a massage of the lower abdomen and lower back. Each of these procedures must be done ten times, twice daily for about 20 minutes. The session must end with breathing exercises (Twycross et al 2000).

Palliative phase: The skin may become hard, tense, indurated, discoloured or inflamed. Gentle support dressing may help. Diuretics are of help if there is a venous component to the swelling. Gentle, active or passive exercises in this phase also enhance lymph flow (Mortimer et al 1997). A pneumatic intermittent compression pump is helpful in shifting venous and hypo-albuminemic edemas.

Intrathoracic metastases: Intrathoracic metastases may present as malignant pleural effusion, parenchymal metastases and nodal/mediastinal metastases with airway compromise. Basic management principles include oxygen, relief of bronchospasm, control of secretions and measures to promote relaxation. In cases with pleural effusion, a thoracocentesis under ultrasonographic guidance gives immediate relief but reaccumulation occurs fast. Repeated thoracocentesis is appropriate for short term management or if needed at longer intervals with a 4% or greater risk of pneumothorax with each procedure (Bartier et al 1993). In patients with longer life expectancy, the option of chemical pleurodesis may be offered. This is done using talc by direct application with video-assisted thoracoscopic surgery (VATS), or through a chest tube with success rates of up to 91% (Kennedy and Sahn 1994; Light 1995). Patients with endobronchial obstruction are not candidates for pleurodesis (Breitbart et al 1995; Sahn 1998). In patients with dyspnea and co-existent emphysema, epidural methadone infusion at chest level at a rate of 6 mg/24 h can effectively palliate dyspnea, improve exercise tolerance and quality of life, without adverse effects upon lung function and respiratory control (Juan et al 2005). Intervention must be done judiciously in patients, in whom chances of alleviating the primary symptoms is possible but we must avoid complications like pneumonitis, arrhythmia and respiratory failure secondary to any procedure.

Cough may be due to conditions unrelated to malignancy such as asthma, chest infection, heart failure, sinusitis or gastro-esophageal reflux which is common in ascitis. Management tailored specially to this includes use of bronchodilators, antibiotics, intranasal or inhaled steroids, antihistamines and proton-pump inhibitors for reflux. Cough due to airway obstruction, responds well to narcotic suppression with morphine or codeine. Humidifiers may be helpful in irritated and dry mucosal linings. Physiotherapy and postural drainage is also an important entity. In cases of suspected fluid overload, diuretics may be tried and of the opiates, morphine is particularly beneficial. Morphine plays a role in decreasing air hunger and dyspnea in these cases (Tucakovic et al 2001). As death becomes imminent, most patients face difficulty in clearing secretions from the upper respiratory tract. Hyoscine, an anticholinergic agent reduces the volume of upper respiratory secretions without compromising respiratory function (Doyle 1987; Bennett 1996).

Bone metastases: Bone metastases are rare in terminal gynecologic cancers, being primarily confined to unusually high grade tumour types such as glassy cell, neuroendocrine tumours, small cell, or clear cell malignancies. The most commonly affected areas are the vertebral bodies secondary to nodal infiltration, pelvis and rarely, the long bones. When they occur, however, the pain associated with bone metastases can be the most excruciating of all the symptoms we encounter. If the metastases are limited in nature, radiation therapy on a palliative basis may supply additional pain relief with a success rate of 50% total pain relief and 80%–90% of patients noting relief of symptoms (Orr et al 1993). Pain is the most frequent symptom (96%) in patients with bone metastasis (Ratanatharathorn et al 1991; Body 1992; Rubens 2000). Approximately 65%–75% of patients with bone metastases will experience pain and impaired mobility (Mauskop and Foley 1988). Bone pain may be nociceptive or neuropathic (Ford and Yarnold 1983; Pecherstorfer and Vesely 2000). Fracture of the weight-bearing long bone occurs in 10%–20% of patients (Mauskop and Foley 1988). This occurs especially in lytic bone metastases.

The majority of patients with bone metastases survive for less than a year and radiotherapy will achieve pain control over this period in the majority of such patients. With short median predicted survival times and achieving pain relief as the end point, a simple short treatment schedule is most appropriate and in the majority of situations, a single treatment delivering a dose of 8 Gy will suffice. There is considerable data in literature supporting the use of single doses in this setting; some patients will receive a more protracted fractionated course of treatment delivering 20–30 Gy over 1–2 weeks which is preferred by some centres where bone strengthening is the main concern. External radiation produces some healing and re-ossification in 65%–85% of lytic lesions in unfractured bone (Harrington 1986; Mauskop and Foley 1988). The treatment techniques used are simple, using a cobalt beam or a linear accelerator. It is particularly important to document carefully the field margins since most patients will have multiple sites of metastases and further treatment with potential overlap of fields may be required. This is of particular importance in the treatment of the spine where metastasis at several levels may require sequential treatment. Overlap of fields in the spine can result in overdosage with the risk of developing radiation myelitis and subsequent neurological deterioration within 6–9 months of treatment. In patients with a short life expectancy, this may not be of significance and a decision to accept the overlap may be done, where the benefit from treatment far outweighs the chances of later myelitis; in other patients where life expectancy is 6 months or more, the risks may become an issue (Hoskin 2004).

There is wide variation in the fractionation schedules reported both in clinical reports and in randomised clinical trials. In a Dutch trial (Streenland et al 1999), 1171 patients were randomised to receive either 8 Gy/1#1/wk or 24 Gy/6#/1 wk (the radiation dose given over six fractions in one week). They found the overall response rates to be similar but re-treatment rates were four times higher in the single fraction group (25% vs 7%, respectively). In a meta-analysis (Wu et al 2003) of seven studies, including 3260 patients with painful bone metastases, comparing a single fraction of 8 Gy to multiple fraction regimens which varied from 20 Gy/5#/1 wk to 30 Gy/10#/2 wk, overall response rates were in favour of single fraction RT (62.1% vs 58.7% for multifraction doses). However, the re-irradiation rate is consistently higher in the single fraction groups (20%–25% vs 7%–12%). It is unclear if this is because radiotherapists are more willing to consider reirradiation after single fraction radiotherapy, or because troublesome pain recurs more frequently in the single fraction group. In a trial by Gaze et al (1997), which included 288 patients, the median duration of pain control in the single fraction group (10 Gy) versus protracted fractionation group (22.5 Gy/5#/1wk) was found to be 13.5 weeks and 14 weeks, respectively.

In choosing between single fraction radiotherapy and a protracted course, one must bear in mind the location, extent of tumour mass and the patient's prognosis. Patients with carcinoma cervix with bone pain due to metastatic nodes infiltrating the vertebrae may require fractionated radiotherapy. A protracted course may also be considered in patients with a better prognosis, where bone strengthening, nerve compression or pathologic fractures is of main concern. For others with bone metastases and severe pain, a single large dose fraction may be given so as to achieve pain relief.

Terminal breathlessness: Major causes of fear at the end of life are the symptoms of dyspnea and chest pain. The pathophysiology of dyspnea is complicated. Normal breathing is maintained by rhythmical activity in the respiratory centre in the brainstem. This is stimulated by mechanical receptors, hypoxia and hypercapnia.

Management (Neighbourhood Network in Palliative Care 2006) includes allowing a cool draught and free flow of air by using fans or by opening windows. Oxygen via nasal prongs may be useful. The sight of attendants may have a calming effect upon the patient. Symptomatic drug treatment includes theophylline and salbutamol, both of which increase muscle strength and are found to be beneficial in the absence of bronchospasms. Morphine reduces the respiratory drive and eases the sensation of breathlessness—if the patient is already on morphine, doses may be increased by 50%. If not on morphine, 2.5–5 mg every 6 hours may be used as a starting dose. Sedatives like diazepam can be given if the patient is very anxious especially in the terminal phase, 5–10 mg stat with lowered doses in the elderly.

A calm, positive, logical approach can do much to alleviate the distress of the patient and their family as well as the palliative caregivers. Occasionally, dyspnea is a very difficult to control symptom despite all the above measures, especially in terminal situations. In such cases, sedation becomes necessary.

Psychologic symptoms in the terminal patient: A terminally ill patient is repeatedly assailed by the interplay of emotions and impending doom. Thus, early recognition of psychological symptoms is important. Physicians must be sensitive to the commonly neglected emotional dimension. Incidence of depression varies from as low as 4.5% to as high as 58% depending upon the population studied (Massie and Holland 1990; Breitbart et al 1995). Anxiety and depression occur in a large proportion of patients, particularly when the disease progresses and cure fails (Breitbart 1995). This may also be attributed to increased physical debility as the patient becomes more and more aware of the futility of treatment and limited life expectancy (Williamson and Schultz 1995; Payne and Massie 2003). Fishbain et al (1997) found a relationship between pain and the development of depression. In a study from University Medical Centre, Utrecht, the Netherlands, the incidence of psychological symptoms in terminal patients with life expectancy ≤3 months was studied (Hotopf et al 2002). In 56 female patients, assessment of anxiety and depression (Hospital Anxiety and Depression Scale (HADS)) and control of symptoms (Edmonton Symptom Assessment Scale) was done. The incidence of self-reported anxiety was at 14%; for self-reported depression it was at 25%. The anxiety and depression were mainly attributed to decreased physical performance. Physical symptoms related to anxiety and depression, were fatigue, drowsiness, impaired well being and dyspnea. Similarly, Massie et al (1990) too found a depression prevalence of 25%. In an extensive review, Hotopf et al (2002) showed that 29% patients scored more than 11 on the HADS depression subscale. The closer a patient is toward dying, the greater is the score for depression, and the lower the score of physical performance.

Psychological symptoms need to be carefully assessed and must be considered important in the overall decision making concerning end of life issues. Management of anxiety, depression along with adequate family support improves the overall feeling of well being in a dying woman.

Care for the medical professional: Within the practice of palliative care and end of life, in particular, there is a tendency for the patient and relatives to demand a more personal approach from the attending physician and nurse. In view of this contact-intensive nature of end of life care, it can be expected that physicians and nurses run the risk of depleting their emotional resources, especially when they cross the crucial line between their professional and personal involvement. This leads to a burnout syndrome. A major stress factor is that oncologists are regularly assailed upon their limited ability to alter the course of the illness. Various other factors posing as major sources of stress are breaking bad news, coping with failure of medical cure, repeated exposure to the death of people with whom we have formed a relationship, involvement in emotional conflicts.

To understand and prevent emotional drain and burnout, team members should be able to share their responses and feelings with others at work. This is made possible by organising support groups at work where they may discuss their experiences and measures for counteracting them (Creagan 1993; Halperin et al 1997). In this way, participants get the opportunity to discuss the emotional aspects of the care of the terminal patient. This is particularly helpful for young and inexperienced personnel. The more experienced senior members of the team can provide perspective and insight into how to manage these difficult situations. Comments, feedback, advice and the mutual help of colleagues is one of the most important factors in staying emotionally and mentally strong as well as to avoid burnout.

The psychosocial burden of cancer on sufferers and their loved ones will continue to increase substantially over the next few decades, as the incidence of malignancy rises. Research agendas are required to bridge the gap between oncologists, gynecologists, psychologists and the palliative care team. End of life care is a very important part of palliative care. It requires the total commitment of the entire healthcare team. It not only includes necessary medical interventions to alleviate suffering, but also psychosocial and emotional support. Physicians need to be sensitive to the needs of a dying woman. Understanding women and their family requirements, how they cope with their daily activities, including stress, and what health services they expect will help professionals improve the quality of life in this vulnerable population. Thus, it is in our hands to make a woman's end of life as peaceful as possible when cure is out of our realm. However, we know that the intensive nature of palliative care in oncology is a risk factor for emotional exhaustion for all healthcare providers. Hence, good end of life care should not only include the patient and their family but also adequate support for the medical team.

References

Aapro MS. 1991. Present role of corticosteroids as antiemetics. In *Recent Results in Cancer Research*. Vol 121. Berlin: Springer-Verlag 91–100.

Arroyo V, M Epstein, G Gallus, P Gentilini, H Ring-Larsen, F Salerno. 1989. Refractory ascites in cirrhosis: mechanism and treatment. *Gastroenterol Int* 2:195–207.

Ashburn MA and AG Lipman. 1993. Management of pain in the cancer patient. *Anesth Analg* Feb 76 (2):402–416.

Aslam N and CR Marino. 2001. Malignant ascites: New concepts in pathophysiology, diagnosis, and management. *Arch Intern Med.* Dec 10-24; 161(22):2733–2737.

Bachwich P, S Chensue, J Larrick, SL Kunkel. 1986. Tumour necrosis factor stimulates interleukin-1 and prostaglandin E, production in resting macrophages. *Biochemical and Biophysical Research Communications* 136:94–101.

Backonja M, A Beydoun, KR Edwards, et al. 1998. Gabapentin for the symptomatic treatment of painful neuropathy in patients with diabetes mellitus: A randomized controlled trial. *JAMA* 280:1831.

Baines MJ. 1997. The pathophysiology and management of malignant bowel obstruction. In *Oxford Textbook of Palliative Medicine*, 2nd edn, ed D Doyle, G Hanks, N Mcdonald. Oxford: Oxford University Press.

Ball ABS, M Baum, NM Breach et al. 2003. Surgical palliation. In: *Oxford Textbook of Palliative Medicine*, eds Doyle D, Hanks GW, Mac Donald N. Oxford: Oxford University Press 282–297.

Banning A, P Sjogren, H Henriksen. 1991. Pain causes in 200 patients referred to a multidisciplinary cancer pain clinic. *Pain* Apr; 45(1):45-48.

Bartier T, PD Mayo, MR Pratter et al. 1993. Lower risk and higher yield for thoracocentesis when performed by experienced operators. *Chest* 103:1873–1876.

Bartlett JG, et al. 1977. Quantitative bacteriology of the vaginal flora. *J Infec Dis* 136(2):271–277.

Beattie GJ, RCF Leonard, JF Smyth. 1989. Bowel obstruction in ovarian cancer: A retrospective study and review of literature. *Palliative medicine* 3:275–280.

Bells RF, C Eccleston, E Kalso. 2003. Ketamine as adjuvant to opioids for cancer pain: A quantitative systematic review. *J Pain Symptom Manage* 26:867–875.

Bennett MI. 1996. Death rattle: An audit of hyoscine (scopolamine) use and review of management. *Pain Symptom Manage* 12:229–233.

Beratis NG, A Kaperonis, MI Eliopoulou, G Kourounis, VA Tzingounis. 2005. Increased activity of lysosomal enzymes in the peritoneal fluid of patients with gynecologic cancers and pelvic inflammatory disease. *J Cancer Res Clin Oncol* Jun; 131(6):371–376.

Bliss JM, B Robertson, PJ Selby. 1992. The impact of nausea and vomiting upon quality of life measures. *British Journal of Cancer* 66:S14–23.

Bodnar R, G Pasternak, P Mann et al. 1989. Mediation of anorexia by human recombinant tumour necrosis factor through a peripheral action in the rat. *Cancer Research* 49:6280–6284.

Body JJ. 1992. Metastatic bone disease: Clinical and therapeutic aspects. *Bone* 13:557.

Body JJ.1992. Metabolic sequelae of cancers (excluding bone marrow transplantation). *Current Opinion in Clinical Nutrition and Metabolic Care* 2:339–344.

Bonica JJ, V Ventafridda, RG Twycross. 1990. Cancer pain. In *The Management of Pain*, 2nd edn, ed JJ Bonica, 400–460. Philadelphia: Lea and Febiger.

Borison HL and C Wang. 1953. Physiology and pharmacology of vomiting. *Pharmacological Reviews* 5:192–230.

Bosnjak S, S Jelic, S Susnjar et al. 2002. Gabapentin for relief of neuropathic pain related to anticancer treatment: A preliminary study. *J Chemother* 14:214.

Bouvier M, JC Grimaud, B Naudy et al. 1987. Effects of morphine on electrical activity of the rectum in man. *J Physiol* 388:153–161.

Breitbart W, E Bruera, HM Chochinov et al. 1995. Neuropsychiatric syndromes and psychological symptoms in patients with advanced cancers. *J Pain Symptom Manage* 9:412–415.

Breitbart W. 1995. Identifying patients at risk for and treatment of major psychiatric complications of cancer. *Support Care Cancer* 3:45–60.

Brescia FJ, D Adler, G Gray, MA Ryan, J Cimino, R Mamtani. 1990. Hospitalized advanced cancer patients: a profile. *Journal of Pain Symptom Management* 5(4):221–227.

Bruera E, E Roca, L Cedaro et al. 1985. Action of oral methylprednisolone in terminal cancer patients: A prospective randomized double- blind study. *Cancer Treatment Reports* 69:751–754.

Bruera E, K Macmillan, J Hanson, N Kuehn, RN MacDonald. 1990. A controlled trial of megestrol acetate on appetite, caloric intake, nutritional status, and other symptoms in patients with advanced cancers. *Cancer* 66:1279–1282.

Bruera E, M Suarez-Almazor, A Velasco et al. 1994. The assessment of constipation in terminal cancer patients admitted to a palliative care unit: A retrospective review. *J Pain Symptom Manage* 9: 515–519.

Caraceni A, E Zecca,C Martini, et al. 1999. Gabapentin as an adjuvant to opioid analgesia for neuropathic cancer pain. *J Pain Symptom Manage* 17:441.

Casilda S and Krishnaswamy M. 2005. Wound care in resource poor settings. *Ind J Palliat Care* 11(2):105–107.

Cassileth PA, GJ Lusk, S Torn, et al. 1983. Antiemetic efficacy of dexamethasone therapy in patients receiving cancer chemotherapy. *Archives of Intern Med* 143:1347–1349.

Chan S, AC Robinson, RJ Johnson. 1980. Percutaneous nephrostomy: Its value in obstructive uropathy complicating carcinoma of the cervix. *Clin Oncol* (R Coll Radiol) May; 2 (3):156–158.

Clarke-Pearson DL, NO Chin, ER DeLong, R Rice, WT Creasman. 1987. Surgical management of intestinal obstruction in ovarian cancer: Clinical features, postoperative complications and survival. *Gynecologic Oncology* Jan; 26(1):11–18.

Cleeland C. 1991. Research in cancer pain. What we know and what we need to know. *Cancer* Feb 1; 67(3 Suppl):823–827.

Coates A, S Abraham, SB Kaye et al. 1983. On the receiving end. Patient perception of the side-effects of cancer chemotherapy. *European Journal of Cancer* 19:203–208.

Coates G, RS Bush, N Aspin. 1973. A study of ascitis using lymphoscintigraphy with 99m Tc-sulphur colloid. *Radiology* 107:577–583.

Cooper S and V Georgior. 1992. The impact of cytotoxic chemotherapy: Perspectives from patients, specialists and nurses. *European Journal of Cancer* 28A:S36–8.

Creagan ET. 1993. Stress among medical oncologists: the phenomenon of burnout and a call to action. *Mayo Clin Proc* 68:614–615.

Curtis EB, R Krech, TD Walsh. 1991. Common symptoms in patients with advanced cancer. *J Palliat Care* 7:25.

Davidson B, Z Xi, TI Klokk, CG Trope, A Dorum, M Scheistroen, F Saatcioglu. 2005. Kallikrein 4 expression is up-regulated in epithelial ovarian carcinoma cells in effusions. *Am J Clin Pathol.* Mar; 123(3):360–368.

Davidson B. 2004. Malignant effusions: from diagnosis to biology. *Diagn Cytopathol.* Oct; 31(4): 246–254.

De Conno F, C Martini, E Zeua et al. 1998. Megestrol acetate for anorexia in patients with far advanced cancer: a double blind controlled clinical trial. *European Journal of Cancer* 34:1705–1709.

De Luca A and IM Coupar. 1996. Insights into opioid action in the intestinal tract. *Pharmacol Ther* 69:103–115

Diehl V and M Marty. 1994. Efficacy and safety of antiemetics. *Cancer Treatment Reviews* 20:379–392.

Doyle D. 1983. Symptom relief in terminal illness. *Medicine in Practice* 1:694–698.

Doyle D. 1987. *Domiciliary terminal care.* Edinburg: Churchill Livingstone.

Editorial. 1978. Cyproheptadine. *Lancet* 1:368.

Fainsinger R, M Miller, E Bruera, et al. 1991. Symptom control during the last week of life on a palliative care unit. *Journal of Palliative Care* 7:5–11.

Farncombe E. 2003. Lymphoedema. In: *Palliative Care and Supportive Oncology* 2nd edn, ed AM Berger, RK Portenoy, DE Weissman. Philadelphia: Lippincott Williams and Wilkins. 333–334.

Farncombe M, G Daniels, L Cross. 1994. Lymphoedema: The seemingly forgotten complication. *J Pain Symptom Manage* 9(4):269–276.

Faull C and R Barton. 2001. Managing complications of cancer. In *Handbook of Palliative Care*, eds Faull C, MCarter Y, Woof R, Panther publishers. 177–201.

Fevery J, G Van Roey, W Van Steenbergen. 1996. Ascites: Medical therapy and paracentesis. *Acta Gastroenterol Belg.* Jul-Sep;59 (3):198–201.

Fishbain DA, R Cutle R, HL Rosomoff, R Steele-Rosomoff. 1997. Chronic pain associated depression: Antecedent or consequence of chronic pain? A review. *Clin J Pain* 13:116–137.

Fogel MR, VK Sawheny, EA Neal, RG Miller, CM Knauer, PB Gregory. 1981. Diuresis in the ascitic patient: a randomized controlled trial of three regimens. *J Clin Gastroenterol* 3:Suppl 1:73–80.

Ford HT and JR Yarnold. 1983. Radiation therapy: Pain relief and medication. In: Stoll BA, Parbhoo S, eds. *Bone metastases: monitoring and treatment.* New York: Raven Press, 343.

Gaze MN, CG Kelly, GR Kerr et al. 1997. Pain relief and quality of life following radiotherapy for bone metastases: a randomised trial of two fractionation schedules. *Radiother Oncol* 45(2):109–116.

Gilstrap LC III et al. 1986. Genital aerobic bacterial flora of women receiving radiotherapy for gynecologic malignancy. *Gynecol Oncol* 23:35–39.

Gines P, L Tito, V Arroyo et al. 1988. Randomized comparative study of therapeutic paracentesis with and without intravenous albumin in cirrhosis. *Gastroenterology* 94:1493–1502.

Glare P and NP Lickiss. 1992. Unrecognised constipation in patients with advanced cancer: A recipe for disaster. *J Pain Symptom Manage* 7:369–371.

Gogos CA, P Ginopoulous, B Salsa et al. 1998. Dietary omega-3 polyunsaturated fatty acids plus vitamin E to restore immunodeficiency and prolong survival for severely ill patients with generalized malignancy. *Cancer* 82:395–402.

Goldberg BB, GA Goodman, HR Clearfield. 1970. Evaluation of ascites by ultrasound. *Radiology* 96:15–22.

Gordon NC, et al. 1989.Response of lower genital tract flora to external pelvic irradiation. *Gynecol Oncol* 35:233–235.

Granda C. 1994. Nursing management of patients with lymphoedema associated with breast cancer therapy. *Cancer Nursing* 17:229–235.

Greenberg DB, OS Surman, J Clarke, A Del Favero. 1987. Alprazolam for phobic nausea and vomiting related to cancer chemotherapy. *Cancer Treat Rep* 71:549–560.

Greenway B, PJ Johnson, R Williams. 1982. Control of malignant ascitis with spironolactone. *Br J Surg* 69:441–442.

Grocott P. 1995. The palliative management of fungating malignant wounds. *J Wound Care* 4(5): 240–242.

Halperin JD, JR Zabora, S Brintzenhofe. 1997. The emotional health of oncologists. *Oncol Issues* 21:20–22.

Harrington KD. 1986. Impending pathologic fractures from metastatic malignancy: Evaluation and management. *Instrct Coursr Lect* 35:357–381.

Harris JT, K Sureshkumar, MR Rajagopal. 2003. Intravenous morphine for rapid control of severe cancer pain. *Palliat Med* 17:248–256.

Hawkey CJ, JA Karrasch, L Szczepanski, et al. 1998. Omeprazole compared with misoprostol for ulcers associated with NSAIDS. Omeprazole versus Misoprostol for NSAID-induced Ulcer Management (OMNIUM) study group. *N Engl J Med* 338:727.

Hawkey CJ. 1998. Progress in prophylaxis against nonsteroidal anti-inflammatory drug-associated ulcers and erosions. Omeprazole NSAID Steering Committee. *Am J Med* 104:67S; Discussion, 79S.

Hernandez-Diaz S and LA Rodriguez. 2000. Association between nonsteroidal anti-inflammatory drugs and upper gastrointestinal bleeding/perforation: An overview of epidemiologic studies published in the 1990s. *Arch Intern Med* 160:2093.

Hirabayashi K and J Graham. 1970. Genesis of ascitis in ovarian carcinoma. *Am J Obstet Gynecol* 106:492–497.

Hoskin PJ. 2004. Radiotherapy in symptom management. In *Oxford Textbook of Palliative Medicine* 3rd edn D Doyle, G Hanks, N Cherny, K Caalman, eds. Oxford University Press: 239–255.

Hoskins PJ and GW Hanks. 1991. Opioid agonist-antagonist drugs in acute and chronic pain states. *Drugs* 41:326.

Hotopf M, J Chidgey, Addington Hall, et al. 2002. Depression in advanced disease: A systematic review. Part I. Prevalence and case finding. *Palliate Med* 16:81–97.

Juan G, M Ramon, JC Valia, et al. 2005. Palliative treatment of dyspnea with epidural methadone in advanced emphysema. *Chest* 128:3322–3328.

Kao HW, NE Rakov, E Savage, et al. 1985. The effect of large-volume paracentesis on plasma volume: A cause of hypovolemia? *Hepatology* 5:403–407.

Kardinal C, C Loprinzi, DJ Shaid, et al. 1990. A controlled trial of cyproheptadine in cancer patients with anorexia. *Cancer* 65:2657–2662.

Kennedy L and SA Sahn. 1994. Talc pleuradesis for the treatment of pneumothorax and pleural effusion. *Chest* 106:1215–1222.

Krebs HB and DR Goplerud. 1983. Surgical management of bowel obstruction in advanced ovarian carcinoma. *Obstet Gynecol* 61(3):327–330.

Kris MG, L Baltzer, KMW Pisters, LB Tyson. 1993. Enhancing the effectiveness of the specific serotonin antagonists. *Cancer* 72:3436–3442.

Lau MW, DE Temperley, S Mehta, et al. 1995. Urinary tract obstruction and nephrostomy drainage in pelvic malignant disease. *Br J Urol* Nov; 76(5):565–569.

Lederle FA, DL Busch, KM Mattox, et al. 1990. Cost-effective treatment of constipation in the elderly: A randomized double-blind comparison of sorbitol and lactulose. *Am J Med* 89:597–607.

Lichter I. 1993. Which antiemetic? *Journal of Palliative Care* 9:42–50.

Lickiss JN. 2001. Approaching cancer pain relief. *European Journal of Pain* 5 Suppl A: 5–14.

Light RW. 1995. Malignant pleural effusion. In: *Pleural Diseases*. 3rd ed, ed RW Light, 90–116. Baltimore: Williams and Wilkins.

Linnik MD, BT Butler, RR Gaddis, NK Ahmed. 1991. Analysis of serotonergic mechanisms underlying benzamide- induced gastroprokinesis. *J Pharmacol Exp Therapeutics* 259:501–507.

Lomen PL, BA Samal, KR Lamborn, et al. 1986. Flurbiprofen for the treatment of bone pain in patients with metastatic breast cancers. *Am J Med* 80:83.

Loprinzi CL, N Ellinson, J Schaid et al. 1990. A controlled trial of megestrol acetate treatment of cancer anorexia and cachexia. *Journal of the National Cancer Institute* 82:1127–1132.

MacDonald N. 1997. The interface between oncology and palliative medicine In *Oxford Textbook of Palliative Medicine*, 2nd edn, ed D Doyle, G Hanks, N Mcdonald. Oxford: Oxford University Press.

Mantovani G, A Maccio, P Lai, et al. 1998. Cytokine involvement in cancer anorexia/cachexia: Role of megestrol acetate and medroxyprogesterone acetate on cytokine deregulation and improvement in clinical symptoms. *Critical Reviews in Oncogenesis* 9:99–106.

Massie MJ and JC Holland. 1990. Depression and the cancer patient. *J Clin Psychiatry* 51[suppl]:12–17.

Mauskop A and KM Foley. 1988. Control of pain In Harrington KD, ed. *Orthopaedic management of metastatic bone disease*. St Louis: CV Mosby, 121–137.

McDonnell FJ, JW Sloan, SR Hamann. 2001. Advances in cancer pain management. *Curr Pain Headache Rep* 5:265–271.

Mercadante S and RK Portenoy. 2001. Opioid poorly-responsive cancer pain. Part 3. Clinical strategies to improve opioid responsiveness. *J Pain Symptom Manage* 21:338–354.

Mercadante S, A Cassucio, A Agnello et al. 1997. Analgesic effects of nonsteroidal anti-inflammatory drugs in cancer pain due to somatic or visceral mechanisms. *J Pain Symptom Manage* 17:351.

Mercadante S. 2001. The use of anti-inflammatory drugs in cancer pain. *Cancer Treat Rev* 27:51.

Michaud MR. 1995. Sonographic detection of peritoneal carcinomatosis: A prospective study of 37 cases. *Abdom Imaging* 20:47–51.

Mortimer PS, C Badger, JG Hall. 1997. Lymphoedema. In: *Oxford Textbook of Palliative Medicine*,2nd edn, ed D Doyle, G Hanks,N Mcdonald, Oxford: Oxford University Press. 407–415.

Neighborhood Network in Palliative Care. 2006. In: *Palliative Care—A handbook for general practitioners*. Harvest Media Services.

Nicholson B. 2003. Responsible prescribing of opioids for the management of chronic pain. *Drugs* 63(1):17–32.

Nobel R. 1989. Effect of cyproheptadine on appetite and weight gain in adults. *JAMA* 209: 2054–2055.

Orr WF, P Kosternick, OH Sanchez-Sweatman, et al. 1993. Mechanisms involved in the metastases of cancer to bone. *Breast Cancer Res Treat* ; 25:151.

Parsons SL, MW Lang, RJ Steele. 1996. Malignant ascites: A 2-year review from a teaching hospital. *Eur J Surg Oncol* 22 (3):237–239.

Pawlowski G. 1975. Cyproheptadine: Weight gain and appetite stimulation. *Current Therapeutic Research* 18:673–678.

Payne DK and MJ Massie. 2003. Anxiety in palliative care In *Handbook of Psychiatry in Palliative Medicine*, ed HM Chochinov, W Breitbart, Oxford: University Press. 63–74.

Pecherstorfer M and M Vesely. 2000. Diagnosis and monitoring of bone metastases: Clinical means. In: Body JJ ed. *Tumor bone disease and osteoporosis in cancer patients*. New York: Marcel Dekker, Inc., 97–129.

Perez-Ayuso RM, V Arroyo, R Planas, et al. 1983. Randomized comparative study of efficacy of furosemide versus spironolactone in nonazotemic cirrhosis with ascites: Relationship between the diuretic response and the activity of the renin-aldosterone system. *Gastroenterology* 84:961–968.

Petouka SJ and SH Synder. 1982. Antiemetics: Neurotransmitter binding predicts therapeutic actions. *Lancet* ii: 658–659.

Philip J, N Lickiss, PT Grant, NF Hacker. 1994. Corticosteroids in the management of bowel obstruction in a gynecological oncology unit. *Gynecologic Oncology* 74:68–73.

Pinto PC, J Amerian, TB Reynolds. 1988. Large-volume paracentesis in nonedematous patients with tense ascites: Its effect on intravascular volume. *Hepatology* Mar-Apr;8(2):207–210.

Planas R, P Gines, V Arroyo, et al. 1990. Dextran-70 versus albumin as plasma expanders in cirrhotic patients with tense ascites treated with total paracentesis: Results of a randomized study. *Gastroenterology* 99:1736–1744.

Pockros PJ and TB Reynolds. 1986. Rapid diuresis in patients with ascites from chronic liver disease: The importance of peripheral edema. *Gastroenterology* 90:1827–1833.

Pockros PJ, KT Esrason, C Nguyen, et al. 1992. Mobilization of malignant ascitis with diuretics is dependent on ascitic fluid characteristics. *Gastroenterology* 103:1302–1306.

Portenoy RK and G Frager. 1999. Pain management: Pharmacological approaches In *Palliative Care and Rehabilitation of Cancer Patients*, ed von Guten CF, 1–29. Boston: Kluwer Academic Publishers.

Portenoy RK, HT Thaler, AB Kornblith et al. 1994. Symptom prevalence, characteristics and distress in a cancer population. *Qual Life Res* 3:183.

Portenoy RK, J Miransky, HT Thaler, J Hornung, C Bianchi, I Cibas-Kong et al. 1992. Pain in ambulatory patients with lung or colon cancer. Prevalence, characteristics and effect. *Cancer* Sep 15; 70(6):1616–1624.

Portenoy RK. 1998. Adjuvant analgesics in pain management In *Oxford Textbook of Pallliative Medicine,* ed Doyle D, Hanks GWC, MacDonald N, 361. Oxford: Oxford University Press.

Prommer EE. 2005. Ziconotide: Can we use it in palliative care? *Am J Hosp Palliat Care* 22(5):369–374.

Rajagopal MR. 1998. Cancer pain emergencies. *J Pain Symptom Manage* 15:5:264–265.

Ratanatharathorn V and WE Power. 1991. Epidural spinal cord compression from metastatic tumors: Diagnosis and guidelines for management. *Cancer Treat Rev* 18:55–71.

Regnard CFB and S Tempest. 1992. *A Guide to Symptomatic Relief in Advanced Cancer* (3rd ed). Manchester: Haigh and Hochland.

Richter I. 1997. Choice of laxative in treatment of constipation. *Home Healthcare Consultant* 4:28–41.

Robert KA. 2004. Palliation of visceral recurrences ans metastases. In *Principles and practice of radiation oncology*, eds Perez CA, Brady LW, Halperin EC, Schmidt-Ullrich RK, Lippincott Williams and Wilkins. 2409–2410.

Rowbotham M, N Harden, B Stacey et al. 1998. Gabapentin for the treatment of postherpetic neuralgia: a randomized controlled trial. *JAMA* 280.

Rowinski EK and RC Donehower. 1998. Microtubule targeting drugs. In *The chemotherapy source book*, ed Perry MC, Baltimore: Williams and Wilkins. 387–414.

Rubens RD. 2000. Clinical aspects of bone metastases. In Body JJ *Tumor bone disease and osteoporosis in cancer patients.* New York: Marcel Dekker 85–96.

Runyon BA, JC Hoefs, TR Morgan. 1988. Ascitic fluid analysis in malignancy-related ascitis. *Hepatology* 8:1104–1109.

Runyon BA. 1994. Care of patients with ascitis. *N Engl J Med* 330:337–342.

Sahn SA. 1998. Malignancy metastatic to the pleura. *Clin Chest Med* 19:351–356.

Schell H. 1972. Adrenal corticosteroid therapy in far-advanced cancer. *Geriatrics* 27:131–141.

Schug SA, D Zech, U Dorr. 1990. Cancer pain management according to WHO analgesic guidelines. *J Pain Symptom Manage* 5:27.

Seal C and A Cartwright. 1994. *The year before death*. Brookfield: Ashgate Publishing Company.

Sears D and SI Hajdu. 1987. The cytologic diagnosis of malignant neoplasms in pleural and peritoneal effusions. *Acta Cytol.* Mar–Apr; 31(2):85–97.

Seynaeve P, PH deMulder, P Lane-Allman et al. 1991. The 5-HT3 antagonist ondansetron re-establishes control in refractory emesis induced by non-cisplatin chemotherapy. *Clin Oncol* 3:199–203.

Shear L, S Ching, GJ Gabuzda. 1970. Compartmentalization of ascites and edema in patients with hepatic cirrhosis. *N Engl J Med* 282:1391–1396.

Sindrup S and T Jensen. 1999. Efficacy of pharmacological treatments of neuropathic pain: An update and effect related to mechanism of drug action. *Pain.* 83:85–90.

Smith EM and GC Jayson. 2003. The current and future management of malignant ascites. *Clin Oncol (R Coll Radiol)* Apr;15 (2):59–72.

Soukop M and D Cunningham. 1987. The Treatment of nausea and vomiting induced by cytotoxic drugs. *Ballieres Clinical Oncology* 1:307–326.

Stadlmann S, A Amberger, J Pollheimer, G Gastl, FA Offner, R Margreiter, AG Zeimet. 2005. Ovarian carcinoma cells and IL-1beta-activated human peritoneal mesothelial cells are possible sources of vascular endothelial growth factor in inflammatory and malignant peritoneal effusions. *Gynecol Oncol* Jun; 97(3):784–789.

Stanley MM, S Ochi, KK Lee et al. 1989. Peritoneovenous shunting as compared with medical treatment in patients with alcoholic cirrhosis and massive ascites. *N Engl J Med* 321:1632–1638.

Steenland E, JW Leer, H van Houwelingen et al.1999. The effect of a single fraction compared to multiple fractions on painful bone metastases: A global analysis of the Dutch Bone Metastasis Study. *Radiother Oncol.*52(2):101–109.

Sureshkumar K, MR Rajagopal, AM Naseema. 2000. Intravenous morphine for emergency treatment of cancer pain. *Palliat Med* 14:183–188.

Swarte NB, JG van der Bom, CH van der Vaart, et al.2003. In *Anxiety and depression in cancer patients prior to death*, ed NB Swarte. Studies on euthanasia. Academic Thesis, Utrecht University.

Swenson RM. 1973. Anaerobic bacterial infections of the female genital tract. *Obstet Gynecol* 42: 538–541.

Tchekmedyian NS, L Hairi, J Siau, et al. 1990. Megestrol acetate in cancer anorexia and weight loss (Abstract). Proceedings of the American Society of Clinical Oncology 9:336.

Thomas S, ed. 1990. *Wound management and dressings.* London: The Pharmaceutical Press.

Tucakovic M, R Bascom, PB Bascom. 2001. Pulmonary medicine and palliative care. *Best Prac Res Clin Obstet Gynecol* 15; 291–304.

Tunca JC, DA Buechler, EA Mack. 1981. The Management of ovarian cancer caused bowel obstruction. *Gynecol oncol* 12:186–192.

Twycross R and A Wilcock. 2001. *Symptom Management in Advanced Cancer,* 3rd edn. Radcliffe Medical Press, Oxford.

Twycross R, K Jeans, J Todd, ed. 2000. *Simple lymphatic drainage.* Oxford: Lymphoedema Radcliffe Medical Press.

Twycross RG and S. Fairfield. 1982. Pain in far advanced cancer. *Pain* 14:303–310.

Twycross RG. 1992. Corticosteroids in advanced cancer. *Brit Med J* 305:969–970.

Tyson LB, RJ Gralla, RA Clark, et al. 1985. Phase I trial of levonantradol in chemotherapy- induced emesis. *Am J Clin Oncol* 8:528–532.

Uys L and S Cameron, eds. 2003. *Home- based HIV/AIDS care.* South Africa: Oxford University Press.

Vadell C, MA Segui, JM Gimenez-Arnau, et al. 1998. Anticachectic efficacy of megestrol acetate at different doses and versus placebo in patients with neoplastic cachexia. *Am J Clin Oncol* 21:347–351.

Vainio A and A Auvinen. 1996. Prevalence of symptoms among patients with advanced cancer: an international collaborative study. *J Pain Symptom Manage* 12:3.

Vane JR, YS Bakhle, RM Botting. 1998. Cyclooxygenase-1 and 2. *Ann Rev Pharmacol Toxicol* 38:97.

Veitch J. 1993. Skin problems in lymphoedema. *Wound Manage* 4(2):42–45.

Ventafridda V, M Tamburini, A Caraceni et al. 1987. A validation study of the WHO method for cancer pain relief. *Cancer* 59:850.

Ventafridda V. 1989. Continuing care: a major issue in cancer pain management. *Pain* 36:137.

Vickers MD, D O'Flaherty, SM Szekely. M Read, J Yoshizumi.1992. Tramadol: Pain relief by an opioid without depression of respiration. *Anaesthesia.* 47:291–296.

Von Roenn JH, CS Cleeland, R Gonin, AK Hatfield, KJ Pandya. 1993. Physician attitudes and practice in cancer pain management. A survey from the Eastern Cooperative Oncology Group. *Ann Intern Med* Jul 15; 119 (2):121–126.

Wald A. 1995. Approach to the patient with constipation. In: Textbook of gastroenterology. 2nd ed, eds Yamada T, Alpers DH, Owyang DH,864-9. Philadelphia: JB Lippincott.

Walker VA, PJ Hoskins, GW Hanks et al. 1988. Evaluation of WHO analgesic guidelines for cancer pain in a hospital-based palliative care unit. *J Pain Symptom Manage* 3:145.

Wallenstein DJ and RK Portenoy. 2002. Non-opioid and adjuvant analgesics. In *Principles and Practice of Palliative Care and Supportive Oncology*, ed Berger AM, Portenoy RK, Weissman DE. Philadelphia: Lipincott-Raven Publishers. 84.

Watanabe S and E Bruera. 1994. Corticosteroids as adjuvant analgesics. *J Pain Symptom Manage* 9:442–445.

Watkinson AF, RP A'Hern, A Jones, et al. 1993.The role of percutaneous nephrostomy in malignant urinary tract obstruction. *Clin Radiol* 47:32–35.

Watson CPN. 2000. The treatment of neuropathic pain: Antidepressants and opioids. *Clin J Pain* 16: S49.

Wilder-Smith C and A Bettiga.1997. The analgesic tramadol has minimal effect on gastrointestinal motor function. *Brit J Clin Pharmacol.*43:71–75.

Williams C. 1999. Clinisorb activated charcoal dressing for odour control. *Br J Nurs* 8:1016–1019.

Williamson GM and R Schulz. 1995. Activity restriction mediates the association between pain and depressed effect: A study of younger and older cancer patients. *Psychol Ageing* 10:369–378.

Wirz S and E Klaschik. 2005. Management of constipation in palliative care patients undergoing opioid therapy: Is polyethylene glycol an option? *Am J Hosp Palliat Care* 22(5):375–381.

Wooldridge JE, CM Anderson, MC Perry. 2001. Corticosteroids in advanced cancer. *Oncology* [Hunting] 15:225–236.

World Health Organization. 1996. *Cancer Pain Relief.* 2nd ed. Geneva: World Health Organization.

Wu JS, R Wong, M Johnston, et al. 2003. Meta-analysis of dose-fractionation radiotherapy trials for the palliation of painful bone metastases. *Int J Radiat Oncol Biol Phys.* 55(3):565–567.

Yavuzsen T, MP Davis, D Walsh et al. 2005. Systematic review of the treatment of cancer-associated anorexia and weight loss. *J Clin Oncol* 23(33):8500–8511.

Yeomans ND, Z Tulassay, L Juhasz et al. 1998. A comparison of omeprazole with ranitidine for ulcers associated with nonsteroidal anti-inflammatory drug. Acid Suppression Trial: Ranitidine versus Omeprazole for NSAID-Associated Ulcer Treatment (ASTRONAUT) Study Group. *N Engl J Med* 338:719.

Yuhasz M, J Laufer, G Sutton, et al. 1985. Radiology of the small bowel in patients with gynecological malignancies. *Am J Radiol* 144:303–307.

Zanon C, M Grosso, F Apra, R Clara, M Bortolini, F Quaglino et al. 2002. Palliative treatment of malignant refractory ascites by positioning of Denver peritoneovenous shunt. *Tumori Genesis*; 88 (2):123–127.

27

Assisted Reproductive Technology

PM Gopinath

Since the first successful in vitro fertilisation (IVF) pregnancy in 1978, the field of assisted reproduction has made tremendous progress. Intracytoplasmic sperm injections (ICSI) and IVF remain the cornerstones of fertility treatment, but there have been many significant clinical and embryological advances which are unique in the field of gynecology. The success rates of treatment continue to improve steadily, with developments such as intracytoplasmic sperm injection, blastocyst transfer and preimplantation genetic diagnosis. Many more couples will benefit from assisted reproductive technologies. Cryopreservation techniques are being improved continually, and with its application to oocyte and ovarian tissue freezing, female fertility preservation is uncovering new horizons.

Newer developments involving in vitro maturation of immature oocytes, preimplantation diagnosis and aneuploidy screening are touched upon and the risks and complications associated with assisted reproductive technologies are highlighted. The newer developments concerning this technology have also been associated with a number of ethical and social dilemmas regarding which society is, in many circumstances, yet to reach a consensus as these are sensitive issues.

The term, assisted reproductive technology (ART), is globally used to describe the advanced infertility treatment options available to help couples with infertility achieve a pregnancy. The techniques of IVF and ICSI and preimplantation genetic diagnosis (PGD) are the cornerstones of ART.

Louise Brown's birth in July 1978, the first successful pregnancy resulting from IVF, uncovered new horizons in the field of infertility. The success followed many years of work by Patrick Steptoe and Robert Edwards (Steptoe and Edwards 1978).

This breakthrough was followed by rapid advances in the use of IVF and other newer assisted reproductive techniques (Tan et al 1990, 1992; Engmann et al 1999). It is estimated that more than a million babies have been born as a result of ART treatment, globally.

Definition: The term ART refers to methods of infertility management which involve the handling of the gametes outside the body. It stems from IVF and includes gamete intra fallopian tube transfer (GIFT), pronuclear stage transfer (PROST), tubal embryo transfer (TET) and ICSI. The most popular and successful methods today are IVF and ICSI.

In vitro Fertilisation: Initially, IVF was developed as a treatment for tubal factor infertility, in particular, after a failed tubal microsurgery. Today it has many more indications, including for male factor infertility.

A variety of IVF protocols are available from which one can choose depending on patient characteristics or clinician preference and the available resources. One of the standard approaches of IVF treatment is outlined below.

Pre-treatment Evaluation

Indications for IVF

- Bilateral blocked fallopian tubes
- Severe endometriosis
- Pelvic inflammatory disease with severe adhesion
- Premature menopause
- Failed reversal of vasectomy/tubectomy
- Obstructive azoospermia
- Oligo-astheno-teratospermia
- Genetic diseases
- Menopause
- Surrogacy (traditional/ gestational)

It is important that couples are counselled appropriately regarding the likely success rates of treatment, as well as associated risks, including multiple pregnancy and ovarian hyperstimulation syndrome (OHSS). From a clinical perspective, the likely response to ovarian stimulation is assessed by the evaluation of early follicular phase levels of follicle-stimulating hormone (FSH) and estradiol, a baseline ultrasound scan to assess the presence or absence of polycystic ovaries (PCO) (MacDougall et al 1993), and measuring the antral follicle count and the intraovarian stromal blood flow velocity (Zaidi et al 1996; Engmann et al 1999)

Pituitary downregulation: Most current IVF treatments use a standard long protocol gonadotrophin-releasing hormone agonist (GnRHa) prior to ovarian stimulation to achieve pituitary suppression (Tan et al 1994). This normally requires seven to 21 days of GnRHa administration. This has the advantage of reducing luteinising hormone (LH) levels during ovarian stimulation, which may, if present in high levels, be detrimental to oocyte quality and subsequent fertilisation and implantation rates (Belen et al 1993). In addition, continuing GnRH agonists during stimulation will minimise the risk of premature LH surge and ovulation (Tan et al 1992).

Controlled ovarian stimulation: Once pituitary suppression is accomplished, ovarian stimulation is achieved by exogenous gonadotrophin (FSH) stimulation. There are a variety of preparations available that are broadly divided into either urinary derived products or recombinant products. Urinary products generally include a variable amount of LH activity, whereas recombinant products are pure FSH. There is ongoing debate regarding the possible deleterious effects and the amount of LH activity required for optimal ovarian stimulation (Shoham 2002). Follicular growth can be assessed accurately by transvaginal ultrasound, with the addition of estradiol evaluation in selected situations (poor or excessive response).

Most protocols continue stimulation until there are at least three follicles with mean diametres of 18 mm or greater.

Ovulation trigger with human chorionic gonadotrophin: Once the leading follicles reach the appropriate dimensions, more than 18 mm size human chorionic gonadotrophin (hCG) 5000 to 10,000 IU is administered as a surrogate for the normal LH surge to induce final oocyte maturation within the follicles.

Oocyte collection: To begin with, the oocytes were recovered by laparoscopy. Nowadays, ultrasound-directed oocyte collection is almost universal. It means that IVF can largely be done as an outpatient procedure, without anesthesia (Tan et al 1990).

With a needle guide attached to a vaginal transducer, a double lumen or single lumen needle is inserted through the posterolateral vaginal fornix into a selected follicle in one ovary. A vacuum pump is used to aspirate follicular fluid into a collecting tube. The tubes are handed over to the embryologist and he examines the aspirate to detect the presence of the oocyte. Each follicle should be emptied completely to ensure maximum oocyte recovery. Flushing of the follicle should be performed sparingly, if at all (Tan et al 1992).

Insemination and embryo culture: Most oocytes are surrounded by a layer of cumulus cells (oocyte cumulus complex). Insemination is performed within 4 to 6 hours following the collection of the oocytes. For routine IVF, a prepared sperm sample with a predetermined count is added to each oocyte cumulus complex. For ICSI, the cumulus cells are stripped away and only metaphase II oocytes are injected with a single sperm under the micromanipulator.

A check is performed for fertilisation, 18 to 20 hours following insemination. The presence of two pronuclei confirms normal fertilisation. Culture is continued for 24 to 36 hours before further assessment for embryo cleavage is performed. At this stage, the embryos are normally between the two to eight cell (blastomere) stages. Embryo quality is assessed depending on blastomere symmetry and the degree of cytoplasm fragmentation before transfer.

Embryo transfer: Classically, embryos are transferred on either day 2 or day 3 following oocyte collection. The number of embryos transferred depends on a variety of factors, including the age of the female patient, number of previous IVF treatments, embryo quality and number, the wishes or concerns of the couple in relation to multiple pregnancies and any legislation relating to the maximum number of embryos that may be transferred. Normally, three embryos are transferred in one sitting and the rest, if any, are cryopreserved. Recent publications suggest a single embryo transfer so that multiple pregnancies may be avoided.

More recently, the use of a sequential culture media has enhanced the rate of formation of blastocysts in the laboratory, and the embryo transfer may be delayed to day 5. Blastocyst culture is an attempt to select embryos with higher implantation potential and to minimise multiple pregnancies.

Luteal support: The secretion of progesterone from the corpus luteum is essential for the support of early pregnancy. There are two main factors that may imply a deficient luteal phase in the context of an IVF cycle. The very nature of follicle aspirations means that many granulose cells may have been removed or disrupted. In addition, there is evidence that the use of a GnRH agonist in IVF treatment has a negative impact on the corpora luteal function.

For these reasons, the luteal phase is supported by the administration of progesterone, either in the form of vaginal pessaries or as daily intramuscular injections. As an alternative, some units will use low dose hCG injections instead of progesterone to support luteal functions. Both are equally efficacious but hCG may increase the risk of OHSS.

The woman normally has a pregnancy test performed 14 days after embryo transfer, and if pregnant, continues luteal support until eight to 12 weeks of gestation.

INTRACYTOPLASMIC SPERM INJECTIONS

Soon after IVF became an established treatment for a variety of fertility problems, it also became apparent that couples with a severe male factor problem were often not helped by traditional IVF. In a situation where the sperm count or motility was very low, or there were high numbers of abnormal sperm, IVF often led to failed fertilisation. A variety of sperm injection techniques were tried, but ultimately, ICSI of sperm proved to be the most successful. It is now practised routinely by many units and is indicated in a number of situations, including severe oligospermia, marked asthenospermia (low motility), elevated numbers of morphologically abnormal sperm (less than 15% normal morphology), previous fertilisation failure with conventional IVF or when epididymal or testicular sperm is used.

In men who produce no sperm (or no viable sperm) in the ejaculate, there are a variety of surgical techniques to retrieve sperm from either the epididymis or from the testicle itself.

CRYOPRESERVATION IN ART

The development of IVF programmes using ovarian stimulation often means that following the transfer of a selected number of fresh embryos, a number of embryos may remain. It was not long before the science of cryobiology was applied and the remaining embryos were frozen for future use. Most embryos are frozen using a slow cooling process with the addition of a cryoprotectant to avoid intracellular ice formation. These embryos may be thawed and replaced at a later date as an alternative to further stimulated cycles of IVF. Embryos may be frozen at pronuclei, cleavage or blastocyst stages of development. When patients have a large number of embryos, it is advisable to consider freezing a portion at the pronucleate phase, because they are less likely to suffer damage to the mitotic spindle, that is, as cleaved embryos. They subsequently yield a higher pregnancy rate following thawing and transfer (Senn et al 2000).

Around 70% to 80% of embryos survive thawing, depending on their initial quality. Once thawed, the embryos are placed in culture, and if frozen at the pronucleate phase, are allowed to cleave before transfer. Transfer of embryos may be done in a natural menstrual cycle, or if the woman has an irregular cycle, pituitary downregulation with GnRH agonists following hormone replacement therapy may be used.

More recently, cryobiology has been applied to the freezing of oocytes and ovarian tissue. The survival of the oocytes following thawing is extremely low compared with that of embryos. There also appears to be an increased risk of aneuploidy when metaphase II oocytes are cooled or warmed. The freezing of immature oocytes has been attempted, but again, the results have been poor. Nevertheless, it is an attractive option for fertility preservation in women undergoing chemotherapy or radiotherapy for various malignancies.

Cryopreservation of ovarian tissue is also an attractive option for women wanting to preserve fertility. The ovarian cortex contains many primordial follicles, but despite the existence of viable follicles following thawing, currently available culture media are inadequate to maintain in vitro maturation (IVM).

Alternatively, it is possible that harvested ovarian tissue may be autografted back to the donor to restore fertility. Some success has been reported in the sheep model (Gosden et al 1994) and there is at least one report of partial restoration of ovarian function in a woman who underwent autologous grafting (Oktay and Karlikaya 2000). There are concerns, however, in transplanting ovarian tissue back to cancer patients, particularly when there may be an etiological link to the ovary (that is, breast cancer).

Vitrification is a cryopreservation technique that is an alternative to the traditional slow freezing method. Essentially, it involves a process of solidification of a solution (within the cytoplasm of a cell) at a low temperature without ice crystal formation. It uses a higher concentration of cryoprotectant that is potentially more toxic to the cell, and it is then cooled at a higher rate. The technique is much simpler and is less expensive than the traditional slow cooling method. It has been used successfully with both oocytes and embryos and may be the method of choice, particularly for oocyte freezing (Kuleshova et al 1999).

Oocyte donation: The first reported pregnancy following the donation of an oocyte fertilised in vitro was in 1983 (Trounson et al 1983). Excellent pregnancy and live birth rates can be expected with the appropriate selection of donors. Initially, it was used as a method of treatment for women with premature ovarian failure, but nowadays it has wider applications, for example, in women who are carriers of specific genetic conditions that are transmitted by the oocyte. It is also often advocated in women with recurrent IVF failures. In theory, there is no age barrier to successful oocyte donation.

Unfortunately, the demand for donor oocytes outweighs the supply; so many units have very long waiting lists of patients requiring donor oocytes. Donors may be altruistic volunteers or known to the recipient (often a friend or relative). Anonymity, even with a known donor, can be achieved using a crossover pairing of two sets of donors and recipients.

Egg sharing is a programme that is increasingly being offered in some units. Patients undergoing IVF may volunteer to donate excess oocyte to an anonymous recipient. The cost of treatment may be shared between the couples.

NEW DEVELOPMENTS IN ART

Assisted reproduction is a rapidly developing area of medicine and the following are the more recent advances.

In vitro Maturation

The collection of immature oocytes from unstimulated ovaries with subsequent IVM and fertilisation is receiving increasing interest as an alternative to traditional IVF.

Initially, pregnancy rates following IVM were low. More recently, pregnancy rates in excess of 25% have been reported particularly in women with PCO (Cha et al 1991; Chain et al 2000; Tan and Child 2002)

The concept of IVM is very attractive for a number of reasons. The cost of treatment is reduced because patients do not require medications for ovarian stimulation. The avoidance of ovarian stimulation also means that side effects due to the use of gonadotrophin are also avoided. Most importantly, the risk of OHSS is avoided and this is especially important to those patients with PCO who are at an increased risk of OHSS with gonadotrophin stimulation. In addition, concern has been expressed over the possible long-term risk of ovarian cancer following repeated cycles of ovarian stimulation (Whittemore 1994), which would not be a concern with IVM treatment.

Patients undergoing an IVM cycle have a baseline ultrasound scan performed between days 2 and 4 of their cycle. At this point, the total number of antral follicles of a size greater than 2 mm to 4 mm is assessed. It has been demonstrated that the success of IVM depends on the number of immature oocytes obtained, which in turn can be predicted on the basis of the antral follicle count (Tan et al 2002). Pregnancy rates comparable with conventional IVF may be obtained when ten or more immature oocytes are collected. Oocytes can be retrieved from about 50% of visible follicles. This implies that patients who have PCO (greater than ten follicles per ovary) visible on ultrasound could be offered IVM treatment as an alternative to IVF (Child et al 2001).

The patient is normally scanned again on day 8, and oocyte retrieval is planned for between days 10 and 14. A subcutaneous injection of hCG is given, 36 hours before oocyte collection. This has been shown to improve the rate of maturation of the immature oocytes and the final number of mature oocyte obtained (Chian et al 1999).

The cycle is normally cancelled if a dominant follicle (greater than 10 mm) is present on day 8, because initial reports have suggested a reduced pregnancy rate (that is, the size of the dominant follicle indicates the pregnancy rate). The collection of immature oocytes is performed under ultrasound guidance with reduced aspiration pressure. Although similar to IVF, it is a more technically challenging procedure.

Following collection, the immature oocytes are cultured for 24 hours before fertilisation (by ICSI) of the metaphase II oocytes. Some oocytes require up to 48 hours to mature. Maturation rates of approximately 80% have been reported. Embryo transfer is performed two to three days later.

The endometrium is also primed with estradiol valerate from the day of collection and progesterone luteal support is given from the day of ICSI.

At present, IVM is most applicable to patients with PCO. With continued improvements, it may also become an option for women with normal ovaries and those who have repeatedly poor quality embryos following conventional IVF. In addition, it may be a viable alternative for egg donors, particularly those with PCO.

Preimplantation diagnosis: Although not strictly a new technique, preimplantation genetic diagnosis (PGD) is gaining more widespread utilisation. The first birth of a child following PGD was over a decade ago (Handyside et al 1990), and the births of more than 500 babies have been reported since then, using this method.

The technique essentially involves removing one or two blastomeres (which are representative of the embryo) from an eight cell embryo, three days after fertilisation. There are two techniques used to analyse the genetic status of the blastomere. First, polymerase chain reaction is used to amplify a particular genetic sequence, and then, with test samples and DNA the cell is subjected to electrophoresis, a mismatch will identify a specific mutation. It can be used for carriers of single gene defects involving autosomes and for sex chromosome-linked disorders.

Second, fluorescent in situ hybridisation is used to determine the ploidy of the blastomere by using probes to bind specific chromosomes. Up to eight chromosomes may be tested using this process (usually X, Y, 13,

15, 16, 18, 21 and 22). The technique has been shown to reduce the rate of trisomic offspring, increase implantation rates and reduce the rate of spontaneous abortion. PGD can be used for aneuploidy screening, sex selection for X-linked disorders and identification of unbalanced translocations from parental carriers (Munne and Well 2002). Once the results of analysis are known, the unaffected embryos are reimplanted. Most embryos survive biopsy; however, pregnancy rates are lower than those achieved with conventional IVF. The remaining embryos are usually retested as a method of quality control. Cryopreservation of embryos following biopsy has not proved to be very successful.

PGD has gained a lot of interest, particularly in relation to aneuploidy screening in women over the age of 37 years undergoing IVF (Munne et al 2002). It is well recognised that the proportion of embryos that have chromosomal abnormalities increases with increasing female age. PGD can be viewed as an adjunct to antenatal diagnosis, although the long term safety is unknown.

One of the limitations of current PGD practice is that two-thirds of the human chromosome complements is untested. Comparative genomic hybridisation is a variation of PGD that allows the visualisation of all 46 chromosomes following amplification of the whole test genome. It is then labelled with one colour and compared with a normal reference sample. Specially developed image processing software can delineate structural differences between the test sample and the control. Although the technique is not yet at a stage to be of practical use, it may well be the way forward for embryo selection before transfer by improving the detection of aneuploidy embryos (Wells and Delhanry 2000).

New drug regimens: Two of the disadvantages of most current IVF drug regimens are the duration of administration of the medications, and that they require subcutaneous or intramuscular injections. More recently, a new variety of medication has become available as an alternative to the traditional GnRH agonist long protocol regimen. GnRH antagonists were developed in the early 1970s, but they were not clinically suitable because they were associated with a significant histamine release at the site of injection. A new generation of GnRH antagonists is now available. They are an improvement over GnRH agonists available earlier in that they cause immediate and transient pituitary suppression. In addition, when used in conjunction with gonadotrophin stimulation, a lower dose of stimulation is often required. The antagonist may be administered as a single or multiple dose protocol. It is commenced normally around day 6 of gonadotrophin stimulation or when the leading follicles are 12–14 mm in diameter. It is continued until the day of hCG administration and appears to be as effective as the GnRH agonist protocols in preventing premature LH surges.

The new drug regimen allows for a more flexible and patient-friendly IVF protocol; however, most studies suggest that, at present, the implantation and pregnancy rate with GnRH antagonists are lower than when the long protocol (when the antagonist is started from the luteal phase of the cycle) GnRH agonists are used. Research is also underway to develop long-acting slow release gonadotrophin preparations and ultimately, an oral form.

Apart from the recombinant FSH, a recombinant LH has also been introduced in the market for triggering the ovulation.

Results of assisted reproduction: There are many variables that affect the chances of a successful outcome for a couple. Of paramount importance is the age of the female partner and success rates of IVF, and all fertility treatments reflect this. Although age is a guide to success rates, other factors such as ovarian reserve, length of infertility, previous treatment history, cause of infertility, the presence of a normal uterine cavity and the number of embryos transferred will have a bearing in individual cases.

Many IVF units now quote clinical pregnancy rates in the order of 35% to 40% per cycle in women up to their mid to late 30s. Women over the age of 40 years may expect success rates of less than 20%. Thereafter, there is a significant reduction, with extremely few women over the age of 44 to 45 conceiving with IVF.

As can be deducted from these figures, the majority of couples will not conceive following a single cycle of treatment. However, a recent study reported that for women younger than 30 years of age, the cumulative pregnancy and live birth rates after three cycles of treatment were 75.5% and 71.8% respectively. For all women treated up to the age of 45 years, the cumulative pregnancy and live birth rates after three cycles were 54.2% and 48.2%, respectively (Engmann et al 1999). With new developments in aneuploidy screening of embryos before replacement, there is potential for significantly improved success rates in the future.

Complications and limitations of ART: There are a number of potential complications that may arise as a result of ART. These complications may occur during the treatment cycle itself or as a result of the pregnancy achieved by treatment.

The development of ovarian cysts during IVF treatment is not uncommon and may occur as a result of pituitary suppression from GnRH agonist use or from previous gonadotrophin therapy. The cysts are generally not a significant health risk and are dealt with relatively easily. When they occur following GnRH agonist therapy, continuing treatment for a further week may lead to resolution or the cysts may be aspirated, particularly if they are large.

The procedure of oocyte collection and embryo transfer can also lead to complications of infection or hemorrhage, although this is not common. Patients with ovarian endometriosis appear to have a higher risk of infection and prophylactic antibiotics should be administered.

The main concern of most IVF practitioners is the development of OHSS. This is a potentially life threatening iatrogenic condition resulting from excessive ovarian stimulation. It is characterised in its most severe form by enlarged ovaries, ascites, pleural effusions and subsequent dehydration and hemoconcentration.

Thromboembolism, which is potentially fatal, may subsequently develop (Stewart et al 1997). Severe OHSS may occur in up to 1% of patients undergoing IVF and a further 10% may have mild to moderate OHSS. It may develop early following oocyte retrieval, or arise a week or so after embryo transfer, when it is often associated with pregnancy. Patients with polycystic ovarian syndrome, lean body mass or a history of OHSS are most at risk. During gonadotrophin therapy, the development of multiple follicles (more than 20), especially medium-sized follicles, 12 mm to 14 mm in diametre, often with a concurrent excessively elevated serum estradiol level (greater than 10,000 pmol/litre) should alert the clinician to the risk of OHSS. Strategies aimed at the prevention of OHSS may include reducing the hCG trigger dose (5000 U), coasting the cycle by withholding stimulation until the estradiol has fallen, and proceeding with collection but freezing all embryos or by cancellation of the cycle. Once OHSS is established, the aims of treatment are essentially supportive, with rehydration and replacement of albumin, ascitic drainage as required and anticoagulation.

Successful ART is often characterised by a higher chance of multiple pregnancy and the incumbent medical, social and economical consequences (Jain et al 2002). At present, the only effective means of reducing multiple pregnancy rates is to limit the number of embryos transferred. There is concern that this will reduce overall pregnancy rates, although some evidence suggests that electively reimplanting only two embryos in young women who produce many good quality embryos reduces triplet pregnancy rates without affecting overall success rates. At our centre, we have adopted this policy for the past six years, and high pregnancy rates have been maintained with a triplet pregnancy rate of less than 4%.

A recent analysis of data from all centres in the United States shows an overall triplet pregnancy rate in excess of 8% (Assisted Reproductive Technology Success Rates 1999). It is hoped that with improved aneuploidy screening techniques, a reduction in the number of embryos being reimplanted can be achieved with either similar or better pregnancy rates.

Pregnancy complications following ART have been well studied. The rates of preterm delivery and low birth weight appear to be more common, even in singleton pregnancies, as a result of ART (Tan et al 1992). However, the majority of problems are a consequence of the increased multiple pregnancy rates associated with treatment, and also most probably the infertility status of these patients (Saimders and Lancaster 1989).

The overall risk of congenital malformations following ART is not significantly different from that of the general population when adjusted for age and multiple pregnancies. However, the incidence of sex chromosomal abnormalities may be increased from 0.2% to 0.7% following ICSI. This is most likely a result of subtle chromosomal abnormalities in the men with severe sperm problems for which ICSI is typically used (Bonduelle et al 2002).

A few years ago, it was suggested that repeated cycles of stimulation (more than 12) without pregnancy may be associated with an increased risk of ovarian cancer. However, it has since been shown that infertility itself is a risk factor for ovarian cancer, and the risk observed may only be a reflection of the infertility status of these patients. Nevertheless, it would be prudent to avoid the unnecessary use of fertility drugs, and the old practice of empirically giving infertility patients months or even years of 'fertility pills' to augment their fertility should be abandoned.

Limitations of ART are not only related to the medical consequences. In most countries, treatment is not funded or at best, partially funded by the government. For the most part, couples have to fund their own treatment, and the costs involved are prohibitive to many. In addition, there are ethical considerations for many couples, whether they are religious or otherwise, that create a barrier to treatment.

The psychological and emotional stress of assisted reproduction should not be underestimated. Significant emotional, financial and temporal commitment is required for a couple to undertake a cycle of treatment. This places their relationship under even more stress than may have existed before commencing treatment. Trained fertility counsellors are an integral part of a treatment programme and couples should be encouraged to make use of them.

Conclusions: The development of IVF and its associated technologies has not only revolutionised the treatment of infertility, but has also created a worldwide industry dedicated to its success. It has become so successful that it is now a relatively rare occurrence when no treatment alternatives are available to a couple. Continued research in this area is likely to lead to higher success rates in the future.

Along with the progress of ART, there have also been associated complications in the form of iatrogenic OHSS and a significant increase in the number of higher order multiple pregnancies. Newer techniques such as IVM and aneuploidy screening may help reduce some of these associated risks and improve outcomes even further.

Access to treatment may be limited by social and economic constraints, and in addition, there have been and will continue to be ethical controversies surrounding some of the available treatments. The speed of development of assisted reproduction has meant that society has, in many cases, not been able to adjust to these ethical situations or develop adequate guidelines.

The success of ART will no doubt continue to improve with higher pregnancy rates, reduced risks and complications, and more affordable and patient-friendly treatment.

References

Assisted Reproductive Technology Success Rates. 1999. <http: //www.cdc.gov/nccdphp/drh/art99 /sample.htm> Version Current at October 2002.

Belen AH, SL Tan, J MacDougall, HS Jacobs. 1993. Miscarriage rates following in-vitro fertilization are increased in women with polycystic ovaries and reduced by pituitary desensitization with buserelin. *Hum Reprod* 8:959–964.

Bonduelle M, I Liebaers, V Deketalaere et al. 2002. Neonatal data on a cohort of 2889 infants born after ISI (1991-1999) and of 2995 infants born after IVF (1983-1999). *Hum Reprod* 17:671–694

Cha K, J Koo, J Ko et al. 1991. Pregnancy after in vitro fertilization of human follicular oocytes collected from nonstimulated cycles, their culture in vitro and their transfer in a donor oocyte program. *Fertil Steril* 55:109–113.

Chain R, W Buckett, T Tulandi et al. 2000. Prospective randomized study of human chorionic gonadotrophin priming before immature oocyte retrieval from unstimulated women with polycystic ovarian syndrome. *Hum Reprod* 15L:165–170.

Chian R, B Gulecki, W Buckett et al. 1999. Priming with human chorionic gonadotrophin before retrieval of immature oocytes in women with infertility due to polycystic ovarian syndrome. *N Engl J Med* 341:1624–1626.

Child TJ, AK Abdul-Jalil, B Gulekli, SL Tan. 2001. In vitro maturation and fertilization of oocytes from unstimulated normal ovaries, polycystic ovaries, and women with polycystic ovary syndrome. *Fertil Steril* 76:936–942.

Engmann L, N Maconochie, JS Bekir et al. 1999. Cumulative probability of clinical pregnancy and live birth after a multiple cycle IVF package: A more realistic assessment of overall and age-specific success rates? *Br J Obstet Gynaecol* 106:165–170.

Engmann L, P Sladkevicius, R Agarwal, JS Bekit, S Campbell, SL Tan. 1999. Value of ovarian stromal blood flow velocity measurement after pituitary suppression in the prediction of ovarian responsiveness and outcome of in vitro fertilization treatment. *Fertil Steril* 71:22–29.

Engmann L, N Maconochie, J Bekir et al. 1999. Cumulative probability of clinical pregnancy and live birth after a multiple cycle IVF Package. A more realistic assessment of overall and age specific success rates? *Br J Obstet Gynecol* 106:165–170.

Gosden RG, DT Baird, JC Wade et al. 1994. Restoration of fertility to oophorectomized sheep by ovarian autografts stored at – 196°C. *Hum Reprod* 9:597–603.

Handyside A, E Kontogianni, K Hardy et al. 1990. Pregnancies from biopsied human preimplantation embryos sexed by Y-specific DNA amplification. *Nature* 344:768–770.

Jain T, BL Harlow, MD Hornstein. 2002. Insurance coverage and outcomes of in vitro fertilization. *N Engl J Med* 347:661–666.

Kuleshova L, Gionaroli L, Magli C, et al. 1999. Birth following Vitrification of a small number of human oocytes: Case report. *Hum Reprod* 14:3077–3079.

Mac Dougall MJ, SL Tan, A Balen, HS Jacobs. 1993. A controlled study comparing patients with and without polycystic ovaries undergoing in vitro fertilization. *Hum Reprod* 8:233–237.

Munne S and D Well. 2002. Preimplantation genetic diagnosis. *Curr Opin Obstet Gynecol* 14:239–244.

Munne S, J Cohen, D Sable. 2002. Preimplantation genetic diagnosis for advanced maternal age and other indications. *Fertil Steril* 78:234–236.

Oktay K and G Karlikaya. 2000. Ovarian function after transplantation of frozen, banked autologues ovarian tissue. *N Engl J Med* 342:1919.

Saimders DM and P Lancaster. 1989. The wider perinatal significance of the Australian in vitro fertilization data collection program. *Am J Perinatol* 6:252–257

Senn A, C Vozzi, A Chanson, et al. 2000. Prospective randomized study of two cryopreservation policies avoiding embryo selection. The pronucleate stage leads to a higher cumulative delivery rate than early cleavage stage. *Fertil Steril* 74:946–952.

Shoham Z. 2002. The Clinical therapeutic window for luteinizing hormone in controlled ovarian stimulation. *Fertil Steril* 77:1170–1177.

Steptoe PC and RG Edwards. 1978. Birth after re-implantation of a human embryo. *Lancet* 8; 2: 366. (Lett)

Stewart JA, PJ Hamilton, AP Murdoch. 1997. Thromboembolic disease associated with ovarian stimulation and assisted conception techniques. *Hum Reprod* 12:2167–2173.

Tan SL and TJ Child. 2002. In vitro maturation of oocytes from unstimulated polycystic ovaries. *Reprod Biomed Online* 4 (Suppl 1):18–23.

Tan SL, C Kingsland, S Campbell S et al. 1992. The long protocol of administration of gonadotrophin-releasing hormone agonist is superior to the short protocol for ovarian stimulation for in vitro fertilization. *Fertil Steril* 57:810–814.

Tan SL, C Steer, P Royston et al. 1990. Conception rates and in-vitro fertilization. *Lancet* 335:299.

Tan SL, J Waterstone, M Wren, J Parsons. 1992. A prospective randomized study comparing aspiration only with aspiration and flushing for transvaginal ultrasound-directed oocyte recovery. *Fertil Steril* 58:356–360.

Tan SL, N Maconochie, P Doyle et al. 1994. Cumulative conception and live- birth rates after in vitro fertilization with and without the use of long, short, and ultrashort regimens of the gonadotrophin-releasing hormone agonist buserelin. *Am J Obstet Gynecol* 171:513–520.

Tan SL, P Doyle, S Campbell, et al. 1992. Obstetric outcome of in vitro fertilization pregnancies compared with normally conceived pregnancies. *Am J Obstet Gynecol* 167:778–784

Tan SL, P Royston, S Campbell, et al. 1992. Cumulative conception and livebirth rates after in-vitro fertilization. *Lancet* 399:1390–1394.

Tan SL, S Bennett, J Parsons. 1990. Surgical techniques of oocyte collection and embryo transfer. *Br Med Bull* 46:628–642.

Tan SL, TJ Child, B Gulekli. 2002. In vitro maturation and fertilization of oocytes from unstimulated ovaries: Predicting the number of immature oocytes retrieved by early follicular phase ultrasonography. *Am J Obstet Gynecol* 186:684–689.

Trounson A, J Leeton, M Besanko et al. 1983. Pregnancy established in an infertile patient after transfer of a donated embryo fertilized in vitro. *Br Med J* 286:835–838.

Wells D and JD Delhanry. 2000. Comprehensive chromosomal analysis of human preimplantation embryos using whole genome amplification and single cell comparative genomic hybridization. *Mol Hum Reprod* 6:1055–1062.

Whittemore AS. 1994. The risk of ovarian cancer after treatment for infertility. *N Eng J Med* 331: 805–806.

Zaidi J, J Barber, A Kyei- mensah et al. 1996. Relationship of ovarian stromal blood flow at the baseline ultrasound scan to subsequent follicular response in an in vitro fertilization program. *Obstet Gynecol* 88:779–784.

28

Gynecological Operative Endoscopy–Indications and Limitations

Kurian Joseph | Vanita Jain

Laparoscopy is used in gynecology for benign as well as malignant conditions. The advantages of laparoscopy over laparotomy include smaller scar, quicker recovery, decreased adhesion formation and decreased cost. A comparison of operative laparoscopy and laparotomy for benign gynecological conditions revealed that the overall risk of minor complications (for example, fever, wound or urinary tract infection) was lower in women undergoing laparoscopic procedures (RR 0.55), while the risk of major complications (pulmonary embolus, transfusion, fistula formation, major additional unplanned surgery) was the same in both groups (Chapron et al 2002).

HISTORY

The concept of endoscopy began in the twentieth century. Professor Kelling, a German, introduced a cystoscope into the abdomen of a dog in 1901. Gynecologists did most of the initial work in the development of laproscopy. Palmer from Paris, and Frangenheim and Semm from Germany were giants in the field who developed several new instruments like the insufflator and morcellator, which made the procedures safer and easier. Better lights and newer concepts in optics rod lens system improved the view. Unipolar electrocautery created problems initially and was supplemented with bipolar cautery by Rioux and Cloutier (1974). Bipolar cauterisation of fallopian tubes gradually developed to emerge as the most common method of tubal sterilisation in the US. Decker (1949) developed culdoscopy, where the scope was introduced through the posterior fornix with the patient in the knee chest position. This technique was gradually replaced by laparascopy, as the surgeon was more familiar with the laparascopic view. The first test tube baby by Steptoe in 1977 also gave prominence to laparascopy as the ovum pickup was done using it (Steptoe and Edwards 1978). The advent video camera revolutionised the field of operative endoscopy as it permitted longer procedures with the surgeon in a comfortable position and involving all the members in the operation room. Recorded films were good for teaching. The development of a suturing technique for laparoscopy by Clarke (1972) enabled more complete surgery. Bruhat et al (1980) and DeCherney and Polan (1983) reported on the use of the laparoscope for ectopic pregnancies. Soon, several other procedures were done successfully through the laparoscope or the hysteroscope. Reich described the first laparoscopic hysterectomy in 1989, and in 1994 Dargent reported laparoscopic radical hysterectomy. Operative endoscopy comprises all operative gynecological work done using an endoscope, chiefly laparoscopy and hysteroscopy. Salpingoscopy and falloposcopy also come in the same group but the indications for their use are limited. Colposcopy does not come under the endoscopic procedures, as no body cavity is entered into with the scope. In the research and experimental field, the procedures of fetoscopy and embryoscopy should be mentioned (Dumez et aI 1992).

LAPAROSCOPY

Preoperative assessment: A history of conditions that are associated with intraabdominal adhesions and anatomic distortion should be carefully elicited. These include previous abdominal surgery, diseases (for example, appendicitis, pelvic inflammatory disease) or radiation therapy. Thorough medical examination to detect any cardiorespiratory compromise should be done. The presence of ventral and umbilical hernias also needs to be noted to avoid needle or trocar insertion at these sites. The risk of bowel or vascular injury, as well as the need to convert to an open procedure, should be discussed with all patients.

Instruments

- The Veress needle is the pneumoperitoneum needle used most frequently. This needle has two working parts—an outer needle with a sharp beveled edge, and an inner, spring-loaded, retractable blunt shaft that extends beyond the end of the needle point.
- Telescopes for laparoscopy are of two basic types, those with and those without an operative channel.
- Cannulas are available in diameters from 3 mm to 12 mm to accommodate laparoscopes and instrumentation of all sizes. They are equipped with either a trumpet or flapper valve to prevent gas leakage. The cannula also helps to control the depth of trocar insertion.
- Trocars have either a pyramidal or conical tip and should be sharp enough to produce the force necessary to penetrate the abdominal wall.
- A variety of uterine manipulators can be used to manipulate the uterus and thereby facilitate visualisation of and access to pelvic structures. Most cannulas also permit injection of a dye solution (chromopertubation) to assess tubal patency.
- Almost all instruments available for laparotomy have been modified for use at laparoscopy. The instruments are modified to fit through a 3 mm to 20 mm port and have to be of sufficient length to reach the pelvis.
- A light source, camera, monitors, gas insuflator and cautery machine.

Technique: Laparoscopy is the most common operative endoscopic technique used. The procedure at laparoscopy has been standardised over the years with the use of the Verress needle to create the pneumoperitoneum. The patient is kept in a horizontal position till adequate carbon dioxide is instilled. The transumbilical port is normally used but when adhesions, previous scars or pathology is suspected, the subcostal or para-umbilical route may be used. Additional ports may be made laterally, taking care to avoid the inferior epigastric artery. The patient is placed in the Trendelenburg position and the peritoneal cavity is first inspected and the pathology assessed. The first decision to be made is whether the procedure could be completed laparoscopically or not. In the presence of incorrect preoperative findings or extensive pathology, it would be wise to convert it to a laparotomy. This decision should be made based on the experience of the operator along with the set up available. Once this decision is made then the location of the other ports to be used are decided. Consider a triangle, the base formed by the two ports with the pathology at the apex. This permits easy traction and dissection. Larger masses require higher ports. If pathology is limited to one side only, then the opposite-side ports facilitate better access. Dissection is carried out with scissors, monopolar electrosurgery or the laser. Hemostasis is secured using bipolar electrosurgery by suturing or by applying stapels. Disposable clip appliers containing both absorbable and nonabsorbable staples are available for laparoscopy. Suction and irrigation are important for all types of laparoscopic surgery. Irrigation is used for removal of char or for visualisation when bleeding is encountered. It can also be used for hydrodissection and creation of tissue planes. Tissue removal at laparoscopy presents a difficult problem. This may be overcome by enlarging the port, morcellating the tissue or by removing it through a colpotomy. At the end of the procedure, hemostasis is achieved. All ports larger than 10 mm require to be closed with a suture through the fascia. Technical advances in laparoscopy include rapid carbon dioxide insufflators, three-chip and high definition cameras that improve picture clarity, ultra-bright light sources, safer energy sources and changes in laparoscopic needle drivers and automated suturing devices

Limitations: There are definite limitations to operative endoscopy. The image viewed is a 2-D image and there will be a loss of depth of perception, hence assessing the location of an object is difficult. The view is unidirectional with a fixed angularity resulting in a lack of spatial awareness. There is a loss of tactile sensation with a restricted force feedback. This may cause problems in judging the effect of surgery on a particular tissue. The instruments used are specially made small and hence their use is limited. The long handles create a fulcrum effect whereby the instrument acts as a lever. The ability to retract is also severely impaired. Yet the single most important limiting factor would be a poorly trained operator with the lack of a thorough knowledge of the anatomy and the structural relations.

Indications: The indications for operative endoscopy have increased many times over the past few years. It has become the gold standard for the diagnosis and treatment of conditions like ectopic pregnancy, benign ovarian cysts, endometriosis and uterine anomalies including septae. The other indications include diagnostic laparoscopy, hysterectomy, myomectomy, lymphadenectomy and repair of pelvic floor defects.

Diagnostic laparoscopy is indicated as part of the infertility evaluation of young women, especially those with a history of pelvic inflammatory disease, ectopic pregnancy, pelvic surgery or chronic pelvic pain. If adhesions or endometriosis are found during diagnostic laparoscopy, an operative laparoscopic procedure for improving fertility can be undertaken at the same time. Distal tubal occlusion can be corrected by fimbrioplasty or terminal salpingoplasty. Laparoscopic salpingectomy for hydrosalpinges is the preferred procedure for improving pregnancy rates in women going in for in vitro fertilisation. Selective tubal catheterisation can be performed in women who appear to have proximal tubal occlusion by hysterosalpingography. Laparoscopy has better results than laparotomy whenever surgery is indicated in infertile patients due to decreased adhesion formation.

Adnexal Surgery

Adnexal mass: It is controversial whether a laparotomy or a laparoscopy should be performed to evaluate **adnexal masses.** The main problem is the difficulty in ruling out a malignant change, the potential risk of tumour spill by rupture of the ovarian capsule during removal of the mass laparoscopically and the potential delay to definitive surgery when complete surgical staging is not performed at the time of diagnosis of an unexpected malignancy.

In a Society of Gynecologic Oncologists member survey, it has been seen that the average delay to definitive surgery was approximately five weeks when a malignant mass was first encountered laparoscopically and not properly staged, and this delay in cases where tumour rupture occurred at the time of laparoscopic evaluation significantly affected survival (Maiman et al 1991).

Malignancy must be suspected before any adnexal ovarian mass is operated upon. A good history and clinical examination supported by an ultrasound scan and tumour marker study would establish the chances of malignancy.

Laparoscopy can be used to assess the cyst for neoplasm, to collect peritoneal fluid for cytology, to inspect the ovary and the peritoneal cavity, to aspirate the cyst, to study the cyst fluid and contents and do a frozen section biopsy. After proper screening, the incidence of malignancy in several large studies was found to be less than 1% (Canis et al 1992). Simple cysts are enucleated and the ovary is left to re-form.

Endometriotic cysts have to be first lifted out of the pelvis, freeing the adhesions from the rectum, bowel and the pelvic sidewall. The cyst cavity is then opened out and the cyst lining peeled out. Occasionally, the wall would be densely adherent; then the lining could be coagulated using laser or electrosurgery. Brosens et al (1996) suggested coagulating only the active areas and permitting the remaining ovarian tissue to involute.

Dermoids present the problem of spillage of the cyst contents. While spillage does not worsen the prognosis, it makes cleaning difficult and time consuming. Small dermoids can be easily shelled out intact. The dermoid can be decompressed in an endobag or removed through a colpotomy with minimal spillage. The peritoneal cavity must be washed with saline or a dilute solution of Povidone iodine. If cysts are many or if the residual ovarian tissue is less than a third, then oophorectomy would be better.

Reich et al (1989) reported the management of **pelvic abscesses** laparoscopically. The procedure was done under antibiotic cover and blunt dissection carried out using the irrigation cannula and an atraumatic forceps. The advantage claimed is that the adhesions being inflammatory are easy to separate earlier rather than later when they have become dense. At oophorectomy, the ovary should be pulled away from the pelvic side wall to avoid injury to the ureter.

In cases of **torsion**, the cyst can be decompressed, 'detorsion' done and the ovary assessed for viability. If viable, then cystectomy tents with a long utero-ovarian ligament oropexy can prevent recurrent torsion.

Ovarian drilling for **polycystic ovaries** is used laparascopically by using the monopolar or bipolar electric current or the carbon dioxide laser. However, medical methods of ovulation induction are the first line of treatment and drilling ovaries is done only in resistant cases (Balen and Jacobs 1995).

Ectopic gestation is managed by salpingectomy if fertility is not required or salpingostomy whenever the tube should be and can be preserved The indication for salpingostomy is in women desiring fertility who are clinically stable with an ectopic less than 6 cm and a β hCG below 20,000 IU/ml. The incision on the tube should be on the antimesentric border adequate to facilitate complete and intact removal of the ectopic. Use of hydro-dissection helps in atraumatic dissection. After the removal, hemostasis is secured by carefully identifying the bleeding points. Occasionally, bleeding is severe and needs salpingectomy.

The presence of live trophoblastic tissue after conservative surgery presents the main problem. All patients should undergo a mandatory hCG assay on the third day to detect persistent trophoblast. A marked fall should be noted. If there is no decline on successive measurements, this should be treated with methotrexate.

Currently, the use of methotrexate is the treatment of choice for unruptured small ectopics. This, however, necessitates monitoring of the patient over the next ten days. Cost studies show that a prolonged hospital stay offsets the cost of surgery. In patients with low initial serum hCG concentrations, systemic methotrexate leads to cost savings compared to laparoscopic salpingostomy (Hajenius et al 2000). In the case of a large ectopic, an unhealthy diseased tube, a grossly distorted tube or if fertility is not required, then salpingectomy is the procedure of choice. Whether salpingectomy or salpingostomy is done, the chance of a subsequent pregnancy depends on a healthy contralateral tube. In a large ectopic pregnancy, removal of the tube and contents from the abdominal cavity often poses problems due to the friable nature of the mass.

Tubal sterilisation became an outpatient procedure with the advent of laparoscopy. The first tubal sterilisation was reported by Ruddock (1934). Many techniques of sterilisation were devised using the monopolar and bipolar current, clips and bands. Mass sterilisation camps were begun as the procedure became more popular.

Monopolar current was found to damage too much of the tube, and it also had the potential to cause visceral bumps. Bipolar was safer and the tube was coagulated at two or three places. The tube was not transected for fear of fistula formation. The clips were more costly and popular in the western world.

The Filshie clip had a low failure rate but laparoscopic application required expensive applicators. The other clips used were the Hulka and Blier clip. The Yoon silastic band has been used in large scale camps in India and in several other countries. Ease of application and the low cost popularised it. Peterson et al (1996) found the cumulative pregnancies were highest with the Hulka clip method (36.5 per 1000) and lowest for monopolar coagulation (7.5 per 1000) after a 10-year follow-up of 10,685 women who underwent tubal sterilisation.

Younger women had a higher rate of failure and this included 53.3 per 1000 for bipolar coagulation and 52.1 per 1000 for Hulka clip application. With the mechanical methods, failures were in the first three to four years following the operation, whereas pregnancies occurred fairly evenly throughout the ten years following bipolar cautery. Electrocoagulation appears to be associated with the highest rate of ectopic pregnancies.

Tubal reanastomosis following sterilisation has been described using the laparoscope. The procedure is long and requires dexterity since thin suture materials need to be used with the long endoscopic instruments.

Uterine procedures: Laparoscopic treatment of uterine problems includes adhesiolysis to mobilise the uterus, myomectomy, excision of a rudimentary horn of the uterus and hysterectomy.

Adhesiolysis of the pelvic structures comprised the first procedures done with the scope. Mobilising the uterus is required for fertility and in chronic backache. The uterus is commonly bound down by adhesions in endometriosis, pelvic infection and after pelvic surgery. The advantage in the laparoscope lies in the magnified view which makes the planes for dissection more visible. Dissection may be done with the scissors, electrosurgery and carbon dioxide laser or with the ultrasound scalpel. The principles of microsurgery, like sharp clean dissection with good hemostasis, should be adhered to. Irrigation for clearing the field of surgery and for moistening the tissue is essential. In the presence of dense adhesions, an adhesion preventing barrier like Interceed may be used. The usefulness of these barriers has still not been established. Congenital anomalies of the uterus, like the functioning non-communicating uterine horn, can be treated laparoscopically with excision of that horn or by hemi-hysterectomy.

Laparoscopic **removal of myomas** is feasible when the myoma is less than 10 cm and when there are not more than 3–4 myomas. Myomectomy is done by incising the capsule of the myoma and applying traction using a myoma screw or a toothed forceps. Hemostasis should be obtained as the myoma is being shelled out. The cavity is then sutured in layers using vicryl. This is a simple procedure for small subserous myomas; but if the myoma is large or situated in the tubo-cornual region, removal may be difficult.

Deep seated myomas and interstitial myomas require to be carefully dissected out using bipolar electrosurgery or ultrasound scalpel to achieve hemostasis. Bleeding from a deep-seated myoma is difficult to control. Recent reports of uterine rupture in pregnancy following laparoscopic myomectomy have cast some doubts on its use in infertile patients (Dubuisson et al 1995; Hockstein 2000). By minimising the use of cautery and with better suturing, this can be prevented. The long term problem of fistulae or wound dehiscence is infrequent. The use of GnRH analogues to decrease the size of the myoma has been used effectively. This is expensive and the effect varies in different myomas.

Myolysis using laser cautery or the cryoprobe involves the coagulation of myomas. This prevents further growth. This procedure is not indicated in the treatment of infertile women for fear of rupture during pregnancy (Arcangeli and Pasquarette 1997). Removal of myoma poses a problem at laparoscopy. An electric motor driven morcellator helps to cut up the myoma into small pieces. If the morcellator is not available, then the tissue could be removed through a colpotomy. The development of effective techniques for uterine artery embolisation may change the need for some of these procedures.

Hysterectomy represents the extreme use of endoscopic technique. The method followed at initial laparoscopic hysterectomy was similar to that of open surgery (Reich et al 1989). Using a three or four port technique, the pedicles were secured using bipolar diathermy or sutures. The aim of the procedure was to convert an abdominal hysterectomy to a vaginal one. Vaginal hysterectomy allows the patient more rapid and less painful recovery than if she were subjected to an abdominal hysterectomy. For this reason, the vaginal approach is preferred over the traditional abdominal approach (Johnson et al 2005). In cases in which vaginal hysterectomy is difficult, laparoscopy can be used to facilitate vaginal removal of the uterus (laparoscopically assisted vaginal hysterectomy or LAVH).

The American College of Obstetricians and Gynecologists has listed the following as potential indications for laparoscopic assistance to facilitate hysterectomy via the vaginal approach—need for adhesiolysis, need for treatment of endometriosis, need for management of large leiomyoma(s) to facilitate uterine extraction and the need for ligation of the infundibulopelvic ligaments to facilitate oophorectomy (ACOG 2005). Hence, if vaginal removal becomes feasible at any stage in the surgery, then it is done. If the uterine arteries are cut laparoscopically then the procedure is called a laparoscopic hysterectomy. The uterosacral ligaments and the parametrial tissue are dissected free. Anterior and posterior colpotomies are done using an obturator or a vaginal tube to distend the fornices. The uterus is then removed vaginally after morcellation, if needed.

The indications for hysterectomy using the laparoscope would be a large uterus up to 16 weeks size, fixed uterus (following previous surgery, PID or endometriosis) adnexal pathology like benign ovarian cysts and associated procedures as in appendicectomy or cholecystectomy. The laparoscope could be used to advantage when the pathology is not clear or the diagnosis is in doubt. It must be emphasised that vaginal hysterectomy has less morbidity than a laparoscopic hysterectomy. In cases of doubt, diagnostic laparoscopy helps to easily complete the procedure vaginally.

There are several contraindications to laparoscopic hysterectomy. In large uteri, over 16 weeks size, very dense adhesions make the procedure very difficult and time consuming. Contraindications for general anesthesia would not permit a laparoscopic procedure. Dissection of the uterine artery is often very difficult as the vessel is covered by dense pelvic fascia, the vessel often divides early and the collaterals in the pelvis are very good. Hence, bleeding from the uterine vessels can be very troublesome. As the ureter is close by, indiscriminate use of cautery may cause injury to it. To decrease problems with this area of dissection the concept of sub-total hysterectomy became popular.

However, the many advantages claimed by its protagonists have not been proved. Releasing the uterosacrals laparoscopically may result in poor support to the vault predisposing a vault prolapse. Laparoscopic hysterectomy with robotic assistance has emerged as a new approach over the past two decades. Two major categories of robotic systems include laparoscope holding systems and laparoscope holders with instrument manipulation systems (Polet et al 2002).

A Cochrane review evaluated 27 randomised controlled trials to determine the most appropriate approach to hysterectomy (Johnson et al 2006).

It showed that major surgical complications occurred more frequently in laparoscopic than abdominal hysterectomy (11% versus 6%). The rate of minor complications was similar (25% to 27%), laparoscopic hysterectomy took longer to perform than abdominal or vaginal hysterectomy, it was associated with less postoperative pain than abdominal hysterectomy, as well as a shorter length of hospitalisation, quicker recovery and better quality of life at six weeks postoperatively. No differences were found in one year.

Radical procedures have been done endoscopically over the last few years. Laparoscopic radical hysterectomy for cancer cervix has been well developed. Several studies have shown that the procedure matches open surgery for its radicality and node clearance. Long term studies of the effectiveness of the procedure are awaited. Further, these operations were performed at centres noted for their ability with the endoscope.

Lymphadenectomy of both pelvic and aortic nodes can be done laparoscopically. The magnified view helps dissection easily with minimal blood loss. If a positive node is obtained then the radical surgery could be abandoned in favour of alternative therapy. In very early cervical cancer in young women desirous of childbirth, radical amputation of the cervix (trachelectomy) with lymphadenectomy has helped in permitting pregnancies in a select group of patients (Dargent 1994). Radical surgery for early ovarian malignancy has been reported with omentectomy, lymphadenectomy and complete tumour removal (Querleu and Leblanc 1994).

The only randomised trial evaluating different approaches to pelvic lymphadenectomy compared laparoscopic to extraperitoneal or transperitoneal lymphadenectomy. The three techniques had similar complication rates, the laparoscopic approach took longer (75 versus 54 and 63 minutes, respectively) and fewer lymph nodes were resected (30 versus 35 and 36, respectively), but recovery was faster (hospitalisation 3.1 versus 3.2 and 5.6 days, respectively) (Kohler et al 2003).

Pelvic floor repair: Repair of stress incontinence by the Burch's technique has been widely used laparoscopically. The dissection into the anterior space is easy and bleeds less. The anatomic landmarks can be easily identified. The problem is to take the suture through the Cooper's ligament. Using Goretex makes the suture slide easily. Care must be taken to dissect carefully in the lateral spaces to avoid damage to the veins. The bladder must be carefully mobilised away from the vaginal wall. If a suture is taken too deep it may enter the bladder or the vagina. The extraperitoneal approach has been used in some cases, but the transperitoneal approach helps to identify any anomaly and also permits the placement of a Moscowitz suture.

The work done by Liu (1996) in the field of laparoscopic pelvic floor repair is commendable. Repair of cystocele, enterocele, rectocele and prolapse of the uterus has been done using the laparoscope. The principles involve the dissection of the bladder and rectum and reinforcing the fascial support with a merselene mesh. In the case of a prolapse uterus or vault prolapse, the mesh is attached to the sacral promontory. In cases of previous surgery, the dissection of the posterior surface of the uterus can often be very difficult. However, it has not been proved that the laparoscopic route offers much advantage over routine techniques in these procedures.

Surgery for pain relief: Pelvic pain is another area where the laparoscope has been used. Severe endometriosis or multiple postoperative adhesions can result in chronic pelvic pain. Laparoscopic uterosacral nerve ablation (LUNA) and presacral neurectomy (PSN) are nerve transection procedures for the treatment of chronic pelvic pain. LUNA involves the destruction of the uterine nerve fibers that exit the uterus through the uterosacral ligament. Most surgeons destroy approximately 2 cm of uterosacral ligament near its attachment to the uterus. Most clinical trials evaluating the efficacy of LUNA in endometriosis-associated pelvic pain fail to demonstrate any efficacy for dysmenorrhea, dyspareunia or nonmenstrual pelvic pain (Johnson et al 2004).

Presacral neurectomy (PSN) has been used to treat women with midline pelvic pain and dysmenorrhoea for almost 100 years (Cotte

1937). Perez (1990) first described laparoscopic presacral neurectomy. PSN significantly reduces midline pelvic pain and pain associated with intractable primary dysmenorrhea but has little effect on adnexal pain (Nezhat and Nezhat 1992). A transverse incision is made in the peritoneum overlying the sacral promontory, extending from the ureter on the right side to the inferior mesenteric and superior hemorrhoidal arteries and sigmoid colon on the left side. Care must be taken to avoid damage to the sigmoid colon and the left common iliac vein.

In a prospective study, Candiani et al (1992) examined the efficacy of PSN with other procedures to provide relief from pain secondary to moderate to severe endometriosis in 78 patients. The study showed good pain relief in 80% of the patients but the relief was primarily of midline pain only. There is a lack of long term studies to observe the pain relief from presacral neurectomy. The problems at presacral neurectomy are chiefly hemorrhage and the side effects of cutting the presacral nerve are bladder dysfunction, constipation, vaginal dryness and backache. Fortunately, these are generally transient and decrease in 3–4 weeks time.

Complications of laparoscopy: Laparoscopy has few complications but those that occur are generally major and require early anticipation and prompt treatment. Around 80% of these are related to entry of the scope. This has lead to the suggestion of using open laparoscopy to prevent these complications. The Verress needle or the scope may be in the wrong tissue plane or puncture into a hollow viscus like the bowel, bladder or a blood vessel. Entry of the needle into the bowel or bladder can be treated conservatively, but a trocar wound will have to be repaired. Injuries to the inferior epigastric, iliac vessels, inferior vena cava and the aorta have been reported. Suspicion, prompt investigation and appropriate repair can be life saving. The importance of keeping the patient horizontal till the scope is introduced has to be further emphasised.

The next major cause of injuries is due to sharp dissection or the use of electrosurgery. Very sharp new instruments and blunt scissors can both cause damage. Extra care should be taken whenever a new instrument is used. Taking care to see that the instruments are in proper working order can minimise electrosurgical injuries. Using a pure cutting current and bipolar when needed, can decrease bowel burns. If bowel injury is suspected, then fill the peritoneal cavity with fluid and move the loops of the bowel. The escape of air bubbles would show a perforation. Repair of the perforation can be done laparoscopically in layers. Incomplete dissection or removal of tissue could cause tissue reaction or lead to pelvic infection. Complete dissection with attention to good hemostasis is essential. When in doubt use a drain. Incisional hernia can occur in ports larger than 10 mm when not sutured (Kadar et al 1993). Chronic discharge and abscess formation in port sites may be due to tissue being retained in the tract of the trocar. Postoperatively, any abdominal distension or pyrexia should be watched for carefully. If needed, a pelvic ultrasonography is done to check hemorrhage, hematoma formation or fluid collection.

Hysteroscopy: This can be performed as a diagnostic or therapeutic procedure, or both. Diagnostic hysteroscopy was slow to develop. It was accepted as a diagnostic tool by 1976. Operative work was developed when Neuwirth used electrosurgery with a urologic resectoscope to remove myomas (Neuwirth and Amin 1976). Goldrath et al (1981) used the Nd YAG laser for endometrial ablation. In 1983, DeCherney did electrosurgical endometrial resection using a resectoscope. Hamou (1980) developed a lens system for magnifying up to 18 times and introduced contact colpomicrohysteroscopy.

Hysteroscopy is often used as an early diagnostic test because it provides direct visualisation of the interior of the uterus. Specific indications for hysteroscopy include evaluation of abnormal uterine bleeding, evaluation of suspected müllerian anomalies, assessment of uncertain or abnormal findings on imaging studies and in conjunction with diagnostic laparoscopy performed during an infertility evaluation.

Operative hysteroscopy allows direct, visual access to the uterine cavity. Indications for operative hysteroscopy include myomectomy of submucous myomas, endometrial polypectomy, removal of an intrauterine device when the string is not accessible, excision of intrauterine adhesions or septa, ablation/resection of the endometrium in women with menorrhagia unresponsive to medical therapy and who want to retain their uterus, sterilisation and tuboplasty

In patients with **Asherman's syndrome,** obtaining a proper plane of cleavage when dense adhesions are present is very difficult. These may be done with a regional anesthesia or even a local block. The main contraindications are the presence of infection, severe bleeding which makes visualisation difficult, pregnancy or malignancy. In large lesions, it is a problem to move the scope in the uterine cavity. The submucous fibroid has to be carefully assessed pre-operatively to determine its myometrial extension. A process of 'hydromassage,' by creating a tissue plane and releasing the myoma by hydrodissection can be followed by distension of the uterus to extrude the myoma. If the removal is still incomplete, then the procedure could be completed in a second session. Subsequent fertility rates after hysteroscopic myomectomy are good and there are no case reports of uterine rupture after hysteroscopic myomectomy (Ubaldi et al 1995).

Septae or intrauterine adhesions are cut with the use of an electro knife. Whether all septae should be cut or not depends on the volume of the uterine cavity available or if there is a history of recurrent abortions. In cases of menorrhagia when fertility is not required, an endometrial resection or ablation could be done using electrosurgery or the laser after ruling out malignancy. Hysteroscopy is done using glycine as the distension media. Good visualisation is achieved using an inflow–outflow system, where the inflow keeps the lens clean and the outflow clears the blood and floating debris.

The main problems at hysteroscopy during transcervical resection of the endometrium (TCRE) are the absorption of glycine causing hyponatremia, perforation of the uterus, hemorrhage and infection. Careful monitoring of the patient and the volume of retained fluid can prevent complications. If at any time, the fluid retained exceeds 2 litres, the procedure should be stopped at once to prevent fluid overload. Constantly remembering the position of the scope and advancing under vision can decrease the chance of perforation of the uterus. Certain workers prefer to monitor the procedure laparoscopically. However, this is difficult as the uterus remains retroverted.

The difficulties at hysteroscopy are due to the size of the uterus. In larger uteri, over 12 weeks size, endometrial resection will be a prolonged procedure resulting in more fluid absorption. Incomplete procedure may result in recurrence of symptoms. In nulliparous women, care is required to dilate the cervix. Severe stenosis may require pre-treatment with a cervical dilator. The results reported vary with the duration of follow-up. Most patients had a decrease in the monthly blood flow. The amenorrhea rate was 40% at 12 months but was only 20% at the end of four years (Magos et al 1989). The failure rate at 12 months following combined resection and roller ball (15.1%) was lower than for resection (19.3%), roller ball alone ((20.7%) 2.2% in the Mistletoe study) (O' Connor et al 1997). The effects on pain relief and on irregular cycles were poor; 8.8% of the patients went in for hysterectomy within three years of TCRE. Coulter (1994) has reported that the introduction of TCRE has had no effect on the hysterectomy rate in Oxford.

Several non-visualisation techniques for endometrial ablation like the balloon ablation (Neuwirth 1994), the microwave ablation (Sharp et al 1995), radio frequency endometrial ablation (Dover 1996) and endometrial laser intrauterine thermotherapy (ELITT) (Donnez et al 1999) have been used which do not have the problems of hysteroscopy. Data show that approximately 10% of women who have an endometrial ablation will eventually have a hysterectomy. Cost data suggest that endometrial ablation is still more cost effective than hysterectomy, even when there is need for repeat procedures or subsequent hysterectomy (Lethaby et al 2000).

Complications from hysteroscopy are rare, but some are potentially life threatening. A multicentre study showed a complication rate of 0.28% (Jansen et al 2000). Diagnostic hysteroscopy had a significantly lower complication rate than operative hysteroscopy. The most common surgical complication was perforation of the uterine cavity (0.76%). The operative procedure with the highest frequency of complications was intrauterine adhesiolysis (4.48% complication rate); other procedures had complication rates less than 1%.

Salpingoscopy and falloposcopy: These two endoscopic techniques are used to assess the Fallopian tubes for fertility. Salpingoscopy is done with the aid of a salpingoscope to assess the distal two-thirds of the tube. Falloposcopy is done transcervically through a hysteroscope to assess the proximal third of the tube. Both these techniques help in determining the state of the tubal epithelium with respect to the presence or absence of rugosity. The falloposcope can be used for cannulation of the tube. Within 12 months of falloposcopy, 6/28 (21%) of the women with at least one apparently normal tube had conceived, 2/22 (9%) of those with mild to moderate disease had conceived and none of the 16 patients with severe disease had achieved a pregnancy (Kerin et al 1992). Salpingoscopic assessment of the condition of the tubal epithelium has been demonstrated to be of significant prognostic value in the surgical treatment of patients with distal tubal disease. Blocks of the tube with amorphous material that are resistant to flushing at hysterosalpingography may be cleared. Severe fibrosis with or without occlusion will not be amenable to surgery. Correct selection of patients for distal surgery should enable post-operative pregnancy rates of 50% or greater (Gomel and Yarali 1992). Some attempts at contraception using the falloposcope with the help of chemical agents or plugs have not been very successful. The main drawback is the cost of the instruments with a small field of vision that has confined it primarily to a research tool.

REFERENCES

ACOG Committee Opinion # 311. 2005. Laparoscopically assisted vaginal hysterectomy. *Obstet Gynecol.* 105:929.

Arcangeli S and MM Pasquarette. 1997. Gravid uterine rupture after myolisis. *Obstet Gynaecol* 89:857.

Balen AH and HS Jacobs. 1995. Conception rates after laparoscopic electrocautery of the ovarian surface. *Fertility and Sterility* 63:1358–1359.

Brosens IA, P Van Ballaer, P Pettemans et al. 1996. Reconstruction of the ovary containing large endometriomas by an extraovarian endosurgical technique. *Fertil Steril* 66:517–521.

Bruhat MA, H Manhes, G Mage et al. 1980. Laparoscopic treatment of ectopic pregnancies by means of laparoscopy. *Fertility and Sterility* 33:411–414.

Candiani GB, L Fedele, P Vercellini et al. 1992. Presacral neurectomy for the treatment of pelvic pain associated with endometriosis: A controlled study. *Am J Obstet Gynecol* 167:100–103.

Canis M, G Mage, A Wattiez et al. 1992. Resultats a court terme et lon terme après traitement coeliscopique des kystes de l'ovaire. *Contraception Fertilite Sexualite*

Chapron C, A Fauconnier, F Goffinet et al. 2002. Laparoscopic surgery is not inherently dangerous for patients presenting with benign gynaecologic pathology. Results of a meta analysis. *Hum Reprod* 17: 1334.

Clarke HC. 1972. Laparoscopy–new instruments for suturing and ligation. *Fertil Steril* 23:274–277.

Cotte G. 1937. Resection of the presacral nerve in the treatment of obstinate dysmenorrheal. *Am J Obstet Gynecol* 1030–1040.

Coulter A. 1994. Trends in gynecological surgery (letter). *Lancet* 344: 1367.

Dargent D. 1994. Pregnancies following radical trachelectomy for invasive cervical cancer. *Gynecol Oncol* 52(1):105.

De Cherney AH and ML Polan. 1983. Hysteroscopic management of intrauterine lesions and intractable uterine bleeding. *Obstet Gynecol* 61:392–397.

Decker A. 1949. Culdoscopy: Its diagnosis and value in pelvic disease. *JAMA* 140:378–385.

Donnez J, R Polet, Squifflet et al. 1999. Endometrial laser intrauterine thermotherapy (ELITT): A revolutionary new approach to the elimination of menorrhagia. *Curr Opin Obstet Gynecol* 11(4):363–370.

Dover R. 1996. Thermoregulated radiofrequecy endometrial ablation. Abstract. British Society for Gynaceological Endoscopy. London

Dubuisson JB, X Chavet, C Chapron, P Morice. 1995. Uterine rupture during pregnancy after laparoscopic myomectomy. *Human Reprod* 10:1475–1477.

Dumez Y, JF Oury, M Dommergues. 1992. Diagnostic embryoscopy: 50 cases of early diagnosis. International Symposium from Gametes to Embryology. Milan, 18–20.

Goldrath MH, TA Fuller, S Segal. 1981. Laser photovaporisation of endometrium in the treatment of menorrhagia. *Am J Obstet Gynecol* 140:14–19.

Gomel V and H Yarali. 1992. Infertility surgery: Microsurgery. *Curr Opin Obstet Gynecol* 4:390–399.

Hajenius PJ, BW Mol, PM Bossuyt, WM Ankum, F Van Der Veen. 2000. Interventions for tubal ectopic pregnancy. *Cochrane Database Syst Rev.* 2: CD000324.

Hamou JE. 1980. Hysteroscopie et microhysteroscopie avec un instrument nouveau: Le microhysteroscope. *Acta Endoscope* 10:415.

Hockstein S. 2000. Spontaneous uterine rupture in the early third trimester after laparoscopically assisted myomectomy: A case report. *J Reprod Med* 45:139–141.

Jansen FW, CB Vredevoogd CB, K Van Ulzen et al. 2000. Complications of hysteroscopy: A prospective, multicenter study. *Obstet Gynecol* 96:266.

Johnson NP, CM Farquhar, S Crossley et al. 2004. A double blind randomized controlled trial of laparoscopic uterine nerve ablation for women with chronic pelvic pain, *BJOG* 111:950.

Johnson N, D Barlow, A Lethaby et al. 2005. Methods of hysterectomy: Systematic review and meta-analysis of randomized controlled trials. *Br Med J*, 330:1478.

Johnson N, D Barlow, A Lethaby et al. 2006. Surgical approach to hysterectomy for benign gynaecological disease. *Cochrane Database Syst Rev* CD 003677.

Kadar N, H Reich, CY Lui et al. 1993. Incisional hernias after major laparoscopic gynecologic procedure. *Am J Obstet Gynecol* 168:1493–1495.

Kerin JF, DB Williams, GA San Roman et al. 1992. Falloposcopic classification and treatment of fallopian tube lumen disease. *Fertil Steril* 57:731–741.

Kohler C, R Tozzi, P Klemm, A Schneider. 2003. Laparoscopic paraaortic left sided transperitoneal infrarenal lymphadenectomy in patients with gynaecologic malignancies: Techniques and results. *Gynecol Oncol* 91:139.

Lethaby A, S Shepperd, I Cooke, C Farquhar. 2000. Endometrial resection and ablation versus hysterectomy for heavy menstrual bleeding. *Cochrane Database Syst. Rev.* CD000329.

Liu CY. 1996. Anatomy and clinical evaluation of pelvic floor defects. In CY Liu ed *Laparascopic Hysterectomy and Pelvic Floor Construction*. Massachusetts: Blackwell Science 299–312.

Magos AL, R Baumann and AC Turnbull. 1989. Transcervical resection of endometrium in women with menorrhagia. *Br Med J* 298:1209–1212.

Maiman M, Seltzer Vand J Boyce. 1991. Laparoscopic excision of ovarian neoplasms subsequently found to be malignant. *Obstet Gynaecol.* 77:563.

Neuwirth R. 1994. Preliminary clinical experience with a thermal balloon endometrial ablation method to treat menorrhagia. *Obstet Gynecol* 83:733–735.

Neuwirth RS and JH Amin. 1976. Excision of submucous fibroids with hysteroscopic control. *Am J Obstet Gynecol* 126:95–99.

Nezhat C and F Nezhat. 1992. A simplified method of laparoscopic presacral neurectomy for the treatment of central pelvic pain due to endometriosis. *Br J Obstet Gynaecol* 166:864–865.

O'Connor H, JA Boradbent, A Magos et al. 1997. Medical Research Council randomized trial of endometrial resection versus hysterectomy in management of menorrhagia. *Lancet* 349:897–901.

Perez JJ. 1990. Laparoscopic presacral neurectomy: Results of the first 25 cases. *J Reprod Med* 35: 625–630.

Peterson HB, Z Xia, JM Hughes et al. 1996. The risk of pregnancy after tubal sterilization: Findings from the US Collaborative Review of Sterilisaton. *Am J Obstet Gynecol* 174(4):1161–1179.

Polet J, M Nisolle M, J Donnez J. 2002. Robotics in endoscopy. In: *An Atlas of Operative Laparoscopy and Hysteroscopy* ed J Donnez and M Nisolle. New York: Taylor and Francis

Querleu D and E Leblanc. 1994. Laparoscopic infrarenal node dissection for restaging of carcinomas of the ovary or the Fallopian tube. *Cancer* 73: 1467–1471.

Reich H, J DeCaprio and F McGlyn. 1989. Laparoscopic hysterectomy. *J Gynecol Surg* 5: 213–216.

Rioux JE and D Cloutier. 1974. A new bipolar instrument for laparoscopic tubal sterilization. *Am J Obstet Gynecol* 119:737–739.

Ruddock JC. 1934. Peritoneoscopy. *Western J Surg* 35:136–139.

Sharp NC, N Cronin, I Feldberg et al. 1995. Microwaves for menorrhagia: A new fast technique for endometrial ablation. *Lancet* 346:1003–1004.

Steptoe PC and RG Edwards. 1978. Birth after reimplantation of a human embryo. *Lancet* 2:366.

Ubaldi F, H Tournaye, M Camus, H Van der Pas, E Gepts, P Devroey. 1995. Fertility after hysteroscopic myomectomy. *Hum Reprod Update* 1:81–90.

Vercellini P, G Aimi, M Busacca et al. 2003. Laparoscopic uterosacral ligament resection for dysmenorrhoea associated with endometriosis: Results of a randomized, controlled trial. *Fertil Steril* 80: 310.

29

Prevention and Treatment of Urinary Tract Injuries in Gynecological Surgery

Javed H Rizvi | Fauzia Haq Nawaz

One of the hazards of surgical procedures in gynecology is injury to the urinary tract. This includes injury to the urethra, the bladder and the pelvic ureter. Gynecologists must familiarise themselves with the identification and treatment of such mishaps, if and when they occur (ACOG 1997; Naru et al 2007).

Opportunity for injury to the bladder is present in all cases where radical surgery is done—in the case of cancer or inflammatory disease, when the lower abdomen is surgically explored or when surgery is performed by the laparoscopic or vaginal route. The frequency of injury to the female bladder and urethra cannot be appreciated by reading of the literature because most of these injuries are unreported and several are recognised and repaired at the time of injury (Brubaker and Willbanks 1991; ACOG 1997). A significant number of lower urinary tract injuries are missed and are discovered only several days after the primary surgical procedure. This produces understandable dismay to the surgeon and patient and a difficult decision as to proper management in some cases.

Injury to the Urethra: Urethral injury during gynecological surgery is uncommon. This is because the urethra is partly protected by the pubic symphysis and is not as firmly anchored as the male urethra.

Injury to the urethra at the time of anterior colporrhaphy or enucleation of a diverticulum is not uncommon. The injury may lead to almost total incontinence. Diagnosis of these injuries is not difficult and is usually made with cystourethroscopy, but a urethrogram may be helpful. If the defect is fresh, a prompt repair is needed. If the injury shows signs of inflammation, diversion of bladder urine with a suprapubic catheter may be needed prior to repair (Brubaker and Willbanks 1991; ACOG 1997; Kostakopoulos et al 1998).

Most urethral injuries require suturing, because of the rich blood supply in this area the lacerations tend to bleed freely. Polyglycolic acid sutures 2/0 or 3/0 or chromic catgut sutures are used. Urethral loss, that is, sloughing of the whole urethra occasionally follows colporrhaphy. For such cases, Chassar Moirs' modification of the Dennis Brown operation is recommended. A strip of anterior vaginal wall is made into a tube over a catheter. It is important to insert plication sutures behind the bladder neck if continence is to be achieved. The inter-position of a Martius graft, between the new urethra and the vaginal wall closure, fills up the potential dead space and improves continence by insuring mobility of the bladder neck. If continence is still not obtained, an artificial urinary sphincter may be needed (Brubaker and Willbanks 1991; ACOG 1997; Kostakopoulos et al 1998; Naru et al 2007).

Martius (1928) was the first to describe the pedicle graft of subcutaneous fat from the labium majus, which has an important place in fistula surgery (Petrous et al 2002). The fibro-fatty tissue is mobilised through a separate vertical incision in the lateral aspect of the labia majora. The blood supply from the superficial external pudendal vessel is preserved when the graft is passed subcutaneous into the vagina to reinforce a repair or obliterate dead space.

INJURY OF THE BLADDER

PREVENTION: A thorough knowledge of anatomy and the common sites where injuries are likely to occur is crucial. This can be accomplished by good exposure through an adequate incision, with careful visualisation and dissection when operating abdominally and with traction, counter traction and palpation of structures when operating vaginally. These techniques increase the margin of safety and security of ligating and cutting the pedicles. Identification of risk factors which may cause distorted anatomy for example, fibroids, endometriosis, previous pelvic surgery, malignancy or urogynecology procedures is important (Kostakopoulos et al 1998; Naru et al 2007; Nawaz and Rizvi 2007).

Preoperative imaging studies are not necessary for every case but one might consider an IVU or contrast-enhanced CT if distorted anatomy is anticipated or previous urinary compromise is suspected (Gilmour et al 1999). Piscitelli et al (1987) reviewed the experience of a university-based gynecology service where IVUs were performed routinely as a preventive preoperative measure. He concluded that previous pelvic surgeries, uterine size of more than 12 weeks and adnexal masses of more than 4 cm are most likely associated with abnormal IVU studies (Piscitelli et al 1987; Simel et al 1988) formulated a decision analysis, using a baseline prevalence of ureteric injury of 0.5% and predicted an extra expense of $166,600 in preventing a single ureteric injury if preoperative IVP were to be used for all patients. Hence, routine use of IVU is questionable. Normal IVU does not dispel the surgeon's responsibility to identify the ureters in all pelvic operations.

The urinary bladder is relatively resistant to injury when collapsed. The first line of defence therefore, is drainage by a catheter, a procedure which should be done in all cases prior to abdominal or vaginal or laparoscopic surgery (Naru et al 2007; Nawaz and Rizvi 2007).

When inflammation, endometriosis or cancer involves the region of the bladder, it becomes fixed, and injury is more common. Loss of normal tissue planes, as in cases where previous surgery has occurred, or injudicious surgical dissection proceeding despite hemorrhage, may traumatise the bladder (Gilmour et al 1999; Naru et al 2007; Nawaz and Rizvi 2007).

Hysterectomy-associated injuries occur during both abdominal and vaginal procedures. Recognition is usually immediate or may be delayed in certain cases. The injury is typically located between the urethral orifices, just posterior to the trigone, but may involve the ureter and may be extensive. If they are recognised at the time of the initial surgical procedure, they can be repaired easily (Piscitelli et al 1987).

Laparoscopic injury to the bladder occurs because of fixation of the bladder from previous surgical procedures or inadequate emptying of the bladder prior to the introduction of the laparoscope. Injury can also occur with the use of diathermy fulguration of Fallopian tubes or endometriotic spots (Oh et al 1998; Simel et al 1988).

In recent years, treating a number of bladder conditions, especially idiopathic detrusor instability and interstitial cystitis by prolonged bladder distention, is in vogue. This procedure has been a cause of bladder rupture. If the rupture is extraperitoneal, management is simple: by continuous bladder drainage. More severe is the intraperitoneal rupture which requires adequate urinary drainage, a prompt and adequate drainage of perivesical space and closure of the defect (Steele et al 2000).

Early recognition of bladder injury: Injury to the bladder can be suspected if there is leakage of urine or hematuria. In these cases, the suspected area must be observed carefully and in case of doubt, the bladder can be filled with methylene blue to identify the site of injury. During vaginal or abdominal procedures, it is a clean cut into the bladder lumen because of distorted anatomy, or it may be a laceration and tearing of the bladder because of difficult dissection. The bladder is composed of three layers—mucosa, muscular layer and an outer adventitial layer that is continuous with the endopelvic fascia. Closure of bladder injury should be performed in a watertight manner, closing the bladder in two layers. The usual material for repairing bladder injuries is either 2/0 or 3/0 polyglycolic acid sutures or chromic catgut. Non-absorbable sutures should not be used as they may cause local irritation and subsequently become a nidus for stone formation. The bladder mucosa should be closed separately from the muscular layer; this minimises bleeding into the bladder. A continuous or an interrupted layer can be used to close the mucosa. The muscular layer can be repaired by continuous locking sutures placed approximately 1 cm apart. This is effective in producing a watertight repair (Steele et al 2000; Naru et al 2007; Nawaz and Rizvi 2007).

Since 1990, intraoperative cystoscopy to detect occult urinary tract injuries has been increasingly used. Gilmour et al (1999) have reviewed the literature and concluded that the frequency of urinary tract injury was 1.6 per 1000 in the group without cystoscopy, but with its use, the incidence rises to 6.2/1000. An analysis of 13 prospective studies reveals that 5.8/1000 ureteric injuries and 10.9 /1000 urinary bladder injuries might be missed without the use of intraoperative cystoscopy. However, intraoperative cystoscopy is not perfect for detecting urinary tract injuries as there have been instances, where despite cystoscopic examination, bladder or ureteric injuries were missed (Steele et al 2000). Recent prospective studies have recommended the use of intraoperative cystoscopy but still there is no consensus of opinion on whether it should be performed during every major gynecological procedure.

If the bladder has been opened and there is any possiblity of injury to the ureter, the incision in the bladder should be enlarged, a catheter should be passed up to the ureteric orifice and the course of the ureter visualised to be sure that no injury to the ureter has occurred (Steele et al 2000).

If the bladder is opened during vaginal surgery, cystoscopy is very helpful in delineating the extent of bladder injury and demonstrating the ureteral orifices and their relationship to the injury. Passage of a catheter up the ureters prior to the closure of the bladder reassures the surgeon that no portion of the ureter is included in the repair. Closure should again be in two layers (Mattingly 1978; Steele et al 2000; Olenvewaju and Roksana 2005).

Filling the bladder with methylene blue solution or sterile milk, may be helpful in demonstrating injuries when they are suspected, but not easily seen.

Following completion of bladder repair, the bladder should be tested for water-tightness. This can be achieved by instilling 300–400 ml of dye stained saline solution. If a leak occurs, it should be closed immediately with interrupted figure of 8 sutures. The bladder should then be drained continuously by a trans-urethral Foley's catheter which should be left in situ for 10 to 14 days. If there is significant infection or the patient has had radiation, the drainage of the bladder may need to be prolonged for two to three weeks (Mattingly 1978; Olenvewaju and Roksana 2005).

Sometimes, a surgical laceration may escape detection and is discovered in the immediate postoperative period. The patient is found to have hematuria and a cystoscopy is performed. Two possible courses of actions are available to the surgeon. The majority of minor lacerations will close up spontaneously, if the bladder is kept on continuous free drainage; the bleeding will usually stop. A three-way Foley's catheter is used so that the bladder can be irrigated in order to avoid clot retention. Only small amounts, 30–50 cc of irrigating fluid should be used. The indwelling catheter should remain for at least two weeks to allow good healing (Brubaker and Willbanks 1991; ACOG 1997; Kostakopoulos et al 1998; Petrous et al 2002; Naru et al 2007; Nawaz and Rizvi 2007).

Occasionally, one may find a non-absorbable suture which has penetrated the bladder. Non-absorbable sutures are used for supra-pubic bladder neck suspensions, as in the Stameys, Marshall Marchetti Krantz operation or the Burch's modification. If a non-absorbable suture is detected penetrating the bladder or urethra, it should be cut transvesically or transurethrally and removed. Sometimes the stitch will retract out of the lumen once it is cut. Failing this, a retro-peritoneal suprapubic cystostomy may be necessary to remove the offending ligature. Leaving a foreign body in situ causes intractable cystitis and leads eventually to stone formation (Mattingly 1978; Olenvewaju and Roksana 2005).

If a large laceration is found at the time of cystoscopy, which sometimes occurs after a difficult vaginal hysterectomy when an enlarged uterus is removed vaginally, this should be repaired immediately by a suprapubic transvesical approach. Whenever doubt exists about the possibility of bladder injury during surgery, continuous urinary drainage should be instituted and continued for seven days. There is no harm in explaining to the patient that this is a safety precaution (Gilmour et al 1999; Naru et al 2007; Nawaz and Rizvi 2007).

Late recognition of bladder injuries: Vesicovaginal fistula may occur as late as 15 days postoperatively, but most commonly, it is discovered between 4 and 8 days after surgery. Total urinary incontinence after surgical trauma suggests that a fistula has formed between the bladder and the vagina. If the patient is incontinent after an operation, but is also able to empty her bladder at regular intervals, a ureteric fistula is more likely (Parra 1994; Michael et al 2002).

When carcinoma of the cervix is treated by intracavitary caesium, the neighboring bladder may receive too high a dosage of Gamma rays, in which case, progressive devitalisation of the bladder wall follows and a urinary fistula develops. This may be delayed for a month or even years after irradiation (Mattingly 1978; Michael et al 2002; Naru et al 2007; Nawaz and Rizvi 2007).

Other cases of delayed trauma may result from the formation of a hematoma under the bladder, which may become infected. If blood is collected at vaginal vault, tension builds up in the cavity and the neighboring bladder wall undergoes necrosis. Ultimately, a urinary fistula may form between the bladder base and the vaginal vault. This sometimes occurs after a straightforward uncomplicated operation (Mattingly 1978; Micheal et al 2002).

When a patient starts leaking urine in the postoperative period, it is usually unwise to make a detailed examination per vaginum to localise the fistula. A cystoscopic evaluation should be avoided and a more simple effort should be made to determine the nature of the fistula. A vaginal tampon is inserted in the vagina and a solution of methylene blue dye is instilled, via a transurethral catheter, into the bladder. Leakage of urine colored by the dye can be confirmed by the presence of dye on the vaginal tampon; this finding suggests that a vesicovaginal fistula is present. If, after a time, the methylene blue has failed to stain the vaginal tampon but the tampon becomes wet with clear urine, a ureteric fistula should be suspected. Another possibility is to inject Indigo Carmine intravenously: this would be excreted through the kidneys and would stain the vaginal tampon reddish pink in colour. Intravenous urography is an essential investigation, to exclude upper urinary tract abnormalities, ureteral involvement and vesical calculi (Mattingly 1978; Olenvewaju and Roksana 2005).

Vesicovaginal fistulas should be treated conservatively in the first instance. Natural healing always reduces their size and some will close spontaneously. This may be encouraged by continuous drainage through a urethral catheter for up to 6 weeks. During catheterisation, the patient can be up and about and even discharged from the hospital. Rest in bed or assuming the prone position usually does not promote healing of the fistula. If most of the urine drains through the fistula rather than through the catheter or the fistula's tract fails to heal within 4–6 weeks, further catheter drainage is unlikely to help. The catheter drainage, however, during this period is annoying to the patient and a difficult problem, as it is a constant reminder to the patient of an undesirable outcome of the surgical procedure.

If the patient continues to leak urine after the catheter has been removed, the catheter should not be re-inserted, so that the irritation and infection that has occurred from prolonged catheterisation can subside. Any consideration of surgical correction of fistula should be deferred for 8–12 weeks. The skin of the vulva and the thighs must be protected from excoriation. A silicon barrier cream, zinc and castor oil cream or paraffin gel is suggested. In this waiting period, edema and infection would have subsided, and the tissues will become soft, pliable and workable. The use of cortisone does not significantly speed up the process. In postmenopausal patients, a short course of estrogen will improve the condition of the vaginal skin and its blood supply (Michael et al 2002).

During this waiting period, the patient's

general health should be built by treatment of any residual sepsis and the correction of anemia. A high protein diet is also desirable and her morale should be sustained by constant encouragement and optimistic counselling. A pregnancy sometimes occurs, in spite of the presence of a vesicovaginal fistula and this should be excluded. A bimanual vaginal examination should precede a speculum examination in order to assess the amount of scaring and stenosis. Sometimes a high fistula is better felt than seen. A Sims speculum of appropriate size should be used, the anterior vaginal wall and the vault of the vagina can then be examined with the aid of a sponge-holding forceps which is used as vaginal retractor. The pelvic examination is not complete without a close scrutiny of the posterior vaginal wall and a digital examination of the rectum (Micheal et al 2002; Naru et al 2007; Nawaz and Rizvi 2007).

In all cases where a genitorurinary fistula is suspected, an intravenous urogram with delayed films in the supine, oblique and lateral position is extremely useful. The methylene blue dye test is a useful manoeuvre to localise small vesicovaginal fistulas (Olenvewaju and Roksana 2005; Naru et al 2007).

Cystourethroscopy helps to determine if there is only one or possibly more than one fistula and to locate the margins of the fistula in relation to the ureteral orifices. However, in large vesicovaginal fistulas, cystoscopy will be impractical. To diagnose vesicouterine fistulas, a hysterosalpingogram and, in exceptional cases, hysteroscopy may be necessary.

Operative repair: It is prudent to remember that the first surgical effort to correct the fistula has the best possibility of success. Thus, one should be certain that the tissues are in absolutely optimal condition before repair is attempted.

Each operator develops her own techniques for repairing fistulas, based on general principles which are well established:

1. Allowing sufficient time for spontaneous healing and maturation of a fistula
2. Examination under anesthesia to evaluate the site and nature of fistula
3. Adequately exposing the fistula surgically prior to closure
4. Repairing of fistula without any tension on the suture line
5. Protection of the ureter with ureteral stents
6. Accomplishing a watertight closure which should be confirmed at the end of operation
7. Maintenance of free postoperative urinary drainage with either a transurethral or a suprapubic catheter

Many gynecologists insist that all vesicovaginal fistulas should be dealt with pervaginum; urologists, however, prefer the abdominal approach. The transvaginal approach is usually preferred for simple fistulas. When dealing with more complicated fistulas (large, complex, multiple or close to ureteral orifices), abdomino-vaginal techniques including transvaginal, transabdominal and transvesical may be needed. If the fistula margin is close to the ureteral orifices, placement of ureteral catheters will facilitate dissection and avoid ureteral injury. There is no one preferred approach for all fistulas. It seems that the vaginal approach is easier as it avoids a cystostomy, involves minimal blood loss and is consequently followed by less postoperative discomfort and a shorter hospital stay.

Preliminary examination under anesthesia is an essential step in the evaluation of a fistula prior to definitive surgery. At this procedure the exact site, size and its relationship to other structures is determined. In a large fistula at the bladder base, the ureteric orifices have to be located because they may be found at the edges of the fistula. The condition of tissue must be carefully assessed and any complicating factors such as vaginal stenosis may be noted.

The final matter to be decided at this examination is the route of repair. In general, bladder fistulas and those involving the urethra should be repaired pergavinum, but if access is poor or the fistula is high, an abdominal approach may be easier. If the fistula is to be repaired by the vaginal route, it is necessary to decide whether the knee-chest or the lithotomy position would provide better access. The knee-chest position provides the best exposure to juxtauretheral fistulas adherent to the back of the pubic bone.

Postoperative management: Postoperative nursing care is almost as important as surgery in the successful treatment of fistula cases. One essential feature is maintenance of good urinary drainage which can be achieved by an indwelling urethral catheter, suprapubic cystostomy, or vaginal cystostomy. In cases where vaginal repair is performed, the urethral catheter should be left in situ for 10–14 days. In cases where an abdominal transvesical approach has been used, the technique recommended is to leave an indwelling urethral catheter as well as a catheter through a suprapubic cystostomy. The supra-pubic catheter is used to irrigate the bladder in order to avoid postoperative retention which can be caused by a blood clot. The urinary output should be measured every hour so that interference with free drainage can be detected before any harm is done to the repair (Trussel 1984; Hudson and Setchell 2003; Naru et al 2007).

Where the abdominal approach has been used, wound drainage from the retroperitoneal space is necessary. Suction drains are favoured; the duration is generally 3–4 days depending on the volume that is drained. The use of broad-spectrum antibiotics is recommended. Continuous urinary drainage into a sterile plastic urinary bag is best. It would still, be necessary to culture the urine once a week (Trussel 1984; Michael et al 2002; Hudson and Setchell 2003).

The patient is mobilised after one week, stool softeners may be given to prevent straining. When the catheter is removed, the patient should be encouraged to micturate frequently. As the bladder capacity would be small at first, the control of micturition may be difficult. Sexual activity should be avoided for at least 3 to 4 months following surgery (Naru et al 2007; Nawaz and Rizvi 2007).

Complications

Early complications: Vaginal bleeding in the immediate postoperative period is uncommon, and therefore, vaginal packs should be avoided. Hemorrhage into the bladder is likely to occur after suprapubic transvesical repair and therefore vigilance is required to prevent blockage of the catheter by a clot. Blockage of the catheter requires immediate investigation and intervention. Urinary infection is rarely a serious problem if close circuit catheter drainage system is used. Breakdown of repair is the most important and distressing complication.

Late complications: Scar tissue formation around the bladder neck following closure of a fistula may lead to stress incontinence of urine. Elevation of the bladder neck would need to be performed surgically using the abdominal route. Only in cases of recurrent failure, a urinary diversion using an ileal conduit, colon conduit or ureterosigmoidostomy is indicated (Hudson and Setchell 2003).

Ureteric Injuries

In gynecological surgery, the ureters are usually injured either at a relatively high level near the pelvic brim, where they lie adjacent to the ovarian vessels, or low down beside the cervix, where they are crossed by the uterine vessels. The ureters may be included in ligatures which are used to tie off these vessels, they may be crushed in clamps and subsequently undergo necrosis, or they may simply be partially or completely divided (ACOG 1997; Naru et al 2007; Nawaz and Rizvi 2007). These complications are most likely to occur in the presence of dense adhesions—as may be produced by pelvic inflammatory disease or endometriosis—or when the normal anatomy of the pelvis is distorted, for example, by fibroids or ovarian tumours growing into the broad ligament, which may displace the ureter from its normal position. Occasionally, the ureter may become devitalised and slough after an extensive pelvic dissection, as in Wertheim's hysterectomy, due to interference with its blood supply, particularly after previous pelvic irradiation. Rarely, the extreme lower end of the ureter may be caught in high stitches inserted besides the cervix during pelvic floor repair or vaginal hysterectomy (Giberti et al 1996; Drake and Noble 1998).

The decision to place ureteric catheters before gynecological surgery should be based on an individual basis. The routine use to prevent ureteric injury is a controversial issue. Proponents of prophylactic ureteric stenting argue that it results in improved prevention and recognition of injury, if it does occur. Detractors cite no advantage in terms of injury prevention and list the possible complications like UTI, ureteral spasm, reflex anuria, injury during catheterisation and hematuria. A review on ureteric catheterisation by Kunok et al (1998) has shown no statistically significant difference in the incidence of operative ureteric injury, but resulted in an additional cost of $ 1,465 per case (Kunok et al 1998).

Injuries recognised or suspected at operation:

Factors which make one suspect ureteric injury at a gynecological procedure are leakage of urine in the field of operation or dilatation of proximal ureter. To detect such injury, one should try and dissect the ureter along its pelvic course. Diuretics can be administered parenterally and the ureter can be observed for peristalsis, proximal dilation or a leak. Unfortunately, only a third of ureteric injuries are detected intraoperatively, the rest of the injuries are diagnosed postoperatively with variable clinical features like fever, peritonitis, paralytic ileus, oliguria or anuria, bilateral flank pain, a mass in the abdomen, hematuria, leakage of urine per vaginum or through intraperitoneal drains (Giberti et al 1996; Drake and Noble 1998; Petrous et al 2002; Naru et al 2007).

If the ureter is injured during operation, or if there are grounds for suspecting that it may have been crushed, divided or included in a ligature, an adequate length of ureter is exposed above and below the injury to define its nature and extent. If injury to the extreme lower end of the ureter is suspected, the bladder should be opened without hesitation by anterior cystostomy, and the appropriate ureteric orifice is catheterised. If the catheter ascends easily and no injury is found, the bladder is simply closed in two layers as described previously. A urethral catheter is left in for 10–14 days. If on the other hand, ureteric injury is found, reconstruction or reimplantation can proceed without delay, using tissues that are fresh and easily identified (Parra 1994; ACOG 1997).

If a high ureteric injury is found, direct

end-to-end anastomosis is performed. The circumference of the cut ends of the ureter is increased by a 1 cm vertical incision, and they are joined using fine chromic catgut or polyglycolic acid sutures. The anastomosis is best performed over a ureteric splint. A double J stent or a fine (8 FG) infant's esophageal feeding tube passed up from the bladder is ideal for this purpose. The most important technical point is to ensure that there is no tension at the site of anastomosis. A suction or a corrugated drain is left near the site of anastomosis and removed after 4 or 5 days. The ureteric splint is usually removed after 10 days (Parra 1994; Rajasekar and Hall 1997).

If a low ureteric injury is found, it is usually possible to reimplant the ureter into the bladder. The lower end of the ureter is dissected out and may be reimplanted directly in the nearest part of the bladder or preferably, the bladder may be opened and the ureter is then reimplanted with a reflux preventing procedure into the posterior or lateral wall (Parra 1994; Drake and Noble 1998).

Injuries recognized in post-operative period: Postoperative symptoms of ureteric injury tend to be variable like flank pain, fever, hematuria, abdominal distention, abscess, paralytic ileus, retroperitoneal urinoma, leakage of urine vaginally and secondary hypertension. Most ureteral injuries are recognised postoperatively. Frequently, the injury is not suspected until obvious urinary fistula occurs (Rajasekar and Hall 1997; Petri 1999).

Where evidence of ureteric damage becomes apparent in the postoperative period, the precise nature of the injury should be defined before deciding on the best approach to repair. A catheter specimen of urine should be sent for bacteriological culture and sensitivity study. Blood urea and electrolytes should be checked routinely and dehydration or electrolyte imbalance should be corrected (Mattingly 1978; Petri 1999).

Because there is very frequently some obstruction at the site of ureteric injury, an intravenous urogram usually shows some dilatation of the ureter—and often of the calyces—on the side of the lesion. If, however, there is no obstruction above the fistula, the ureter and kidney may look normal (Mattingly 1978; Parra 1994; Petri 1999).

The most reliable method of identifying the injured side is by cystoscopy and observation of the presence of efflux from the ureteric orifice of the intact side, and the absence of efflux on the injured side. This test is facilitated by adequate hydration by giving intravenous fluids and then intravenous diuretic with or without indigo carmine. Further confirmation of the site of the lesion may be obtained by attempting to pass a catheter up the non-effluxing side. Failure to pass the catheter up the ureter may be because it is arrested at the site of the injury or it may be due to the angle of the ureteric orifices or a mucosal fold. It is therefore not as reliable a test as simply observing the absence of ureteric efflux from one side (Rajasekar and Hall 1997; Naru et al 2007; Nawaz and Rizvi 2007).

The level of the site of the injury can be recognised with the help of a high dose intravenous urogram with screening or delayed films which usually show the lower limit of the intact ureter and will sometime demonstrate the exact site of the leakage and may show filling of the vagina. If the site of injury is not clearly seen on the intravenous urogram, cystoscopy and ascending uretrography will show it more exactly (Rajasekar and Hall 1997; Naru et al 2007; Nawaz and Rizvi 2007).

Once the nature of the lesion has been

defined, a decision on the best form of management can be reached. In some early cases, simple ureteric drainage with a double J stent may allow a small fistula to heal. If it does not dry up quickly, some form of operative intervention is necessary and there is little point in further delay. If the ureter is completely obstructed, reconstruction or reimplantation should be undertaken as soon as possible if worthwhile kidney function is to be preserved (Parra 1994).

The operative approach to the repair of ureteric injuries proceeds along similar lines as described earlier. The ureter is generally approached extraperitoneally and either repaired or reimplanted, with or without a Boari's flap. If a considerable defect has to be bridged, it may occasionally be necessary to do a high transuretero ureterostomy (Parra 1994; Naru et al 2007).

Over the years, medico-legal aspects of urinary tract injuries have increasingly become a major area of concern. If an individual sustains a urinary tract injury, there is 90-fold increase in the chance of medical litigation. Patients may commence litigation procedure against a surgeon for a variety of reasons including physical and psychological suffering from unexpected surgical outcome. Search of the literature reveals a litigation rate of 3% in gynecological surgeries with urological injuries versus 0.03 % with no injuries (Mattingly 1978; Parra 1994).

COMMENTS: There are three levels of prevention needed in order to avoid urinary tract injuries in gynecological surgery. Primary prevention consists of keeping the bladder empty and avoiding lower urinary tract injuries by employing careful surgical techniques, including identifying the ureters and bladder during major gynecological surgery. Secondary prevention involves the intraoperative recognition and repair of injury. Tertiary prevention or minimising the morbidity and sequelae, once urinary tract injuries become symptomatic in the postoperative period, usually involves further diagnostic and surgical intervention to confirm and manage the injuries. When compared with tertiary prevention, primary and secondary prevention are often easier, more successful and less morbid (Donna et al 2005).

In gynecological surgery, if the injury to the bladder or the ureter is recognised at the time, primary repair will give the best results. If the damage only becomes evident later, extreme care must be exercised to locate the injury accurately, and then to choose the optimum timing and surest technique for repair. Marshall's statement (1979) 'Try the best operation the first time' should be remembered.

REFERENCES

ACOG Technical Bulletin. 1997. Lower urinary tract operative injuries. No. 238.

Brubaker LT and GD WillBanks.1991. Urinary tract injuries in pelvic surgery. *Surg Clin North Am* 71:21–26.

Drake MJ and JG Noble. 1998. Ureteric trauma in gynaecological surgery. *Int Urogynaecol J* 9:108–117.

Donna Gilmour T, and Thomas F. Baskett. 2005. Disability and litigation from urinary tract injuries at benign gynaecologic surgery. *Canada Obstet Gynaecol* 105:109–114.

Giberti C, F Germinale, M Lillo, P Bhottino, A Simonotano, G Carmignani. 1996. Obstetric and gynaecology ureteric injuries: Treatment and results. *Br J Uron* 77:21–26.

Gilmour DT, PL Dywer, MP Carey. 1999. Lower urinary tract injury during gynecologic surgery and its detection by intraoperative Cystoscopy. *Obstet Gynaecol* 94:883–889.

Hudson CN and ME Setchell. 2003. Risk management: Avoidance and management of surgical complications. In: Shaw's *Textbook of Operative Gynaecology*. 6th ed. New Delhi: Elsevier

Kostakopoulos A, Deliveliotis C, Louras G.1998. Early repair of injury to the urethra or bladder after hysterectomy. *Int Urol Nephrol* 30(4):445–450.

Kunok K, A Menzin, HH Kauder et al 1998. Prophylactic ureteric catheterization in gynaecologic surgeries. *Urology* 52(6):1004–1008.

Marshall FV. 1979. Vesicovaginal Fistulas on one Urological Service, *Am J Urol* 121:25–29.

Mattingly RF. 1978. Acute operative injury to the lower urinary tract. *Clin Obstet Gynecol* 5:123–149.

Michael P, Arouson, Teresa M. Bose. 2002. Urinary tract injury in pelvic surgery. *Clin Obstet Gynaecol* 45(2):428–438.

Naru T, F Haq, J Rizvi. 2007. Urinary incontinence following gynecological surgery. *Obstet Gynecol Reprod Med* 17(9):266–271.

Nawaz FH and J Rizvi. 2007. Urinary tract injuries during obstetrics and Gynaecology Procdures at Aga Khan University Hospital Karach Pakistan. A 20 year review. *Urol Int* 78:106–111.

Oh BR, DD Kwon, KM Park. 1998. Bladder injury during laparoscopic surgery. *Obstet Gynecol* 95(3): 175–180.

Olenvewaju S and B Roksana. 2005. Prevention and management of ureteric injuries. *Hospital Medicine* 66:329–334.

Parra RO. 1994. Laparoscopic repair of intraperitoneal bladder perforation *J Urol* 151:1003

Petri E. 1999. Urogical trauma in gynecological surgery: diagnosis and management. *Curr Opinion Obstet Gynecol* 11(5):495–498.

Petrous S, J Jones, R Parra. 2002. Matius Flap Harvest site: Patient Self Preception. *J Urol* 167(5): 2098–2099.

Piscitelli JT, DL Simel, WA Addison. 1987. Who should have intravenous pyelogram before hysterectomy for benign disease? *Obstet Gynaecol* 69:541–545.

Rajasekar D and M Hall. 1997. Urinary tract injuries during obstetric intervention. *Br J Obstet Gynaecol* 104 (6):731–734.

Simel DL, DM Matchar, JT Piscitelli. 1988. Routine intravenous pyelogram before hysterectomy in cases of benign diseases: Possibly effective, definitely expensive. *Am J Obstet Gynaecol* 159:1049–1053.

Steele AC, S Wassar, MM Karram. 2000. Failure of intraoperative Cystoscopy to identify partial ureteric obstetrical. *Obstet Gynaeocol* 96:847.

Trussel R. 1984. Gynecological urology in the third world In *Clinical Gynecologic Urology* ed SL Stanton 29:364–377.

30

Breast and the Gynecologist

Rekha Kurian | Sarala Gopalan

The breast is a part of the reproductive system and a careful systematic breast examination is necessary to complete any gynecological examination. Adequate knowledge of breast disease including breast cancer is required to advice patients and to request appropriate referral. Simple diagnostic studies like aspiration of cysts and possibly fine needle aspiration (FNA) can be performed by the gynecologist. The follow-up of a breast cancer patient may also be undertaken, in consultation with the oncologist, as also issues like contraception and estrogen replacement therapy in these patients. In its guidelines, the American College of Obstetricians and Gynecologists (1998) has stated that physicians should encourage their female patients to do a monthly breast self-examination. Physicians should be encouraged to do clinical breast examination of all female patients during every periodic examination. A baseline mammogram should be obtained between the ages of 35 and 40 years. Thereafter, mammography is suggested every one or two years for women aged 40–50 years and annually for women over 50 years of age. At least 75% of patients seen in breast clinics do not have breast cancer and are treated for a variety of breast conditions.

Female breast development: In a term pregnancy, by the time of birth, the mammary ducts in the neonate are formed and colostrum appears in up to 90% of newborn term babies during the first week. In male babies, the ducts regress and only a rudimentary nipple and areola remain. In female babies, the epithelial ducts lengthen and ramify slowly. At puberty, in females, the breast develops at an extraordinary pace, in response to the increased estrogen and progesterone levels. In addition, genetic, nutritional and environmental factors may influence breast development.

In 1962, Tanner described the sequential development of breasts in pubertal girls, and its relation to pubic and axillary hair development and menarche as follows.

Stage I: Infantile stage, from birth to puberty

Stage 2: Budding stage when breast papilla elevates and areola enlarges

Stage 3: Breast areola increases in size and the shape of an adult female breast is seen

Stage 4: The areola and nipple continue to develop to form a secondary elevation of the apex of the breast cone.

Stage 5: Typical adult stage with a smooth shape and with disappearance of the secondary areolar and nipple elevation

The largest part of the breast's volume is fatty tissue. The breast size is unrelated to breast function in normal females.

Anatomy: The adult mammary gland is

composed of 15–20 irregular lobes or tubulo-alveolar glands which are modified epidermal sweat glands. The breast tissue often extends into the anterior axillary fold in the adult female, known as the axillary tail of Spence. The upper half of the breast, particularly the upper outer quadrant, contains more glandular tissue than the rest of the breast. The circular areola has underlying sebaceous, sweat and accessory areolar glands of Montgomery which lubricate the nipple during lactation. The nipple normally lies opposite the fourth interspace, but during lactation it becomes pendant. The nipples protrude spontaneously on touch by the action of circular muscle fibres at the base and longitudinal fibres attached to the lactiferous ducts.

The female breast has three components—epithetilial tissue, adipose tissue and connective tissue. Fibrous bands of connective tissue which separate the lobes from each other and connect with the dermis of the breasts are the suspensory ligaments of Cooper. Abundant adipose tissue occupies the dense connective tissue of the interlobular spaces. The more tenuous intralobular connective tissue contains little fat.

The main duct of each lobule exits at the nipple. Each lactiferous duct, as it approaches the base of the nipple, presents a fusiform or ampullary enlargement (the lactiferous sinus) which acts as a temporary reservoir for the secretion of the gland. The duct narrows beyond the sinus and passes into the nipple.

The epithelial lining of the ducts are made of a single layer of columnar or cuboidal cells, except in the lactiferous sinus where two layers of cuboidal cells are found. The myoepithelial cells below the epithelial cells form a basket-like network around the larger ducts.

Changes during Menstrual Cycle: The inactive breast undergoes slight changes during the menstrual cycle in response to estrogen and progesterone. Early in the menstrual cycle, the ductules appear to be cords with unimpressive lumens. The secretory cells increase in height at the time of ovulation and then the lumens become evident as secretions, fluid and lipid materials accumulate. In the luteal phase of the menstrual cycle, there is marked proliferative activity in the epithelium of the breast, the mitotic peak occurring on day 25, unlike in the endometrium.

In the follicular phase, the progressive rise in estrogen stimulates epithelial proliferation with sprouting and cellular mitosis. A second proliferative peak occurs during the mid luteal phase when progesterone peaks, causing dilatation of the ducts and changes in the glandular epithelium. Fat droplets are produced and there is some intraluminal secretion. Specific receptors are present on the cell membrane for estrogen, progesterone as well as prolactin. The histamine-like action of the endogenous estrogens raises the blood flow which along with the presence of the interlobular edema causes an increase in the volume and tenderness of the breasts.

Changes during Pregnancy and after Childbirth: During pregnancy, the ductules branch and alveoli begin to develop and become more pronounced as pregnancy progresses. Alveolar hypertrophy and accumulation of alveolar secretions lead to subsequent breast enlargement at term. The protein and the lipid components of milk are released separately by the cells into the cavity of the alveoli.

The breast releases colostrum in the first few days after childbirth, which is an important source of antibodies for the newborn along with the IgG which crosses the placenta. Eventually, the concentration of lymphocytes and plasma cells that supply antibodies to the colostrum decrease and milk production commences.

The connective tissue parenchyma undergoes varying degrees of softening and atrophy as the glandular elements increase; the pendulous breasts of multiparous women are a result of this and some diminution of fat.

Arterial and venous supply: The arterial supply to the breast is from the following:

1. Perforating rami of the internal mammary artery
2. Lateral thoracic branch of the axillary artery
3. Direct rami from the axillary artery
4. Branches of the subclavicular artery

All these branches anastamose en route to their convergence at the nipple.

Venous drainage is important because these are routes of tumour embolisation to the lungs, bones and distant organs. The groups of deep veins are:

1. Perforating branches of the internal mammary vein which is the largest vein
2. Axillary vein
3. Intercostal veins

These veins empty into the azygous veins. It is possible that they may transport metastatic emboli to the pulmonary network and to the skeleton.

Lymphatic drainage: The main lymphatic drainage of the breast to the axilla is by the external and internal trunks which arise from the circumareolar plexus. The subareolar plexus drains into the circumareolar plexus. The external trunk arises from the lateral edge of the circumareolar plexus and also receives drainage from the upper half of the breast. The internal trunk arises from the medial edge of the circumareolar plexus and receives tributaries from the lower half of the breast, as it travels downwards and laterally to eventually terminate in the axillary lymph nodes.

There are two accessory routes of lymphatic drainage from the breast to the apex of the axilla—the transpectoral route and the retropectoral route. The transpectoral route begins as a retromammary plexus in the loose areolar tissue between the breast and pectoral fascia, then perforates the pectoralis major, the coracoid fascia and ends in the axillary nodes. The lymph nodes of this route that lie between the pectoralis major and minor are known as Rotter's nodes.

The retropectoral route is found in a third of women and drains the superior and internal portion of the breast. It runs laterally to the outer edge of the pectoralis major and then on its undersurface to the apex of the axilla and empties into the subclavicular group of nodes. This is a direct pathway and explains the bad prognosis of carcinoma situated in the upper inner aspect of the breast.

The central and medial lymphatics of the breast empty into the internal mammary chain of nodes in the interspaces between the costal cartilages, 3 cm from the sternal edge.

Once emboli filter through the axillary lymph nodes and reach the subclavian trunk, their route to the venous circulation at the base of the neck is short and easy, as is spread from the internal mammary group. In such a case, even the most careful and radical surgical attack has little chance of curing carcinoma of the breast.

Physiology of lactation: During pregnancy, glandular changes occur under the effect of luteal and placental steroids, placental lactogen, chorionic gonadotrophins and prolactin. Blood levels of prolactin peak during the second and third trimester and lactation can occur as early as 16–18 weeks, if premature delivery occurs.

After delivery, there is a lowering of sexual steroids and placental lactogen which act as antagonists of the prolactinemic effect. There is also a temporary decrease in hypothalamic secretion of the prolactin inhibiting factor. The production of colostrum is followed first by transitional milk and then true milk. The process of lactation, that is, the synthesis, secretion and ejection of the milk is triggered by complex neuroendocrine interactions (let down reflex) and this is stimulated by suckling, and the sight and sound of the newborn along with the production of oxytocin by the neurohypophysis.

Breastfeeding confers passive immunity to the baby and also provides the best condititions for the maturation of the immune system resulting in a dramatic fall in hospitalisation during the first year of life. The emotional and intellectual development of the child is also better. To the mother, prolonged breastfeeding provides protection against mammary cancer and also acts a contraceptive.

History in relation to breast examination: A family history of breast disease makes it 2–3 times more likely for a person to develop a malignancy than the general population; further, this is much more likely to occur in premenopausal women than in postmenopausal women.

A woman with a history of breast cancer has a ten-fold risk of developing a contralateral lesion. The malignant potential of benign processes is inconclusive. However, there is no increasing risk factor with fibroadenoma, fibrosis, sclerosing adenosis macro or microcysts, ductectasia and mastitis. A moderate risk factor is associated with atypical epithelial hyperplasia. An obstetric and gynecological history, especially of reproduction and breastfeeding may be of help.

Psychological, educational and socioeconomic factors also affect a patient's comprehension and compliance. A systematic enquiry should be made into the presenting complaints. If pain is the main complaint, information about the onset, duration and periodicity along with location, aggravating and alleviating factors should be obtained. Telorrhea may be the presenting complaint and enquiry should be made into whether it is bilateral, multiductal, the type and colour of secretion, onset, periodicity, duration and presence/absence of any associated mass. Other presentations may be as a lump, pathology of the nipple (for example retraction) or cutaneous alteration.

Clinical examination: This includes inspection, palpation and staging and is the basis for choosing the appropriate complementary test so as to make the best decision between no further action, repeated check up, biopsy or surgery.

Inspection and palpation are performed with the patient standing, then sitting with the arms along the body, with the hands raised over the head, supine and bending forwards.

Inspection: It requires varying optimal tangential light. Inflammatory signs like redness, edema with or without peau d'orange or a visible tumour or ulceration are to be looked for. Modification of nipple and areola, especially retraction of the nipple which becomes more pronounced on raising the arm, are important. So is the outline of the whole breast, especially if asymmetrical.

Palpation: Both static and dynamic palpation with fingers, extending to the clavicle and under the mammary fold is important. The location, size and shape of the tumour and whether it is well-defined, are precisely recorded. The consistency may be fluctuant as in a cyst, elastic as in fibroadenosis or firm and hard as in a malignancy. Mobility is the most important differentiating sign in benign tumours. Nipple discharge is observed by expressing, to check the nature of the discharge and whether it is bilateral or monoductal. The axillary nodes are palpated with muscle relaxation and the clavicular nodes are also examined. Routinely, it is better to do the examination standing and after menstruation when the breasts are painless and soft.

The sensitivity of the clinical examination is 70% and the specificity about 80%. Clinical examination is the basis for clinical international classification (TNM classification) of breast cancers.

Breast self-examination: In developing countries, breast cancer mortality is increasing, the main reason being late diagnosis. Some countries have shown that 90% of cases are diagnosed in stage II or later and only 2.8% of cases were diagnosed in preclinical stages. Therefore, breast self-examination (BSE) has been suggested as a practical solution for early detection.

Medical and paramedical personnel must educate women about how to perform this examination and what to look for during a BSE. From the second decade of life, women should be encouraged to routinely perform BSE a week after menstruation, or the first week of every month in postmenopausal women. This includes:

1. Visual inspection in front of the mirror with hands pressed at the hips
2. Breast examination while standing up during a bath, using fingertips with light pressure, clockwise starting in 12 o' clock until the entire breast and nipples are examined. Repeat on the other breast.
3. While lying down a similar examination is again completed including the axilla on both sides. If there is any abnormality, nodularity, mass or abnormal discharge from the nipple, a physician should be consulted without delay.

Investigating modalities: These modalities are screening tests that help in diagnosis.

Screening: Clinical examination of the breast and mammography are basic detection methods and are complementary; both are necessary to achieve maximum detection rates.

A large breast is an indication for mammography to augment what in most cases is an inadequate physical examination. It is recommended that these screening processes begin by the age of 40 years and consist of annual clinical examination with screening mammography at 1–2 year intervals. The sensitivity of screening is 90% in women older than 50 years, but reduces to 56% under this age. The specificity is 94%–99%.

The frequency and type of examination will vary for the individual with symptoms and should be determined by her physician. For a patient who is at high risk for breast cancer, the screening process should begin by the age of 35 years or even 30 years and continue annually thereafter.

A major problem with the frequent use of mammography is the discovery of the nonpalpable occult lesion. This may be as an asymmetric density or a geographic cluster of microcalcifications. A decision must be made at this point, whether to repeat the films to clarify the diagnosis or repeat the film after several months to assess stability or to recommend localisation and biopsy. Most of these lesions are benign, although 15% to 20% may represent early cancer. Consultation with a radiologist is essential and the decision to perform a biopsy is made by the radiologist. Organising programmes for early breast cancer detection is important, with consideration for practicality and cost effectiveness.

Once a dominant mass has been noticed, diagnosis must be resolved. Attempts should be made to aspirate the mass with a fine gauge

Table 30.1: Pathological staging of the disease according to the TNM classification

T	***Primary tumour***
Tx	Primary tumour cannot be assessed.
T0	No evidence of primary tumour.
Tis	Carcinoma-in-situ: Clinical Paget's disease of the nipple with no tumour mass. Pathological intraductual carcinoma, lobular carcinoma-in-situ or Paget's disease with no invasive component.
T1	2 cm or smaller in greatest dimension.
T1a	0.5 cm or smaller in greatest dimension.
T1b	Larger than 0.5 cm but not larger than 2 cm in greatest dimension.
T1c	Larger than 1 cm but not larger than 2 cm in greatest dimension.
T2	Larger than 2 cm but not larger than 5 cm in greatest dimension.
T3	Larger than 5 cm in greatest dimension.
T4	Of any size with direct extension to the chest wall or the skin. The chest wall includes ribs, intercostal muscle and serratus anterior but not the pectoral muscle.
T4a	Extension to the chest wall.
T4b	Edema (peau d'orange or ulceration of the skin, tumour of the breast or satellite skin nodules confined to the same breast.
T4c	Both a and b above.
T4d	Inflammatory carcinoma.
N	***Regional nodes***
Nx	Regional nodes cannot be assessed.
N0	No regional lymph node metastasis.
N1	Metastasis to movable ipsilateral axillary lymph nodes.
N2	Metastasis to ipsilateral axillary nodes which are fixed to one another or to another structure.
N3	Metastasis to ipsilateral mammary lymph nodes.
M	***Distant Metastasis***
MX	Presence of distant metastasis cannot be assessed.
M0	No distant metastasis.
M1	Distant metastasis (include metastasis to ipsilateral supraclavicular nodes).

needle; local anesthesia is not always required. If the mass remains immediately following the aspiration, or if the fluid is bloody, or if there is a residual mass on the first follow-up visit in one month, open biopsy is recommended. If the mass is solid, open biopsy is recommended, except in teenagers for whom an excision biopsy can be performed on an elective basis.

Fine needle aspiration biopsy: It is useful only if positive; a negative finding is unreliable and it is therefore recommended that except in very special circumstances, fine needle aspiration should be confirmed by open biopsy. In a study done by Tiwari (2007), sensitivity and specificity of FNAC of the breast was found to be 83.3% and 100% respectively. The study concluded that FNAC is a simple procedure, cost effective and less traumatic than biopsy.

Mammography: This may be used to confirm the findings of physical examination, but it is important to realise that the presence of a dominant mass and a negative mammogram do not preclude the necessity for an open biopsy.

Ultrasonography: It is useful in confirming the presence or absence of a macrocyst, particularly if these lesions are discovered by mammography and are nonpalpable; MRI, thermography and diaphonography are experimental and should not be used for routine screening for breast cancer.

Biopsy: The major indication for an open biopsy is a solid mass and in most cases it can be performed on an outpatient basis and under local anesthesia. Because of the advent of conservative treatment, biopsy often becomes part of treatment and therefore it must be meticulously planned and performed by a team consisting of surgical, medical and radiation oncologists.

Though formerly the treatment consisted of radical mastectomy and regional lymph node clearance, it is now individualised and varies from lumpectomy to radical mastectomy depending on the case and age of the patient. Postoperative chemotherapy plays an important role. In estrogen receptor positive tumours, tamoxifen gives good results.

Benign Breast Diseases

Puerperal mastitis: This is localised inflammation with tenderness and slight elevation of temperature. Treatment includes continuation of breastfeeding or emptying of the breast with a pump and the use of appropriate antibiotics. If fever and tenderness persist, a breast abscess is suspected. Adequate drainage under general anesthesia followed by 7–10 days of full therapeutic dose of antibiotics is instituted.

Nonpuerperal mastitis: The usual history is the presence of a multicoloured discharge either through the nipple or near a Montgomery follicle. It is not clear whether infection occurs first followed by squamous metaplasia or if the squamous metaplasia initiates obstruction with subsequent infection. Successful treatment requires complete excision of the involved duct system under general anesthesia.

Galactorrhea: Secretion of milk from the breast may be due to excessive secretion of prolactin by a pituitary tumour, either a microadenoma or a macroadenoma. Treatment with bromocriptine 2.5 mg twice daily usually brings down prolactin levels. If the patient is not able to tolerate bromocriptine or if a high dose is needed, cabergoline 2.5 mg weekly is advised. In case of microprolactinoma associated with infertility due to anvoluation produced by hyperprolactinemia, bromocriptine should be continued till pregnancy is confirmed; subsequently it is stopped. In macroprolactinoma, the risk of enlargement of the tumour in pregnancy is much higher (16–36%); therefore, these macroadenomas should be treated surgically or with radiation before pregnancy (Randeva et al 2000). Drugs like metaclopromide, cimetidine, phenothiazines, reserpine and monoamine oxidase inibitors may also increase prolactin levels and on cessation of therapy, galactorrhea stops. Renal disorders and hypothyroidism may also cause elevated prolactin levels.

Breast Pain and nodularity: Mastalgia is the most common breast symptom and it may be cyclic or noncyclic. Cyclic mastalgia occurs at about the age of 30 years, is bilateral, diffuse, with a dull ache, and 80% respond to hormonal manipulation. Noncyclic breast pain occurs after 40 years of age and sometimes even after menopause. It is unilateral, well localised, sharp and presents with a stabbing pain. In fibrocystic disease, the pain becomes worse in the luteal phase of the cycle.

Almost all patients with pain and nodularity suspect breast cancer and therefore a dominant mass has to be excluded. If physical examination reveals a breast mass or abnormal thickening, further evaluation and management in the form of FNAB and/or excision biopsy are indicated. If ultrasonographic and mammographic examination reveals a cystic lesion, evaluation of the lesion wall by the injection of air after fine needle aspiration cytology is undertaken. If the cyst wall is irregular, excision biopsy is indicated.

Treatment of breast pain begins with simple measures like reassurance, change in undergarments being used, dietary education, non-steroidal analgesics, danazol, bromocriptine and surgical treatment. Supplementation with vitamin E and gamma linoleic acid are also effective measures. Breast pain associated with hyperprolactinemia responds to bromocriptine. Surgical treatment should be avoided in the absence of a dominant mass or ductectasia.

Nipple discharge: Nipple discharge may be unilateral or bilateral; clear, yellow/greenish, watery, serosanguinous or frankly bloody. Most physiological discharges are white, greenish or rarely yellowish. If serosanguinous or bloody, it may be due to carcinoma 17%–70% of the time; the risk is greater if it is associated with a palpable mass. Most common cause is intraductal papilloma when the bloody discharge is from the nipple (Marchant 1994). Mammography should be performed in every case. Cytology has very little predictive value and ductography has a very high failure index. Surgery in these cases includes catheterisation and resection of the involved duct system.

Fibroadenoma: This is the most common benign lesion, seen predominantly in young women (18–30 years) and presents as a firm, painless and mobile mass. They tend to be multiple and bilateral in 20%–30% of cases. It is recommended that these lesions be removed for the following reasons:

1. They do not disappear and once discovered produce anxiety
2. Although they do not dramatically increase in size, they do grow, making their removal more difficult and less cosmetic.

Pain is not frequent unless there is rapid growth, trauma, hematoma or ischemic necrosis. The use of hormonal contraceptives does not have any influence on this lesion.

- Physical examination is the ideal method for diagnosis.
- Ultrasonography may be useful for differentiating the solid mass from the cystic mass. The echogenicity of the fibroadenoma differs from carcinoma, due to the internal brim regularity and lack of mean shadow. In a study by Smith and Burrows (2008), they concluded that the majority of patients in the 25 years and under age group have benign breast pathology, most commonly fibroadenoma. Modern ultrasound is a reliable technique to diagnose fibroadenoma in the hands of experienced breast radiologists. Therefore, in this age group, it was proposed that a palpable lump that has ultrasound characteristics entirely consistent with a fibroadenoma need not be biopsied unless there is overriding clinical concern. The patient should be reassured, discharged and advised to return for further evaluation only if she detects a change in the palpable mass, noted by increased size.
- Mammography is not advisable for patients under the age of 30 years. Fine needle aspiration may be indicated since it allows diagnostic precision in about 80% of cases.

Surgical as well as conservative treatment

has been described for fibroadenomas. Both have disadvantages. A minimally invasive treatment, ultrasound-guided, vacuum-assisted percutaneous excision has been shown to facilitate the removal of all imaged evidence of benign breast lesions, including fibroadenomas up to 3 cm in diameter (Grady et al 2008). A retrospective review of 69 consecutive fibroadenomas treated with ultrasound-guided percutaneous excision was carried out. The overall recurrence rate was 15% with an actuarial recurrence rate of 33% at 59 months. All of the recurrences were in lesions which were larger than 2 cm in size at initial presentation. The data suggested that the mechanism of recurrence is the regrowth of retained lesion fragments too small to be detected by ultrasound, not the incomplete excision of all imaged lesion evidence. Despite successful percutaneous excision, fibroadenomas do recur. Lesions smaller than 2 cm in size, so treated, do not need additional therapy or surveillance. Fibroadenomas larger than 2 cm are prone to recurrence and require additional treatment.

Fibrocystic disease of the breast: It occurs mainly in women between 30 and 50 years and presents as painful breast (mastodynia) or lumpy breast, mostly seen in the upper outer quadrant of the breast. Pain and tenderness fluctuate with the menstrual cycle and become progressively worse till menopause. The risk may be more in women of higher socioeconomic status. Treatment is symptomatic with analgesics, vitamins and danazol, 100–400 mg for 4–6 months. Mammography helps in the diagnosis when in doubt. Cytological evaluation of cyst fluid is not recommended as a routine examination. The smear from nipple discharge may be examined for cytology. In case of doubt, a biopsy could be done. In cases of atypical hyperplasia, risk of cancer is five times more than in the general population.

Phyllodes tumour: These uncommon tumours of the breast account for 1% of breast tumours and occur in women of 40–90 years of age. It is a well-defined, rapidly growing swelling usually 5–8 cm in size. The tumour is lobulated and fleshy with a firm nodularity. They have a tendency to recur in 30% of patients. Histologically, they may be benign or malignant. Malignant tumours are rare and are called sarcomas. The treatment of choice for this lesion is local tumour excision with enough tumour-free margins of normal breast tissue.

The breast is the most common site of cancer in women in the developed countries and the next in importance to cervical cancer in India and other developing countries. The incidence of breast cancer in different countries is shown in Table 30.2. According to the National Cancer Registry (ICMR, 1992), age-adjusted incidence of carcinoma of breast in Indian women is about 20 per 10,00,000 women. In India, one in 50 women may develop carcinoma of the breast during their lifetime. The risk is higher when there is familial or genetic disposition. Other risk factors are early menarche, late menopause, delayed full pregnancy (after 30 years), history of ovarian or endometrial cancer, postmenopausal obesity and the use of exogenous sex hormones (as in combined oral contraceptives or in HRT).

The tumour is mostly in the upper outer quadrant of the breast. Before surgical interference, excision biopsy and histology should be done in all cases. In 60%–70% of the cases, it is intraductal carcinoma. The spread occurs mainly by the lymphatics sometimes through the bloodstream. Regular self-examination of the breast, periodic screening by the physician and mammography help in early diagnosis.

Over the last decade, dramatic advances have been made in our understanding of the molecular changes that underlie both the development of sporadic cancer and the inheritance in familial cancer. The most significant of these are related to breast, ovarian and colorectal cancer.

Although all cancers are genetic mutations in a single somatic cell, the genetic changes in sporadic cancers are confined to a particular tissue; while in inherited cancers a predisposing genetic mutation is present in all somatic and germline cells. Mutations in BRCAI and BRCA2 (situated on chromosome 17) are inherited in an autosomal dominant fashion but show incomplete penetrance, that is, not all people who have a mutation develop the disease. Additional genetic, environmental and hormonal factors determine the ultimate development of cancer in BRCA mutation carriers.

Screening the general population for BRCA mutation is not appropriate because such mutations are rare (1 in 600), and with the current technology would take considerable time. Moreover, if a mutation is found, its significance is uncertain in the absence of a family history. The alternative is to first identify individuals who are at higher risk as given in the box.

Various computer programmes have been introduced including even more factors in the family history, so as to derive the risk level of the individual.

Studies of high risk families for BRCAI and BRCA2 mutations showed a prevalence of 12%–16% carriers. Uncertainty about the penetrance of BRCA1 and BRCA2 mutations adds to the difficulties of counselling an

High risk

1. Breast or ovarian cancers in families with four or more relatives on the same side affected at any age.
2. Breast cancer in three affected relatives with average age at diagnosis being below 40 years.
3. Breast/ovarian cancers in families with three affected relatives with average age at diagnosis being below 60 years.
4. Families with one relative with both breast and ovarian cancer.

Such patients should be referred to a genetic centre for genetic testing.

Moderate risk

1. One first degree relative with breast cancer below 40 years of age.
2. Two first or second degree relatives with breast or ovarian cancer at any age.
3. One first degree relative with bilateral breast cancer diagnosed at the age of below 60 years.
4. One first degree male relative with breast cancer at any age.

Patients aged between 35–49 years in this group should be referred for annual mammography and those above 50 years once every 18 months.

Table 30.2: Cancer of the breast—incidence rate per 100,000 person years

Country	Rate
Algeria	9.5
China	11.2
France	85.9
India	21.3
Israel	90.5
Japan	19.1
Korea	7.1
Thailand	14.6
USA	103,7

Source: IARC, 1997

individual accurately about their risk of developing cancer. In certain founder populations (for example, Ashkenazi Jews and Icelanders), the penetrance may be 40%–70%, in various families (Struewing et al 1997; Fodor et al 1998; Thorlacius et al 1998).

Diagnostic testing is performed on the individuals who have already developed cancer and have a family history suggestive of an autosomal dominant mutation. If such a mutation is identified, then predictive testing, in which only that specific mutation is sought, can be offered to the unaffected relatives. Only those found to possess the same mutation will be at significantly higher risk of cancer.

BRCA1 testing has potential psychological benefits for carriers and non-carriers. Non-carriers can alter their intention concerning prophylactic mastectomy and oophorectomy (Lerman et al 1996). The ultimate beneficial effect of prophylactic surgery in carriers is not reported.

Reducing the risk of breast cancer

Chemoprevention: Chemoprevention offers a potentially more attractive alternative and several large randomised controlled trials are going on. The risk of breast cancer is related to levels of endogenous and exogenous hormones. Tamoxifen and raloxifene are selective estrogen receptor modulators.

Tamoxifen is active against advanced breast cancer and is used as adjuvant therapy. Treatment with tamoxifen for 5 years reduced the annual odds of recurrence and contralateral breast cancer both by 47% regardless of the receptor status of the initial tumour. Various trials evaluated whether 20 mg of tamoxifen daily for 5 years could reduce the incidence of breast cancer in women at increased risk. In April 1998, the Breast Cancer Prevention Trial (BCPT) conducted in the USA was stopped early after finding a 45% reduction in the incidence of breast cancer among those on tamoxifen (Fisher et al 1998). However, the Italian and British Chemopreventive Trials showed no evidence of a beneficial effect, a possible explanation being that smaller numbers were included in these countries (Veronesi et al 1998). The women in the British and Italian studies will continue to be followed up to provide long term data on the effectiveness and safety of tamoxifen. The International Breast Cancer Intervention Study (IBCIS) currently in progress in Europe should provide additional evidence. FDA approval has been obtained for the use of tamoxifen for reduction of breast cancer risk in women at increased risk of this disease.

Tamoxifen is generally well tolerated with a well defined toxicity profile based on many years of clinical use, but in rare circumstances it can cause vascular events like deep vein thrombosis, (RR 1.5) or endometrial cancer (RR 2.5). Tamoxifen maintains bone density in postmenopausal women but its effect on coronary heart disease is controversial. However, the reduction in breast cancer outweighs its risks and benefits. For women at very high risk of breast cancer, the absolute benefit is greater.

Raloxifene has FDA approval for the prevention and treatment of osteoporosis in postmenopausal women. Raloxifene may be an alternative preventive agent following a trial in postmenopausal women for osteoporosis, which demonstrated a 76% reduction in the incidence of breast cancer during 3 years of treatment (Powles et al 1998; Cummings et al 1999). The clinical trials are now comparing the efficacy of raloxifene with that of tamoxifen in reducing the risk of breast cancer (Armstrong et al 2000). A review done by Moen and Keating (2008) concluded that there was no significant difference between raloxifene and tamoxifen in the reduction in the risk of invasive breast cancer achieved in postmenopausal women at high risk of such cancer.

Prophylactic surgery: A recent retrospective study of 639 women at high risk for breast cancer found that prophylactic mastectomy reduced the risk by over 90% (Hartmann et al 1998). However, in women who were carriers of BRCA1 or BRCA2 mutations, the benefit of prophylactic mastectomy differed depending on the breast cancer risk conferred by the mutations. Bilateral mastectomy is a reasonable option for women identified as being at high risk of over 85% as it is an irreversible procedure, potentially disfiguring, and therefore requires careful consideration of the risks and benefits.

The degree of breast cancer risk reduction after surgery in women who carry these mutations has been studied by Rebbeck et al (2004): 483 women with disease-associated germline BRCA1/2 mutations were studied for the occurrence of breast cancer. Breast cancer was diagnosed in two (1.9%) of 105 women who had bilateral prophylactic mastectomy and in 184 (48.7%) of 378 matched controls who did not have the procedure, with a mean follow-up of 6.4 years. Bilateral prophylactic mastectomy reduced the risk of breast cancer by approximately 95% in women with prior or concurrent bilateral prophylactic oophorectomy and by approximately 90% in women with intact ovaries. Bilateral prophylactic mastectomy reduces the risk of breast cancer in women with BRCA1/2 mutations by approximately 90%.

Lifestyle changes and other interventions: Increased dietary fat intake, obesity, alcohol intake and decreased exercise have been associated with increased breast cancer risk in preclinical and observational studies. Therefore, lifestyle changes should be encouraged rather than interventions like drugs and surgery.

Other interventions in carriers of BRCA1 mutation could be mammography annually and MRI breast screening. CA125 and transvaginal ultrasound for ovarian cancer screening and combined oral contraceptive pill for chemoprevention of ovarian cancer may be helpful. Combination therapy with a gonadotrophin-releasing hormone agonist and tamoxifen is also suggested. Also under evaluation is a combination of tamoxifen with feretinide and monotherapy with novel selected estrogen receptor modulators (EM-652 and LY353381) and aromatase inhibitors.

The diagnosis and treatment of breast conditions is the responsibility of the obstetrician and gynecologist. FIGO has advised obstetricians and gynecologists worldwide to include mastology as a routine part of gynecological education and practice (Bonilla-Musoles 1993). The teaching programme should include all aspects of physiology and pathophysiology of breast disease, epidemiology, screening procedures and follow-up of breast diseases. Every gynecologist should follow the guidelines for screening and early detection of breast cancer, and should be able to perform simple diagnostic procedures. Only when adequately trained should the gynecologist perform breast biopsies or surgical treatments.

References

American College of Obstetricians and Gynecologists. 1991. Carcinoma of the breast. *Technical Bulletin* 158:1–3.

Armstrong K, A Eisen, B Weber. 2000. Assessing the risk of breast cancer. *N Eng J Med* 342: 564–571

Bonilla-Musoles F. 1993. The role of the gynaecologist/obstetrician in the diagnosis and management of breast disease. *Int J Gynecol Obstet* 43:1–2.

Cummings SR, S Eckert, KA Krueger et al. 1999. The effect of Raloxifene on risk of breast cancer in postmenopausal women: Results from the MORE randomized trial. Multiple outcomes of Raloxifene Evaluation. *JAMA* 281: 2189–2197

Fisher B, JP Constantino, DL Wickerham et al. 1998. Tamoxifen for prevention of breast cancer: Report of the National Surgical Adjuvant Breast and Bowel Project P-1 Study. *J Nat Cancer Inst* 90: 137–188.

Fodor FH, Weston A, Bleisweiss IJ et al. 1998. Frequency and carrier risk associated with common BRCA1 and BRCA2 mutations in Ashkenazi Jewish breast cancer patients. *Am J Hum Genet* 63:45–51.

Grady I, H Gorsuch, S Wilburn-Bailey. 2008. Long-term outcome of benign fibroadenomas treated by ultrasound-guided percutaneous excision. *The Breast Journal* Vol 14, 3:275–278.

Hartmann LC, DJ Schaid, JE Woods et al. 1998. Efficacy of bilateral prophylactic mastectomy in women with a family history of breast cancer. *N Eng J Med* 340:77–84.

Lerman C, S Narod, S Schulman, K Hughes et al. 1996. BRCA1 testing in families with hereditary breast-ovarian cancer. A prospective study of patient decision making and outcomes. *JAMA* 275: 1885–1892.

Marchant DJ. 1994. Fibrocystic disease: Diagnosis and treatment In DR Popkin and LJ Peddle eds *Women's Health Today*. London: The Parthenon Group, 313–320.

Moen MD and GM Keating. 2008. Raloxifene: A review of its use in the prevention of invasive breast cancer. *Drugs* 68(14):2059-2083.

Powles T, R Eeles, S Ashley et al. 1998. Interim analysis of the incidence of breast cancer in the Royal Marsden Hospital tamoxifen randomised chemoprevention trial. *Lancet* 352:98–101.

Randeva HS, M Davies, GM Prelevic. 2000. Prolactinoma and pregnancy. *Br J Obstet Gynecol* 107: 1064–1068.

Rebbeck TR, Friebel T, Lynch HT, Neuhausen SL, van 't Veer L, Garber JE, Evans GR, Narod SA, Isaacs C, Matloff E, Daly MB, Olopade OI, Weber BL. 2004. Bilateral prophylactic mastectomy reduces breast cancer risk in BRCA1 and BRCA2 mutation carriers: the PROSE Study Group. .*J Clin Oncol* 15;22(6):981-983.

Smith GE and P Burrows .2008. Ultrasound diagnosis of fibroadenoma: Is biopsy always necessary? *Clin Radiol* 63(5):511-515; discussion 516-7. Epub 2008 Jan 14.

Struewing JP, P Hartge, S Wacholder et al. 1997. The risk of cancer associated with specific mutations of BRCA1 and BRCA2 among Ashkenazi Jews. *N Engl J Med* 336:1401–1408.

Struewing JP, P Watson, DF Easton, BAJ Ponder et al. 1995. Prophylactic oophorectomy in inherited breast/ovarian cancer families. Heriditary breast, ovarian and colon cancer. *Journal of the National Cancer Institute* Monographs. No.17. Washington DC: Government Printing Office (NIH Publication No. 94–03837), 33–35.

Thorlacius S, JP Struewing, P Hartge et al. 1998. Population based study or risk of breast cancer in carriers of BRCA2 mutation. *Lancet* 352:93–97.

Tiwari M. 2007. Role of fine needle aspiration cytology in diagnosis of breast lumps. *Kathmandu Univ Med J (KUMJ).* 2007. 5(2):215-217.

Veronesi U, P Maisonneuve, A Costa et al. 1998. Prevention of breast cancer with tamoxifen: Preliminary findings from the Italian randomised trial among hysterectomied women. Italian tamoxifen prevention study. *Lancet* 352:93–97.

31

GnRH Analogues in Gynecology

Siya S Sharma | Sucheta Jindal

NATIVE GONADOTROPHIN RELEASING HORMONE (GNRH)

Gonadotrophin releasing hormone (GnRH) is a decapeptide produced in the mediobasal hypothalamus by neurons located in the arcuate nucleus. Green and Harris (1947) first postulated its existence in 1947 and it was identified and isolated in 1971 (Amoss et al 1971; Schally et al 1971).

In native GnRH, the amino acid sequence at position 2 and 3 facilitates the release of gonadotrophins, while the sequence at position 6 is involved in enzymatic cleavage. The residues 1, 6 and 10 are important for the three-dimensional structure and thus for receptor binding. GnRH binds to specific transmembrane receptors in the gonadotrophic cells in the anterior pituitary. The receptors then undergo a dimerisation process and initiate a cascade of intracellular events that culminate in the synthesis and secretion of follicle stimulating hormone (FSH) and luteinising hormone (LH). Once the dimer has completed its signal transduction, it is internalised into the cell. The dimer then breaks and the receptors recycle to the surface and allow a subsequent pulse of GnRH to repeat the cycle (Cornea et al 1999). This physiological pattern of pulsatile release also maintains GnRH receptor numbers as well as the functional intracellular transduction pathways.

GONADOTROPHIN RELEASING HORMONE (GNRH) ANALOGUES—AGONISTS AND ANTAGONISTS

Physiology of GnRH agonists: The GnRH agonist group include buserelin, goserelin, leuprorelin acetate, nafarelin and triptorelin. Natural GnRH has a short half life of only a few minutes, so a new analogue was synthesised with a longer half life of a few hours, increased binding affinity and decreased peptidase degradation aiming to increase biological activity (Geiger et al 1971).

This is achieved by changes in amino acid sequence, particularly substitution at position 6 and alteration or deletion at position 10, which produces more potent analogue. GnRH agonists have 100 to 200 times higher binding affinity for the GnRH receptors than does the native molecule. These analogues have proportionately high potency to release luteinising and follicle stimulating hormones from the pituitary. The substitution at position 6 helps protect against enzymatic degradation of analogues.

The short term effects of GnRH agonists are similar to GnRH. Once the dimer is internalised, this dimer form of receptor is favoured because of the abundance of agonist with long half life. Now receptors are incorporated into the cell and are unable to return to the cell membrane. The cell cannot therefore respond to a subsequent pulse of

GnRH. This process of desensitisation is achieved by a decrease in the number of GnRH receptors (down-regulation) (Gordon and Hodgen 1992).

Mechanism of action of agonists: Administration of agonists initially induces the liberation of high amounts of LH and FSH from pituitary and an increase in the number of GnRH receptors (up-regulation). This 'flare-up' effect is observed within 12 hours of administration and lasts up to 7 days, when there is a five-fold increase of FSH, ten-fold rise in LH and four-fold elevation of estradiol (Lemay et al 1984).

Continuous use (not pulsatile) of agonists causes opposite effects, internalisation of agonist–receptor complex and a decrease in the number of receptors (down-regulation). This causes paradoxical suppression of the pituitary gonadotrophin synthesis and release. The decreased levels of FSH and LH result in arrest of follicular development and maturation and cause a fall in ovarian steroid levels. It may take up to 21 days before complete down-regulation is established and estradiol levels are reached at postmenopausal levels. This is the basis for the clinical use of agonists.

During the agonist treatment, the pituitary blockade persists and is completely reversible after cessation of therapy. A normal menstrual cycle is re-established in about 6 weeks.

Physiology of GnRH antagonists: The GnRH antagonist group include cetrorelix and ganirelix. These antagonists are associated with side effects related to histamine release due the presence of GnRH receptors in mast cells (Kiesel and Runnebaum 1992). The ideal antagonist with high potency, long half life and clinically insignificant side effects is developed by modifications in amino acids sequences at position 1, 2, 3, 6, 8 and 10. These potent GnRH antagonists have high aqueous solubility.

The substitutions in amino acid sequences at positions 1, 2 and 3 confer antagonistic properties. The substitution in position 6 prolongs the half life by protecting against enzymatic degradation. The elimination of the histamine-release activity is achieved by substitutions at positions 8 and 10 (Brogden et al 1990).

Mechanism of action of antagonists: The antagonists act by blocking GnRH receptors competitively and block the ability of GnRH to initiate dimer formation and signal transduction leading to complete blockade of endogenous gonadotrophins secretion. This results in an immediate suppression of FSH and LH, and consequently in a quicker drop of ovarian steroid levels.

The use of antagonists is advantageous over agonists in some circumstances. Since antagonists act by competitive binding of receptors, it is possible to modulate the degree of hormonal suppression by variation in the dose of antagonists. This may help in avoiding or reducing menopausal side effects (Bouchard et al 1990). Also, antagonists do not cause pituitary exhaustion, so gonadotrophs can respond to an adequate stimulus almost immediately. The duration of treatment is much shorter than for agonists, and this reflects in reduced duration of gonadotrophin treatment in controlled ovarian hyperstimulation. Also after discontinuation, a rapid recovery of pituitary function is established due to the relative short elimination half life of about 12 hours.

Clinical Indications

In gynecology, many clinical indications of GnRH analogues have been investigated and therapeutic applications determined, either as single or in combination with other agents. GnRH analogues are indicated in endometriosis, fibroids, precocious puberty, infertility, polycystic ovarian syndrome (PCOS), preparation of endometrium for ablation methods and carcinomas. The effective delivery systems for GnRH analogues include parenteral (subcutaneous and intramuscular) and intranasal routes.

The disadvantage associated with the use of GnRH agonists is that because of long term treatment, unpleasant menopausal symptoms such as headache, hot flashes, mood changes and a reduction in bone mineral density occur. Generally, these effects last for some time, even after stopping the medication in case of agonists. On the contrary, with GnRH antagonists, the side effects are reversed rapidly after discontinuation of treatment (Ganirelix Study Group 1998, Oberyé et al 1999). There is some evidence to suggest that side effects can be reduced by 'add-back' therapy for a period of 6–12 months. The addition of hormonal add-back therapy to reduce side effects does not reduce efficacy of analogues (Leather et al 1999; Wyatt et al 2004).

Assisted Reproduction

GnRH analogues are used in ART in conjunction with gonadotrophins to achieve ovarian stimulation. Raised basal levels of LH have a negative impact on the quality of oocytes and embryos, and subsequently on pregnancy rates. So, the treatment with analogues significantly decreases the occurrence of premature LH surge and this has reduced the incidence of cancellation of stimulated in-vitro fertilisation (IVF) cycles from 20% to 2%. Also, fertilisation and implantation rates have improved (Loumaye 1990; Diedrich et al 1994).

GnRH agonist in assisted reproduction: Use of agonists induces a pharmacological state of hypogonadotrophic hypogonadism prior to controlled ovarian hyperstimulation in IVF cycles. This ensures an improved clinical control over the process of ovulation induction and prevents premature luteinisation. Pituitary desensitisation is achieved in about three weeks of agonist use. Agonists are used in IVF cycles for controlled ovarian hyperstimulation as well as in frozen embryo transfer cycles when hormone replacement is required.

Their use improves oocyte yield, quality, helps in oocyte pickup planning and results in higher pregnancy rates. However, their use necessitates luteal phase support (Ron-El et al 1991; Maroullis et al 1991; Hughes et al 1992).

In a long, down-regulation protocol, the agonist is administered to achieve complete pituitary suppression and place ovaries in a quiescent state prior to stimulation with exogenous gonadotrophins. Short-acting agonists are most commonly used via the subcutaneous or the intranasal route on a daily basis until satisfactory down-regulation is achieved. Long-acting agonists are used monthly via the subcutaneous or the intramuscular route which are more convenient for patient compliance but have a potential disadvantage in that they produce more profound down-regulation resulting in the need for higher doses of gonadotrophins. However, studies have shown that the use of long-acting agonists provides success rates similar to the short-acting agonists (Dada et al 1999; Neuspiller et al 1998; Yim et al 2001).

In the short and ultra-short protocols, 'flare-up' effect is utilised. The long protocol is generally most effective and is most often used. The disadvantages with long protocol are long duration of treatment, relatively high cost due to increased requirement of gonadotrophins and requirement of luteal phase support with progesterone or human chorionic gonadotrophin (hCG) due to pituitary desensitisation (Smitz et al 1992).

GnRH antagonist in assisted reproduction: The antagonists allow a short and simple treatment regimen for IVF patients undergoing ovarian stimulation. The antagonists are indicated for women undergoing ovulation induction with poor response to agonists, especially with marginally elevated FSH levels (>10–14 IU). These antagonists are used in single or multiple doses during gonadotrophin use, once adequate follicular response (about 14 mm diameter follicles) and elevation in estradiol levels has been observed around day 6 or 7 of controlled ovarian hyperstimulation to prevent premature LH surge (Borm and Mannaerts 2000; Shapiro 2003). The advantages of antagonist use are reduction in dose of gonadotrophin required for ovulation induction and a lower risk of developing ovarian hyper stimulation syndrome (OHSS).

The pregnancy rates appear to be a little lower with antagonists than agonists though not statistically significant (Shapiro 2003). With further experience, this difference is being eliminated and similar pregnancy rates are achieved in both agonists and antagonist groups (Albano et al 2000). The clinical outcome, that is, pregnancy rates and ongoing pregnancy rates (20%–25%), metaphase II oocyte (80%–85%), fertilisation rate (60%–65%) are similar with GnRH agonists and antagonists (Borm and Mannaerts 2000).

Polycystic Ovarian Syndrome (PCOS)

GnRH agonists: In PCOS, it is demonstrated that luteinising hormone levels are increased (Speroff et al 1999). In such cases, GnRH agonists inhibit pituitary gonadotrophins, particularly LH and cause a reduction in ovarian androgen and estradiol secretion improving the endocrinology in PCOS. In assisted reproduction once complete down-regulation has been achieved, exogenous gonadotrophins are used for adequate follicular development. In resistant PCO cases, combined use of GnRH analogues with gonadotrophins induce ovulation and pregnancy in up to 75% cases. This regimen eliminates premature luteinisation, ensures ovarian endometrial synchrony and improves oocyte and embryo quality (Coutts et al 1988).

The agonist treatment produces significant decreases in the hirsutism score (Ferriman Gallwey scores) after 6 months (Shaw and Williams 1991). In some women, there may not be improvement in hirsutism, although there is a significant decline in androgen levels (Szilagyi 2000). The improvement in hirsutism may persist up to 3 years with normal circulating testosterone levels, despite the return of gonadotrophins to pretreatment levels (Efstathiadou 2001). However, there is no significant decrease in body weight and body mass index (BMI) by agonist treatment (Shaw and Williams 1991).

GnRH antagonists: The antagonists have the advantage of immediate suppression of gonadotrophins and a greater suppression of LH compared with FSH secretion, especially in short term treatment. This may be beneficial in women with high LH/FSH ratio (Reissmann et al 1995).

Induction of endogenous LH surge for oocyte maturation: To prevent and reduce the risk of severe ovarian hyperstimulation syndrome (OHSS) in high risk women (such as PCOS), in intrauterine insemination (IUI) and IVF cycles, GnRH agonists are used instead of commonly used hCG to induce endogenous LH surge for oocyte maturation and ovulation. The agonist administration induces quick endogenous LH surge resulting in early ovulation, thereby reducing the risk of OHSS in controlled ovarian hyperstimulation in particular (Sharma et al 2001). The use of agonists for this purpose in IVF cycles is relevant only where there has not been previous desensitisation with GnRH agonists (Buckett et al 1998).

Endometriosis

Uterine Fibroids Endometriosis causes pelvic pain, dyspareunia and infertility. If left untreated it is progressive in extent and symptoms. Agonists are safe and effective in inducing hormonal, menstrual and endometrial suppression.

The aim of treatment with GnRH agonists is to suppress or abolish secretion of estradiol hormones from the ovaries. The treatment with agonists for 3–6 months is effective in symptom relief and lowering the extent of disease. In severe endometriosis, there is greater reduction in the extent of disease (Dmowski et al 1989; Raitz von Frentz and Schweppe 1990). The agonists are also indicated for preoperative preparation for surgical treatment of endometriosis.

Uterine Fibroids

GnRH agonists in fibroids: The agonists induce a sustained and reversible hypoestrogenic state. It helps in decreasing the size of fibroids with marked reduction in uterine volume (25%–60%) and relief of symptoms. This instils a sense of well being by causing reduced menstrual blood loss and improving anemia. The re-enlargement of fibroid volume occurs after 4–6 months of discontinuation of therapy (Matta et al 1989).

The appropriate indication for agonists use is prior to myomectomy for a pre-operative period of 3–4 months, when maximum reduction is achieved. Longer duration of use brings only a little further reduction in size. Doppler studies of uterine and fibroid vasculature confirms the increase in resistance leading to reduction in blood flow. These changes are beneficial during surgery by easing operative procedure, reducing operating time, and decreasing blood loss with low risk of anemia postoperatively.

Although evidence is scarce, there is a tendency to believe that pre-treatment with agonists makes endoscopic myomectomy or hysterectomy more feasible (Friedman et al 1989; Lethaby et al 2002). A midline incision can be avoided in many women after treatment with anlogues and the resultant reduced fibroid size. Also, an abdominal hysterectomy can be converted to vaginal procedure or laparoscopic assisted vaginal hysterectomy following the use of these agents (Stovall et al 1991; Lethaby et al 2002).

About 10% of fibroids do not seem to respond to the GnRH agonists induced hypoestrogenic state. This phenomenon can probably be ascribed to the fact that fibroids vary in the expression of receptor level and type (Cirkel et al 1994).

The agonists have been used for 2–3 months before IVF treatment in women with moderate sized uterine fibroids (Akagbosu and Awonuga 2005). This reduces fibroid volume and thus easier access to the ovaries at transvaginal ultrasound guided oocyte retrieval.

GnRH antagonists in fibroids: In view of the direct suppressive effect of antagonists on gonadotrophins and consequently on ovarian steroid secretion, it is anticipated that their use has advantages over conventional agonist treatment, because a shorter treatment duration is required which enables to schedule the surgery much earlier and a rapid recovery from adverse effects is anticipated after cessation of treatment. One drawback of antagonists is the need for daily administration.

Treatment with the antagonists results in a rapid and substantial reduction in fibroid volume (25%–40%) within only three weeks, unlike agonists which requires 3–4 months (Felberbaum et al 2001; Flierman et al 2005).

Endometrial Ablation Methods

Preparation of the endometrium with GnRH agonists for 3–4 months induces a thinner endometrium. This facilitates its complete removal, reduces operating time and fluid absorption and has better compliance. It helps in organising the operation without dependence on the menstrual cycles (Cooper et al 1996).

Precocious Puberty

When precocious puberty occurs, there is disturbance of the normal sequences of changes and evidence of dissociation between adrenarche and gonadarche. The aim of the treatment is to remove gonadotrophic or estrogen stimulus. The agonists are particularly used in constitutional precocious puberty (Swaenepoel et al 1991). This results in regression of the breast, uterine and ovarian development and cessation of menstruation which delays the bone maturation. Long term follow up after treatment with agonists is still limited but a high rate of ovulation (90%) is observed in treated girls after menarche (Jay et al 1992).

Premenstrual syndrome

The agonists provide effective therapy for physical and psychological symptoms of premenstrual syndrome by suppressing ovarian steroidogenesis (Leather et al 1999). The agonists offer a significantly superior therapeutic effect compared with vitamin B6, progesterone or selective serotonin reuptake inhibitors. Although these are effective, the menopausal side effects preclude long term use.

Chronic pelvic pain

The reported incidence of this condition is 1%–3%. The main symptoms are cyclical or constant chronic pelvic pain and deep dyspareunia. Examination may reveal tenderness in the lower abdomen and at the vault of the vagina, and occasionally a tender, palpable ovary may be palpated. Pelvic ultrasonography frequently reveals normal ovaries.

Chronic pelvic pain may be observed due to presence of ovaries or residual ovary syndrome. The correct diagnosis based on clinical grounds is made in only 30% of cases. The diagnosis is made with certainty only with the resolution of symptoms after oophorectomy. So before surgery analogues are used to establish the diagnosis of pelvic pain due to ovarian origin which helps in predicting the effectiveness of surgery. The continuous exposure to GnRH analogues induces suppression of the hypothalamo-pituitary-ovarian axis. One to two monthly depot subcutaneous injections are needed to see the response (Carey and Slack 1996).

Carcinomas

GnRH analogues display antitumour effects in women with steroid hormone dependent carcinomas such as endometrial, ovarian and breast carcinomas (Emons and Schally 1994). The agonists have been used in postmenopausal women with recurrent endometrial cancer because of their direct antiproliferative antitumour action on the endometrial neoplastic tissue (Jeyarajah et al 1996). However, analogues are not used routinely for oncological indications as antitumour effects are not universally seen which may be due to variation of receptor expression (Chatzaki et al 1996). Further research is required for a better understanding of receptor expression to facilitate the development of suitable and effective therapy in this field (Albano et al 2001).

References

Akagbosu FT and AO Awonuga. 2005. The use of gonadotrophins releasing hormone agonist and antagonist in infertility. In *Textbook of in vitro fertilization and assisted reproduction*, ed PR Brinsden, London: Taylor and Francis. 165–176.

Albano C, RE Felbernaum, J Smitz et al. 2000. Controlled ovarian stimulation with HMG: Results of a prospective randomized phase III European Study comparing the LHRH-antagonists cetrorelix (Cetrotide) and the LHRH agonist buserelin. *Hum Reprod* 15:526–531.

Albano C, P Platteau and P Devroey. 2001. Gonadotrophins releasing hormone antagonist: How good is the new hope? *Curr Opin Obste Gynecol* 13:257–262.

Amoss M, R Burgus, P Blackwell et al. 1971. Purification, amino acid composition and N-terminus of hypothalamic luteinising hormone releasing factor (LRF) of ovine origin. *Biochem Biophys Res Commun* 44:205–210.

Borm G and B Mannaerts. 2000. Treatment with the gonadotrophins releasing hormone antagonist ganirelix in women undergoing ovarian stimulation with recombinant follicle stimulating hormone is effective, safe, and convenient: Results of a controlled, randomized, multicentre trail. *Hum Reprod* 15;7:1490–1498.

Bouchard P, A Caraty, D Medalie. 1990. Mechanism of action and clinical uses of GnRH antagonists in women. In *Recent progress on GnRH and gonadal peptide,* ed P Bouchard, F Haour, P Franchimont, B Schatz. Paris: Elsevier, 209.

Brogden RN, MT Buckley, A Ward et al. 1990. Buserelin. A review of the pharmacodynamic and pharmacokinetic properties, and clinical profile. *Drug* 39:399–437.

Buckett WM, B Bentick, RW Shaw. 1998. Induction of endogenous gonadotrophins surge for oocyte maturation with intra-nasal gonadotrophins-releasing hormone analogue (buserelin): Effective minimum dose. *Hum Reprod* 13;4:811–814.

Carey MP and MC Slack. 1996. GnRH analogue in assessing chronic pelvic pain in women with residual ovaries. *Br J Obstet Gynecol* 103:(2), 150–153.

Chatzaki E, Bax CMR, Eidine KA et al. 1996. The expression of gonadotrophins releasing hormone and its receptors in endometrial cancer and its relevance as an antitumor growth factor. *Cancer Res* 56:2059–2065.

Cirkel U, H Ochs, A Roehl. 1994. Estrogen and progesterone receptor content of enucleated uterine myomata after luteinising hormone-releasing hormone analogue depot therapy. *Acta Obstet Gynecol Scand* 73:328–332.

Cooper KG, SB Pinion, S Bhattacharya, DE Parkin. 1996. The effects of the gonadotrophin releasing hormone analogue (goserelin) and prostaglandin E_1 (misoprostol) on cervical resistance prior to transcervical resection of the endometrium. *Br J Obstet Gynecol* 103:(4), 375–378.

Cornea A, JA Janovich, X Lin, et al. 1999. Simultaneous and independent visualization of gonadotrophins releasing hormone receptor and its ligand: Evidence for independent processing and recycling in living cells. *Endocrinology* 140:4272–4280.

Coutts JRT, S Finnie, C Conaghan, WP Black, R Fleming. 1988. Combined buserelin and exogenous gonadotrophin therapy for the treatment of infertility in women with PCO disease. *Gynecol Endocrinol* 2 (Suppl):Abstract 61.

Dada T, O Salha, HS Baillie, V Sharma. 1999. A comparison of three gonadotrophins releasing hormone analogues in an in vitro fertilization programme: A prospective randomized study. *Hum Reprod* 14:288–293.

Diedrich K, C Diedrich, E Santos, et al. 1994. Suppression of endogenous luteinising hormone surge by the gonadotrophin releasing hormone antagonist cetrorelix during ovarian stimulation. *Hum Reprod* 9:788–791.

Dmowski WP, I Tummon, E Radwanska, P Pepping, Z Binor. 1989. Ovarian suppression induced with buserelin or danazol in the management of endometriosis: A randomised comparative study. *Fertil Steril* 51:395–400.

Efstathiadou Z and A Tsatsoulis. 2001. Long-term remission of ovarian hyperandrogenism after short-term treatment with a gonadotrophin-releasing hormone agonist. *Fertil Steril* 75:59.62.

Emons G and V Schally. 1994. The use of luteinising hormone releasing hormone agonists and antagonist in gynecological cancers. *Hum Reprod Update* 91:364–370.

Felberbaum RE, W Kupker, M Krapp, B Gehl, M Ludwig, K Diedrich. 2001. Preoperative reduction of uterine fibroids in only 16 days by administration of a gonadotrophin-releasing hormone antagonist (Cetrotide). *Reprod Biomed Online* 3:14–18.

Flierman PA., JJL Oberyé, VPM Van der Huls, S de Blok. 2005. Rapid reduction of leiomyoma volume during treatment with the GnRH antagonist ganirelix. *Br J Obstet Gynecol* 112; 5:638.

Friedman AJ, MS Rein, D Harrison-Atlas, JM Garfield, PM Doubilet. 1989. A randomized, placebo-controlled, double-blind study evaluating leuprolide acetate depot treatment before myomectomy. *Fertil Steril* 52:728–733.

Ganirelix Dose-Finding Study Group. 1998. A double-blind, randomized, dose-finding study to assess the efficacy of the GnRH antagonist ganirelix (Org 37642) to prevent premature LH surges in women undergoing controlled ovarian hyperstimulation with recombinant FSH (Puregon). *Hum Reprod* 13: 3023–3031.

Geiger R, W Konig, H Wissam et al. 1971. Synthesis and characterisation of a decapeptide having LH-RH-FSH-RH activity. *Biochem Biophys Res Commun* 45:767–773.

Gordon K and GD Hodgen. 1992. GnRH agonists and antagonists in assisted reproduction. *Bailliere's Clin Obstet Gynecol* 41:863–871.

Green JD and GW Harris. 1947. The neurovascular link between the neurohypophysis and adenohypophysis. *J Endocrinol* 5:136–146.

Hughes EG, MA Sagle, DM Federkow et al. 1992. The routine use of GnRH-a prior to IVF and GIFT: A meta analysis of RCT. *Fertil Steril* 58:888–896.

Jay N, J Mansfield, RM Blizzard, et al. 1992. Ovulation and menstrual function of adolescent girls with central precocious puberty after therapy with gonadotrophins releasing hormone agonist. *J Clin Endocrinol and Metab* 75:890–894.

Jeyarajah AR, CJ Gallgher, PR Blake et al. 1996. Long-term follow up GnRH: A treatment for recurrent endometrial cancer. *Gynecol Oncol* 63:47–52.

Kiesel L and B Runnebaum. 1992. Gonadotrophin-releasing hormone and analogues. Physilogie and pharmakogie. *Gynakol Geburtsh Rundsch* 32:22–30.

Leather AT, JWW Studd, NR Watson, EFN Holland. 1999. The treatment of severe premenstrual syndrome with goserelin with and without 'add-back' estrogen therapy: A placebo-controlled study. *Gynecol Endocrinol* 13(1):48–55.

Lemay A, R Maheux, N Faure et al. 1984. Reversible hypogonadism induced by a leutinising hormone-releasing hormone (LHRH) agonist (buserelin) as a new therapeutic approach for endometriosis. *Fertil Steril* 41:863–871.

Lethaby A, B Vollenhoven, M Sowter. 2002. Pre-operative GnRH analogue therapy before hysterectomy or myomectomy for uterine fibroids. Oxford (UK): *Cochrane Review Library*.

Loumaye E. 1990. The control of endogenous secretion of LH by gonadotrophins releasing hormone agonist s during ovarian hyperstimulation for in-vitro fertilization and embryo transfer. *Hum Reprod* 5:357–376.

Maroullis GB, A Saphier, M Emery et al. 1991. Prospective randomised study of human menotropin versus a follicular and a luteal phase gonadotropin-releasing hormone analogue: Human menotropin stimulation protocols for IVF. *Fertil Steril* 55:115–164.

Matta WHM, RW Shaw, M Nye. 1989. Long term follow up of patients with uterine fibroids after treatment with the LHRH agonist buserelin. *Br J Obstet Gynecol* 86:200–206.

Neuspiller F, M Levy, J Remohi, A Ruiz, C Simon, A Pellicer A. 1998. The use of long- and short-acting forms of gonadotrophin-releasing hormone analogues in women undergoing oocyte donation. *Hum Reprod* 13:(5);1148–1151.

Oberyé J, B Mannaerts, J Huisman, CJ Timmer. 1999. Pharmacokinetic and pharmacodynamic characteristics of ganirelix (Orgalutran). Part II: Dose-proportionality and gonadotropin suppression after multiple doses of ganirelix in healthy female volunteers. *Fertil Steril* 72:1006–1012.

Raitz von Frentz M and KW Schweppe. 1990. Ovarian suppression by the GnRH analogue buserelin in the treatment of endometriosis. Clinical, biochemical and pelviscopic studies. *Geburtshilfe Frauenheilkd* 50:634–639.

Reissmann T, R Felberbaum, K Diedrich et al. 1995. Development and application of luteinising hormone releasing hormone antagonists in the treatment of infertility: An overview. *Hum Reprod* 10:1974–1981.

Ron-El R, A Herman, A Golan et al. 1991. Gonadotrophins and combined gonadotrophins releasing hormone agonist—gonadotrophins protocol in a randomized prospective study. *Fertil Steril* 55: 574–578.

Schally AF, A Arimura, Babay et al. 1971. Isolation and properties of FSH and LH-releasing hormone. *Biochem Biophys Res Commun* 43:393–399.

Shapiro DB. 2003. GnRH antagonists symposium: Introduction. *Fertil Steril* 80:S1–7.

Sharma Siya, P Kumar, S Jindal. 2001. Induction of an endogenous LH surge by GnRH-a. *J Obstet Gynecol India* 51 (5), 134–138.

Shaw RW and I Williams. 1991. The effects of long-term administration of GnRH analogues in the treatment of polycystic ovarian syndrome. *Adv Reprod Endocrinol* 3:121–133.

Smitz J, R Ron-El, BC Tarlatziz. 1992. The use of gonadotrophins releasing hormone agonists for in vitro fertilization and other assisted procreation techniques: Experience from three centres. *Hum Reprod* 7:(Suppl1) 49–66.

Speroff L, RH Glass, NG Kase eds. 1999. Anovulation and polycystic ovaries. In *Clinical gynecologic endocrinology and infertility*, 6th edn, 487–521. Philadelphia: Lippincott

Stovall TG, FW Ling, LC Henry. 1991. A randomised trial evaluating leuprolide acetate before hysterectomy as treatment for leiomyomas. *Am J Obstet Gynecol* 164:1420–1425.

Swaenepoel C, JL Chaussain, M Roger M. 1991. Long term results of long acting luteinising hormone releasing hormone in central precocious puberty. *Hormone Res* 36:126–130.

Szilagyi A, J Homoki, S Bellyei, I Szabo. 2000. Hormonal and clinical effects of GnRH agonist treatment in PCOS. *Gynecol Endocrinol* 14:337–341.

Wyatt Katrina M and Paul W Dimmock, MK Kahled Ismail, Peter W Jones et al. 2004. The effectiveness of GnRH-a with and without 'add-back' therapy in treating premenstrual syndrome: A meta analysis. *Br J Obstet Gynecol* 111:(6), 585–593.

Yim SF, IH Lok, LP Cheung, CM Briton-Jones, TTY Chiu. 2001. Haines CJ. Dose-finding study for the use of long acting gonadotrophins-releasing hormone analogues prior to ovarian stimulation for IVF. *Hum Reprod* 16:3:492–494.

32

Prostaglandins

Pankaj Desai | Sarbani Ghosh

Introduction: Prostaglandins are members of the lipid class of biochemicals and are known for their potent physiological properties. Prostaglandins vary from one another and may exhibit subtle differences in their chemical structure, for example, in the side-chain substitutions. These small variations are believed to be responsible for the immense diversity of effects characteristic of prostaglandins. Also, the same prostaglandins act differently in different tissues.

History: Prostaglandins were first discovered in semen in the 1930s by the Swedish scientist, Ulf von Euler. They derived their name from the prostate gland, from where they were first thought to originate. Early studies of prostaglandins carried out by Euler and other researchers revealed that these substances were active, capable of lowering blood pressure and instigating the contraction of uterine tissue. Synthesis takes place in the membranes of various cells. Its ultrastructure is shown in Fig. 32.1

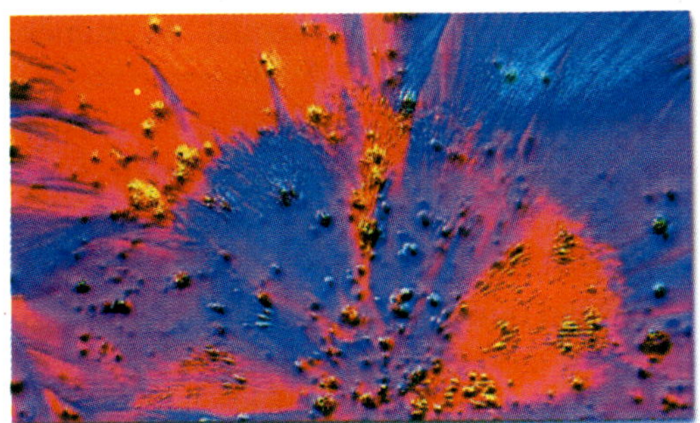

FIGURE 32.1: PHOTOMICROGRAPH: PROSTAGLANDIN B_1

Physiology: About a dozen different prostaglandins have been identified, each of which is associated with different kinds of activities, with different effects on various tissues. Prostaglandins are found in virtually all tissues and organs. They have a wide variety of actions but most prostaglandins cause muscular constriction and mediate inflammation. Other effects include calcium movement, temperature control, hormone regulation, cell growth control, lipolysis and immune system response.

Thromboxane is created in platelets and causes vascular constriction and platelet aggregation. Working in conjunction with thromboxanes, prostaglandins play an important role in blood clotting, the balance between the two controls, whether or not coagulation occurs.

BIOCHEMISTRY

Arachidonic acid is released from membrane phospholipids by hydrolysis, by the enzyme phospholipase A_2. There are multiple phospholipase A_2 enzymes, subject to activation through different signal cascades. For instance, the inflammatory signal molecule platelet-activating factor is involved in activating some variants of phospholipase A_2, whereas corticosteroids are anti-inflammatory because they inhibit phospholipase A_2, reducing arachidonate release as shown in Fig. 32.2

Cyclic pathway: Prostaglandin H_2 Synthase (PGH_2 Synthase) catalyses the important step in the 'cyclic pathway' that leads to the production of prostaglandins, prostacyclins and thromboxanes. PGH_2 Synthase exhibits two catalytic activities—cyclo-oxygenase and peroxidase. The enzyme expressing both activities is sometimes referred to as cyclo-oxygenase and abbreviated as COX as shown in Fig. 32.3

Non-steroidal anti-inflammatory drugs (NSAIDs), such as aspirin and derivatives of ibuprofen, inhibit the cyclo-oxygenase activity of PGH_2 Synthase. They inhibit the formation of prostaglandins involved in fever, pain and inflammation. They also inhibit blood clotting by blocking thromboxane formation in blood platelets.

Aspirin acetylates a serine residue near the cyclo-oxygenase active site. This prevents the binding of arachidonate. The anti-clotting effect of aspirin is attributed to the inhibition of thromboxane formation in blood platelets. Ibuprofen and related compounds act by

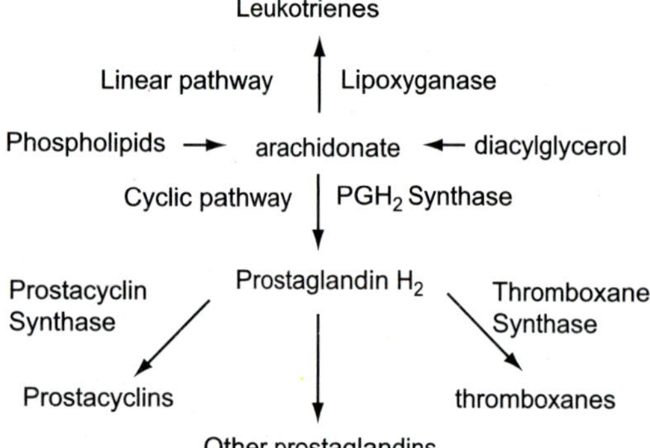

FIGURE 32.2: CYCLO-OXYGENASE PATHWAY

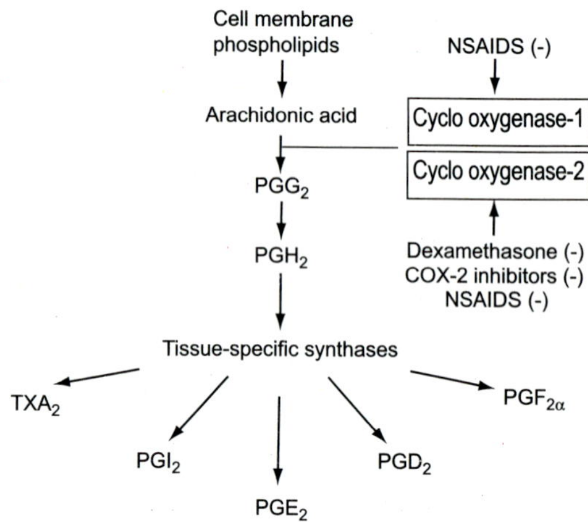

FIGURE 32.3: PROSTAGLANDIN SYNTHESIS

blocking the hydrophobic channel by which arachidonate enters the cyclo-oxygenase active site. Two isoforms of PGH_2 synthase are COX-1 and COX-2 (cyclo-oxygenase I and II).

COX-1 is constitutively expressed at low levels in many cell types. COX-1 is known to be essential for maintaining the integrity of the gastrointestinal epithelium. COX-2 expression is stimulated by growth factors, cytokines and endotoxins. Inflammation is associated with upregulation of COX-2 and increased formation of prostaglandins. COX-2 levels increase in inflammatory disease states such as arthritis. Increased expression of COX-2 is seen in some cancer cells. Angiogenesis (blood vessel development), essential to tumour growth, requires COX-2. Overexpression of COX-2 leads to an increase in the expression of the vascular endothelial growth factor (VEGF). Regular use of NSAIDs has been shown to decrease the risk of developing colorectal cancer.

Most NSAIDs inhibit both COX-1 and COX-2. Recent evidence suggests the existence of a third isoform, designated COX-3, with roles in mediating pain and fever, and subject

(Lipitz et al 1997). Dinoprost a synthetic analogue of $PGF_2\alpha$, has also been tried in the intra-amniotic route, the limitations being the need for repeated instillation and the high cost of the preparation (Krofta et al 1998).

Extra-amniotic $PGF_2\alpha$ has been widely used (Munthali and Moodley 2001) and so has intracervical PGE_2. In fact, the intracervical application of PGE_2 gel appeared to be the most successful and physiological method for cervical ripening. The synthetic PGE_1 compounds currently used are gemeprost and misoprostol.

Misoprostol: In combination with mifepristone, misoprostol is a safe and effective regimen for mid trimester medical abortion. Various doses, frequency of administration and routes have been studied to achieve maximum efficacy with minimal side effects and patient acceptance. Misoprostol, 400 µg given vaginally every three hours (Ngai et al 2003) is probably the optimal regimen for second trimester abortion. It is more effective than the regimen of vaginal misoprostol every 6 hours (Wong et al 2001). It is generally recommended that a maximum of five doses be used in 24 hours. However, there is an increased incidence of fever in this group (Pongsatha et al 2005), and some workers have observed that misoprostol (600 µg) administered at 12 hour intervals was associated with fewer adverse effects and was as effective as at 6 hour intervals (Tang et al 2004).

Vaginal misoprostol should be the regimen of choice but sublingual misoprostol is also an effective alternative (Gonzalez et al 2001). Outpatient initiation of second trimester medical termination with self-administered misoprostol has also been found to be effective and it decreased the time of hospitalisation. Vaginal misoprostol tablets, 200 µg every 6 hours, were used in one study (Gonzalez et al 2001).

Role of misoprostol in women with previous cesarean section: In second trimester abortions, the use of misoprostol in women with prior cesarean delivery was not associated with an excess of complications compared with women with unscarred uteri. The most commonly used regime was 400 mg six hourly (Dickinson 2005; Daskalakis et al 2005).

Role of misoprostol as a cervical priming agent before surgical abortion: Of all available agents, misoprostol has been found to be safe, effective, cheap and easily applicable (Gronlund et al 2002). Vaginal misoprostol 400 µg, 3–4 hours before vacuum aspiration appears to be the most effective regimen.

Role of misoprostol in missed abortion: Vaginal misoprostol, 400 to 600 μg, is effective in most patients with missed abortion. Pretreatment with mifepristone did not increase the success rate (Gronlund et al 2002).

ROLE OF PROSTAGLANDINS IN INDUCTION OF LABOUR

Induction of labour is a common obstetric intervention occurring in about 15% of all deliveries. Induction with an unfavourable cervix (Bishop's score <5) is associated with increased risk of prolonged labour to the mother and the fetus, as well as a high cesarean section rate. Prostaglandins undoubtedly play an important role in the control of cervical ripening. The pharmacological effects of prostaglandins on the cervix and the subsequent induction of labour have also been extensively studied. Various forms and various routes of administration have been tried and tested and some like the intravenous route abandoned because of the high incidence of side effects.

Until the advent of misoprostol, the popular choices were intracervical PGE_2 gel, (Dinoprostone) as 1 mg or 2 mg inserts and vaginal PGE_2 pessaries or tablets, varying between 2–10 mg; extra amniotic inserts of PGE_2 and $PGF_{2\alpha}$ have also been used.

Role of misoprostol in cervical ripening and induction of labour: A meta analysis of 62 trials in the Cochrane database has surmised that:

- Compared to placebo, misoprostol was associated with increased cervical ripening. It was also associated with reduced failure to achieve vaginal delivery within 24 hours. Uterine hyperstimulation, without fetal heart rate changes, had increased (Hofmeyr and Gulmezoglu 2001; Hofmeyr et al 2000; Alfirewic 2000; Sanchez-Ramos 2005).
- Compared with vaginal prostaglandin E2, intracervical prostaglandin E2 and oxytocin labour induction using vaginal misoprostol was associated with less epidural analgesia use, fewer failures to achieve vaginal delivery within 24 hours and more uterine hyperstimulation.
- Compared with vaginal or intracervical prostaglandin E2, oxytocin augmentation was less common, it was more common with misoprostol and meconium-stained liquor.
- Compared with intracervical prostaglandin E2, unchanged or unfavourable cervix after 12 to 24 hours was less common with misoprostol.
- Lower doses of misoprostol compared to higher doses were associated with more need for oxytocin augmentation, less uterine hyperstimulation, with and without fetal heart rate changes and a non-significant trend to fewer admissions to a neonatal intensive care unit.
- Use of a gel preparation of misoprostol versus tablet was associated with less hyperstimulation and more use of oxytocin and epidural analgesia.
- Doses, not exceeding 25 μg four-hourly, appeared to have similar effectiveness and posed the same risk of uterine hyperstimulation to conventional labour inducing methods.
- Until the optimum dose and timing intervals of misoprostol administration are established, increased abnormalities of the CTG remain an area of concern (Ramsey et al 2003; Lokugamage et al 2003) and misoprostol should be used with careful monitoring of the fetal heart rate and uterine activity.

Dosage schedule of misoprostol: Vaginal misoprostol, in its currently recommended dose of 25 µg seems to be more efficacious to be repeated every 4 hours up to a maximum of five doses (Shetty et al 2003). Tachysystole and hyperstimulation syndrome appear to occur less frequently among women who received 25 µg of misoprostol than with 50 µg. However, neonatal outcomes appear to be comparable with the two doses. Intravaginal misoprostol at doses of 50 µg for cervical ripening and labour induction is more efficacious but it is unclear whether it is as safe as the 25 µg dose (Meydanli et al 2003).

Oral versus vaginal misoprostol: There is consensus among practitioners that compared with oral misoprostol, vaginal misoprostol for the induction of labour at term results in a shorter induction-to-delivery time, with fewer doses required per patient. Vaginal misoprostol may be associated with higher rates of cesarean sections. There were no differences between the two routes of administration with respect to rates of hyperstimulation or neonatal asphyxia (Fisher et al 2001).

Higher rates of tachysystole were noted with the use of vaginal misoprostol (Paungmora et al 2004; le Roux et al 2002) except in studies where a higher dose of oral misoprostol was used; oral misoprostol, though found to have a similar efficacy as that of the vaginal misoprostol, was associated with a higher frequency of excessive uterine contractility and intervention (Wing et al 2000; Carlan et al 2001).

Another study noted that stepwise oral misoprostol (50 µg. followed by 100 µg.) appears to be as effective as vaginal misoprostol (25 µg.) for cervical ripening with a low incidence of hyperstimulation, no increase in side effects, a high rate of patient satisfaction, and was associated with a lower cesarean section rate (Colon et al 2005).

Outpatient cervical ripening: A single dose of 25 µg misoprostol administered vaginally in the outpatient setting significantly decreases oxytocin use, largely due to labour within the ripening period. No patient had hyperstimulation or required cesarean delivery for non-reassuring fetal assessment during the ripening period (Meyer et al 2005).

Vaginal prostaglandin (PGE_2 and PGF_{2A}) for induction of labour at term: There were insufficient data to make meaningful conclusions for the comparison of vaginal PGE_2 and PGF2α. PGE_2 tablet, gel and pessary—each of these appears to be as efficacious as the other. Lower dose regimes, as defined in the review, appear as efficacious as higher dose regimes (Kelly et al 2003).

Prostaglandins after cesarean section: The issues related to safety of induction of labour in women with previous cesarean section remain controversial. In women with previous cesarean section and no vaginal deliveries, induction of labour carries a relatively high risk of uterine rupture/dehiscence despite all precautions, including intrauterine pressure monitoring. This risk was estimated to be about 2.4%, in a tertiary referral centre, with approximately 6000 births per annum in the UK (Kayani and Alfirevic 2005).

A recent study proposed that prostaglandins induce local, biochemical modifications that weaken the scar, predisposing it to rupture. Women treated with prostaglandins experienced rupture at the site of their old scar more frequently than women in the oxytocin-alone group in whom the rupture tended to occur at a location remote from their old scar (Buhimschi et al 2005).

The few studies which found prostaglandins safe to be used for induction, advise that it be used with caution, following a strict protocol (Locatelli et al 2004).

Prostaglandins in premature rupture of membranes (PROM): Premature rupture of membranes (PROM) occurs in 8% of term deliveries. In this situation, labour induction with prostaglandins, compared with expectant management, results in a reduced risk of chorioamnionitis, neonatal antibiotic therapy, neonatal intensive care (NICU) admission and increased maternal satisfaction. The use of prostaglandins is associated with an increased rate of diarrhea and use of analgesia/anesthesia (Crane and Young 2003). It appears to be an effective method of labour induction with term PROM.

Active management with oral misoprostol resulted in more women going into labour and delivering within 24 hours of the prelabour rupture of membranes with no increase in maternal or neonatal complications. Women tended to view active management of prelabour rupture of membranes more positively. Oral misoprostol might be an option to consider in those wishing active management (Shetty et al 2002). However, a multicentric randomised controlled trial has produced results that have refuted this view as have other researchers. Oral misoprostol does not offer any advantage in terms of time taken from induction to vaginal delivery or the risk of cesarean section (Wing et al 2005).

Prostaglandins for prevention of postpartum hemorrhage: Review of current literature shows that oral misoprostol in the dose of 600 µg shows, clinically and statistically, significantly more blood loss compared with conventional injectable uterotonics. Rigour and elevated body temperature are the main side effects of misoprostol and are dose related. Injectable prostaglandins are associated with reduced mean blood loss in the third stage of labour when compared to conventional injectable uterotonics but have more side effects. In conclusion, neither intramuscular prostaglandins nor misoprostol are preferable to conventional injectable uterotonics as part of the active management of the third stage of labour especially for low-risk women. Future research on prostaglandin use after birth should focus on the treatment of postpartum hemorrhage rather than prevention where they seem to be more promising (Gülmezoglu et al 2004).

PROSTAGLANDINS IN PRE-ECLAMPSIA

Pre-eclampsia is characterised by an imbalance between two cyclo-oxygenase metabolites of arachidonic acid—thromboxane and prostacyclin—with an increase in the amount of thromboxane. In the maternal circulation, this imbalance is primarily manifested by decreased production of prostacyclin by endothelial cells, prostacyclin being a potent vasodilator and preventing platelet aggregation. This is then followed by increased secretion of platelet thromboxane synthesis but this is seen only in severe pre-eclampsia.

In the placenta and in the leukocytes, the imbalance is exacerbated by increased production of thromboxane coupled with decreased production of prostacyclin in both mild and severe pre-eclampsia. The thromboxane/prostacyclin imbalance predates the onset of clinical symptoms of pre-eclampsia (Mills et al 1999; Walsh 2004).

This imbalance between thromboxane and prostacyclin is most likely caused by oxidative stress, which is manifest in pre-eclampsia by increased lipid peroxidation and decreased antioxidant protection. Decreased placental antioxidant enzyme protection leads to a cascade of events in the placenta, of uncontrolled lipid peroxidation with increased thromboxane production and increased tumour necrosis factor (TNF-alpha) production (Walsh 1998).

Pyridoxine, 300 mg orally twice daily, has been found to increase the prostacyclin production and inhibit thromboxane and leukotriene synthesis and might be beneficial in such disorders (Saareks et al 2002). A thromboxane synthetase inhibitor, pirmagrel, strongly inhibited thromboxane production in a dose-related manner, with reciprocal increase in prostacyclin production occurring in cytotrophoblasts and may therefore warrant further investigation as a treatment for pre-eclampsia (Ding et al 2002).

Aspirin is an inhibitor of the cyclo-oxygenase system. Low-dose aspirin therapy (50–150 mg/day) has been considered for the prevention of pre-eclampsia because it selectively inhibits thromboxane synthesis without affecting prostacyclin synthesis. Although low-dose acetylsalicylic acid (ASA) restores the balance in favour of prostacyclin, the clinical results of administering ASA remain uncertain (Vainio et al 2005). Early randomised trials reported on promising reductions in pre-eclampsia risk and possible fetal growth retardation. But subsequent multicentric trials during the nineties like the CLASP, ECCPA, BLASP trials and the Jamaican low dose aspirin study group failed to confirm a large benefit, which may in part be explained by lack of strict criteria for inclusion, late initiation of treatment, low dosages, low patient compliance, different timing of aspirin ingestion, wide inclusion of women with concomitant disorders such as chronic hypertension, diabetes mellitus and kidney disease and use of ill-defined end points (Dekker 1995; Klokenbusch and Rath 2002). There is now growing evidence that the earlier ASA treatment is started, the greater is the reduction in the risk of pre-eclampsia. The crucial time for starting treatment may be before 16 weeks and daily ingestion before bedtime appears useful.

A recent trial by the ERASME collaborative group suggests that aspirin at a dose of 100 mg does not reduce the incidence of pre-eclampsia in nulliparous women and is associated with an increase in bleeding complications (Subtil et al 2003).

In view of all the available literature, we can say that although aspirin is no longer considered the miracle drug, it is still too early to write it off totally. The Paris Collaboration (2005) has been formed to undertake the review of all available literature to date, analysing existing individual patient data, rather than designing yet another trial. It will examine the uncertainties regarding whether some women (in terms of risk) benefit more than others, what dose of aspirin is best and when in pregnancy treatment should ideally start. Final results were expected by 2006–07 (Paris Collaboration 2005).

PROSTAGLANDINS AND DYSFUNCTIONAL UTERINE BLEEDING

Dysfunctional uterine bleeding (DUB) or primary menorrhagia has been defined as menstrual blood loss in excess of 80 ml in the absence of any organic disease in the genital tract or outside it. In primary menorrhagia, the levels of total prostaglandins are raised and there is a comparatively increased amount of vasodilator prostaglandins like the PGE_2 as compared to $PGF_{2\alpha}$ which cause vasoconstriction and platelet aggregation. The reason for this is not quite clear. In fact, it has also been reported that median PGE receptor concentrations were significantly higher in the women with menorrhagia than in the women with normal menstrual blood loss, and correlated with the menstrual blood loss (Adelantado et al 1988). Other factors have also been implicated in causing the increased blood loss. Endothelin-1(ET-1) may play a role in the local control of the endometrial vascular bed either directly, or through the release of $PGF_{2\alpha}$ (Cameron et al 1991).

Vasoactive substances like leukotrienes and cytokines have also been implicated. The role of nitric oxide has also been under observation, which acts as a potent vasodilator and inhibitor of platelet aggregation and also appears to mediate the vasodilatory actions of both PGE_2 and estrogen (Telfer 1995).

DUB SECONDARY TO INTRA UTERINE CONTRACEPTIVE DEVICE (IUD): The imbalance of PGI_2/TXA_2 ratio may be the direct cause of IUD-induced menorrhagia. Excessive production of leukotrienes causing vasoconstriction, followed by plasma leakage and by the extravasation of erythrocytes, has also been suggested.

NONSTEROIDAL ANTI-INFLAMMATORY DRUGS (NSAIDS) IN THE MANAGEMENT OF DUB: NSAIDs reduce menstrual blood loss by inhibiting the cyclo-oxygenase system thereby reducing the production of endoperoxides. The fenamates—mefenamic acid, meclafenamate—also block myometrial PGE_2 receptors. Although NSAIDs are effective in about 25% of cases (Anderson et al 1976), the degree of reduction is proportionate to the initial blood loss (Fraser and McGarron 1991).

Although mefenamic acid has been studied extensively, other compounds like naproxen, ibuprofen and flurbiprofen have also been found to be effective. Because of their analgesic action, these drugs are also helpful in treating any concurrent dysmenorrhea, and as such, form an effective first-line therapy in the treatment of DUB.

ROLE OF PROSTAGLANDINS IN ENDOMETRIOSIS

Endometriosis is a disease characterised by the occurrence of ectopic endometrium, and occurs most frequently in the pouch of Douglas and the ovaries. Prostaglandin E_2 has been shown to stimulate steroidogenesis in ectopic endometriotic stromal cells and may be involved in the development of endometriosis since this disorder is highly estrogen dependent. The biosynthesis of PGE_2 is controlled by the rate-limiting enzyme termed cyclo-oxygenase (COX). Elevated expression of both COX-1 and COX-2 in peritoneal macrophages may contribute to increased peritoneal fluid PGE_2 concentrations and may thus play an important role in the development of endometriosis (Wu et al 2002).

Aromatase activity is absent in the normal endometrium. In contrast, aromatase is expressed aberrantly in endometriosis, which gives rise to strikingly high levels of aromatase activity in this tissue. Both aromatase expression and activity are stimulated by PGE_2. This results in local production of estrogen, which induces PGE_2 formation and establishes a positive feedback cycle. The clinical relevance of these findings resulted in the successful treatment of an unusually aggressive case of postmenopausal endometriosis using an aromatase inhibitor (Bulun et al 2002).

Prostaglandins, produced in large amounts in the pelvis, might interfere with fertility through various mechanisms like alterations in the egg implantation, follicle genesis, luteinisation, sperm motility as well as tubal disorders (Pungetti et al 1987). It has been shown that in patients with endometriosis, the isthmus and ampulla produced much more PGE and PGF in the proliferative phase than in normal controls (Nabekura et al 1994). This along with the significant increase in the amount of prostaglandins released by peritoneal macrophages might alter uterine and tubal contractility, thereby affecting fertility (Karck et al 1996). Prostaglandins released by the ectopic implants do not synchronise with their release by the uterus and are produced at the wrong time sending the wrong message. For instance, there is a normal surge in prostaglandin F production at the end of the menstrual cycle, causing the corpus luteum of the ovary to die down and signaling the start of a new menstrual cycle. The implants of endometriosis produce their own prostaglandin surge several days after that produced by the womb lining. This may be one of the main causes of very early miscarriage. If a woman is a few days pregnant, then the endometriosis implants producing prostaglandin F would incorrectly signal the ovary to start a new menstrual cycle, causing the womb lining with the implanted egg to be expelled and the consequence is an early miscarriage. Increased prostaglandins can also produce an altered immune response or a luteal phase defect and thus produce rejection of the implanted embryo.

It has been postulated that one of the reasons for infertility in women with endometriosis may involve the increased number of activated macrophages and their ability to interfere with sperm–egg interaction, causing a significant decrease in ovum penetration (Chacho et al 1986). Also, peritoneal fluid from infertile women with endometriosis has been shown to immobilise spermatozoa in minutes or hours (Dorez et al 1985). Thus, it appears that the factors involved in the pathophysiology of endometriosis are probably multiple and interrelated and prostaglandins play an important role in the disease process.

PROSTAGLANDINS AND GYNECOLOGICAL MALIGNANCIES

Cyclo-oxygenases (COX-1 and COX-2) catalyse the conversion of arachidonic acid to prostaglandins. Prior to the discovery of cyclo-oxygenase-2 (COX-2), a beneficial association was shown between chronic usage of non steroidal anti-inflammatory drugs (NSAIDs), that non-selectively inhibit both cyclo-oxygenase-1 (COX-1) and COX-2, and the prevention of colorectal cancer.

Epithelial ovarian cancers: Increased COX-2 expression significantly correlated with histologic type (mucinous 5.6% vs. non-mucinous 65.2%), stage, tumour grade, residual disease status and the presence of ascitis. Survival was lower in patients with high COX-2 expression, although only tumour grade and stage were found to be independent prognostic indicators. But others have found COX-2 expression to be an independent prognostic factor in ovarian carcinoma. Expression of COX-2 also correlates well with expression of p53 and VEGF. In animal models, selective inhibition of COX-2 activity is associated with the enhanced radiation sensitivity of tumours without appreciably increasing the effects of radiation on normal tissue, and preclinical evidence suggests that the principal mechanism of radiation potentiation through selective COX-2 inhibition is the direct increase in cellular radiation sensitivity and the direct inhibition of tumour neovascularisation. Therapies that combine COX-2 inhibitors and radiation will need to enter randomised clinical trials (Choy and Milas 2003).

While overwhelming evidence suggests a role for COX-2 in epithelial ovarian cancers, the contribution of COX-1 remains much less explored. Prostacyclin PGI_2 is the major prostaglandin generated downstream of COX-1 in these cells, and SC-560, a COX-1-selective inhibitor, was found to dramatically inhibit PGI_2 production. Clinical studies testing the efficacy of COX inhibition as adjuvant therapy for ovarian cancer may see more beneficial effects with adjuvant therapy with either a COX-1 selective or nonselective cyclo-oxygenase inhibitor as compared with a COX-2 selective drug (Gupta et al 2003).

Endometrial cancer: There is an upregulation of COX-2 and PGE_2 in endometrial adenocarcinoma. PGE_2 may regulate neoplastic cell function in an autocrine/paracrine manner through the two subtypes of PGE_2 receptors, namely EP2 and EP4. Expression of EP2 and EP4 receptors was detected in adenocarcinomas from all grades of differentiation and was significantly higher than that detected in normal secretory phase endometrium (Sales et al 2002). Thus, COX-2 inhibitors have potential as therapeutic (and possibly, chemopreventive) agents for endometrial cancers that over express COX-2.

Cervical cancer: *In vitro* models have shown that COX-1 upregulation resulted in an induced expression of cyclo-oxygenase-2 (COX-2) and prostaglandin E synthase (PGES) concomitant with increased prostaglandin E(2)

TABLE 32.1: USE OF SYNTHETIC PROSTAGLANDINS
Synthetic prostaglandins are used:
To induce abortions and labour (PGE_2 or $PGF_{2\alpha}$, with mifepristone)
To prevent/treat postpartum hemorrhage
For cervical softening before gynecological procedures
To treat male erectile dysfunction
To close a patent ductus arteriosus in newborns
To prevent and treat peptic ulcers (PGE)
As a vasodilator in severe Raynaud's phenomenon or ischemia of a limb
In pulmonary hypertension

PGE_2 synthesis, which possibly acted in an autocrine/paracrine manner to enhance and sustain tumourogenesis in neoplastic cervical epithelial cells. The upregulation of COX-2, EP2 and EP4 expression and PGE_2 synthesis might be controlled in an autocrine/paracrine manner via the EP2/EP4 receptors (Sales et al 2001).

In cervical cancer, COX-2 was expressed in a greater proportion of adenocarcinoma of cervix (ADC) patients than in squamous cell carcinoma (SCC) patients. The overall positive expression of COX-2 and the quantity of PGs, especially PGE_2 in inflammation, CIN and cervical carcinoma was higher than in normal cervix. Therefore, testing the expression of PGs may be a prognosis marker for clinical diagnosis (Dai et al 2005).

Breast cancer: Markedly increased levels of cyclo-oxygenase-2 (COX-2) mRNA, protein and prostaglandin E(2) synthesis were detected in breast cancer tissues (Subbaramaiah et al 2002). The increased secretion of prostaglandins such as PGE_2 from constitutive COX-1 and inducible COX-2 isozymes present in epithelial and stromal cell compartments appear to result in both autocrine and paracrine actions to increase aromatase expression in the tissues, the increased aromatase activity (and subsequent increased estrogen biosynthesis) influencing breast cancer growth.

COX-2 expressed in the epithelial cell compartment regulates angiogenesis in the stromal tissues of the mammary gland. Microvessel density is increased before visible tumour growth and exponentially during tumour progression. Upregulation of COX-2 enzyme resulting in the accumulation of PGE_2 in a cancer cell environment is a marker for progression of breast cancer. COX-1 is detected in both metastatic and nonmetastatic tumours but only tumours resulting from the transplantation of metastatic cell lines express COX-2 in vivo. Thus, eventhough cell lines express both isoforms, the majority of the prostaglandin synthesis stems from the activity of the inducible, COX-2 isoform. Likewise, cell growth is inhibited by both indomethacin and the selective COX-2 inhibitor NS398 in a dose-dependent manner (Kundu et al 2001).

REFERENCES

Adelantado JM, MC Rees, A Lopez Bernal, AC Turnbull. 1988. Increased uterine prostaglandin E receptors in menorrhagic women. *Br J Obstet Gynaecol* 95(2):162–165.

Alfirevic Z. 2000. Oral misoprostol for induction of labour. *Cochrane Database Syst Rev.* (4): CD001338.

Anderson ABM, PJ Haynes, J Guillebaud, AC Turnbull. 1976. Reduction in menstrual blood loss by prostaglandin synthetase inhibitors. *Lancet* i:774–776

Ashok PW, Flett GM, Templeton A. 1998. Termination of pregnancy at 9–13 weeks' amenorrhoea with mifepristone and misoprostol. *Lancet* 353.542–543.

Breitbart V. 2000. Counseling for medical abortion. *Am J Obstet Gynaecol* 183:S26–S33.

Buhimschi CS, IA Buhimschi, S Patel, AM Malinow, CP Weiner. 2005. Rupture of the uterine scar during term labour: contractility or biochemistry? *Br J Obstet Gynaecol* 112(4):451–455.

Bulun SE, S Yang, Z Fang, B Gurates, M Tamura, S Sebastian. 2002. Estrogen production and metabolism in endometriosis. *Ann N Y Acad Sci*–955:75-85; Discussion 86-8, 396–406.

Cameron IT, AP Davenport, MJ Brown, SK Smith. 1991. Endothelin-1 stimulates prostaglandin F2 alpha release from human endometrium. *Prostaglandins Leukot Essent Fatty Acids* 42(3):155–157

Carlan SJ, S Bouldin, D Blust, WF O'Brien. 2001. Safety and efficacy of misoprostol orally and vaginally: A randomized trial *Obstet Gynecol* 98(5 Pt 1):875–876.

Chacho KJ, MS Chacho, PJ Andresen, A Scommegna. 1986. Peritoneal fluid in patients with and without endometriosis: Prostanoids and macrophages and their effect on the spermatozoa penetration assay. *Am J Obstet Gynecol* 154(6):1290–1299.

Choy H and L Milas. 2003. Enhancing radiotherapy with cyclo-oxygenase-2 enzyme inhibitors: A rational advance? *J Natl Cancer Inst* 95(19):1440–1452.

Colon I, K Clawson, K Hunter, ML Druzin, MM Taslimi. 2005. Prospective randomized clinical trial of inpatient cervical ripening with stepwise oral misoprostol vs vaginal misoprostol. *Am J Obstet Gynecol* 192 (3):747–752.

Crane JM and DC Young. 2003. Induction of labour with a favourable cervix and/or pre-labour rupture of membranes. *Best Pract Res Clin Obstet Gynaecol* 17(5):795–809.

Dai Y, X Zhang, Y Peng, Z Wang. 2005. The expression of cyclo-oxygenase-2, VEGF and PGs in CIN and cervical carcinoma. *Gynecol Oncol* 97(1):96–103.

Daskalakis GJ, SA Mesogitis, NE Papantoniou, GG Moulopoulos, AA Papapanagiotou, AJ Antsaklis. 2005. Misoprostol for second trimester pregnancy termination in women with prior caesarean section. *Br J Obstet Gynaecol* 112(1):97–99.

Dekker GA. 1995. The pharmacological prevention of pre-eclampsia. *Baillieres Clin Obstet Gynaecol* 9(3):509–528.

Dickinson JE. 2005. Misoprostol for second-trimester pregnancy termination in women with a prior cesarean delivery. *Obstet Gynecol* 105 (2):352–356.

Ding ZQ, J Rowe, B Ng, MJ Sinosich, ED Gallery. 2002. Modulation of prostacyclin and thromboxane secretion by cytotrophoblasts from normal and pre-eclamptic human pregnancies *Placenta* 23(8-9): 594–599.

Dorez F, P Wahl, F Bajolle, C Quereux. 1985. Immobilization of spermatozoa by peritoneal fluid in sterile women. Preliminary results. *J Gynecol Obstet Biol Reprod* 14(3):295–299.

Ellertson C, B Elul, S Ambardekar, L Wood, J Carroll, K Coyaji. 2000. Accuracy of assessment of pregnancy duration by women seeking early abortions. *Lancet* 355(9207):877–911.

Fisher SA, VP Mackenzie, GA Davies. 2001. Oral versus vaginal misoprostol for induction of labor: A double-blind randomized controlled trial. *Am J Obstet Gynecol* 185(4):906–910.

Fraser IS and G McGarron. 1991. Randomized trial of 2 hormonal 2 prostaglandin inhibiting agents in women with a complaint of menorrhagia. *Aus NZ Obstet Gynaecol* 31:66–70.

Gonzalez JA, SJ Carlan, MW Alverson. 2001. Outpatient second trimester pregnancy termination. *Contraception* 63(2):89–93.

Gronlund A, L Gronlund, L Clevin et al. 2002. Management of missed abortion: Comparison of medical treatment with either mifepristone+misoprostol or mosoprostol alone with surgical evacuation. A multi-center trial in Copenhagen County, Denmark. *Acta Obstet Gynaecol* 42(2): 161–163.

Gülmezoglu AM, F Forna, J Villar, GJ Hofmeyr. 2004. Prostaglandins for prevention of postpartum hemorrhage. *The Cochrane Database of Systematic Reviews* Issue 1. Art. No.: CD000494.pub2. DOI: 10.1002/14651858.CD000494.pub2.

Gupta RA, LV Tejada, BJ Tong, SK Das, JD Morrow, SK Dey, RN DuBois. 2003. Cyclo-oxygenase-1 is overexpressed and promotes angiogenic growth factor production in ovarian cancer. *Cancer Res* 63(5):906–911.

Hofmeyr GJ, AM Gulmezoglu, Z Alfirevic. 2000. Misoprostol for induction of labour: A systematic review *Br J Obstet Gynaecol* 107 (4):576–577.

Hofmeyr GJ, AM Gulmezoglu. 2001. Vaginal misoprostol for cervical ripening and induction of labour. *Cochrane Database Syst Rev* (3):CD000941.

Kahn JG, BJ Becker, L MacIssa, JK Amory, J Neuhas, J Olkin, MD Creinin. 2000. The efficacy of medical abortion: a meta-analysis. *Contraception* 61(1):29–40.

Karck U, F Reister, W Schafer, HP Zahradnik, M Breckwoldt. 1996. PGE2 and PGF2 alpha release by human peritoneal macrophages in endometriosis. *Prostaglandins* 51(1):49–60.

Kayani SI and Z Alfirevic. 2005. Uterine rupture after induction of labour in women with previous caesarean section. *Br J Obstet Gyneacol* 112 (4):528.

Kelly AJ, J Kavanagh, J Thomas. 2003. Vaginal prostaglandin (PGE2 and PGF2a) for induction of labour at term. *Cochrane Database Syst Rev.* 3:(4):CD003101.

Klockenbusch W and W Rath. 2002. Prevention of pre-eclampsia by low-dose acetylsalicylic acid--A critical appraisal Z *Geburtshilfe Neonatol* 206(4):125–130.

Krofta L, P Calda, Z Zikka, H Hruskova, J Kapras. 1998. Termination of pregnancy in the second trimester using intraamniotic administration of prostaglandins. *Ceska Gynaecol* 63(5):414–417.

Kulier R, AM Gulmezoglu, GJ Hofmeyr, LN Cheng, A Campana. 2004. Medical methods for first trimester abortion. *Cochrane Database Syst Rev* (1):CD002855.

Kundu N, Q Yang, R Dorsey, AM Fulton. 2001. Increased cyclo-oxygenase-2 (cox-2) expression and activity in a murine model of metastatic breast cancer. *Int J Cancer* 93(5):681–686.

le Roux PA, JO Olarogun, J Penny, J Anthony. 2002. Oral and vaginal misoprostol compared with dinoprostone for induction of labor: a randomized controlled trial. *Obstet Gynecol* 99 (2):, 201–205.

Lipitz S, D Grisaru, A Libshiz, Z Rotstein, E Schiff, A Lidor, R Achiron. 1997. Intraamniotic prostaglandinF_2 alpha for pregnancy termination in the second and early third trimester of pregnancy, *J Reprod Med* 42(4):235–238

Locatelli A, AL Regalia, A Ghidini, E Ciriello, A Biffi, JC Pezzullo. 2004. Risks of induction of labour in women with a uterine scar from previous low transverse caesarean section. *Br J Obstet Gynaecol* 111(12):1394–1399.

Lokugamage AU, SF Forsyth, KR Sullivan, H El Refaey, CH Rodeck. 2003. Dinoprostone versus misoprostol: A randomized study of nulliparous women undergoing induction of labor. *Acta Obstet Gynecol Scand* 82 (2):133–137.

Meydanli MM, E Caliskan, F Burak, MA Narin, R Atmaca. 2003. Labor induction post-term with 25 µg.rams vs. 50 µg.rams of intravaginal misoprostol. *Int J Gynaecol Obstet* 81(3):249–255.

Meyer M, J Pflum, D Howard. 2005. Outpatient misoprostol compared with dinoprostone gel for preinduction cervical ripening: A randomized controlled trial. *Obstet Gynecol* 105(3):466–472.

Mills JL, R DerSimonian, E Raymond, JD Morrow, LJ Roberts II, JD Clemens, JC Hauth, P Catalano, B Sibai, LB Curet, RJ Levine. 1999. Prostacyclin and thromboxane changes predating clinical onset of preeclampsia: A multicenter prospective study. *JAMA* 282(4):356–362.

Munthali J and J Moodley. 2001. The use of misoprostol for mid-trimester therapeutic termination of pregnancy. *Trop Doct* 31(3):157–161.

Nabekura H, H Koike, T Ohtsuka, M Yamaguchi, Miyakawa I, Mori N. 1994. Fallopian tube prostaglandin production with and without endometriosis. *Int J Fertil Menopausal Stud*39 (1):57–63.

Ngai SW, OS Tang, PC Ho. 2003. Prostaglandins for induction of second-trimester termination and intrauterine death. *Best Pract Res Clin Obstet Gynaecol* 17(5):765–775.

Orioli IM and EE Catilla. 2000. Epidemiological assessment of misoprostol teratogenecity. *Br J Obstet Gynaecol* 107 (4):519–523.

Paungmora N, Y Herabutya, P O-Prasertsawat, P Punyavachira. 2004. Comparison of oral and vaginal misoprostol for induction of labor at term: A randomized controlled trial *J Obstet Gynaecol Res* (5):358–362.

Pongsatha S, T Tongsong, O Suwannawut. Y Herabutya, B Chanrachakul, P Punyavachira. 2005. A randomized controlled trial of 6 and 12 hourly administration of vaginal misoprostol for second trimester pregnancy termination. *Br J Obstet Gynaecol* 112(9):1297–1301.

Pungetti D, M Lenzi, D Travisani, D Cantiero, G Maurizio, G Sarti, E Zanardi, P Andreone, M Baraldini, G Gasbarrini. 1987. Prostanoids in peritoneal fluid of infertile women with pelvic endometriosis and PID. *Acta Eur Fertil* 18(3):189–192.

Ramsey PS, DY Harris, PL Ogburn Jr, RH Heise, PM Magtibay, KD Ramin. 2003. Comparative efficacy and cost of the prostaglandin analogs dinoprostone and misoprostol as labor preinduction agents. *Am J Obstet Gynecol* 188(2):560–565.

Saareks V, P Ylitalo, I Mucha, A Riutta. 2002. Opposite effects of nicotinic acid and pyridoxine on systemic prostacyclin, thromboxane and leukotriene production in man. *Pharmacol Toxicol* 90 (6): 338–342.

Sales KJ, AA Katz, M Davis, S Hinz, RP Soeters, MD Hofmeyr, RP Millar, HN Jabbour. 2001. Cyclo-oxygenase-2 expression and prostaglandin E(2) synthesis are up-regulated in carcinomas of the cervix: A possible autocrine/paracrine regulation of neoplastic cell function via EP2/EP4 receptors *J Clin Endocrinol Metab* 86(5):2243–2249.

Sales KJ, AA Katz, B Howard, RP Soeters, RP Millar, HN Jabbour. 2002. Cyclo-oxygenase-1 is up-regulated in cervical carcinomas: Autocrine/paracrine regulation of cyclo-oxygenase-2, prostaglandin e receptors, and angiogenic factors by cyclo-oxygenase-1. *Cancer Res*15;62(2):424–432.

Sanchez-Ramos L. 2005. Induction of labor. *Obstet Gynecol Clin North Am* 32(2):181–200.

Shannon CS, B Winikoff, R Hausknecht, E Schaff, PD Blumenthal, D Oyer, H Sankey, J Wolff,

R Goldberg. 2005. Multicenter trial of a simplified mifepristone medical abortion regimen. *Obstet Gynecol*105(2):345–351

Shetty A, K Stewart, G Stewart, P Rice, P Danielian, A Templeton. 2002. Active management of term prelabour rupture of membranes with oral misoprostol. *Br J Obstet Gynaecol* 109(12):1354–1358.

Shetty A, I Livingstone, S Acharya, P Rice, P Danielian, A Templeton. 2003. Oral misoprostol (100 ugm.) versus vaginal misoprostol (25 μg) in term labor induction: A randomized comparison. *Acta Obstet Gynecol Scand* 82 (12):1103–1106.

Subbaramaiah K, L Norton, W Gerald, AJ Dannenberg. 2002. Cyclo-oxygenase-2 is overexpressed in HER-2/neu-positive breast cancer: Evidence for involvement of AP-1 and PEA3. *J Biol Chem* 277(21):18649–18657. Epub 2002 Mar

Subtil D, P Goeusse, F Puech, P Lequien, S Biausque, G Breart, S Uzan, P Marquis, D Parmentier, A Churlet. 2003. Essai Regional Aspirine Mere-Enfant (ERASME) Collaborative Group Aspirin (100 mg) used for prevention of pre-eclampsia in nulliparous women: The Essai Regional Aspirine Mere-Enfant study (Part 1). *Br J Obstet Gynaecol* 110 (5):475–484.

Tang OS, WN Lau, CC Chan, PC Ho. 2004. A prospective randomized comparison of sublingual and vaginal misoprostol in second trimester termination of pregnancy. *Br J Obstet Gyneacol* 111(9):1001–1005.

Telfer JF, F Lyall, JE Norman, IT Cameron. 1995. Identification of nitric oxide sythetase in the human uterus. *Human Reprod* 10(1):19–23.

The Perinatal Antiplatelet Review of International Studies (PARIS) Collaboration Steering Group on behalf of the PARIS Collaboration; The PARIS Collaboration. 2005. Antiplatelet agents for prevention of pre-eclampsia and its consequences: A systematic review and individual patient data meta-analysis. *BMC Pregnancy Childbirth*5 (1):7.

Vainio M, A Riutta, AM Koivisto, J Maenpaa. 2005. Prostacyclin, Thromboxane A2, and the Effect of Low-Dose ASA in Pregnancies at High Risk for Hypertensive Disorders. *Obstet Gynecol Surv* 60(5):281–282.

Walsh SW. 1998. Maternal-placental interactions of oxidative stress and antioxidants in preeclampsia. *Semin Reprod Endocrinol* 16 (1):93–104.

Walsh SW. 2004. Eicosanoids in preeclampsia. *Prostaglandins Leukot Essent Fatty Acids*. 70 (2):223–232.

Wing DA, C Guberman, M Fassett. 2005. A randomized comparison of oral mifepristone to intravenous oxytocin for labor induction in women with prelabour rupture of membranes beyond 36 weeks' gestation. *Am J Obstet Gynecol* 192 (2):445–451.

Wing DA, MR Park, RH Paul. 2000. A randomized comparison of oral and intravaginal misoprostol for labor induction. *Obstet Gynecol* 95 (6 Pt 1):905–908.

Wong KS, CS Ngai, EL Yeo, LC Tang, PC Ho. 2001. A comparison of two regimens of intravaginal misoprostol for termination of second trimester pregnancy: A randomized comparative trial. *Hum Reprod* 16(2):393

Wu MH, HS Sun, CC Lin, KY Hsiao, PC Chuang, HA Pan, SJ Tsai. 2002. Distinct mechanisms regulate cyclooxygenase-1 and -2 in peritoneal macrophages of women with and without endometriosis. *Mol Hum Reprod* 8 (12):1103–1110.

33

Genetics in Infertility and Prenatal Diagnosis

Mandakini Pradhan

Prenatal diagnosis refers to the detection of a structural, chromosomal or genetic abnormality in the fetus before birth. The potential benefits of prenatal diagnosis include providing

a. Reassurance to 'at risk' families when the results are normal
b. Risk information to couples for whom termination of an affected pregnancy is an option
c. Risk information to couples who would not have a child without such assurance
d. To couples to prepare for the birth of an affected child and
e. Allowing the medical provider to plan for the delivery and postnatal care of an affected infant.

The detection of an abnormality before birth has several medical, legal and ethical implications. From the medical perspective, it offers several management options such as termination of pregnancy, intrauterine treatment and optimising delivery and postnatal care. Although terms like 'prenatal diagnosis' and 'prenatal screening' are sometimes used interchangeably, these have different meanings.

Prenatal screening is defined as the methods to identify a couple at risk of having a baby with chromosomal, metabolic or single gene disorder. It does not diagnose the condition in the fetus per se. A couple found to be at higher risk after prenatal screening may opt for a prenatal diagnosis which diagnoses the condition in the fetus with certainty. For example, maternal serum screening in a young woman in the first trimester (that is, PAPP-A and β-hCG) may indicate a higher risk of the fetus having chromosomal aneuploidy which can be confirmed by doing chromosomal analysis of the fetus after obtaining fetal tissue by invasive methods like chorionic villous sampling, amniocentesis or cordocentesis.

This chapter aims to cover indications, techniques and pitfalls of prenatal screening, prenatal diagnosis methods, ethical issues involved and recent advances.

Candidates for prenatal diagnosis: The frequency of chromosomal abnormalities differs in different situations (Table 33.1). Similarly, the incidence of single gene disorder differs in different populations and ethnic groups. For example, cystic fibrosis is more common in Ashkenazi Jews, and Beta thalassemia in Mediterranean countries. To diagnose single gene disorder in the fetus, it is essential to obtain fetal tissues in 'at risk' pregnant women, whereas to diagnose chromosomal abnormalities, a pregnant woman can be screened and offered prenatal testing only if she is found to be at higher risk.

Table 33.1: Frequency of chromosome anomalies

Live births	0.6%
Mentally retarded, institutionalised	12%
Mentally retarded with congenital anomalies	23%
First trimester pregnancy losses	50%
Second trimester pregnancy losses	15%–20%
Third trimester pregnancy loss (stillbirth)	6%
Major fetal malformation (USG)	35%
Prenatal diagnosis for maternal age ≥35 years	1%–3%

Table 33.2: Screening tools to detect pregnancies at high risk of fetal genetic disorders

Maternal age
Family history of genetic disorder
Maternal serum screening
Screening for common genetic disorders such as hemoglobinopathies
Ultrasound

Invasive procedures such as chorionic villous sampling and amniocentesis cannot be offered at every pregnancy, as the risks of such procedures far outweigh the benefits in most of them. The use of prenatal screening methods enables detection of pregnancies with high risk of diagnosable fetal disorders.

Prenatal screening: Prenatal screening implies routine evaluation for the presence or absence of a given condition in apparently normal individuals. Table 33.2 lists the screening tools which should be used in every pregnancy.

a. Maternal age: The risk of chromosomal abnormality increases with advancing maternal age (Table 33.3). Every singleton pregnant woman, 35 years or more at the time of delivery; should be offered antenatal cytogenetic studies. A cut-off point of 35 has been chosen as the risk from invasive tests is supposed to be equal to the risk of a positive result at this age. With the use of maternal age alone as a screening tool, up to 30% of pregnancies affected with Down syndrome can be detected.

Table 33.3: Maternal age and risk of autosomal trisomy

Maternal age	*Risk at amniocentesis*	*Risk at birth*
20	1:1000	1:1000
25	1:900	1:1350
30	1:600	1:900
35	1:250	1:380
40	1:75	1:100
45	1:20	1:25

b. Genetic history: An obstetrician must attempt to determine whether a couple or anyone in their family has a heritable disorder or is at risk of having an abnormal offspring. A systematic genetic history should be taken in every pregnancy. Table 33.4 provides a questionnaire for eliciting genetic history. Family history of a known genetic disease warrants risk assessment in the couple and the provision of prenatal diagnosis. A detailed obstetric history should be obtained and the presence of adverse perinatal outcome such as recurrent spontaneous abortions, stillbirths and anomalous infants should prompt cytogenetic evaluation of the couples for the presence of balanced chromosomal translocations.

c. Maternal serum screening: During pregnancy, critical biochemical markers in

TABLE 33.4: A SAMPLE QUESTIONNAIRE FOR GENETIC HISTORY

Section 1. Patient Information

Name Date of Birth Occupation
Address
Phone number:
Referring Physician's Name Phone Number

Section 2. Information about the husband

Name Date of Birth Occupation

Section 3. Have you, your husband or anyone in your families ever had the following conditions?

	Yes	No		Yes	No
Down syndrome			Polycystic kidney disease		
Other chromosome problems			Huntington disease		
Mental retardation or autism			Heart defect at birth		
Spina bifida (open spine)			Cleft lip/cleft palate		
Anencephaly (opening in head/brain)			Blindness/deafness.		
Blood disorder, such as hemophilia or sickle cell . .			Baby who died after birth or within the first year . . .		
Muscular dystrophy or neuromuscular disease . . .			Stillborn or two or more pregnancy losses		
Neurofibromatosis.			Any birth defect not listed above		
Thalassemia			Any other inherited (genetic) condition		
Skeletal disorder, like dwarfism			Any other serious medical condition or surgery		

Are you and your partner related to each other, other than by marriage?. . . . .
Is there a history of infertility in you and/or your partner?. . . . .
Please specify the cause of infertility, if known . . . .
Have you and/or your partner had carrier testing for beta thalassemia?. . . . .
Have you and/or your partner had carrier testing for any other genetic disorder?. . . . .
Have you and/or your partner had blood chromosome testing? . . . .

Section 5. Please complete the following patient information:

Do you have diabetes, PKU or lupus? . . . . Yes/ No
Current medications . . . .
Please list: Are you considering or have you used: Yes/no
Recreational drugs . . . .
Alcoholic drinks. . . . .
Cigarette smoking. . . . .

Section 6. If you are currently pregnant, have you had any of the following?

Due Date: . . . .

Yes/No

1. Rashes, infections, fever . . . .
2. Have you had maternal serum screening? . . . . .

(such as AFP blood screen, triple marker screen, first trimester screen) spotting, bleeding or any other complications . . .

3. Exposure to x-rays

I have answered these questions to the best of my knowledge.

Patient's signature **Date**

combination with ultrasound can be used to provide a statistical risk assessment for fetal chromosomal anomalies, like Down syndrome (trisomy 21), Edward syndrome (trisomy 18) and for nonchromosomal anomalies such as Neural tube defect (Ager and Oliver 1987; Haddow et al 1992; Phillips et al 1992). Determining the risk of these disorders is dependent on many factors including maternal age, weight, gestational period, number of fetuses and requires relating this information to the concentration of certain hormones as measured against their gestational age specific median that is, expressed as multiples of median or MoM. The objective of a screening test is to maximise detection at an acceptable false-positive rate. Maternal serum screening tests, expressed as MoMs are used in combination

TABLE 33.5: CAUSES OF ABNORMAL MSAFP

Increased:
- Incorrect gestational age
- Threatened abortion or fetal death in utero
- Decreased maternal weight
- Multiple pregnancy (twin gestation)
- Fetal malformations

1. Neural tube defect
   - Anencephaly
   - Open spina bifida
2. Sacrococcygeal teratoma
3. Exomphalos
4. Gastroschisis
5. Cystic hygroma
6. Placental abnormalities
7. Renal abnormalities
   - Polycystic kidney or absent kidney
   - Urinary obstruction
   - Congenital Nephrosis

Decreased :
1. Incorrect gestational age
2. Trisomy 21 (Down syndrome)
3. Trisomy 18 (Edward syndrome)
4. Hydatiform mole
5. Increased maternal weight

to calculate likelihood ratios from normal and affected distributions. Combined with the pregnant woman's age-related risk, they estimate the risk of her fetus being affected.

The hormones tested are:

Alpha fetoprotein (AFP): AFP is the major globulin in fetal serum produced by the yolk sac, gastrointestinal tract and liver of the fetus.

- Normal level of AFP in non-pregnant female is ≤10 ng/ml.
- Maternal serum AFP level rises steadily and peaks in the third trimester.
- There are a number of conditions associated with high or low MSAFP concentrations (table 33.5).
- In the absence of diagnosable causes, elevated MSAFP concentrations have also been associated with adverse pregnancy outcomes such as low birth weight and stillbirth, pregnancies in which concentrations are elevated may be monitored more closely than those with normal concentrations (Hsieh et al 1997).

Human chorionic gonadotrophin (hCG): hCG is a glycoprotein produced exclusively by syncytiotrophoblast cells of the placenta.

- Normal levels in non-pregnant women are ≤5 mIU/ml.
- Maternal serum hCG peaks at 8–10 weeks and then slowly declines.
- An increased hCG level appears to be the most sensitive marker for detecting trisomy 21.

Uncongugated Estriol (uE_3): Although placenta is the source of estriol, this hormone reflects fetal steroidogenesis. Unlike total estriol, unconjugated estriol is produced almost entirely by the fetal–placental unit and is, therefore, a more sensitive indicator of fetal condition.

- Maternal serum unconjugated estriol level increases as the fetus develops and reaches 15 ng/ml at term.

Pregnancy-associated plasma protein A (PAPP-A): This is a glycoprotein produced by trophoblast.

- Maternal serum PAPP-A levels are detectable as early as eight weeks of gestation, the levels then rise throughout pregnancy.
- PAPP-A is a screening marker for Down syndrome pregnancy and has the advantage of being used in the first trimester.
- Maternal serum PAPP-A levels, when measured between 8 and 13 weeks of gestation are significantly reduced.
- Interestingly, maternal serum PAPP-A levels return to normal value between 17 and 19 weeks of gestation even in Down syndrome pregnancies.

Free β-subunit hCG: A glycoprotein secreted by placental trophoblast and can be detectable after 10 post-fertilisation days. Initially, it doubles every 1.5–2 days and peaks at 8–10 weeks.

- Maternal free β-hCG levels are elevated in Down syndrome pregnancies and it is used for first trimester serum screening marker.

First trimester maternal serum screening: The first trimester maternal screening test includes maternal age, serum screening like PAPP-A and free β-hCG and ultrasound demonstration of fetal nasal bone and nuchal translucency measurement (Wapner et al 2003). It is done at 11–14 weeks of gestation. First trimester screening has the advantage of a higher detection rate of fetal Down syndrome (Table 33.7). A negative result can reduce maternal anxiety earlier in the pregnancy, positive results can lead to earlier diagnosis and when pregnancy termination is elected, there is more privacy and reduced maternal morbidity.

Second trimester maternal serum screening: After the advent of MSAFP screening for NTDs, it was recognised that low second trimester MSAFP concentrations were associated with an increased risk of Down syndrome. Since that time, additional serum markers that increase the detection rate for Down syndrome have been identified. At 16–18 weeks gestation, MSAFP and unconjugated estriol (uE_3) levels tend to be lower in Down syndrome pregnancies than in normal pregnancies, whereas the level of maternal serum human chorionic gonadotrophin (hCG) is usually elevated. When second trimester MSAFP testing is combined with the measurement of β-hCG and uE_3, these three proteins constitute the 'triple screen' for fetal aneuploidy. None of these parameters gives absolute discrimination, but taken together they provide a means of modifying a woman's prior age-related risk to give an overall probability that the fetus is affected. When this probability exceeds 1 in 250, invasive testing in the form of amniocentesis or chorionic villous sampling is done to confirm or exclude fetal aneuploidy.

The triple test will also detect approximately 50% cases of trisomy 18. In this condition, all the three parameters are low (table 33.6).

Using age alone as a screening parameter, if all pregnant women aged 35 years and over opt for fetal chromosome analysis, approximately 35% of all Down syndrome pregnancies will be detected. If the aforementioned three biochemical markers are also included, 60% of all Down syndrome pregnancies will be detected. It has been found that another biochemical marker, inhibin-A, is also increased in maternal serum in Down

Table 33.6: Levels of the triple screen parameters in different conditions

Condition	*MSAFP*	*uE*	HCG
Neural tube defect	Increased	Normal	Normal
Trisomy 21	Low	Low	Increased
Trisomy 18	Low	Low	Low
Molar pregnancy	Low	Low	Very High
Multiple gestation	Increased	Normal	Increased
Fetal death (stillbirth)	Increased	Low	Low

Table 33.7: Detection rate of Down syndrome using different screening strategies

Screening test	*DR (%)*	*FPR (%)*
MA	30	5
MA +NT at 11–14 weeks	75	5
MA + NT + NB at 11–14 weeks	90	5
MA + NT + NB + PAPP-A + β hCG at 11–14 weeks	97	5
MA +PAPP-A + β hCG at 11–14 weeks	60	5
MA + Triple screening at 15–18 weeks	60–70	5
MA+ Quadruple screening at 15–18 weeks	75	5
USG for fetal defects and markers at 16–23 weeks	75	10–15

MA: Maternal age, NT: Nuchal translucency, NB: Nasal bone, DR: Detection rate, FPR: False positive rate

syndrome pregnancies. Some screening programmes have added inhibin A to the triple screen to improve the sensitivity and specificity of the test (quadruple test) (Wald et al 2003). Inclusion of inhibin A increases the detection rate from 60% to 75% (table 33.7)

d. Ultrasound: The use of routine ultrasound in pregnancy is controversial. However, it is common practice to offer a 'dating scan' at around 12 weeks of gestation. At this time, there is a strong association between chromosome abnormalities and the abnormal accumulation of fluid behind the baby's neck—increased fetal nuchal translucency (NT). This applies to Down syndrome, the other autosomal trisomy syndromes, that is, trisomy 13 and trisomy 18, Turner syndrome, triploidy, as well as a wide range of other fetal abnormalities and rare syndromes.

There appears to be a clear association between the absence of the fetal nasal bone (NB) on first trimester ultrasound examination and Down syndrome, especially in the high-risk group. Although there are conflicting reports on the use of NB as a screening tool in the general population, it is an independent marker and by combining information on maternal age with the results of fetal NT thickness measurements, together with maternal serum markers, it is possible to detect more than 90% of fetuses with trisomy 21 (Cicero et al 2005). In addition to increased nuchal translucency, important sonographic markers for chromosomal abnormalities include fetal growth restriction, tachycardia, abnormal flow in the ductus venosus, megacystis, exomphalos and single umbilical artery.

Apart from the dating scan, a detailed fetal anomaly scan is suggested for all pregnant women at 18 weeks. A large number of fetal malformations can be identified. Proper intervention can be taken depending upon the malformation identified. Ultrasound as a screening test is far less accurate with specificity as high as 99%, but sensitivity varies from 9%–85% depending upon the expertise of the operator, the machine and the organ system involved (Table 33.8).

Although chromosome abnormalities cannot be diagnosed directly, their presence can be suspected by the ultrasound detection of an abnormality such as exomphalos. The chromosomal abnormality is also suspected by the presence of 'soft markers' (Table 33.9).

Table 33.8: Sensitivity of ultrasound by type of anomaly (Grandjean et al 1999)

Anomaly	*Sensitivity (%)*
Central nervous system	88
Cardiovascular	28
Musculoskeletal	37
Urinary tract	88
Digestive system	54
Cleft lip and palate	18

E. Screening of common genetic disorders such as hemoglobinopathies:

Beta thalassemia is the most common single gene disorder in many countries, including India. It is a major public health problem. Approximately 300,000 children with thalassemia major are born each year worldwide (ACOG Bulletin 78). About 1

Table 33.9: Major and Minor Markers of Aneuploidy (Benacerraf et al 1992)

Organ System	*Major*	*Minor/Soft Markers*
CNS	Ventriculomegaly Holoprosencephaly Microcephaly Dysgenesis of corpus callosum Abnormal posterior fossa—Dandy Walker complex	Choroid plexus cyst
Musculoskeletal	Hand and feet anomalies—syndactyly, clinodactyly, clenched fist, radial ray aplasia, clubfoot and rocker-bottom foot	Short long bones
Face	Cleft palate and lips, micrognathia, macroglossia, hypo- and hypertelorism, low set ears, small ear	–
Neck	Cystic hygroma	Nuchal fold thickening
Cardiac	Endocardial cushion defect, ventricular septal defect, hypoplastic left heart syndrome, tetralogy of Fallot, and other complex cardiac anomalies	Echogenic focus within heart
Gastrointestinal tract	Esophageal and duodenal atresia, small bowel obstruction, diaphragmatic hernia and omphalocele	Echogenic bowel
Genitourinary tract	Moderate to severe hydronephrosis, dysplastic renal disease and renal agenesis	Mild pyelectasis
Others	Intrauterine growth retardation in second trimester, hydrops	Two-vessel cord, single umbilical artery

to 2 per 1000 couples, are at increased risk of having a child with thalassemia major. Since it is an autosomal recessive disorder, if both the partners are carriers of thalassemia minor (trait) the fetus in utero is at 25% risk of having thalassemia major. Screening for thalassemia minor is by red cell indices and hemoglobin electrophoresis. Indications of thalassemia minor are low MCV, low MCH with increased HbA2 (≥3.5%). Hemoglobin electrophoresis can also be detected from other abnormal structural hemoglobin variants like HbS, HbE etc. If a pregnant lady is found to be a carrier, her husband should be tested for the carrier status (or vice versa). If both of them are carriers, molecular studies to detect the status of the unborn child should be done.

Indications for prenatal diagnosis: After a thorough genetic history and results of screening tests, those pregnancies at high risk of fetus with abnormality can be identified. These pregnancies should be pursued further with more diagnostic tests depending upon the condition.

Indications for invasive tests can be broadly divided into three categories.

1. Indications for fetal chromosomal analysis: The most commonly cited reason for prenatal diagnosis is advanced maternal age, which is considered to be 35 years or older at the time of delivery. Amniocentesis or CVS is offered to such women because of the increased risk of aneuploidy. Other indications of fetal chromosomal analysis are

a. Abnormal maternal serum screen
b. Major or minor markers on ultrasound c. a chromosome abnormality in a previous offspring
d. One of the parents with balanced chromosomal translocation and
e. A previous offspring with multiple malformations in whom no chromosomal study was obtained. Amniotic fluid, chorionic villi and cord blood can be used to do the fetal chromosomal analysis; but amniotic fluid is used widely (ACOG Bulletin 2007).

2. Indications for biochemical studies: Biochemical studies are undertaken most often when a known abnormality is present in a family and the disorder can be diagnosed by a specific biochemical test. The number of biochemical disorders that can be diagnosed prenatally is growing rapidly, so that many common inborn errors of metabolism can be diagnosed through biochemical testing for enzyme deficiency or an abnormal metabolite. Conditions such as Tay-Sachs disease, mucopolysaccharidoses and peroxisomal diseases may be diagnosed by biochemical tests on amniocytes, or chorionic villi. However, facilities for such advanced testing are at present very limited in our country.

3. Indications for molecular genetic studies: Similar to biochemical studies, molecular genetic studies are undertaken because there is a positive family history of a specific genetic disease or prenatal findings point to a possible single-gene disorder that can be diagnosed by molecular techniques. The list of available molecular genetic studies have grown considerably in the last several years, and many of the common single-gene disorders can be diagnosed rapidly and conclusively by molecular techniques. Examples of disorders that are diagnosed by molecular methods include β thalassemia, sickle cell disease, spinal muscular atrophy, fragile X syndrome, cystic fibrosis, Duchenne and Becker muscular dystrophy and hemophilia. In each case, it is important that the clinician first know the specific mutation that is being sought in the case of a positive family history.

TECHNIQUES OF PRENATAL DIAGNOSIS

1. Amniocentesis: Transabdominal amniocentesis is the most commonly used procedure for obtaining fetal cells that can be analysed for chromosomal, biochemical or molecular abnormalities. In addition, amniotic fluid can be analysed separately for α-fetoprotein and acetylcholinesterase concentrations associated with open NTDs. The procedure is most commonly performed at a gestational age of 15 to 18 weeks. Amniocentesis in the second trimester is associated with a low rate of complications and provides an accurate sample for analysis in more than 99% of cases. Fetal chromosome analysis is the most common laboratory study performed on samples obtained by amniocentesis. Results are usually available two to three weeks after the procedure. Fluorescence in situ hybridisation studies are performed for rapid detection of fetal aneuploidy or for microdeletion syndromes such as 22q11 deletions in fetuses with conotruncal heart defects. Risks of amniocentesis include fetal loss, chorioamnionitis, fetal injury and maternal Rh sensitisation, each of which is very uncommon. Amniocentesis is an outpatient procedure performed under ultrasonographic guidance, by putting a spinal needle of 20G which minimises the risk of direct fetal injury. Twenty millilitres of amniotic fluid is aspirated under aseptic precaution in plain syringes. The risk of fetal loss in most large series is less than 0.5%.To prevent Rh isoimmunisation, Rh immune globulin is administered at the time of the procedure to nonsensitised Rh-negative women.

2. Chorionic villous sampling (CVS): This is usually performed at 10 to 12 weeks gestational age. The procedure involves transcervical placement of a catheter or transabdominal placement of an 18G spinal needle, under ultrasonographic guidance, into the developing placenta. A sample of the chorionic villus is removed by aspiration with a 20 ml syringe containing 2–3 ml of culture media and producing a negative pressure. Once removed, the fetal villi are dissected from the maternal decidual tissue. Chromosomal, molecular and some biochemical studies can be performed on CVS samples. The advantage of CVS is earlier diagnosis. Earlier diagnosis provides additional time for counselling and decision-making, and in the circumstance in which termination of pregnancy is elected, termination can be performed more safely for the mother. The risk of fetal loss rate is 1%–2% in most series.

3. Fetal blood sampling: In some circumstances, it is desirable to obtain a sample of fetal blood. This technique, referred to as cordocentesis or percutaneous umbilical blood sampling, may be used to assess fetal blood disorders, fetal infections or isoimmunisation or may be used for rapid fetal karyotyping. It has also been used for fetal treatment such as transfusions. Percutaneous umbilical blood sampling is usually performed with a 20- or 25-gauge spinal needle inserted into the umbilical vein or artery, preferably near the insertion of the cord into the placenta. Fetal loss or spontaneous abortion is reported in approximately 1% to 2% of cases.

4. Fetoscopy: This involves visualisation of the fetus by means of an endoscope (Cullen et al 1990). Increasingly, this technique is being superseded by 3D and 4D ultrasound scanning, although occasionally, fetoscopy is still undertaken during the second trimester, to try to detect the presence of subtle structural abnormalities that would point to a serious underlying diagnosis. Fetoscopy has also been used to obtain samples of tissue from the fetus that can be analysed as a means of achieving the prenatal diagnosis of several rare disorders such as electron microscopy from skin biopsy for epidermolysis bullosa. Fetoscopy is associated with a 3% to 5% risk of miscarriage. Due to this relatively high risk, coupled with the increasing sensitivity of ultrasound scanning, fetoscopy is used only infrequently and in highly specialised prenatal diagnostic centers.

5. Fetal echocardiogaraphy: This option is considered when there is an increased risk of congenital heart disease because:

1. There is an extracardiac malformation identified by ultrasonographic examination
2. There has been prenatal exposure to a teratogenic agent
3. There is a family history of congenital heart defects, especially in a parent or sibling
4. A fetal chromosome abnormality or genetic disease associated with heart defects is suspected
5. A maternal disease associated with fetal structural heart defects, such as diabetes or phenylketonuria, or maternal disease associated with fetal cardiac arrhythmia, such as lupus erythematosus, has been identified
6. A cardiac defect is suspected by findings on routine ultrasonography or
7. A fetal arrhythmia has been detected on auscultation or examination (Copel et al 1987)

Fetal echocardiography is usually performed after 20 weeks of gestation.

Recent advances in prenatal diagnosis: Chromosomal analysis requires culture of amniocytes, which takes two to three weeks time. For quick results, chromosomal analysis was tried with uncultured cells. Fluorescence in situ hybridisation (FISH) can be done to check for a specific chromosomal abnormality in two to three days. To reduce parental anxiety, several DNA based techniques have been developed to detect aneuploidy and other chromosomal abnormalities like QF-PCR. These tests use DNA from uncultured cells and hence the results are rapidly available. These are quantitative PCR, multiplex ligation dependent probe amplification MLPA, and microarray based comparative genome hybridisation.

Cell free fetal DNA circulates in maternal plasma (Lo et al 1997). It is now being used to determine the fetal Rh D status in Rh negative pregnant women (Lo et al 1998). This DNA can also be used to diagnose or exclude fetal transmission of some inherited diseases.

Ethical issues: Nothing in medical science raises more ethical concerns and dilemma than prenatal diagnosis. For those situations in which a couple comes in for prenatal diagnosis because of a known genetic disorder running in their respective families, the situation is straightforward. However, the problem arises when a minor or uncertain abnormality is detected during routine testing. To avoid complexity, the following principles should be taken care of.

Informed consent: None of the prenatal diagnostic tests (screening or diagnostic) should be done without explaining it to the patient. The purpose of the test, possible results and the implications of the results should be clearly explained to the patient. There are no routine tests in prenatal diagnosis. It is necessary that the person ordering the test is informed about the test. Sometimes, a triple test is suggested but the practitioner may not be able to interpret it. Such instances only bring anxiety to the pregnant woman and her family.

Termination of pregnancy: This is the most controversial issue in prenatal diagnosis. While in the case of serious congenital malformation and a genetic disorder which is likely to result in a lifelong handicap, the termination of pregnancy seems a reasonable option, sometimes parents opt for termination even for a relatively mild abnormality such as surgically correctable heart disease. The issues of the rights of the mother, physician and the unborn baby arise here. This issue is very delicate and needs discussion.

Conclusion: Up until the early 1970s, prenatal diagnosis of congenital anomalies was primarily aimed at detecting chromosomal abnormalities by amniocentesis. Over the last two decades, prenatal diagnosis has greatly benefited from advances in ultrasound technology and our ability to detect more and more single gene disorders and microscopic and sub-microscopic chromosomal abnormalities. At present, invasive prenatal diagnosis continues to be the gold standard for pregnancy at higher risk for chromosomal anomaly or other genetic disease, with chorionic villous sampling being the procedure of choice for the first trimester; whereas mid-trimester amniocentesis continues to be the most common form of invasive procedure for prenatal diagnosis. Invasive techniques are restricted to subgroups of patients at risk of anomalies, for whom such time consuming procedures are believed to be cost effective and accounts for procedure related abortion risk. In a low risk population, prenatal diagnosis generally consists of a screening procedure which includes ultrasound and maternal serum biochemistry.

References

ACOG Committee on Obstetrics. 2007. Hemoglobinopathies in pregnancy. ACOG Practice Bulletin No. 78: *Obstet Gynecol* 109(1):229–237.

ACOG Practice Bulletin No. 88. 2007. Invasive prenatal testing for aneuploidy. *Obstet Gynaecol* 110(6):1459–1467.

Ager RP and RW Oliver. 1987. Screening for Down syndrome. *Lancet* 2(8558):566–567.

Benacerraf BR, D Neuberg, B Bromley, FD Frigoletto Jr. 1992. Sonographic scoring index for prenatal detection of chromosomal abnormalities. *J Ultrasound Med* 11(9):449–458.

Cicero S, K Spencer, K Avgidou, S Faiola, KH Nicolaides. 2005. Maternal serum biochemistry at 11–13(+6) weeks in relation to the presence or absence of the fetal nasal bone on ultrasonography in chromosomally abnormal fetuses: An updated analysis of integrated ultrasound and biochemical screening. *Prenat Diagn* 25(11):977–983.

Copel JA, G Pilu, J Green, JC Hobbins, CS Kleinman. 1987. Fetal echocardiographic screening for congenital heart disease: The importance of the four-chamber view. *Am J Obstet Gynecol* 157(3):648–655.

Cullen MT, EA Reece, J Whetham, JC Hobbins. 1990. Embryoscopy: Description and utility of a new technique. *Am J Obstet Gynecol*162(1):82–86.

Grandjean H, D Larroque, S Levi. 1999. The performance of routine ultrasonographic screening of pregnancies in the Eurofetus Study. *Am J Obstet Gynecol* 181:446–454.

Haddow JE, GE Palomaki, GJ Knight, J Williams, A Pulkkinen, JA Canick et al. 1992. Prenatal screening for Down's syndrome with use of maternal serum markers. *N Engl J Med* 327(9):588–593.

Hsieh TT, TH Hung, JJ Hsu, WY Shau, CW Su, FJ Hsieh. 1997. Prediction of adverse perinatal outcome by maternal serum screening for Down syndrome in an Asian population. *Obstet Gynecol* 89(6):937–940.

Lo YM, N Corbetta, PF Chamberlain, V Rai, IL Sargent, CW Redman, JS Wainscoat. 1997. Presence of fetal DNA in maternal plasma and serum. *Lancet* 350(9076):485–487.

Lo YM, NM Hjelm, C Fidler, IL Sargent, MF Murphy, PF Chamberlain, PM Poon, CW Redman, Wainscoat JS. 1998. Prenatal diagnosis of fetal RhD status by molecular analysis of maternal plasma. *N Engl J Med* 339(24):1734–1738.

Phillips OP, S Elias, LP Shulman, RN Andersen, CD Morgan, JL Simpson. 1992. Maternal serum screening for fetal Down syndrome in women less than 35 years of age using alpha-fetoprotein, hCG, and unconjugated estriol: A prospective 2-year study. *Obstet Gynecol* 80(3 Pt 1):353–358.

Wald NJ, WJ Huttly, AK Hackshaw. 2003. Antenatal screening for Down's syndrome with the quadruple test. *Lancot* 361(9360):835–836.

Wapner R, E Thom, JL Simpson, E Pergament, R Silver, K Filkins et al. 2003. First Trimester Maternal Serum Biochemistry and Fetal Nuchal Translucency Screening (BUN) Study Group: first-trimester screening for trisomies 21 and 18. *N Engl J Med* 349(15):1405–1413.

34

Induced Abortion

Rupinder Kaur Ruprai

The International Federation of Gynecology and Obstetrics (FIGO) Ethics Committee defines induced abortion as 'the termination of pregnancy using drugs or surgical intervention after implantation and before the conceptus has become independently viable' (Abortion Statistics, 2002). The World Health Organization (WHO) defines abortion as the termination of pregnancy before 22 weeks of gestation, when birth weight is approximately 500 g. The upper limit for induced abortion in India is 20 weeks. The term 'abortion' is used throughout this chapter to refer to the induced termination of an established pregnancy (after implantation). It does not include the use of emergency hormonal contraception. All current methods of emergency contraception work prior to implantation, and therefore are not abortifacients.

INDICATIONS FOR THERAPEUTIC ABORTION

Maternal indications for abortion

Pre-existing maternal disease

- Moderately severe cardiac disease in a woman who does not desire any/more children
- Severe degree of chronic hypertension, especially if associated with myocardial or renal damage
- Kidney disease with impaired renal function
- Pulmonary disease: pulmonary insufficiency (vital capacity of 1500 ml is necessary)
- Disease of GIT: impaired liver function, pancreatitis, ulcerative colitis
- Disease of CNS: intracranial aneurysm
- Psychiatric disorders: when caused or made worse by pregnancy
- Malignant disease
- Others: severe diabetes with retinopathy, sickle cell disease, autoimmune disease, metabolic disease

Diseases of pregnancy: Examples are, hyperemesis gravidarum, liver necrosis, bilateral uncontrollable pyelonephritis and pregnancy psychosis.

Fetal indications for abortion

- Fetal death
- Major fetal anomalies
- Genetically transmitted disease
- Inherited metabolic defect
- Viral disease:
  - o Rubella within the first three months of pregnancy can be lethal to the embryo.
  - o Chicken pox: exposure in the first three months can lead to significant anomalies, especially of the CNS.
- Exposure to heavy irradiation/noxious drugs in first trimester

THE MTP ACT

The MTP Act (Act No. 34 of 1971) is defined as 'an Act to provide for the termination of certain pregnancies by registered medical practitioners and for matters connected therewith or incidental thereto'. It was passed by Parliament on August 10, 1971, and implemented on April 1, 1972. Voluntarily 'causing miscarriage' to a woman with child, other than in 'good faith for the purpose of saving her life' is a crime, punishable by simple or rigorous imprisonment and/or fine.

When Pregnancies may be terminated:

Duration of Pregnancy: Pregnancies not exceeding 12 weeks may be terminated based on a single opinion formed in good faith, those beyond 12 weeks till 20 weeks require the opinion of two clinicians. Since use of medical methods governed by guidelines issued by the Drug Controller is presently up to 49 days, single clinical opinion is necessary and sufficient.

Grounds for termination

1. If pregnancy would involve a risk to life of the pregnant woman or of grave injury to her physical and mental health
   - Pregnancy alleged by the pregnant woman to have been caused by rape
   - Pregnancy resulting from failure of any device used by any married woman or her husband for the purpose of limiting children
2. If there is a substantial risk that the child, if born, would suffer physical or mental abnormalities as to be seriously handicapped.

It is important to note that the MTP Act does not permit induced abortions on demand. The responsibility rests with the medical practitioner to opine in good faith regarding the presence of a valid legal indication. These indications are also mandatory with medical methods.

Valid legal consent: The MTP Act mandates the presence of a valid informed legal consent for both medical and surgical methods, recorded in Form C recommended in Rule 8 of the MTP Rules.

1. In minors (under 18 years of age) or lunatics with consent of guardian, in writing.
2. In adult women, their valid consent alone is sufficient. An adult woman requires no other person's consent except her own.

Where pregnancies may be terminated:

1. A hospital established or maintained by the Government
2. A place approved for the purpose of the Act by the Government

The following facilities should be provided:

1. An OT table and instruments for abdominal and gynecological surgery.
2. Anesthetic, resuscitation and sterilisation equipment.
3. Drugs and parenteral fluids for emergency use.

By whom pregnancies may be terminated: It may be terminated by a person with the following qualifications and/ or experience

1. Postgraduate degree or diploma in gynecology and obstetrics
2. Hospital or medical establishment registered before commencement of the Act with over three years experience in the practice of obstetrics and gynecology
3. Registered after commencement of the Act if the person has
   - Six months of house surgeonship in gynecology and obstetrics

- Experience in any hospital of over one year in the field of gynecology and obstetrics
- Assisted in performing 25 MTP's in a government hospital or a recognised training institute

Documentation and records: All approved centres are required to maintain an Admission Register (MTP Register) which is a mandatory confidential document.

Amendment to the MTP Act 1971

- The word 'lunatic' is substituted by 'mentally ill person' defined as 'a person who is in need of treatment by reason of any mental disorder other than mental retardation'.
- No termination of pregnancy shall be made in accordance with this Act at any place other than a hospital established or maintained by Government, or a place for the time being approved by Government or by the Chief Medical Officer or District Health Officer.
- Termination of pregnancy by a person who is not a registered medical practitioner/ owner of a place which is not approved shall be punishable with imprisonment for a term not less than two to seven years.

PREABORTION CARE AND MANAGEMENT

Assessment before medical abortion includes: Ascertainment of the woman's desire for termination of pregnancy; evaluation for absolute or relative contraindications; assessment of gestational duration; Rh-status; pregnancy options counselling, physical examination, tests for sexually transmitted infections, hemoglobin level or other laboratory tests and contraception counselling may also be appropriate. Gestational age should be established. Ideally, an ultrasonography should be performed to confirm intrauterine gestation and its age.

Physical: A brief physical examination is usually conducted prior to an abortion procedure. The focus is on dating the pregnancy, ensuring the absence of other gynecologic pathology (particularly STI's). Active vaginal infection, if any, must be treated.

PATIENT SELECTION CRITERIA

Cases at risk for MTP include: known morbidity from prior procedure (for example, CS, or previous attempts at MTP), large fibroids, congenital anomaly of uterus, and period of gestation (POG) not known/uterine size disproportionate to POG.

Contraindications: Absolute contraindications are virtually unknown; the only absolute contraindication in India is abortion for sex selection. In the face of significant maternal risk of medical or psychiatric morbidity/mortality, continuation of pregnancy usually presents far greater risk than termination of pregnancy.

Medical abortion is contraindicated in patients with: Coagulopathy or concurrent anticoagulation (increased risk of hemorrhage), inherited porphyries (progesterone has been implicated in pathogenesis of acute attacks of porphyria; mifepristone could increase attacks), severe liver disease/renal disease, concurrent systemic corticosteroid use/adrenal failure (mifepristone has antiglucocorticoid effects), severe asthma, glaucoma, medical conditions or the use of medications that preclude use of abortion medications, misplaced IUD/IUD in place (strong uterine contractions against an IUD is a theoretical risk), undiagnosed adnexal masses/ectopic pregnancy, or known allergy to one of the medications (allergy to mifepristone or PG is extremely rare).

Relative Contraindications: Pregnancy with large fibroids distorting the endometrial cavity (can cause heavy bleeding and interfere with uterine contractility), pregnancy with valvular heart disease, unwilling to undergo a surgical abortion if required (continuing pregnancies are exposed to teratogens), severe anemia, poorly controlled bowel disease (PGs increase bowel motility and may cause diarrhea), significant cardiovascular/cerebrovascular disease (inappropriate for outpatient abortion; mifepristone, misoprostol, gemeprost and methotrexate have no known direct cardiovascular effects), uncontrolled seizure disorder (inappropriate for outpatient abortion and self-care), breastfeeding (no studies have addressed breastfeeding; both misoprostol and mifepristone are excreted in breast milk; mifepristone is undetectable after 11 days and misoprostol is cleared in less than two days (Meckstroth and Darney 2003). Surgical abortion is preferred if the patient desires concurrent tubal ligation.

Medical abortion should be performed with caution in patients with: Severe anemia, poorly controlled bowel disease (as it may cause an exacerbation of symptoms), complicated diabetes mellitus, concurrent anticoagulation, concurrent use of anti-tubercular drugs (decreases the efficacy of medical abortion pills), uterine scar (single/ multiple) of cesarean, hysterotomy or myomectomy: women with a scarred uterus from a prior cesarean section or other surgery. Bronchial asthma is not a contraindication as misoprostol is a weak bronchodilator.

Sulprostone is contraindicated in women over the age of 35 years who are obese, who smoke, or who have other cardiovascular risk factors, because the drug is associated with heart failure in such women (Ulmann et al 1992). These restrictions do not apply to gemeprost and misoprostol. Women given methotrexate should not take any medication containing folate, as it interferes with the action of methotrexate.

Instillation abortion techniques are contraindicated in patients with: Active pelvic infections, inability to tolerate a solute load (saline only), asthma, glaucoma, epilepsy, hypertensive cardiovascular disease, pulmonary hypertension ($PGF_{2\alpha}$) and fetal demise (saline, urea).

Surgical abortion is contraindicated in patients with: Hemodynamic instability, profound anemia, and/or profound thrombocytopenia, anesthetic contraindication, uncontrolled seizures, active genital herpes, large or symptomatic uterine fibroids, undiagnosed adnexal masses, ectopic pregnancy.

Multifetal reduction of pregnancy has inherent risks of rupture of membranes, preterm labour, preterm delivery, and infection, which must be balanced against the benefits of the procedure. Special circumstances, such as the selection of the presenting fetus for reduction, may present a greater risk of loss of the entire pregnancy and must be considered in the risk–benefit analysis.

Assessment of pregnancy and gestational age: When providing medical abortion, accurate dating of pregnancy is important to achieve the highest efficacy and to avoid complications.

Ancillary Technique: Ultrasound enables the accurate determination of gestational duration, as well as diagnosis of ectopic pregnancy, uterine myomas and hydatidiform moles, which may affect the outcome of medical abortion.

Blood Tests

- Pregnancy tests to confirm the pregnancy
- Hemoglobin concentration, to identify patients with significant anemia
- ABO and rhesus blood groups. Rh-negative women are given anti D to prevent Rh-sensitisation in subsequent pregnancies. It is not cost-effective routinely to cross-match women undergoing induced abortion, as only 0.2% of clients may require blood transfusion. When blood bank facilities are remote, availability of O-negative blood may be considered. In about 50% of women beyond 15 weeks of gestation, hemorrhage will be associated with disseminated intravascular coagulation (DIC) (RCOG, 2004)
- Screening for hemoglobinopathies, HIV, and hepatitis B and C, if indicated. HIV prevalence is up to three times higher in women seeking abortion
- In cases of methotrexate use, platelet count, electrolytes, liver function tests and blood urea nitrogen (BUN) and creatinine levels are required. Thrombocytopenia and chemical hepatitis are rare (in the doses used for medical abortion) but known complications of methotrexate use
- Electrolyte assays are necessary in patients who develop significant vomiting associated with the use of medical abortion techniques
- Platelets, coagulation studies, liver function tests and renal function tests are recommended as baseline testing for instillation methods because of the risk of coagulopathy, vomiting and diarrhea associated with this method

Genetic testing: In the case of an abnormal pregnancy, genetic testing may be done either preoperatively or at the time of the abortion procedure. At the time of the procedure, either the fetus or the placenta may be tested, but these tests have to be pre-arranged and may be expensive.

Cervical cytology: Women who have not had a cervical smear within the interval recommended may be offered one within the abortion service.

Ultrasound scanning: All services must have access to scanning, as it can be a necessary part of pre-abortion assessment, particularly where gestation is in doubt or where extra-uterine pregnancy is suspected. However, it is not an essential prerequisite.

CONSENT

Women must be furnished with written material that would outline alternatives to abortion and potential risks of the procedure and receive preabortion counselling. The MTP Act mandates the presence of a valid legal consent:

1. In minors (under 18 years of age) or lunatics with consent in writing of guardian
2. In adult women, their valid consent must be obtained

Rights of the spouse or partner: The decision to terminate a pregnancy rests with the woman and her doctors. Legally, the woman's spouse and/or the putative father of the child have no rights to demand or refuse a termination.

FIRST TRIMESTER ABORTION PROCEDURES

- Up to 9 weeks of gestation, pregnancy termination can be safely performed using vacuum aspiration (VA), or by using medications such as a combination of mifepristone and misoprostol or misoprostol alone, or in combination with mtx where mifepristone is not available. (Kulier et al 2004; Stubblefield et al 2004).

- At 9–12 weeks, both surgical and medical methods are safe, effective and acceptable.

MEDICAL METHODS OF INDUCED ABORTION IN FIRST TRIMESTER

Medical abortion has a success rate that ranges from 75%–95%, with approximately 2%–4% of failed abortions requiring surgical abortion and 5%–10% of incomplete abortions, depending on the stage of gestation and agents used. The process involves bleeding, often heavy, which must be differentiated from hemorrhage. Regardless of the amount of tissue passed, the patient must be seen for evaluation of completeness of the procedure. Blood transfusion rates with medical abortion are approximately 0.2% (Spitz et al 1998).

Antiprogestins (mifepristone: RU 486): Mifepristone binds to the progesterone receptor and blocks its action. It causes the trophoblast to separate from the decidua. An efficacy rate of 64%–85% when 200–600 mg of mifepristone alone is administrated at gestational age of 63 days or less is seen (Couzinet et al 1986). Mifepristone can also be used to trigger cervical softening and dilatation before surgical abortion. (Lefebvre et al 1990). Addition of low dose of PG improves its efficacy.

Prostaglandin analogues: Prostaglandins increase uterine activity and can be used by various routes for the expulsion of products of conception (POC). The success rate as assessed by complete abortion is relatively low with PG alone.

Misoprostol, a PGE_1 analogue, is the medication of choice for medical abortion. It has largely replaced PGE_2 and $PGF_{2\alpha}$ as it is equally effective, stable at room temperature, and less expensive with fewer gastrointestinal side effects. It is safer than other methods for medical abortion (Autry et al 2002).

- In early gestation: A single vaginal dose of 800 µg misoprostol is used
- In late first trimester: 800 µg misoprostol daily for three days is used

Routes and pharmacokinetics: Misoprostol is well absorbed after oral, sublingual, vaginal and rectal administration and is excreted in colostrum in low concentrations. The peak serum concentrations achieved are highest after sublingual administration compared to the oral, vaginal and rectal routes (Tang et al 2002a). Vaginal and sublingual routes are more effective and faster, with decreased ongoing pregnancy and fewer gastrointestinal side effects as compared to the oral route (Grimes, 1997).

- After oral administration, plasma concentration begins rising at two minutes, reaching peak serum level between 12.5–60 minutes and declining steeply to 12% of peak concentrations at 120 minutes. The decrease in serum concentrations by the second hour is seen in both the sublingual and the oral routes. This supports the rationale of misoprostol application at two hourly intervals. The typical effect of a single oral dose is an increase in uterine tonus. It is only following repeated doses that regular uterine contractions appear.
- The effect of sublingual administration is the same as in vaginal treatment and it is significantly more pronounced than after oral treatment.
- The buccal route is a safe alternative for administration for cervical ripening in first trimester and second trimester surgical abortions (Todd et al 2002).

Misoprostol is active with oral administration through seven weeks of pregnancy (Spitz et al 1998). Beyond that period of gestation, it remains effective only when administered vaginally at a dose of 800 μg when it results in a successful abortion rate of almost 99% and a complete abortion rate exceeding 90% (Ashok et al 1998a; Schaff et al 2000a).

Dose and timing of misoprostol

- Vaginal misoprostol 1, 2 or 3 days after mifepristone, has no difference in efficacy (Schaff et al 2000b)
- The incidence of side effects increases with the dose and is maximal at 600 μg. Because side effects increase with dose, the lowest effective dose for each route of administration is ideal

Misoprostol used alone has a success rate of 40–60% up to nine weeks (Koopersmith and Mishell Jr., 1996). Improved success is seen when tablets are moistened and placed vaginally. Up to three doses of 800 μg of misoprostol, placed vaginally after moistening achieves a success rates over 90% (800 μg vaginally, followed three hours later by a second dose of 800 μg vaginally).

Combination of mifepristone and PG analogues: The combined treatment of mifepristone and misoprostol is safe and effective for the termination of early first trimester pregnancy. During pregnancy, progesterone maintains the uterus in a quiescent state. When the action of progesterone is blocked from the pregnant uterus, the excitability of the myometrium increases, and the gap junctions between myometrial cells permit coordinated uterine contractions. Mifepristone also induces cervical ripening, probably due to an increase in endogenous PG (Baird, 2000). The resulting cervical ripening, uterine contractions and decidual necrosis lead to abortion.

Mifepristone alone achieves complete abortion in only 60%–80% of women, even with high doses. Continuing pregnancies after mifepristone alone range from 7%–40% (Kovacs et al 1984; Couzinet et al 1986). The success rate increases to 90%–98% (with failure rate of 0.3%–1.5%) if a PG (sulprostone 0.25–0.5 mg i.m., or gemeprost 1 mg vaginal pessary or misoprostol 800 μg vaginally) is administered 36–48 hours later to mifepristone (Christin-Maitre et al 2000). The interval between mifepristone and misoprostol administration can be shortened from two days to one day without loss of efficacy (Schaff et al 2000b).

Misoprostol alone vs. combination of mifepristone and mispostol: Misoprostol alone has a success rate of 88%, while a combination of 200 mg mifepristone and 800 μg vaginal, has a success rate of 95.7% (Jain et al 2002). The time taken to complete the abortion is slower, and additional doses of misoprostol are required more frequently with misoprostol alone.

Simultaneous 200 mg oral mifepristone and 800 μg vaginal misoprostol: This is a promising regimen for abortion up to nine weeks. The success rates appear higher in pregnancies up to seven weeks with a 24 hour expulsion rate of 90% and a complete abortion rate of 98% (Murthy et al 2005).

Mifepristone and misoprostol, both administered vaginally: Mifepristone administered vaginally bypasses hepatic first-pass (when the products of conception are expelled) effect and therefore should improve tissue bioavailability and response. However, complete abortion rate of 61% is lower than that with standard medical regimen (Sharma et al 2006).

Combination of methotrexate (MTX) and misoprostol: Methotrexate is effective when given in combination with misoprostol. Compared with mifepristone, it is slightly less effective, takes longer for abortion with a longer interval of bleeding. It may be used in countries where mifepristone is unavailable. However, it is not recommended for inducing abortion, because it increases the risk of fetal malformation in a future pregnancy (UNDP/UNFPA/WHO 1997; Yedlinsky et al 2005).

Oral or i.m. mtx followed 3–7 days later by vaginal 800 µg misoprostol has a success rate of 88%-97%. Efficacy is optimal if misoprostol is given seven days after mtx. (Grimes 1997). There is no difference in failure to achieve complete abortion when i.m. was compared with oral mtx. Combination of mtx 50 mg/m^2.m. on day one followed by 800 µg misoprostol vaginally on day 7, repeated if required on day 8, is safe and effective up to nine weeks. Complete abortion occurs in 93%–94% of cases (Creinin and Darney 1993; Carbonell et al 1998; Pai and Ruprai 2002).

Gestational Duration Limits

In early first trimester (Up to 9 weeks): Mifepristone plus PG is the most effective method of abortion at gestations of less than 7 weeks and continues to be appropriate for women in the 7–9 weeks band (Ashok et al 1998b; Schaff et al 2000a, 2002). It is less effective between 7–9 weeks when misoprostol is administered orally (Spitz et al 1998; Creinin et al 1999). A dose of 200 mg of mifepristone is appropriate.

In late first trimester (9–13 Weeks): The following is a safe, effective and acceptable alternative to surgical abortion between 9–13 weeks:

- Mifepristone, 200 mg orally followed, 36–48 hours later by misoprostol 800 µg vaginally. A maximum of four further doses of misoprostol 400 µg may be administered at three hourly intervals, vaginally or orally (depending on the amount of bleeding). The median induction interval with misoprostol is 5 hours, with a range of 2–28 hours. It results in a complete abortion of 95% (Gouk et al 1999).
- Mifepristone, 200 mg, followed by gemeprost 1 mg to a maximum of five doses at 9–12 weeks of gestation has a complete abortion rate of 96% (Vyjayanthi and Piskorowskyj 2002).

OUTLINE OF EVENTS FOR MEDICAL TERMINATION

Visit 1: Day 1

- Counselling and signing of informed consent
- Medical history and physical examination
- Blood samples taken for hemoglobin level and Rh-factor, RBS (if required)
- Pregnancy dating with ultrasound or hCG level if no gestational sac is seen
- Administer 50 µg Anti-D if patient is Rh-negative
- Administer mifepristone 200 mg orally
- Instruct on self care and clinic emergency contact information and schedule next visit

Visit 2: Day 3

- Use ultrasound to check if patient has aborted (6% may abort prior to misoprostol)
- Administer 2–4 misoprostol tablets for a total dose of 400–800 µg
- Observe patient for four hours (~50% will abort during this time period) after half an hour of rest
- Give a prescription for pain medication

- Instruct patient on self care for expectant cramping, bleeding and gastrointestinal side effects and schedule next visit

Visit 3: Day 15

- Confirm abortion by sonography or hCG level (> 50% decrease)
- Assess level of bleeding since last visit
- Advice contraception

VARIATIONS OF PROTOCOL

- Using a lower dose (200 mg) of oral mifepristone. More than 200 mg of mifepristone provides no additional benefit (Meckstroth and Darney 2003)
- Administering 800 µg of misoprostol vaginally instead of orally. Vaginal misoprostol is superior to oral, especially between 7–9 weeks gestation. Buccal and sublingual routes of administration of misoprostol are also promising
- Allowing the patient to use misoprostol at home on day 2, 3, or 4
- Following up sooner than 14 days

Patient instructions

- Patients are given instructions and an emergency telephone number to contact in case of questions or concerns. They are told to expect bleeding and cramps, especially after misoprostol is administered. The heaviest bleeding should stop 1–2 hours after passing the pregnancy (when the products of conception are expelled). The mean number of days of bleeding using mifepristone and misoprostol is 14 (Davis et al 2000) and 3–4 days following a surgical abortion
- Patients are instructed to take pain medication as needed for cramps
- Patients are instructed that up to nine weeks of gestation, usually only the placenta and blood are visible to the eye when the products of conception are expelled
- Before leaving the medical centre, all women should receive information on contraception and, if they so request, contraceptives or referral to contraceptive services should be done
- Instruct the patient that follow-up is important

PATIENT FOLLOW-UP

During the second visit, to receive misoprostol, patient should be asked about the symptoms of pregnancy, bleeding and cramping over the two days preceding the visit. Unless abortion is complete at this time, the patient is given a dose of misoprostol at this visit.

During the third visit, the patient is again asked about the symptoms and an ultrasound is done. If at this time the pregnancy has not been terminated successfully or is incomplete, either give another dose of misoprostol or proceed to surgical termination.

SURGICAL METHODS OF INDUCED ABORTION IN FIRST TRIMESTER

Selection of the surgical procedure primarily depends on gestational age. Options include:

- Menstrual regulation (up to 7 weeks)
- MTP
  - o Dilatation and Vacuum Aspiration (VA) (till 12 weeks)
  - o Electric VA (EVA)
  - o Manual Vacuum Aspiration (MVA)
  - o Dilatation and Evacuation (D and E)
  - o Combined method: priming cervix followed by either dilatation and EVA/ MVA or dilatation and evacuation (D and E)

Early (first trimester) abortions are best undertaken by MVA or EVA up to 12 weeks, or medical combination of oral mifepristone and vaginal or oral misoprostol, for up to 9 weeks. If aspiration or medical methods are unavailable, dilation and curettage (D and C) should be used. For pregnancies of over 12 weeks, preferred methods are D and E using VA and forceps, mifepristone followed by repeated doses of PG, or PG alone in repeated doses.

- At gestations below 7 weeks, conventional suction termination should be avoided as the failure rate is higher than for medical abortion and are three times more likely to fail than those between 7-12 weeks (Kaunitz et al 1985)
- At 7–15 weeks, conventional suction termination is appropriate, although the skills and experience of the practitioners may make medical abortion more appropriate at gestations above 12 weeks. Suction curettage is preferable to sharp curettage for surgical abortion (Kulier et al 2001). The risk of sharp curettage includes Asherman's syndrome and routine intra-operative ultrasound obviates the need for sharp curettage
- Between 10–12 weeks of gestation, WHO recommends VA. In many parts of the world, the main method used for up to 12 weeks is D and C. However, VA is associated with fewer complications and less pain than D and C and at present, there is general agreement that D and C should be replaced by VA (Greenslade et al 1993; WHO 2003)
- Between 10–14 weeks is the grey zone. Vacuum aspiration can be done but the risk of blood loss and trauma to the genital tract increases. Termination in this period may also be done by PG

CERVICAL PRIMING FOR SURGICAL ABORTION

Cervical priming is the most critical step as most cervical and uterine injuries are due to forceful dilatation of the cervix. The WHO's Technical and Policy Guidance on Safe Abortion recommends 'cervical preparation before surgical abortion for durations of pregnancy over 9 weeks for nulliparous women, for women younger than 18 years old, and for all over 12 weeks (WHO 2003). The RCOG Recommendation is cervical preparation should be routine if the woman is aged less than 18 years or at a gestation of more than 10 weeks (RCOG 2004). For optimal cervical preparation prior to first or second trimester surgical abortion:

- Misoprostol, 400 µg vaginally, three hours prior to surgery
- Mifepristone, 600 mg orally, 36–48 hours prior to surgery
- Nitric oxide donors and danazol for cervical priming, is the subject of current research

Between 7–14 weeks gestation:

Hygroscopic Agents/Osmotic Dilators Hygroscopic agents act by extracting water from the stroma and swell without lengthening, resulting in gradual, atraumatic and reversible dilatation of the cervix. Osmotic dilators reduce the risk of cervical laceration and uterine perforation five fold, although they do not completely prevent it (Schulz et al 1983; Grimes et al 1984).

Mifepristone: is more effective than an intracervical laminaria tent 12 hours before induction (Ho et al 1995).

Nitric oxide: relaxes myometrial smooth muscles and has an upregulation with advanced gestation (Ekerhovd et al 1999; 2000). It ripens the uterine cervix before first-trimester suction termination of pregnancy but is less effective than PG (Thomson et al 1997; 1998).

Prostaglandins (PG): Pharmacological ripening is preferable to laminaria as it reduces trauma and increases operative ease. They are easy to administer and are very effective. Gemeprost use is restricted because it is expensive and requires refrigeration for storage. Vaginal, oral and buccal administration of misoprostol has proven successful for cervical preparation in first and second trimester surgical and medical abortions.

Recommended dose of misoprostol: 400 μg misoprostol vaginally, orally or sublingually, three hours prior to surgery. The time interval of three hours allows both the pretreatment and the surgery to be performed as an outpatient procedure. The short pretreatment period will reduce the risk for excessive bleeding and abortion prior to surgery, which has been reported to occur when the pretreatment time was 12 hours (Lawrie et al 1996).

Vaginal route produces cervical dilation superior to laminaria, and oral misoprostol produces dilation equivalent to that produced by laminaria (MacIsaac et al 1999). It produces adequate dilation, with few side effects in over 95% of women before first trimester surgical termination (Meckstroth and Darney 2003).

Sublingual vs. buccal (800 μg) misoprostol: Sublingual misoprostol results in higher bioavailability compared with the buccal route.

Sublingual misoprostol vs. 15-methyl-PGF$_{2A}$ prior to surgical abortion: 15-M-PGF$_{2\alpha}$ administered vaginally 3–12 hours prior to VA results in significant dilation of the cervix and a decrease in operative complications (Bygdeman et al 1980). However, sublingual misoprostol is more effective than vaginal 15-M-PGF$_{2\alpha}$ for cervical priming prior to VA. It is more acceptable to women than the i.m. administration of 15-M-PGF$_{2\alpha}$. In addition, misoprostol is inexpensive and convenient to use (Vimala et al 2005).

MEDICATION IN SURGICAL ABORTION

Premedication with injection Pentazocine and Promethazine and injection Atropine (to prevent vasovagal attack) is given.

Medication for pain management: In general, LA affords the greatest safety. GA for surgical abortions is associated with greater overall risk of anesthesia complications and hemorrhage.

Paracervical anesthesia: A PCB is effective in alleviating the pain associated with the application of a tenaculum to the cervix, and with cervical dilatation, but offers limited relief for the pain associated with suction and curettage. The choice of local anesthetic for the PCB does not change effectiveness.

MENSTRUAL REGULATION (MR)

It is a procedure for the removal of uterine contents, within two weeks after a missed period, without confirming whether the woman is pregnant or not. A small-bore plastic cannula is inserted into the uterus with suction applied through a 50 ml syringe. Other names for this procedure are menstrual extraction, mini suction, menstrual aspiration, interception and uterine aspiration. This procedure can be done between 35–49 days gestation; prior to 35 days gestation, more than 50% cases are found not to be pregnant leading to an increased failure rate. The procedure can be performed quickly in the outpatient department, without dilatation and without anesthesia. The blood loss associated with the procedure is negligible and the complication rate is low.

MANUAL VACUUM ASPIRATION

This is an in-office procedure. The MVA can be used for the termination of pregnancy up to 12 weeks gestation with 99.5% efficacy with no major complications, minor complications including RPOC and infection. Gestations in excess of 10 weeks are associated with relatively increased amounts of blood loss (>250 ml). It is performed using a syringe that can hold vacuum and appropriate size flexible plastic cannulae (Karman's cannula).

Advantages:

- It is a simple technique that is safe and effective in completely evacuating the uterus in more than 98% of cases
- It is not dependent on the availability of electricity and can be performed in any facility with basic facilities for minor surgery/normal delivery as it is portable, low cost, easy to use, reusable and quiet
- It can be performed without any anesthesia In selected cases, local infiltration may be required
- There is high patient and provider satisfaction

The MVA set includes:

1. MVA syringe is a double valve 60 cc. syringe (polyethylene) with a capacity to hold a vacuum of 25–26 inches/600–650 mm Hg which is equivalent to the vacuum created in an electric suction pump. The parts of the syringe include—a barrel with calibrations, a double or single valve set that fits the tip of the barrel (tip of the syringe is fashioned to hold the cannula tight), a plunger with arms that snap out when the plunger is pulled back, a collar-stop that holds and locks the plunger inside the syringe when fully pulled back out of the barrel.
2. Flexible plastic cannulae (Karman's cannula) that can also be used as dilators of different sizes corresponding to the period of gestation.
   - 4–7 mm (dilatation): thickness of wall is 0.03 inches
   - 8–12 mm (evacuation): thickness 0.05 inches

   Each cannula has a closed rounded tip with two opposing openings with an overhanging convex hood that acts as a curette and an adaptor.

Preliminary steps: Empty the bladder and perform a vaginal examination to note the size and position of the uterus. Visualise the cervix and swab it with an antiseptic solution. The cervix is held with volsellum/tenaculum.

Preparation of vacuum syringe and cannulae: Inspect the syringe for any visible cracks and defects to ensure that that it can hold vacuum to its maximum capacity. Inspect the cannulae for any visible cracks or defects as broken cannulae can cause tissue injury. Close the pinch valve by pushing the buttons down and forward towards the syringe tip. Create a vacuum in the syringe (called charging the syringe). Pull back on the plunger until the arms of the plunger snap outward at the end of the syringe barrel holding the plunger in place. Check the stable positioning of the plunger arms (the plunger arms must be fully extended to the sides and secured over the edge of the barrel).

Dilation of the cervix: Excessive force in dilation of the cervix can cause cervical or uterine injury. In addition, overdilation should be avoided with MVA because it can compromise the vacuum pressure. Women undergoing termination of an early pregnancy may be dilated using metal dilators or misoprostol.

The procedure: The size of the dilator

used should be 2 mm > POG, and size of cannula is 2 mm < POG. Insert the cannula through the cervix into the uterine cavity just past the internal os by rotating the cannula while gently applying pressure. Start with a cannula of size 4 and gradually increase to the size that corresponds with POG. Push the cannula slowly into the uterine cavity just beyond the os until it touches the fundus. Note the uterine depth (the dot nearest to the tip of the cannula is 6 cm from the tip and each dot is at a 1 cm interval). Withdraw the cannula slightly. Attach the prepared syringe to the cannula. Release the pinch valve on the syringe to release the vacuum into the uterine cavity. Bloody tissue and bubbles should begin to flow through the cannula into the syringe. Evacuate any remaining contents of the uterine cavity by gently rotating the syringe and then moving the cannula gently and slowly back and forth within the uterine cavity (do not rotate the cannula more than 180 degrees, but half turn). The syringe must be emptied an average of 1–3 times to complete the procedure.

Caution:

- Do not remove the cannula from the uterus while the vacuum in syringe aspirates the endocervical canal
- Do not advance the plunger of the syringe while the cannula is connected and within the uterus (air embolism)
- The cannula should not be pushed in too much to avoid perforation. Strong force employed in using the cannula against vacuum resistance may perforate the uterus. Every two-week increase in gestational age is associated with 1.4 times increased risk of perforation.
- While the vacuum is well established and the canuula is in the uterus, ensure that the syringe is not grasped by the plunger as it may cause the plunger arms to become unlocked and slide back into the syringe pushing the contents back into the uterus. Remember to put a collar stop, else the plunger will come out.

Check for signs of complete evacuation:

- The appearance of red or pink foam and no more tissue are seen in the canuula.
- A gritty sensation is felt as the canuula passes over the surface of the evacuated uterus.
- The uterus grips the cannula.

Inspect the tissue removed from the uterus. Note its volume. Immerse the tip of the canuula in a container of water and flush the syringe two or three times. The villi/sac will be seen floating. If the POC are not seen, then the women may have passed the products completely before the procedure or the procedure is not successful or the pregnancy is an ectopic pregnancy.

Possible MVA complications: It is important to be able to diagnose and manage possible complications of MVA, as described below:

- Incomplete evacuation: Using a cannula that is too small or stopping the aspiration too soon can result in retained tissue, subsequent hemorrhage and infection
- Uterine perforation: This is most likely to occur during dilation. Careful examination to determine the position of the uterus and cervix is essential to avoid this complication
- Cervical laceration: This may require surgical repair
- Pelvic infection: Treatment depends on location and type of infection
- Hemorrhage: Heavy bleeding, soaking of a maxi-pad every 20 minutes for one hour is rare but can occur following MVA

- Hematometra: This fosters continued bleeding. The uterus may be larger than before the procedure and extremely tender. This condition is treated by re-aspirating the uterus
- Unrecognised ectopic pregnancy: Absence of villi, gestational sac, or both, upon inspection uterine contents may indicate an ectopic pregnancy. Careful tissue inspection is essential to confirm the aspiration of an intrauterine pregnancy

DILATATION AND ELECTRICAL VACUUM ASPIRATION (EVA)

Empty the bladder and perform a vaginal examination to note the size and position of the uterus. Visualise the cervix and swab it with an antiseptic solution. Insert the Sim's speculum. Wipe the external os with an antiseptic solution. Cervix is held with volsellum/tenaculum. Pass a uterine sound to note the length of uterine cavity and then pass dilators gradually. Insert a Karman's cannula till it reaches the fundus. Connect it to the suction apparatus. Create a vacuum (600–650 mm Hg) and aspirate contents after giving oxytocics. Examine the collected products upon completion of the procedure.

SUCTION CURETTAGE

Mechanical cervical dilatation: Forcible dilatation with tapered rods is the standard. Place a single tooth tenaculum/volsellum to provide traction near the internal os. Traction straightens the angle between the cervix and the uterus, helping to avoid perforation. Then the dilators are inserted slowly. The dilator tip must negotiate a curve where the cervix and the uterus join. The direction is reversed if the uterus is retroverted. If the cervical os is very small, use misoprostol treatment. Dilate the internal os of the cervix with graduated, tapering metal dilators. Hold the dilator with a 'pen grip'. Generally, it is approximately 1.0 mm more than the POG. The tip of each successive dilator should go no further than just beyond the internal os.

Introduce the suction cannula with an external diameter equal to the number of weeks of gestation, into the uterine cavity, until it touches the fundus, and then withdraw the cannula slightly. The cannula most commonly used is a Karman's cannula of 6–8 mm size. Connect the cannula to the suction machine. Activate suction, raising the negative pressure to 70 cm of mercury. In case of a metal cannula, suction is activated by pressing against the hole on the thumb grip. Evacuate the uterine contents by rotating the cannula from side to side as well as to and fro, with slow controlled motion, till the cavity is completely evacuated. The endometrium is curetted and the fragmented conceptus is sucked into a container.

DILATATION–EVACUATION

In this method, commonly known as D and E, the uterine contents are evacuated using an ovum forceps or a blunt curettage alone, after rapid instrumental dilatation of the cervix. However, it is no longer recommended as a procedure of choice, as it is a time consuming process and is associated with more blood loss.

COMBINED METHOD

Prime the cervix with prostaglandin (15 methyl $PGF_{2\alpha}$, 120 μg), three hours before and 120 μg one hour before, or with Misoprostol 400 μg (vaginally) followed by evacuation. Advantages of the combined method include:

- Decreased chances of cervical tear and injury to the internal os. Dilatation becomes easier.
- Uterine contraction is better and therefore avoids the need for oxytocics

Signs of complete evacuation

- Foamy bubbles without tissue in the cannula
- Gritty feeling of cannula against the myometrium
- Uterus contracts around the cannula
- Internal os contracts

Examination of aspirated products: If POC cannot be identified, re-evaluate with sensitive UPT or Beta human chorionic gonadotrophins (β-HCG) or ultrasonography (USG). Failure to identify could imply a recent spontaneous abortion, failed attempted abortion, perforation with aspiration outside uterus, ectopic pregnancy, or uterine anomaly. Beyond nine weeks, gestation fetal parts can be easily identified. At less than nine weeks gestation, chorionic villi and membranes can be identified after washing with water/white vinegar. Villi appear as soft, fluffy, feathery, discernible finger-like projections. Decidua appears coarse, shaggy and translucent, while the amnion and chorion appear filmy and transparent.

Decontaminate the cannula for 10 minutes, in 0.5% chlorine solution for 10 minutes. Hot water should not be used (it can coagulate protein such as blood, making it hard to remove) and soap is not recommended (it can leave a residue, which is difficult to remove). Do not use brushes or other small objects to remove matter as they can scratch the inside of the cannulae, creating crevices where organic material can get trapped.

Sterilisation/High level disinfection (HLD): Submerge the decontaminated and cleaned syringe and cannulae in 2% activated glutaraldehyde (Cidex) or 0.5% chlorine for 20 minutes (ensure that the solution fills the cannulae). Remove and rinse with sterile water/boiled cool water. Do not use iodine or formalin. Do not boil or autoclave.

MID-TRIMESTER ABORTION PROCEDURES

Choice of mid-trimester procedure: At all gestations up to 20 weeks, abortion can be performed by either surgical or medical methods. Methods for abortion beyond 20 weeks would usually be undertaken on the grounds of fetal abnormality, and are out of the scope of this chapter. The complication rate is lower for surgical than medical second trimester abortions as chances of an incomplete abortion are higher by medical methods; however, of the medical methods used, misoprostol is the better choice. The advantage of D and E is for procedures performed at 13–16 weeks. Thereafter, the risks for major complications and death are comparable (Kafrissen et al 1984). The psychological impact on the patient is much greater with labour induction abortion than with D and E (Kaltreider et al 1979).

MEDICAL METHODS

Intra-amniotic instillation of various solutions was a popular method of terminating pregnancies after the 14th week.

Hypertonic saline: Amnioinfusion of hypertonic saline (200 ml of a 20% solution) has mean time from instillation to abortion of 33–35 hours (Berger and Edelman 1975). There are serious hazards unique to hypertonic saline—cardiovascular collapse, pulmonary and cerebral edema, and renal failure if the solution is injected iv and all patients are at risk for DIC.

Hypertonic urea: It is an alternative to saline because of its greater safety. A combination of 5 mg of $PGF_{2\alpha}$ and 80 g of urea instilled into the amniotic sac produces abortion in a mean time of 17.5 hours, with 80% of patients aborting within 24 hours (Burkeman et al 1981). The presence of renal disease or hypertension is a contraindication for use of saline or urea and before the latter is given, blood urea estimation is essential.

Prostaglandins: PGE_2 is used to produce cervical dilatation and $PGF_{2\alpha}$ to stimulate the uterine myometium. Intravenous PG infusion produces abortion, but this route is avoided because of associated vomiting and diarrhea. Side effects are much reduced given by the intra-amniotic route.

Intra-amniotic PG: Prostaglandins injected into the amniotic sac by abdominal amniocentesis are safer than 20% saline and other solutions. After withdrawing 10 ml of liquor under aseptic precautions, 2.5 mg (10 ml) 15-methyl $PGF_{2\alpha}$ is instilled intra-amniotically under ultrasound guidance. There are fewer adverse effects compared to parenteral administration of the drug. Vasovagal collapse, or more usually, transient hypotension can be an immediate reaction; occasionally, cardiovascular collapse and death occurs. Pyrexia, vomiting and diarrhea may occur.

Systemic PG

15-METHYL $PGF_{2\alpha}$: Injections of 250 μg are administered im every 2–3 hours up to a maximum of 10 doses. The mean induction to abortion interval is 16 hours and 87% of patients abort successfully within 24 hours.

DINOPROSTONE: A PGE_2 derivative, has been used as 2 mg vaginal suppository every three hours. The mean induction to abortion interval in mid-trimester is 12 hours and 90% abort within 24 hours. However, it is expensive and needs refrigeration. It is contraindicated in patients with glaucoma and bronchial asthma.

GEMEPROST: is a PGE_1 analogue used for mid-trimester abortion, but is not widely available and is expensive.

MISOPROSTOL: Before misoprostol's widespread use, other PG such as PGE_2 vaginal suppositories and $PGF_{2\alpha}$ injections were commonly used. These agents are associated with side effects such as severe nausea, vomiting, diarrhea and fever in a high percentage of patients. Pre-medication with antiemetics, antipyretics and antidiarrheals is often required. In addition, the dosing regimen of these requires a vaginal examination by a physician or a painful im injection every three hours throughout the induction process. Side effects of misoprostol are much better tolerated than other PG for pregnancy termination in the second trimester. The optimal dosage and route of administration of misoprostol, however, are yet to be defined.

PROTOCOL: A 400 μg oral dose 3-hourly up to five doses has a mean induction to abortion interval of 12 hours. A 200 μg dose used vaginally can produce the same effect.

Misoprostol works well in pregnancies complicated by intrauterine fetal demise (IUD). Three-hourly oral doses of 400 μg have been used in such patients. The induction to abortion interval in those with mid-trimester pregnancies is shorter in those with IUD (10.4 hours) than in those with live fetus (15.4 hours).

Vaginal misoprostol followed by repeated doses of oral misprostol has higher abortion rates: (Dilbaz et al 2004). The initial vaginal application of misoprostol is based on the possible direct effect of misoprostol on cervical softening. Vaginal misoprostol

400 μg administered every three hours is more effective than every six hours (Wong et al 2000).

400 μg misoprostol every four hours up to 24 hours vaginally vs. orally: Mean time to delivery is 18 hours in the vaginal group and 31 hours in the oral group. The vaginal group has less nausea and vomiting (Hollander 2004).

Vaginal misoprostol vs. intra-amniotic PG (IAPG): There is no difference in complication rates between intra-amniotic $PGF_{2\alpha}$ and intravaginal misoprostol for induction in the second trimester (Perry et al 1999).

Ethacridine lactate (Emcredil): It is an acridine derivative with uterotonic and antiseptic properties. The exact mechanism of action is unknown. A no. 16 Foley's catheter is used to introduce 0.1% ethacridine into extra-amniotic space in a dose of 10 ml per week of gestation to a maximum of 150 ml. The bulb of the catheter is inflated with 10–15 ml of saline to seal the internal os. The catheter is removed after six hours and an oxytocin infusion of 50 mIU/ minute started to expedite the procedure. Alternatively, the catheter is left in place until it is expelled on its own once cervical dilatation occurs. However, misoprostol is largely replacing its use now.

High-Dose Oxytocin: PGE_2 suppositories and high-dose oxytocin protocol at 17–24 weeks have equal efficacy, with fewer side effects from oxytocin (Winkler et al 1991).

Mifepristone and PG mid-trimester regimen

For mid-trimester abortion (13–24 weeks of gestation) medical abortion with mifepristone followed by PG is safe and effective, with shorter induction to abortion intervals than methods using PG alone or supplemented by oxytocin infusion. The use of 200 mg of mifepristone prior to PG significantly reduces the time between first administration of PG to expulsion of fetus (Urquhart and Templeton 1990).

The following regimen appears to be optimal for mid-trimester medical abortion (RCOG 2004):

- Mifepristone, 200 mg orally, followed 36–48 hours later by 800 μg misoprostol vaginally, then 400 μg misoprostol orally, three-hourly, to a maximum of four oral doses. In all cases, follow-up visit is required two weeks after misoprostol use to check that abortion is complete and there are no complications
- Mifepristone, 600 mg orally, followed 36–48 hours later by gemeprost 1 mg vaginally every three hours, to a maximum of five pessaries

SURGICAL METHODS OF SECOND TRIMESTER ABORTION

Cervical Priming: Various methods have been tried to shorten the induction–abortion interval and therefore lessen the cumulative amount of PG needed. Mifepristone is more effective than intracervical laminaria tent 12 hours before induction (Ho et al 1995).

Buccal misoprostol for cervical ripening before second-trimester abortion is effective (Todd et al 2002).

Laminaria as an adjunct to PG in mid-trimester is not used much in modern times.

Dilatation And Evacuation (D And E): Cervical priming is done and the uterus is evacuated under PCB with light sedation, short-acting intravenous barbiturates or GA. The fetus can be removed by the intact or non-intact procedure.

Hysterectomy: This may be indicated if

there is uterine disease, as well as a pregnancy, to be removed (for example, fibroids). It carries a much higher morbidity rate than hysterotomy or tubal resection.

Pregnancy Termination After Fetal Death In Utero: After fetal death, laminaria treatment may result in the onset of labour. The amniotic sac may be more permeable after fetal death, and intra-amniotic injection becomes technically more difficult. Systemic reactions from hypertonic saline or intra-amniotic PG are more common in such cases. The response to PG is faster than with intact gestations, and treatment-to-expulsion times are shorter (Gabbe 2002).

Selective Termination Of Anomalous Twins And Reduction Of Multifetal Pregnancies: The techniques available for selective reduction include the following:

- Intracardiac injection (potassium chloride or digoxin)
- Cord occlusion techniques: Embolisation with alcohol, enbucrilate gel; Nd: YAG laser photocoagulation, fetoscope cord ligation, bipolar cord coagulation, monopolar cord coagulation.

POST ABORTION CARE AND FOLLOW UP

- Prophylactic antibiotics reduce post abortion infection rates to less than 1%–2%. Most use doxycycline at 100 mg b.i.d, with erythromycin for those who are allergic
- Analgesia: During the first 24 hours, a non-aspirin analgesic, such as acetaminophen, is recommended. After that time, patients can switch to an NSAID, such as ibuprofen or naproxen. Most patients have a short period of intense cramping during the process of evacuation.
- Rhesus Prophylaxis: The incidence of isoimmunisation with first trimester abortion is unknown. Anti-D immunoglobulin G (50 µg in first and 100 µg in second trimester) should be given, by injection into the deltoid muscle, to all non-sensitised Rh-D negative women within 72 hours following abortion.

COMPLICATIONS

Mortality from abortion: Mortality rates are highest with the most invasive procedures and with increasing gestational age. Causes of death include infection, hemorrhage, pulmonary embolism, anesthesia complications and amniotic fluid embolism.

Hemorrhage: Bleeding can occur as a result of atony, cervical laceration, uterine perforation, incomplete abortion, placental implantation abnormalities, coagulopathy, cervical pregnancy, pregnancy of more advanced gestational age than anticipated, or infection. General anesthesia increases the risk of atony. Excessive bleeding (hemorrhage) does happen in a small number of women.

MANAGEMENT:

- The need for transfusion (seen in 2%–5%) is rare. Initial hemorrhage should be evaluated by ensuring complete uterine evacuation. Gentle exploration of the uterine cavity is done with a curette or forceps to confirm that there is no perforation. Abortion is completed under iv oxytocin cover (10–20 mIU/L running at 100–200 mL). Aspiration (or curettage) is necessary to stop excessive bleeding, but for treating incomplete abortion, where bleeding is not excessive, it may not be necessary as an additional dose of misoprostol may suffice.
- Intracervical administration of 10 units

of vasopressin diluted to 10 ml, or im. Methergine at 0.2 mg, helps reduce bleeding and produces strong uterine contractions. Administration of dilute vasopressin in PCB is associated with decreased blood loss beyond 15 weeks. Vasopressin given as part of the cervical block is more effective with fewer side effects than methylergonovine maleate in preventing hematometra (Keder 2003).

- Misoprostol, 800 μg rectally, can be given as an adjunct. Intrauterine inflation of a Foley balloon can also be used. Balloons of 5 mL inflated with 30 mL, or 30 mL balloons inflated up to 100 mL of sterile saline may be used. The inflation should correlate with uterine size.
- When these measures fail, begin fluid resuscitation. Uterine artery embolisation or selective embolisation of bleeding vessels can be used if placenta accreta, cervical pregnancy and low cervical perforation are encountered. If bleeding persists, rule out DIC and prepare for laparoscopy.

DIC is rare after first trimester vacuum curettage (8 per 100,000) as opposed to mid-trimester D and E (191 per 100,000), and highest for saline instillation procedures (658 per 100,000). DIC must be considered whenever post-abortal hemorrhage is seen (Kafrissen et al 1983).

Post-abortal syndrome (hematometra): This occurs when the uterus fails to remain contracted after an induced abortion, a type of uterine atony. The patient complains of increasing lower abdominal pain half hour or so after abortion and may develop tachycardia and diaphoresis, cramps, bleeding, open cervix. The uterus is large, appears softer than expected, globular and tense, and could be mistaken for a broad ligament hematoma except that the mass is midline and arises from the cervix. Treatment is immediate re-evacuation with suction curettage and antibiotic therapy. Pretreatment with ergot, 0.1 mg im reduces the incidence.

Retained POC/incomplete abortion: Retained placenta accounts for 77% of complications associated with medical abortion. Patients who undergo second trimester medical abortion should be advised of a significant risk (21%) of requiring surgery for retained POC. The retained POC rate is less than 1%. Patients with misoprostol are less likely to require a D and C for retained placenta (Goldberg et al 2001).

Failed abortion and continuing pregnancy: All methods of first-trimester abortion carry a small risk of failure. The risk for surgical abortion is 2.3 in 1000 and for medical abortion 1–4 in 1000 (depending on the regimen used). The rate of failure with suction termination performed at 12 weeks or below is increased for multiparous women, for abortions at six weeks or below, when small cannulae are used, by the presence of uterine abnormalities or if the procedure is performed by a junior doctor.

Ectopic pregnancy: When no chorionic villi are found, ectopic pregnancy is a risk.

Coexistent ectopic pregnancy: With residual positive hCG titers one needs to be vigilant in order to avoid missing an ectopic pregnancy. The presence of significant tenderness during the postoperative examination, history of continued pain and the elevation or plateau of hCG titers should raise suspicion. Heterotropic pregnancies should be ruled out.

Post-abortion infection: Genital tract infection, including pelvic inflammatory disease (PID), occurs in up to 10% of cases (Heisterberg and Petersen 1985). Surgically induced abortions have a rate of 12 in 1000 (Zhou et al 2002). Endometritis and PID occur in less than 1% of cases. These are usually due to pre-existing infections or a failure of antibiotic prophylaxis.

Prophylactic Antibiotics

The following regimens are suitable for peri-abortion prophylaxis:

- Metronidazole, 1 g rectally, at the time of abortion plus doxycycline, 100 mg orally, bd for seven days, commencing on the day of abortion or
- Metronidazole, 1 g rectally, at the time of abortion plus azithromycin, 1 g orally, on the day of the abortion

Choice of antibiotics for post-abortal infection

- A combination of three drugs: ampicillin (2–3 g intravenously every six hours), clindamycin (900 mg intravenously every eight hours), and gentamicin (loading dose of 2 mg/kg of body weight, followed by 1.5 mg/kg every eight hours) may be used (Stubblefield and Grimes 1994)
- For the management of victims of sexual assault, either the seven day doxycycline regimen or the immediate-dose azithromycin regimen is recommended (CDC 2002)

Management of septic abortion: Clostridial sepsis, a common complication of illegal abortion, is occasionally seen as a complication of legal abortion. This is suspected when tachycardia seems out of proportion to the fever, and when hematuria and shock develop rapidly. Patients can rapidly develop severe adult respiratory distress syndrome. Initial treatment requires high-dose penicillin, vacuum aspiration (VA) of the uterus and fluid management. If hemolysis is present, prompt hysterectomy may be necessary.

- Supportive care: requires intensive care unit management with cardiovascular support. Monitor with arterial line, central venous pressure, dopamine and dobutamine as needed. Monitor tissue oxygenation, ventilation if oxygen saturation falls below 90% or if pulmonary compliance decreases
- Treat the infection: obtain cultures, start high-dose, broadspectrum antibiotics
- Empty the uterus
  First trimester: vacuum curettage under LA with conscious sedation.
  Mid-trimester: D and E, with ultrasound guidance or PG induction (carboprost 250 µg im every two hours or misoprostol 200 µg vaginally every 12 hours) or high dose oxytocin regimen.
- Laparotomy, if there is no response to uterine evacuation and adequate medical therapy, or perforation with suspected bowel injury, pelvic abscess or clostridial myometritis. Total abdominal hysterectomy for severe myometritis. Copious irrigation of abdominal cavity, drainage, closure with stay sutures and delayed primary closure.

Post-abortal triad: The most common post-abortal problem is the triad of pain, bleeding and low-grade fever. Although these may be managed by oral antibiotics and ergot preparations, many reveal some retained gestational tissue or clot in the uterine cavity. The management includes repeat uterine evacuation.

Complications of medical abortion

- There is a risk of heavy bleeding, especially if the abortion is incomplete. Surgical evacuation of uterus helps stop the bleeding; about 1 in 100 women require this.
- If a woman develops fever above 100.4°F lasting for more than four hours, or if fever starts 6–8 hours after misoprostol, infection may have developed. However, infection risk after medical abortion is less than 1% (Shannon et al 2004). Death from complications of sepsis following medical abortion is extremely rare, about 1 per 100,000 women (US FDA 2005).
- About 5%–15% of patients who undergo medical abortion are treated with narcotics, and about a third to half report vomiting and diarrhea, but these are limited to the duration of the medication regimen and usually do not require more than symptomatic treatment (Westhoff et al 2000; Creinin et al 2001b).
- Exposure to teratogens: Mifepristone has no known teratogenic effects. Exposure to misoprostol in early pregnancy has been associated with multiple congenital defects.

Complications of surgical abortion: The more advanced the gestational age, and the more invasive the procedure, the higher the complication rate. Minor abortion complications include infection, repeat suction, cervical stenosis, cervical tear, seizure and underestimation of dates. MVA complications include-infection, 0.7%; perforation, 0.05%; retained POC, 0.5%; and repeat aspiration, 0.5-0.25% (Roche 2004). In D and E, the skill of the provider is the most important factor in maintaining a low complication rate. Coagulopathy is a rare complication in D and E.

Perforation: The rate of perforation is 0.9 per 1000 (Grimes et al 1984). It can be recognised when an instrument passes endlessly without resistance, heavy or persistent vaginal bleeding occurs, signs of peritoneal irritation appear, or fat or other tissue appears in the specimen. It can occur with sound, dilators, curette, suction tip, forceps, or passive dilators and may cause injury to major blood vessels, bowel, or bladder and endanger the patient's life. In the first trimester, most perforations are in the body of uterus, usually fundal. Risk factors for perforation are previous uterine surgery such as, previous TOP, lower-segment cesarean deliveries (20-fold increase in risk) (Chapman et al 1996) and grand multiparity.

Management: Suspected perforation can be confirmed by inserting a sterile blunt instrument through the cervix into the suspect area with ultrasound guidance. Fundal perforations require only observation. If the extent of perforation cannot be determined, if the patient is medically unstable, if suction was applied at the time of perforation, or if bowel or fat content was obtained by forceps at the time of perforation, surgical evaluation by laparoscopy or laparotomy is necessary where mesentery and intestines must be examined from the jejunum to the rectum. Abortion can be completed under laparoscopic guidance.

Cervical trauma: The risk of damage to the external cervical os at the time of surgical abortion is moderate (less than 1 in 100). Perforation of the cervix, either at the junction of the cervix and lower uterine segment, or lower down the canal, produces two different clinical syndromes depending on the anatomic location of perforation.

Uterine rupture: may occur when saline, urea or PG are augmented with high-dose oxytocin infusion. PG abortions are frequently incomplete causing late bleeding. Oxytocin should be used with caution in PG-treated patients in order to avoid uterine rupture. More recent reviews of women undergoing first and second trimester medical abortion with various regimens have not identified any cases of uterine rupture (Debby et al 2003).

Bowel injury: If perforation is not recognised, the bowel may be grasped with the vacuum cannula or forceps and lacerated or stripped off its mesentery. A suspected bowel injury must be completely visualised. Laparotomy is indicated if the site of injury cannot be completely visualised on laparoscopy.

Bladder injury: The evaluation of a major perforation includes catheterisation of the bladder to look for gross hematuria and laparoscopy to confirm the injury.

Complications of local anesthesia: Intravascular injection or an overdose can produce a severe systemic response—convulsions, cardiorespiratory arrest and death (Stubblefield 1998).

Cervical shock: Vasovagal syncope produced by stimulation of the cervical canal can be seen even after PCB.

Remote Physical Complications

- Menstrual disturbances
- Asherman syndrome: Post-abortion uterine synechiae (or adhesions)
- Rhesus isoimmunisation: 5%–10% can develop antibodies if not immunised with Anti D
- Cervical conditions: Ectropion, chronic cervicitis and cervicovaginal fistula

Second trimester and the risk of subsequent preterm delivery: Although D and E is categorised as a risk factor for future spontaneous preterm birth, studies have not documented an association (Kalish et al 2002).

Infertility is not a consequence of uncomplicated induced abortion (Daling et al 1985). There may be an association between induced abortion complicated by pelvic infection and tubal infertility. The risk of placenta previa might increase in a dose-response fashion with sharp curettage abortions, but VA does not confer an increased risk (Johnson et al 2003). Both induced abortion and prior cesarean delivery increase the risk of placenta previa.

References

Abortion Statistics. 2002. Legal abortions carried out under the 1967 Abortion Act in England and Wales. London: Office for National Statistics, Department of Health, Office for National Statistics.

Ashok PW, GM Flett, A Templeton. 1998a. Termination of pregnancy at 9–13 weeks' amenorrhoea with mifepristone and misoprostol. *Lancet* 352:542–543.

Ashok P, G Penney, G Flett, A Templeton. 1998b. An effective regimen for early medical abortion: A report of 2000 consecutive cases. *Hum Reprod* 13:2962–2965.

Autry AM, EC Hayes, GF Jacobson, RS Kirby. 2002. A comparison of medical induction and dilation and evacuation for second-trimester abortion. *Am J Obstet Gynecol* 187:393–397.

Baird DT. 2000. Mode of action of medical methods of abortion. *J Am Med Wom Assoc* 55(3):121–126.

Berger GS and DA Edelman. 1975. Oxytocin administration, instillation to abortion time, and morbidity associated with saline instillation. *Am J Obstet Gynecol* 121:941.

Burkeman RT, TM King, MF Atienza. 1981. Hyperosmolar urea. In Berger GS, Brenner WE, Keith LG eds. *Second Trimester Abortion: Perspectives after a Decade of Experience.* Boston, John Wright, PSG, Inc.

Bygdeman M, K Bremme, NJ Christensen, V Lundstrom, K Green. 1980. A comparison of two stable prostaglandin E analogues for termination of early pregnancy and for cervical dilatation. *Contraception* 22:71–83.

Carbonell JL, L Varela, A Velazco et al. 1998. Oral methotrexate and vaginal misoprostol for early abortion. *Contraception* 57: 83–88.

Centers for Disease Control and Prevention. 2002. Sexual assault and STDs. Sexually transmitted diseases treatment guidelines. *MMWR Recomm Rep* 51(RR-6):69–74.

Chapman SJ, M Crispens, J Owen et al. 1996. Complications of midtrimester pregnancy termination: The effect of prior cesarean delivery. *Am J Obstet Gynecol* 175:889– 892.

Christin-Maitre S, P Bouchard, IM Spitz. 2000. Medical termination of pregnancy. *N Engl J Med* 342:946–956.

Couzinet B, N Le Strat, A Ulmann et al. 1986. Termination of early pregnancy by the progesterone antagonist RU 486 (mifepristone). *New Eng J M* 315:1565–1570.

Creinin MD and PD Darney. 1993. Methotrexate and misoprostol for early abortion. *Contraception* 48:339–348.

Creinin MD, JL Carbonell, JL Schwartz et al. 1999. A randomized trial of the effect of moistening misoprostol before vaginal administration when used with methotrexate for abortion. *Contraception* 59:11–16.

Creinin MD, HC Pymar, JL Schwartz. 2001b. Mifepristone 100 mg in abortion regimens. *Obstet Gynaecol* 98:434–439.

Daling JR, NS Weiss, L Voigt, LR Spadoni, R Soderstorm, DE Moore et al. 1985. Tubal infertility in relation to prior induced abortion. *Fertil Steril* 43:389–394.

Davis A, C Westhoff, L De Nonno. 2000. Bleeding patterns after early abortion with mifepristone and misoprostol or manual vacuum aspiration. *J Am Med Womens Assoc* 55(3 suppl):141–144.

Debby A, A Golan, R Sagiv, O Sadan, M Glezerman. 2003. Mid-trimester abortion in patients with a previous uterine scar. *Eur J Obstet Gynecol Reprod Biol* 109:177–180.

Dilbaz S, E Caliskan, B Dilbaz, BG Kahraman. 2004. Frequent low-dose misoprostol for termination of second-trimester pregnancy. *Eur J Cont Reprod Health Care* 9, 1; *Health & Medical Complete.* pg. 11.

Ekerhovd E, M Brannstrom, B Weijdegard, A Norstrom. 1999. Localization of nitric oxide synthase and effects of nitric oxide donors on the human Fallopian tube. *Mol Hum Reprod* 5:1040–1047.

Ekerhovd E, M Brannstrom, B Weijdegard, A Norstrom. 2000. Nitric oxide synthases in the human cervix at term pregnancy and oxide on cervical smooth muscle contractility. *Am J Obstet Gynecol* 183: 610–616.

Gabbe SS. 2002. Surgical procedures in pregnancy, in *Obstetrics: Normal and Problem Pregnancies. Fertility Control and Health,* Gabbe 4th ed. pp.625–637.

Goldberg AB, MB Greenberg, PD Darney. 2001. Misoprostol and pregnancy. *N Engl J Med* 344: 38-47.

Gouk EV, K Lincoln, A Khair, J Haslock, J Knight, DJ Cruickshank. 1999. Medical termination of pregnancy at 63 to 83 days gestation. *Br J Obstet Gynaecol* 106:535–539.

Government of India (GOI). 2001. Guidelines for medical officers for medical termination of pregnancy up to eight weeks using manual vacuum aspiration technique. Maternal Health Division. Ministry of Health and Family Welfare (Department of Family Welfare).

Greenslade FC, J Benson, J Winkler, V Henderson, M Wolf, A Leonard. 1993. Summary of clinical and programmatic experience with manual vacuum aspiration. IPAS (Carrboro, NC). 3:1–4.

Grimes DA, KF Schulz, WJ Cates Jr. 1984. Prevention of uterine perforation during curettage abortion. *JAMA* 251:2108–2111.

Grimes DA. 1997. Medical abortion in early pregnancy: A review of the evidence. *Obstet Gynecol* 89: 790-796.

Heisterberg L and K Petersen. 1985. Metronidazole prophylaxis in elective first trimester abortion. *Obstet Gynecol* 65:371–374.

Ho PC, SS Tsang, HK Ma. 1995. Reducing the induction to abortion interval in termination of second trimester pregnancies: A comparison of mifepristone with laminaria tent. *Br J Obstet Gynaecol* 102: 648–651.

Hollander D. 2004. For Second-Trimester Abortion, Women Given Misoprostol Vaginally Report the Greatest satisfaction as compared to oral. Perspectives on Sexual and Reproductive Health; 36, 3; *Health & Medical Complete* pg. 133.

Jain JK, C Dutton, B Harwood, KR Meckstroth, DR Mishell Jr. 2002. A prospective randomized, double-blinded, placebo-controlled trial comparing mifepristone and vaginal misoprostol alone for elective termination of pregnancy. *Hum Reprod* 17:1477–1482.

Johnson LG, BA Mueller, JR Daling. 2003. The relationship of placenta previa and history of induced abortion. *Int J Gynaecol Obstet* 81:191–198.

Kafrissen ME, MW Barke, P Workman et al. 1983. Coagulopathy and induced abortion methods: Rates and relative risks. *Am J Obstet Gynecol* 147:344.

Kafrissen ME, KF Schulz, DA Grimes, W Cates Jr. 1984. Midtrimester abortion: Intra-amniotic instillation of hyperosmolar urea and prostaglandin F2-alpha vs dilatation and evacuation. *JAMA* 251:916–919.

Kalish RB, ST Chasen, LB Rosenzweig, WK Rashbaum, FA Chervenak. 2002. Impact of midtrimester dilation and evacuation on subsequent pregnancy outcome. *Am J Obstet Gynecol* 187:882–885.

Kaltreider NB, S Goldsmith, AJ Margolis. 1979. The impact of midtrimester abortion techniques on patients and staff. *Am J Obstet Gynecol* 135:235.

Kaunitz AM, EZ Rovira, DA Grimes, KF Schulz. 1985. Abortions that fail. *Obstet Gynecol* 66:533–537.

Keder LM. 2003. Best practices in surgical abortion. *Am J Obstet Gynecol* 189:418–422.

Koopersmith TB and DR Mishell Jr. 1996. The use of misoprostol for termination of early pregnancy. *Contraception* 53:238–242.

Kovacs L, M Sas, BA Resch et al. 1984. Termination of very early pregnancy by RU 486—an antiprogestational compound. *Contraception* 29:399–410.

Kulier R, A Fekih, GJ Hofmeyr, A Campana. 2001. Surgical methods for first trimester termination of pregnancy. *Cochrane Database Syst Rev* 4.

Kulier R, A Gulmezoglu, G Hofmeyr, L Cheng, A Campana. 2004. Medical methods for first trimester miscarriage. *Cochrane Database Syst Rev* 2:CD002855.

Lawrie A, G Penney, A Templeton. 1996. A randomized comparison of oral and vaginal misoprostol for cervical priming before suction termination of pregnancy. *Br J Obstet Gynecol* 103:1117–1119.

Lefebvre Y, L Proulx, R Elie et al. 1990. The effects of RU38486 on cervical ripening. *Am J Obstet Gynecol* 162:61.

MacIsaac L, D Grossman, E Balistreri, P Darney. 1999. A randomized controlled trial of laminaria, oral misoprostol and vaginal misoprostol before abortion. *Obstetrics and Gynecology* 93:766–770.

Meckstroth KR and PD Darney. 2003. Prostaglandins for first-trimester termination. *Best Pract Research Clin Obstet Gynaecol* 17(5):745–763.

Murthy AS, MD Creinin, B Harwood, C Schreiber. 2005. A pilot study of mifepristone and misoprostol administered at the same time for abortion up to 49 days gestation. *Contraception* 71:333–336.

Pai M and RK Ruprai. 2002. Single dose methotrexate followed by vaginal misoprostol for early abortion-non-surgical method. *J Obst Gyn of India* 52(6):50–55.

Perry KG Jr, BK Rinehart, DA Terrone, RW Martin, WL May, WE Roberts. 1999. Second-trimester uterine evacuation: A comparison of intra-amniotic (15S)-15-methyl-prostaglandin F2α and intravaginal misoprostol. *Am J Obstet Gynecol* 181:1057–1061.

RCOG. 2004. Royal College of Obstetricians and Gynaecologists Evidence-based Clinical Guideline Number 7: The Care of Women Requesting Induced Abortion. London: RCOG.p104. http://www.guideline.gov/summary/summary. aspx? ss = 15 and doc_id = 7668 & nbr = 4467.

Roche NE. Therapeutic Abortion eMedicine.com. http//www.emedicine.com/med/topic 3311.htm. Updated: September 28, 2004.

Schaff EA, SL Fielding, C Westhoff. 2002. Randomized trial of oral versus vaginal misoprostol 2 days after mifepristone 200 mg for abortion up to 63 days of pregnancy. *Contraception* 66:247–250.

Schaff EA, SL Fielding, SH Eisinger et al. 2000a. Low-dose mifepristone followed by vaginal misoprostol at 48 hours for abortion up to 63 days. *Contraception* 61:41–46.

Schaff EA, SL Fielding et al. 2000b. Vaginal misoprostol administered 1, 2, or 3 days after mifepristone for early medical abortion: A randomized trial. *JAMA* 284:1948–1953.

Schulz KF, DA Grimes, W Cates Jr. 1983. Measures to prevent cervical injury during suction curettage abortion. *Lancet* 1:1182–1184.

Shannon C, LP Brothers, NM Philip et al. 2004. Infection after medical abortion: A review of the literature. *Contraception* 70:183–190.

Sharma S, H El-Refaey, H Mitchel, O Ozturk, C Rodeck. 2006. Mifepristone vaginally in an early medical abortion regimen: A pilot study. *Contraception* 73:261–264.

Spitz IM, CW Bardin, L Benton, A Robbins. 1998. Early pregnancy termination with mifepristone and misoprostol in the United States. *New Engl J Med* 338:1241–1247.

Stubblefield PG and DA Grimes. 1994. Septic abortion. *N Engl J Med* 331:310.

Stubblefield PG, S Carr-Ellis, L Borgatta. 2004. Methods for induced abortion. *Obstet Gynecol* 104: 174–185.

Stubblefield PG. 1998. Complications of induced abortion. In Pearlman MD, Tintinalli JE eds. *Emergency Care of the Woman*. New York: McGraw-Hill, p 37.

Tang OS, H Schweer, HW Seyberth, SWH Lee, PC Ho. 2002a. Pharmacokinetics of different routes of administration of misoprostol. *Hum Reprod* 17:332–336.

Thomson AJ, Cl Burnett, IT Cameron, IA Greer, JE Norman. 1997. Nitric oxide donors induce ripening of the human cervix: A randomized controlled trial. *Br J Obstet Gynaecol* 104:1054–1057.

Thomson AJ, CB Lunan, M Ledingham et al. 1998. Randomised trial of nitric oxide donor versus prostaglandin for cervical ripening before first trimester termination of pregnancy. *Lancet* 352: 1093–1096.

Todd CS, M Soler, L Castleman et al. 2002. Buccal misoprostol as cervical preparation for second trimester pregnancy termination. *Contraception* 65: 415–418.

Ulmann A, L Silvestre, L Chemama et al. 1992. Medical termination of early pregnancy with mifepristone (RU 486) followed by a prostaglandin analogue: Study in 16,369 women. *Acta Obsta Gynecol Scand* 71:278–283.

UNDP/UNFPA/WHO/World Bank Special Programme of Research, Development and Research Training in Human Reproduction. 1997. Methotrexate for the termination of early pregnancy: A toxicology review. *Reproductive Health Matters* 5(9):162–166.

Urquhart DR and A Templeton. 1990. The use of mifepristone prior to prostaglandin induced mid-trimester termination. *Hum Reprod* 5:883–886.

US Food and Drug Administration. 2005. FDA Alert for Healthcare Professionals: Mifepristone (marketed as Mifeprex), 22 July 2005. At: <http://www.fda.gov/cder/ drug/InfoSheets/HCP/MifepristoneHCP.pdf> and <http://www.fda.gov/cder/drug/infopage/mifepristone/mifepristone-qa20050719.htm>. Accessed 29 August 2005.

Vimala N, S Mittal, V Dadhwal. 2005. Cervical priming with sublingual misoprostol vs. 15-methyl-prostaglandin F2A prior to surgical abortion. *Int J Gynaecol Obstet* 88:134–137.

Vyjayanthi S and N Piskorowskyj. 2002. Medical termination of pregnancy at 9–12 weeks of gestation. *J Obstet Gynaecol* 22:669–671.

Westhoff C, R Dasmahapatra, B Winikoff, S Clarke. 2000. Mifepristone Clinical Trials Group. Predictors of analgesia use during supervised medical abortion. *Contraception* 61:225–229.

WHO. 2003. *Safe Abortion: Technical and Policy Guidance for Health Systems* Geneva: WHO.

Winkler CL, SE Gray, JC Hauth JC et al. 1991. Mid-second-trimester labor induction: Concentrated oxytocin compared with prostaglandin E2 suppositories. *Obstet Gynecol* 77:297.

Wong KS, CS Ngai, EL Yeo, LC Tang, PC Ho. 2000. A comparison of two regimens of intravaginal misoprostol for termination of second trimester pregnancy: A randomized comparative trial. *Hum Reprod* 15:709–712.

Yedlinsky NT, FC Morgan, PW Whitecar. 2005. Anomalies associated with failed methotrexate and misoprostol termination. *Obstet Gynecol* 105(5/Pt 2):1203–1205.

Zhou W, GL Nielsen, M Møller, J Olsen. 2002. Short-term complications after surgically induced abortions: A register-based study of 56,117 abortions. *Acta Obstet Gynecol Scand* 81:331–336.

35

Recent Trends in Contraceptive Technology

Gita Arjun

From vaginal sponges to homemade condoms, several contraceptives have been tried over the centuries. The introduction of hormonal contraceptives in the twentieth century, have made it easier for a woman to maintain control and exert choice over her reproductive function.

This chapter will focus on those advances in contraception which provide more effective and less expensive options. The improvements expected in a new contraceptive are that it should be more user-friendly and have fewer side effects compared to contraceptive methods that are already available.

New contraceptives for developing countries: The US Agency for International Development (USAID) is one of the largest suppliers of contraceptives in the developing world. Regulatory decisions made by agencies like the US Food and Drug Administration (US FDA) and the European Medicines Evaluation Agency (EMEA) play an important role in the introduction of new contraceptive methods in developing countries as well. After new contraceptive methods are approved by these agencies, they reach people in developing countries, either through national family planning programmes or through private pharmaceutical companies (Upadhyay 2005).

The contraceptives that will be discussed in this chapter are new advances in

- Intrauterine devices
- Condoms: male and female
- Vaginal barriers
- Transdermal contraception
- Spray-on contraceptive
- Contraceptive implants
- Vaginal rings

New intrauterine devices (IUD)

The improvements expected in a new IUD are:

- Ease of insertion and removal
- Reduction of expulsion rates
- Reduction of side effects like bleeding and pain

Levonorgestrel intrauterine system: (Mirena, Schering) is a type of IUD that slowly releases 20 µg per day of levonorgestrel into the uterine cavity. The ideal candidate for levonorgestrel intrauterine system (LNG-IUS) use is a woman who has had at least one child and has no history of pelvic inflammatory disease.

As with oral contraceptive pills, particularly the progestin-only pill, the thickening of the cervical mucous and inhibition of sperm motility and function are considered to be the primary means of preventing pregnancy. The presence of a foreign body in the uterus prompts the release of leukocytes and prostaglandins by the endometrium, substances that are hostile to both sperm and ova. Although endometrial concentrations of LNG are initially high, systemic concentrations are uniformly low. Ovulation is rarely suppressed after the first year, and even women who experience absence of bleeding using the LNG-IUS have the same incidence of ovulation as those who continue menstruating (Nilsson et al 1984).

The LNG-IUS causes an initial increase in spotting or bleeding during the first few months of use. After about three to six months, however, a significant reduction in both the amount and length of menstrual bleeding occurs. There is also a significant reduction in dysmenorrhea. About 15%–20% of women can become amenorrheic. It is important to warn women about the amenorrhea so that they do not worry that they are pregnant.

The LNG-IUS has not been associated with any serious side effects. There has been an increased association of benign follicular cysts in women using the LNG-IUS. As with any intrauterine device, perforations, misplacement, expulsions and pelvic inflammatory disease may occur as complications of the LNG-IUS.

The LNG-IUS is also associated with several non-contraceptive benefits. Endometrial suppression and decreased menstrual flow caused by LNG comes in useful for the non-surgical management of menorrhagia (Kumar et al 2005). The LNG-IUS is highly effective in reducing menstrual bleeding and has been shown to reduce the numbers of patients proceeding to hysterectomy (Hurskainen et al 2004).

Frameless IUDs: The frameless IUD consists of several copper cylinders tied together on a string. It is anchored one centimetre deep into the fundus of the uterus. This design is intended to cause less pain and bleeding than framed devices (Van Kets et al 1995; Masters and Everett 2005). GyneFix®, a frameless IUD was introduced in Europe in the early 1990s, to improve ease of insertion and attachment to the uterine wall (Van Kets et al 1995).

Promising results were reported for GyneFix® in minimising menstrual blood loss and discontinuation (Dennis and Hampton 2002; Andrade et al 2004). However, a Cochrane review found that symptoms of bleeding and pain, and contraceptive efficacy did not improve with the frameless device. The review also stated that there was insufficient data to show that problems of early expulsions have been overcome with the modified introducer used in GyneFix (O'Brien and Marfleet 2004). Expulsion rates have been higher than found in early clinical trials. The frameless IUD is less likely to be expelled when inserted by an experienced provider (Wildemeersch et al 2001; Wildemeersch 2003).

Another frameless IUD in development, FibroPlant-LNG, releases the progestin, levonorgestrel. Based on the design of the GyneFix® IUD, it too is anchored into the fundus of the uterus. FibroPlant-LNG delivers 14 μg of levonorgestrel daily and prevents pregnancy for at least three years (Wildemeersch et al 2002).

Vaginal barriers: In recent years, there has been a re-examination of the role of female-controlled barrier methods. The awareness of the need for protection against sexually transmitted disease, including HIV/AIDS along with the need for good contraception has fuelled the research for an effective barrier method for women.

The improvements expected in an effective barrier method are:

- Ease of use
- Protection against pregnancy
- Protection against sexually transmitted infections, including HIV/AIDS

It is hoped that cervical barrier methods will protect against infection by limiting access to cells in the cervix. There is enough biological evidence to suggest that the cells of the cervix are particularly susceptible to infection by HIV and other organisms causing sexually transmitted infections. Conversely, cervical barriers could also reduce the amount of viral shedding into vaginal secretions, thereby protecting partners of infected women.

It seems reasonable that cervical barrier methods will be more effective when used with a microbicide. Microbicides are gels, creams or other substances that are designed, when applied vaginally, to reduce transmission of HIV or other sexually transmitted infections. Unfortunately, there is no effective microbicide yet.

Diaphragm-like devices: The improvements expected in the new diaphragm-like devices are:

- More effectiveness
- More comfort
- Ease of insertion and removal

Lea's shield: is a cup-shaped device made of soft silicone rubber. Its advantage over the conventional diaphragm is that it comes in one size designed to fit most women. The shield is placed over the cervix and features a one-way valve designed to allow air and cervical secretions to pass out, while continuing to maintain a tight fit. It also contains a loop at the front end for ease of removal. It covers the cervix, blocking sperm from reaching the cervical canal. It has been designed to hold a spermicide or microbicide. Data on effectiveness are limited. Pregnancy rates in one study compared favourably with other studies of barrier contraceptive methods including the cervical cap, diaphragm and sponge (Mauck et al 2006).

SILCS intravaginal contraceptive device (SILCS): is a silicone device placed in the vagina to cover the cervix. Its shape makes insertion and removal easy. A preliminary acceptability trial of a fourth-generation prototype of the device and a phase I study comparing postcoital testing and safety of the SILCS diaphragm and the Ortho All-Flex diaphragm (both used with spermicide) supported the safety, comfort and ease of insertion, use and removal of the device (Schwartz and Gabelnick 2002).

Cervical caps: Two new contraceptive cervical caps, FemCap™ and Ovès™, are on the market in several countries. However, the acceptability among women has been poor because it requires fitting by a physician and few physicians are trained in the procedure.

FemCap is a silicone rubber device that fits snugly over the cervix and blocks the passage of sperm. FemCap was designed to dislodge less often than other cervical caps and to put less pressure on the urethra than the diaphragm. It has been available for several years in several European countries and recently was approved by the USFDA for use with spermicide. In a multicentric, randomised study, more women reported problems with the FemCap with regard to insertion, dislodgement and especially removal when compared to the Ortho Flex diaphragm (Mauck et al 1999). Pregnancy rates for the FemCap are 18 per 100 women per year of use.

Ovès: is a disposable cervical cap, first introduced in France in 1997. Ovès is made of thin silicone instead of latex. Like FemCap, it comes in three sizes and must be fitted by a provider. The thin dome of the cap resembles a membrane and adheres to the cervix like a film, a feature intended to make it comfortable and undetectable in use. Its effectiveness has not yet been established.

Condoms: Though condoms currently offer the best protection against sexually transmitted diseases and HIV infection, they have a high failure rate. Latex condoms deteriorate if exposed to heat, light or humidity. Oil-based lubricants used at the time of intercourse can cause damage and failure of condoms. To encourage usage and to reduce contraceptive failure, newer condoms, both male and female, have been developed.

Male condoms: Newer forms of male condoms include synthetic non latex condoms. New condom materials include polyurethane and styrene ethylene butylene styrene (SEBS). Polyurethane condoms have been available in the US since 1995, but the availability of non latex condoms in developing countries is limited.

Polyurethane and SEBS condoms have several advantages over latex condoms. They have a longer shelf life and can be used with oil-based lubricants, which can damage latex condoms. Some users also say non latex condoms have fewer odours, fit more comfortably and are less constricting, and transfer body heat better than latex condoms.

Several synthetic non-latex condoms, however, break or slip more often during intercourse or withdrawal than latex condoms. Despite the greater breakage and slippage rates, most were as effective as latex condoms in preventing pregnancy (Gallo et al 2003).

Female condoms: With consistent and correct use, the method failure rate for female condoms is 5%, while the typical use failure rate is 21% (Trussel 2004). Gross cumulative pregnancy rates of 12.4% (USA) and 22.2% (Latin America) at 6 months were found in a large multicentre study (Farr et al 1994). Higher contraceptive efficacy rates were identified in a Japanese study (Trussel 1998).

Breakage rates for female condoms are very low (<1 in 100 female condoms used). The slippage rate (slipping out of the vagina or being pushed up into the vagina) for female condoms is 5.6%. A randomised trial found a total clinical failure rate (breakage during sex, turned completely or partially inside out, slipped completely out, outer ring displacement, penetration outside the condom) of 5.24% (Beksinska et al 2006)

Men and women can be advised that when used consistently and correctly, female condoms are 95% effective at preventing pregnancy

FC2 Female condom: This is a second-generation female condom. It is made from synthetic latex, which is softer than polyurethane.

VA feminine condom, also known as the Reddy female condom or V-Amour, contains a soft sponge to hold it in place inside the vagina rather than a ring as used in the female condom. It also has a V-shaped external rim.

PATH woman's condom: This has been under development since 1998. The goal is to have a female condom with ease of insertion, comfort, stability, design and cost. The final product consists of a dissolving capsule intended to make insertion easier. A polyurethane condom pouch and a soft outer ring, allows for an almost universal fit. Once inserted, sections of urethane foam on the condom pouch allow the condom to cling lightly to the vaginal walls so that it does not move during use.

Transdermal contraception: Delivering a combination of estrogen and progestin, and 99% effective in preventing pregnancy, transdermal contraception offers the benefits of a low-dose oral contraceptive pill without the daily pill-taking routine that many women find difficult to maintain.

The transdermal contraceptive patch is a thin, beige square patch (4.45 x 4.45 cm), consisting of three layers—an outer protective layer of polyester, a medicated adhesive middle layer and a clear polyester release liner, which is removed before application. The patch releases a continuous level of 20 μg ethinyl estradiol and 150 μg norelgestromin transdermally into the bloodstream. It can be applied to the outer upper arm, upper torso (back and chest, but not breasts), abdomen or buttocks and must be changed every seven days for three weeks. The fourth week is patch free, and bleeding will occur in that time. Women may be able to use the patch continuously, using a fourth patch in the fourth week, skipping the withdrawal bleeding period. Studies are in progress to evaluate continuous use.

The patch adheres well to the skin, allowing women to perform regular daily activities such as bathing, swimming, working and exercising without interruption even in warm, humid climate (Zacur et al 2002). In about 2% of cases, the patch may fall off entirely, especially if women place it where they have applied creams, oils, powder or make-up. Women must be warned about this problem and properly counselled about application.

Recent study results indicate that the contraceptive patch is comparable to a combination pill in pregnancy prevention and cycle control, and compliance is better with the patch than with the pill (Audet et al 2001; Smallwood et al 2001).

The risks of transdermal contraception are also similar to those associated with the use of oral contraceptive pills and include an increased risk of blood clots (which remains less than half the risk of blood clots associated with pregnancy).

In clinical trials comparing patch users with oral contraceptive pill users, the incidence of breakthrough bleeding and spotting (one of the common reasons women discontinue hormonal contraceptives), was found to be significantly higher only in the first two cycles with the patch group, but the incidence of breakthrough bleeding alone was comparable between patch users and pill users in all cycles. Both methods were found to be similarly well tolerated. Application site reactions and breast tenderness were more common in the patch group, the latter side effect largely resolving after the first two cycles.

Younger women who have trouble following rules for correct use of oral contraceptive pills may find it easier to use the patch correctly. One study comparing correct use among patch users and oral contraceptive pill users found that patch users under age 20 years reported using it correctly in 89% of cycles. This compares very favourably to the fact that oral contraceptive pill users under age 20 reported taking their pills correctly in only 68% of cycles.

Even when not used correctly all the time, the patch is still highly effective. In typical use, 0.8 of every 100 women (8 per 1000) become pregnant in the first year of use. When the patch is used correctly, 0.6 of every 100 women (6 per 1000) become pregnant in the first year of use according to pooled data from three clinical studies. Another international multicentre study found a correct-use pregnancy rate of 1.1 per 100 women and a typical-use rate of 1.3 per 100 women, a rate lower than for women in the control group using combined oral contraceptive pills (Audet et al 2001).

Spray-on contraceptives: Once-a-day dosing of the contraceptive spray, Nestorone® Metered Dose Transdermal System® (MDTS®), provides sustained delivery of the contraceptive agent, Nestorone. Mean serum concentrations of Nestorone were maintained in the target range expected to be effective for contraception. In clinical trials, the spray was well tolerated, with no serious adverse events recorded.

The spray-on approach is a new technique for transferring a preset dose of fast-drying hormones onto the skin. The spray is absorbed almost instantaneously, so there is no risk of washing it off. The hormone collects as a reservoir within the skin, from which it then slowly diffuses into the bloodstream.

Potential advantages of the Nestorone MDTS over existing methods of contraception, such as pills and patches, are:

- Suitability for breastfeeding mothers and women who cannot tolerate combined oral contraceptives containing estrogen
- Increased flexibility in dosing time compared to progestogen-only pills
- Reduced skin irritation compared to patches
- Convenient daily dosing of the spray, which leaves no visible residue on the skin.

Contraceptive implants: In an effort to improve acceptance of implantable contraceptive devices, the focus has moved to reducing the number of rods or capsules implanted. Rods are filled with a mixture of steroid crystals and polymer. Capsules are hollow polymer tubes filled with free steroid crystals.

Different progestins have been used to minimise side effects, particularly bleeding disturbances. Safety during breastfeeding is also an important issue. Norplant® implant, the first implant available, was approved by the USFDA in 1990. Norplant implants employ six capsules to deliver the progestin levonorgestrel. They provide excellent contraceptive protection but in some countries also have high discontinuation rates due to bleeding disturbances. Bleeding disturbances are cited as the most common reason for discontinuation by women using the implants (Glasier 2002).

The newer implants offer several improvements. The new implants consist of one or two rods or capsules. Like Norplant, they are inserted just under the skin of the upper arm to deliver progestins into the bloodstream. Most use rods rather than capsules. Unfortunately, the new implants are expensive to develop and market and they require provider training in techniques of insertion and removal.

New implants deliver the progestin levonorgestrel (Jadelle®), etonogestrel (Implanon®) or ST-1435 (Elcometrine and Nestorone implant). Implants prevent pregnancy by thickening cervical mucous so that it is impenetrable to sperm, preventing ovulation in many cycles and suppressing endometrial growth.

The newer implants are inserted using a specially designed preloaded applicator that eliminates the need for a separate incision. Most insertions of Jadelle® take less than five minutes, and for trained providers using a preloaded disposable applicator, Implanon® insertion takes less than one minute (Walling 2000). Rates of complications and removal are about half those for Norplant implants.

A review of studies reported that infection or pain at the implant site occurred in less than 7% of users. The most frequent side effects that are probably related to implant use are headaches and acne, both reported by less than 30% of users. Weight gain, dizziness and mood changes are mentioned by less than 20% of users. Rates of these problems are similar among users of the different implants (Brache et al 2002).

Vaginal rings: These rings, offer a new way to deliver hormones into the bloodstream to prevent pregnancy. Hormone-releasing vaginal rings are kept in the vagina and remain in place day and night for three weeks or one year, depending on the formulation. Unfortunately, the cost of the vaginal rings might prevent their being available in developing countries.

Vaginal rings come both as combined formulations (containing a progestin and an estrogen) and as progestin-only formulations. Vaginal rings work by releasing progestin with estrogen or progestin alone. They prevent ovulation, cause thickening of cervical mucous, and suppress endometrial growth. Combined estrogen and progestin rings offer good cycle control and deliver hormones more steadily than combined oral contraceptives. Studies in developed countries have found that women follow rules for correct use at rates higher than those seen in studies of combined oral contraceptives (Bjarnadottir et al 2002).

Vaginal rings have proved effective and result in 1.2–1.5 pregnancies per 100 women in the first year as typically used.

To use the vaginal ring, a woman inserts it into the vagina with her fingers, placing it anywhere that feels comfortable. It fits best in the higher part of the vagina. The ring remains in place all day and night. Hormones diffuse continuously from a reservoir within the ring. Passing through the vaginal tissues, they reach the bloodstream. The ring can be removed for up to three hours for comfort during sexual intercourse, for cleaning or for any other reason.

Combined vaginal rings: The combined formula NuvaRing® is the first vaginal ring to be widely introduced. NuvaRing releases 120 µg of the progestin, etonogestrel and 15 µg of the estrogen, ethinyl estradiol, per day. Women use NuvaRing for three weeks, then remove it for a week, during which time they have withdrawal bleeding. A new NuvaRing is needed for each four-week cycle. Thus, a woman would require 13 rings per year. A single ring can last up to 35 days (Mulders et al 2002). Small studies suggest that women may be able to safely use combined vaginal rings consecutively for four weeks at a time, skipping the withdrawal bleeding. Results of larger studies are needed to evaluate continuous use.

Another ring, still in clinical trials, releases a combination of 150 µg of a different progestin, Nestorone®, and 15 µg of the estrogen ethinyl estradiol per day. This ring is being developed specifically for use in developing countries. It will be effective for over 12 months, making it more cost-effective than NuvaRing. Users would keep the ring in place for three weeks, remove it for the fourth week to allow a withdrawal bleed, and then reinsert the same ring for another three weeks (Johansson and Sitruk-Ware 2004).

Bleeding problems are less frequent among users of combined vaginal rings than among users of combined oral contraceptives or of progestin-only rings. Breakthrough bleeding can occur, but this side effect is not common (Roumen et al 2001).

Progestin-only rings: These prevent pregnancy mainly by thickening cervical mucous to prevent sperm penetration. They also have some effect on preventing ovulation and build-up of the endometrium (Mishell 1993).

Progestin-only rings are less effective than rings containing both a progestin and an estrogen. However, they are highly effective in breastfeeding women because breastfeeding itself provides some protection from pregnancy. Bleeding disturbances, a common side effect of all progestin-only methods, is less likely to be noticed while a woman is breastfeeding. Usually, women will switch to more effective contraception after they stop breastfeeding.

Progesterone rings: These release 10 mg of progesterone daily and last for three months. Women can use these rings continuously for up to one year, after which effectiveness declines.

In clinical trials, women using the progesterone ring reported experiencing vaginal problems related to discharge, urinary discomfort, bleeding disturbances and reproductive tract infection However, in a Chilean study of breastfeeding women, less than 5% of users experienced any one of these side effects.

Nestorone rings: These are similar to progesterone rings but rely on ST-1435, a more potent synthetic progestin that has unique properties. This ring will release 50, 75 or 100 µg of Nestorone per day. Nestorone-releasing rings provide effective protection from pregnancy for lactating women for up to one year, even if weaning takes place earlier.

References

Andrade AT, JP Souza, GN Andrade, PJ Rowe, D Wildemeersch. 2004. Assessment of menstrual blood loss in Brazilian users of the frameless copper-releasing IUD with copper surface area of 330 mm^2 and the frameless levonorgestrel-releasing intrauterine system. *Contraception* 70(2):173–177.

Audet MC et al. 2001. Evaluation of contraceptive efficacy and cycle control of a transdermal contraceptive patch vs an oral contraceptive: A randomized controlled trial. *JAMA* 285 (18): 2347–2354.

Beksinska M, J Smit, Z Mabude, G Vijayakumar, C Joanis. 2006. Performance of the reality polyurethane female condom and a synthetic latex prototype: A randomized crossover trial among South African women. *Contraception* 73:386–393.

Bjarnadottir RI, M Tuppurainen, SR Killick. 2002. Comparison of cycle control with a combined contraceptive vaginal ring and oral levonorgestrel/ethinyl estradiol. *Am J Obstet Gynecol* 186(3): 389–395.

Brache V, A Faundes, F Alvarez, L Cochon. 2002. Nonmenstrual adverse events during use of implantable contraceptives for women: Data from clinical trials. *Contraception* 65(1):63–74.

Dennis J and N Hampton. 2002. IUDs: Which device? *J Fam Plann Reprod Health Care* 28(2):61–68.

Farr G, H Gabelnick, K Sturgen, L Dorflinger. 1994. Contraceptive efficacy and acceptability of the female condom. *Am J Public Health* 84:1960–1964.

Gallo MF, DA Grimes and KF Schulz. 2003. Non-latex versus latex male condoms for contraception. *Cochrane Database of Systematic Reviews* (2): CD003550.

Glasier A. 2002. Implantable contraceptives for women: Effectiveness, discontinuation rates, return of fertility, and outcome of pregnancies. *Contraception* 65(1):29–37.

Hurskainen R, J Teperi, P Rissanen, AM Aalto, S Grenman, A Kivelä et al. 2004. Clinical outcomes and costs with the levonorgestrel-releasing intrauterine system or hysterectomy for treatment of menorrhagia. Randomised trial 5-year follow-up. *JAMA* 291:1456–1463.

Johansson ED and R Sitruk-Ware. 2004. New delivery systems in contraception: Vaginal rings. *Am J Obstet Gynecol* 190(Suppl 4): S54–59.

Kumar S, ZK Antony, V Mohindra, A Kapur. 2005. Therapeutic use of LNG intrauterine system (Mirena) for menorrhagia due to benign lesions: An alternative to hysterectomy? *J Obstet Gynecol India* Vol. 55, No. 6: 541–543

Masters T and S Everett. 2005. Intrauterine and barrier contraception (a practical review of recent developments). *Curr Obstet Gynaecol* 15(1):31–37.

Mauck C, LH Glover, E Miller et al.1996. Lea's Shield: A study of the safety and efficacy of a new vaginal barrier contraceptive used with and without spermicide. *Contraception.* 53(6):329–335.

Mauck C, M Callahan, DH Weiner, R Dominik. 1999. A comparative study of the safety and efficacy of FemCap, a new vaginal barrier contraceptive, and the Ortho All-Flex diaphragm. The FemCap Investigators' Group. *Contraception.* 60(2):71–80.

Mishell DR. 1993. Vaginal contraceptive rings. *Annals of Medicine* 25(2):191–197.

Mulders TM, TO Dieben, HJ Bennink. 2002. Ovarian function with a novel combined contraceptive vaginal ring. *Hum Reprod* 17(10):2594–2599.

Nilsson CG, PL Lahteenmaki and T Luukkainen. 1984. Ovarian function in amenorrheic and menstruating users of a levonorgestrel-releasing intrauterine device. *Fertil Steril.* 41(1):52–55.

O'Brien P and CC Marfleet. 2004. Frameless versus classical intrauterine device for contraception. *Cochrane Database of Systematic Reviews*, Issue 4. Art. No. CD003282. DOI: 10.1002/14651858.CD003282. pub2

Roumen FJ, D Apter, TM Mulders, TO Dieben. 2001. Efficacy, tolerability and acceptability of a novel contraceptive vaginal ring releasing etonogestrel and ethinyl oestradiol. *Hum Reprod* 16(3):469–475.

Schwartz JL and HL Gabelnick. 2002. Current Contraceptive Research. *Perspect Sex Reprod Health* Volume 34, Number 6

Smallwood GH et al. 2001. Efficacy and safety of a transdermal contraceptive system. *Obstet Gynecol* 30 (5):799–805

Trussell J. 1998. Contraceptive efficacy of the Reality female condom. *Contraception* 58:147–148

Trussell J. 2004. Contraceptive efficacy. In: Hatcher RA, Trussell J, Stewart F, Nelson A, Cates W, Guest F et al. (eds), *Contraceptive Technology.* New York, NY: Ardent Media.

Upadhyay UD. 2005. *New Contraceptive Choices. Population Reports*, Series M, No. 19. Baltimore: The Johns Hopkins Bloomberg School of Public Health, The INFO Project.

Van Kets H, M Vrijeus, Y Van Trapper et al. 1995. The frameless GyneFix® intrauterine implant: A major improvement in efficacy, expulsion and tolerance. *Adv Contraception* 11:131–142

Walling M. 2000. Development of contraceptive implants. *Brit Fam Plann* 26(1):12–13.

Wildemeersch D, I Batar, B Affandi, A Andrade, W Shangchun et al. 2003. The 'frameless' intrauterine system for long-term, reversible contraception: A review of 15 years of clinical experience. *J Obstet Gynaecol Res* 29(3):164–173.

Wildemeersch D. 2001. Further information and recommendations to prevent perforation with the frameless GyneFix IUD. *J Fam Plann Reprod Health Care* 27(4): 241.

Wildemeersch D, E Schacht, P Wildemeersch, D Janssens, M Thiery. 2002. Development of a miniature, low-dose, frameless intrauterine levonorgestrel-releasing system for contraception and treatment: A review of initial clinical experience. *Reprod Biomed Online* 4(1): 71-82.

Zacur HA, B Hedon, D Mansour, GA Shangold, AC Fisher, GW Creasy. 2002. Integrated summary of Ortho Evra/Evra contraceptive patch adhesion in varied climates and conditions. *Fertil Steril* 77(2 Suppl 2): S32–35.

36

Hormonal Contraceptives: Current Problems and Developments

A Padma Rao

Oral contraceptives, the first of the series of hormonal contraceptives, marked the fortieth year of its usage in 2000. 'The pill' as the oral contraceptive is called is the most extensively studied medication in medical history. Over the last 40 years or more, the 'pill' has undergone continuous changes in its composition and dosage in order to solve many of its debated problems. Many non-oral methods of hormonal contraceptives have been introduced and still more are being researched for introduction to improve user compliance and to reduce problems. Some major benefits of hormonal contraceptives have also been identified.

The following are discussed in this chapter:

1. Hormonal contraceptives
2. Health benefits of hormonal contraceptives
3. Current problems
4. Current developments
5. Tentative conclusions

The hormones in contraceptives are steroids. The term 'steroid' is derived from Greek, meaning 'like a sterol'. Sterols are certain solid alcohols that occur widely in plants and animals, the best known being cholesterol. The story of oral contraception cannot be written without mentioning the name of Russel Marker who paved the way for others to synthesise many other steroids to be supplied the world over at affordable rates. A brilliant but eccentric chemist, he extracted injectable progesterone—diosgenin—from a yam by a simple process—tons of the plant, were boiled in an old building in Mexico before he succeeded. Marker showed the world a new source of steroids in the 1940s. The first oral progesterone, Norethisterone, also known as norethindrone, was synthesised in 1951 by Carl Djerassi, and since then it has been incorporated into 50% of hormonal contraceptives. The name progestin (also progestogen) was suggested by Djerassi (1981) to mean a 'progesterone-like' substance.

The first 'pill' launched in 1960 after nine years of clinical trial, contained 10 mg of progestin and 150 μg of estrogen. The high dose proved to be effective in preventing ovulation. However, it became clear that it also induced some undesirable side effects. Therefore, newer pills were developed. The doses of progestin and estrogen were drastically reduced. The current pill contains a little over 1% of the progestogen and less than 20% of the estrogen contained in the first pill.

The estrogen component is ethinyl estradiol

in almost all the pills available currently. In the earliest pill, the estrogen component was mestranol, which is a weaker estrogen compared to ethinyl estradiol. Mestranol had to be converted in the body to ethinyl estradiol before it functioned. The progestogens in the pill vary. Thus, three generations of progestogens and three generations of oral hormonal contraceptives have emerged.

Norethisterone (Norethindrone), norethynodrel, norethindrone acetate, lynestrenol and ethynodiol diacetate are first generation progestins. All of them are derived from 19 nortestosterone and are converted to norethisterone in the body (Djerassi 1981). Norethindrone enanthate, norgestimate and norgestrel belong to the second generation. Norgestrel is more potent than the first generation progestins. It has two racemic forms, dextro and levorotatory. The levorotatory form is the active isomer and is known as levonorgestrel, sometimes written as dl-norgestrel.

Desogestrel and gestodene are third generation progestins. Etonogestrel, an active metabolite of desogestrel, is used in implants and in the vaginal ring. The other progestins of the third generation are dionogest and drosperinone. Dionogest has antiandrogenic properties and is used in the pill; it has the property of preventing acne. Drosperinone is also used in the pill and is useful for dealing with the premenstrual syndrome (Brown et al 2002).

Types of hormonal contraceptives

1. Oral hormonal contraceptives

- Combined oral hormonal contraceptive (COC)
- Progestin-Only Pill (POP)
- Multiphasic Pill

2. Non-oral hormonal contraceptives

- Injectables
- Implants (Intradermal)
- Transdermal
- Hormone-releasing intra uterine system

Combined Oral Hormonal Contraceptives (COC)

There are three generations of combined oral hormonal contraceptives:

- First generation contains 50 µg or more of estrogen
- Second generation contains second generation progestins and 20, 30 or 35 µg of estrogen
- Third generation contains third generation progestins and 20, 25 or 30 µg of estrogen.

The COC pill is to be started within five days of the first day of menstruation. It is to be taken every day for three weeks leaving one pill-free week. Whether there should be a seven-day free interval before starting the next pack of pills is a point of debate. Utilising a four-day pill-free interval rather than the usual seven days is associated with greater ovulation suppression (Sullivan et al 1999). Research by Yeshaya and colleagues compared the effect of starting COC on the first day of menses verses the last day (up to day 5). They found that the incidence of breakthrough bleeding was reduced when the pill was started on the last day of menses, which may be day 3, 4 or 5 (Yeshaya et al 1998).

Missed pill: If one pill is missed, a pill is to be taken as soon as remembered and the course must be continued as usual. A back-up, such as a condom, may be used for the rest of the cycle. If two pills are missed, two pills are to be taken as soon as remembered and again two more pills the next day and thereafter, continue with one pill every day. However, another back-up method of contraception must be used for the rest of the cycle. If more than three pills are missed, the patient must stop taking the pills and use another method of contraception till the next menstruation.

The mechanism of action: The action of progesterone in the pill precedes that of estrogen, the cervical mucus gets thick and impermeable to sperms, the endometrium becomes thin, glands atrophy and become unreceptive to ovum implantation. The progesterone component also suppresses LH surge, thus preventing ovulation.

The estrogen component suppresses the action of FSH and thus prevents the emergence of a dominant follicle. Estrogen also provides stability to the endometrium to prevent irregular shedding (breakthrough bleeding). Estrogen also potentiates the action of progestin by increasing the intracellular progestational receptor, thus making it possible to reduce the progestin dose in the pill.

Effectiveness of COC: 'Method effectiveness' is 99.9% when the COC is used correctly as prescribed.

'Use effectiveness' is 85% to 90% when the COC is used irregularly.

Some 'beliefs' of the past clarified

1. It was believed that all derivatives of 19-nortestosteronewerametabolisedwithin the body to estrogenic compounds. This question was restudied and it was argued that the previous evidence for metabolism to estrogenic compounds was due to an artifact in the laboratory analysis. More recent studies indicate that norethindrone can be converted to ethinyl estradiol; however, this rate of conversion is so low that an insignificant amount of ethinyl estradiol can be found in the circulation or urine following administration of the commonly used doses of norethindrone (Stanczyk and Roy 1990).
2. **The pill and antibiotics:** It was believed that antibiotics such as ampicillin, quinolone, tetracycline and metranidazole lowered the effectiveness of the pill. Studies indicate that the plasma levels of contraceptives are unchanged and that there is no evidence of ovulation with the use of the above-mentioned antibiotics (Speroff and Fritz 2005). The only exception is rifampicin, which lowers the efficacy of the pill.
3. **The pill and breakthrough bleeding:** Prolonged breakthrough bleeding was treated in the past by administering two or three COC pills. But the current thought is to administer, in such situations, a short course of exogenous estrogen, conjugated estrogen 1.25 mg or estradiol 2 mg for seven days instead of two or three COC pills. The pill-taking schedule should not be disturbed (Speroff and Fritz 2005).
4. **The pill and amenorrhea:** The idea that the pill causes amenorrhea has now been dispelled. There is no cause and effect relationship between oral hormonal contraceptive use and secondary amenorrhea. Women who have not resumed their menses within 12 months should be evaluated as any other patient with secondary amenorrhea.

Progestin-only pill or minipill: The progestins used in the minipill are norethindrone, levonorgestrel, lynestrenol, ethinodiol diacetate and desogestrel. The minipill does not provide full protection against ovulation. But in a breast-feeding patient, the minipill together with lactation provides dual contraception.

The lactating mother who initially chooses to rely on the Lactational Amenorrhea Method (LAM) is advised to begin POPs

- When her menses returns or

- When she is no longer fully or nearly fully breastfeeding or
- At six months postpartum whichever comes first

Lactating women who took COC did not experience much change in the quantity of milk. However, they stopped lactation by six months, whereas those using POP could continue lactation like those who did not use any pill. For breast-feeding women, delaying POP initiation for six weeks after delivery avoids exposing the newborn to exogenous steroids during the time of greatest neuroendocrine development. Approximately 12% of maternal serum levonorgestrel (from implants) transfers to breast milk and 75% of this amount transfers to infant serum (Shikary et al 1987).

In an 8-year follow-up study of children breastfed by mothers using oral contraceptives, no effect could be detected on diseases, intelligence or psychological behaviour (Nilsson et al 1986). The minipill should be started on the first day of menses, it should be taken daily at the same time of the day and without a pill-free period. The change in the cervical mucus requires 2–4 hours to take effect. It is important to note that impermeability lasts for 22 hours after the intake of the minipill and ceases by 24 hours. Therefore, the minipill has to be taken at the same time of the day, preferably late afternoon or 4 to 5 hours before the usual time of sexual activity and if there is a delay of more than 3 hours in taking the pill, a back-up method should be used for 48 hours.

A progestin-only pill with desogestrel 75 µg (Cerazette) affords more effective prevention of ovulation.

To summarise, the minipill is:

1. To be started on the first day of menses and taken daily without a pill-free period.
2. To be taken at the same time of the day, it should not be delayed by more than three hours. This disadvantage is overcome by using implants and other non-oral hormonal methods with progestins.
3. If there is a 3 hour delay in taking the pill, a back-up method should be used for 48 hours.
4. Irregular menstrual bleeding is a major problem seen more here than with COC.
5. Amenorrhea occurs in 10% of users. It is a major reason to discontinue the pill (Broome and Fotherby 1990).
6. Development of acne is common.
7. If pregnancy occurs, it is more likely to be an ectopic pregnancy
8. There is an associated risk—the likelihood of a three-fold increase in the risk of diabetes in lactating women with recent gestational diabetes (Kjos et al 1998).
9. The minipill is ideal for lactating women because lactation provides additional contraception

Multiphasic pill (triphasic pill): Like other low-dose COCs, the multiphasic pill appears to provide highly effective contraception, if used correctly. Some clinical trials have observed that multiphasics produce minimal breakthrough bleeding, spotting and amenorrhea. There is little evidence that the risk of serious health problems are less with multiphasics than with other low-dose pills (Speroff et al 1988).

HEALTH BENEFITS OF HORMONAL CONTRACEPTIVES

Reduced risk of epithelial ovarian cancer: Epithelial ovarian cancer forms 90% of all ovarian cancers. Risk factors of epithelial ovarian cancer are nulliparity, family history and genetic factors like BRCA1/BRCA2 mutation. The protective effect of OC in reducing the risk of epithelial ovarian cancer is being investigated since 1980. The Cancer and

Steroid Hormone Study (CASH) conducted by the Centres of Disease Control, between 1980 and 1982, provided the initial evidence for this protective effect. It is also the largest study. It demonstrated a 40% reduction in risk after as little as 3 to 6 months of OC use. The degree of protection increased progressively with prolonged duration of use up to 80% at 10 or more years suggesting a biological gradient (Anonymous 1987). The CASH study also demonstrated that the protective effect persisted for at least 15 years after last use (Gross and Schlesselman 1994).

Hankinson et al (1992) confirmed the findings of the CASH study through a meta-analysis of 20 studies. They also noted that the protection persisted for at least 10 years after the last use. Surveillance, Epidemiology and End Results (SEER) network also confirmed this protective effect, that five years of oral hormonal contraceptive use reduced the risk of epithelial ovarian cancer in nulliparous women to that of parous women. The Hereditary Ovarian Cancer Clinical Study Group (HOCSG) conducted a transnational case-control study. They demonstrated that OC produced risk reduction even in BRCA mutation subjects (Rosenberg et al 1994). Women in the study who had used OC 20 years earlier demonstrated persistence of the effect for up to 19 years. The protective effect on epithelial ovarian cancer is also documented with low-dose pills. On the basis of this compelling information, OC use should be continued in appropriate women during the later reproductive years, it should be offered to women at high risk for ovarian cancer, as a primary indication for protection against ovarian cancer, even if a contraception benefit is not required (Jenson et al 2000).

Protection against endometrial cancer: The CASH study by Centres of Disease Control and Prevention confirmed a significant protective effect, of OCs, against endometrial cancer that persisted at least 15 years after stopping OC use. Twelve months of OC use reduced the risk of endometrial cancer by 40%. The protection increased with longer duration of use, a significant 60% reduction by 10 years of use (The CASH Study 1987).

A study by WHO noted that high-estrogen/ high-progestin formulations offered the most protection. A large US population-based case-control study found equal protection against endometrial cancer for OCs containing either low or high doses of progestin (Voigt et al 1994). A study in Sweden found that subsequent use of hormone replacement during menopause did not modify the protective effect against endometrial cancer (Weiderpass 1999).

Reduction of colorectal cancer: There was a reduction of almost 40% in the risk of colorectal cancer among women who had used OC for 96 months or longer, the possible explanation being the favourable action of estrogen on bile synthesis and excretion and the reduction of bile acid concentration in the colon. A review of available literature indicated a reduced risk of colorectal cancer in ever-users of oral contraceptives (Franceschi and La Vecchia 1998).

Reduction of pelvic inflammatory disease: There is strong evidence that COC not only reduces the risk but also the severity of pelvic inflammatory disease (Wolner-Hanssen 1996). However, lower genital tract chlamydia infection is not reduced. The exact cause is not clear. In spite of more susceptibility to lower genital tract infection with chlamydia, COC users are less likely to experience acute symptomatic chlamydeal salpingitis than women using non-hormonal methods of contraception (Spinillo et al 1996).

Better bone density: A retrospective study of 2297 perimenopausal women found that women who had used COC had better bone density than those who had not used COC (Kleerekoper et al 1991).

Fewer fibroids: In the past it was believed that fibroids of the uterus enlarged in pregnancy and also with the use of COC. But this belief has since been dispelled. It has been found that low doses of COC do not increase the size of fibroids; such doses also reduce symptoms such as menorrhagia. Long-term use of COC prevents the formation of fibroids. Protection increased with duration of use (Chiaffarino et al 1999). This indeed is a great benefit, because the incidence of fibroids has increased now, with increased use of birth control measures.

Prevention of anemia: As menstrual bleeding is reduced with COC, iron stores improve and the risk of iron deficiency anemia is substantially reduced. A Danish study revealed that serum ferritin levels were noted to be higher in COC users (Milman et al 1998). This is a welcome benefit in developing countries.

Menstrual benefits: Regular menstrual cycles, relief from dysmenorrhea and tailoring one's menstrual cycle to one's convenience are all well known.

CURRENT PROBLEMS

1. Noncompliance
2. Cardiovascular accidents
3. Diabetes
4. Breast cancer
5. Cervical cancer

Noncompliance: This is the major problem in our country. Only 1.2% of eligible couples were using hormonal contraception in India in 1993 (Population Report 2000), and it is no better now. Minor side effects like nausea, vomiting and breakthrough bleeding may be the cause, but not the only reasons. Magnified reports by the media on the side effects of the pill could be one of the reasons for non-compliance by women.

It is time to recollect the story of the pill. Gregory Pincus, a research biologist was requested by Margaret Sanger, the birth control pioneer, at a dinner party at New York in the residence of a philanthropist, Katherine McCormick, to find a new approach to contraception. Sanger never thought of a pill. Pincus was promised US $ 2100 to cover the expenses of the first year's research. Driving alone from New York to Shrewsbury, Massachusetts, Pincus analysed the problem with quick and incisive clarity and the idea flashed in his brain as he arrived at his doorstep that 'progesterone is the answer, it worked in rabbits to stop ovulation in the Pennsylvania research of 1937, so why not in women?' Pincus used large doses of progesterone injection for his preliminary research (Vaughan 1972).

Later, when oral progestins were available he used for his clinical trials, high doses of progestins (10 mg and 5 mg) in the pill, for he believed that the pill should create a pregnancy-state. Thus, the side effects of the earlier pill were those occurring in pregnancy; for example nausea, vomiting, urinary tract infection, vaginal candidiasis, altered carbohydrate metabolism (diabetes), hypercoagulable state (thrombosis). Unfortunately, the major side effects of the original high-dose pills were researched and reported years after the high-dose pill was withdrawn and a very low-dose pill had been introduced. Women remembered the side effects of the high-dose pill, of the past and disregarded the merits of the new low-dose pill. Another reason for not using the pill is that the remarkable health benefits of hormonal contraception are not widely known to women. Perhaps Djeressi's remark that 'Politics rather than science will shape the future of birth control' may be true (McBride 2002).

Cardiovascular accidents: Two types of cardiovascular accidents can occur.

Venous Thromboembolic disease (VTE): This problem can occur in the form of venous thromboembolic disease, fatal pulmonary embolism, and rarely, cerebral venous thrombosis. Venous thromboembolic disease is the most common cardiovascular event among users of oral contraceptives. However, it contributes very little to any increase in the number of deaths since the associated mortality is relatively low, compared to that associated with arterial diseases. Long-term disability from nonfatal venous thromboembolic disease is also low. The risk is probably highest in the first year of use—ten-fold, which falls to a two-fold increase in subsequent years (Suissa et al 1997) and declines thereafter, but persists until discontinuation. Important risk factors for arterial disease such as cigarette smoking, hypertension and diabetes do not appear to be risk factors for venous thromboembolic disease. However, age is a risk factor. The absolute risk of venous thromboembolic disease increases with age. Women with hereditary clotting defects such as factor V Leiden mutation, protein C deficiency, protein S deficiency or antithrombin III defect, are at a much higher risk of venous thromboembolism, if they use oral contraceptives. The relative risk of deep vein thrombosis is 35 compared with nonusers without this mutation. Even with such high relative risk, the absolute risk was still low (Vandenbroucke et al 1994).

Please note that relative risk is the association between exposure to the factor and the development of the disease; absolute risk or attributable risk depends on the size of relative risk and the incidence of the disease.

Arterial cardiovascular complications (Table 36.1)

1. Acute myocardial infarction
2. Ischemic stroke
3. Hemorrhagic stroke

1. Acute Myocardial Infarction (AMI): The incidence of fatal and non-fatal myocardial infarction is very low in women of the reproductive age. Cigarette smoking carries a higher risk for myocardial infarction than oral contraceptives, but there is no evidence that non-smoking users of oral contraceptives are at an increased risk (Lewis et al 1997). The overall incidence of myocardial infarction in the reproductive age is 5 per 1,00,000 per year (Petitti et al 1997). The incidence of MI in less than 35 years and non-smokers is 4/100,000/year and in non-smokers and OC users too it is 4/100,000/year. But the incidence doubles in smokers using OC-8/100,000/year. As age advances, the incidence of MI increases in those over 35 years. The incidence of MI in non-smokers, non-smokers using OC, smokers and smokers using OC are 10/100,000/year, 40/100,000/year, 88/100,000/year and 485/100,000/year respectively. These include undetected cardiovascular risk factors like hypertension, diabetes etc which were not screened in the study (WHO 1997). In a Danish case-control study, statistically significant increase in the risk of MI was noted in current users of 50 µg ethinyl estradiol (Lidegaard and Edstrom 1996).

TABLE 36.1: ARTERIAL AND VENOUS COMPLICATIONS COMPARED

Arterial	Venous
AMI and Stroke	VTE and cerebral venous thrombosis
Less common	More common
Mortality more	Mortality negligible Morbidity also negligible
Smoking, hypertension and diabetes are confounding factors	Smoking, hypertension and diabetes are not confounding factors
Increases with age	Increases with age
Hereditary clotting defects such as factor V Leiden mutation are not risk factors	Hereditary clotting defects such as factor V Leiden mutation are risk factors Relative risk is high, but absolute risk is very low.
Risk is constant throughout the duration of use. No risk in past users	Risk is highest in the first year of use and declines thereafter but persists until discontinuation.

2. Stroke: The incidence of fatal and non-fatal ischemic and hemorrhagic stroke is very low in women of reproductive age. Risks are similar to that noted for acute myocardial infarction.

Diabetes (impaired glucose tolerance): Plasma levels of insulin as well as blood sugar were elevated with the use of the very early high-dose pills, which contained a high dose of progestin. Insulin sensitivity is affected mainly by the progestin component of the pill. The glucose intolerance is dose related and the insulin and glucose changes are so minimal with the low-dose pill that it is now believed they are of no clinical significance (Troisi et al 2000).

Breast cancer: Development of breast cancer is a major fear among pill users. Surveys have shown that nearly a third of respondents incorrectly believed that oral contraceptive use is associated with an increased risk for breast cancer (Peipert and Gutmann 1993). In an attempt to clarify this misconception, a reanalysis of epidemiological data was done. The study did reveal that breast cancer risk was slightly increased in young oral contraceptive users. A study by Rosenberg et al (1996) likewise found a small increase in the risk of breast cancer in young (25–34 years) and recent (at least a year) oral contraceptive users, but no other risk among other women. The collaborative group study also demonstrated that the breast cancer developed in pill users was less advanced and more amenable to treatment and more likely to be cured. It is not yet known whether the incidence of breast cancer diminishes with the introduction of genetic screening for BRCA 1/BRCA 2.

Cancer of the cervix: Studies have indicated that the risk for dysplasia and carcinoma in situ of the uterine cervix increases with the use of oral contraceptives (Brinton 1991). There has been an increase in the incidence of adenocarcinoma of the cervix (10% of all cervical cancers) in young women over the last 20 years. There is concern that this increase reflects the use of oral contraceptives. Other risk factors such as multiple partners, age at first coitus, human papilloma virus (HPV) and smoking will have to be studied. Therefore, no conclusions can be drawn regarding the incidence of cervical cancer in pill users.

EMERGENCY CONTRACEPTION WITH STEROID HORMONES

These are contraception methods to deal with unprotected intercourse at any point in the menstrual cycle.

The various methods are:

1. The Yuzpe's method that is used currently is 100 μg of ethinyl estradiol and 1.0 mg of levonorgestrel given twice, 12 hours apart within 72 hours of intercourse (Yuzpe and Lancee 1977).
2. Levonorgestrel-only regimen: A single dose of 1.5 mg levonorgestrel is to be taken as soon as possible. Alternatively, a single dose of 0.75 mg levonorgestrel to be taken as soon as possible followed by the same dose 12 hours later (International Medical Advisory Panel 2004).
3. High-dose oral contraceptive pill, the dose matched with Yuzpe's combination regime is equally effective. For example, two tablets of Ovral (levonorgestrel 0.25 mg and EE 0.05 mg) as soon as possible and two tablets, 12 hours later. Alternatively, Ovral L (Levonorgestrel (0.25 mg and EE 0.03 mg) 4 tablets + 4 tablets may be taken.
4. Danazol has been tried without success.
5. Mifepristone in lower doses (10 mg) would provide emergency contraception without significantly compromising effectiveness (WHO 1999).

Mechanism of action of emergency contraception: If administered before ovulation, the estrogen–progestin combination delays ovulation. If administered after ovulation it may suppress the hormone receptors and asynchronise maturation of the endometrium, rendering it unsuitable for implantation. There is no evidence of emergency contraception acting as an abortifacient.

Points to remember

1. Emergency contraception cannot be availed of more than twice in a cycle.
2. Progestin-only regime (levonorgestrel) is found to be more effective and has fewer side effects.
3. As ovulation may be delayed by emergency contraception, another birth control measure should be adopted (abstinence or some effective contraception) in that cycle.
4. If vomiting occurs within two hours of taking either dose of emergency contraception, a further dose and an anti-emetic, or an IUCD is advised.
5. Contraception is more effective if taken within 24 hours.

NON-ORAL HORMONAL CONTRACEPTIVES

Non-oral routes offer continuous and steady steroid levels for several years and avoid the first-pass peak effect through the hepatic portal system, thereby avoiding the peak plasma levels of steroids associated with oral dosing. Further higher bioavailability leads to a lower dose of steroid being administered with a possible parallel reduction in the occurrence of adverse effects.

Implants: The first implant, Norplant, consisted of six capsules containing levonorgestrel. Because of the difficulty in insertion and removal, this device is replaced by a single rod implant system containing etonogestrel, known as Implanon, which is now used in most of the major European countries, Australia, Mexico and Brazil (Table 36.2).

Before the introduction of Implanon a two-rod levonorgestrel releasing contraceptive implant (Jadella) was developed by the Population Council. Insertion and the removal of the two-rod implant is easier than with multiple implants. Otherwise its profile is the same.

An implant is useful

- To postpone the first pregnancy
- To space childbirth
- To use as a reversible alternative to sterilisation
- For those who need an estrogen-free contraceptive

Injectable contraceptives

1. Progestin only Injectables (Table 36.3)

- Medroxyprogesterone acetate 150 mg (DMPA or Depo-Provera) aqueous microcrystalline suspensions
- Norethisterone enanthate NET-EN 200 mg

2. Combined Injectable Contraception (CIC)

- MPA 25mg+ estradiol cypionate 5 mg (Brand name: Cyclofem or Lunelle)
- Norethisterone enanthate 50 mg + estradiol valerate (Brand name: Mesigna)
- Dihydroxyprogesterone Acetophenide 150 mg + Estradiol enanthate 10 mg (Brand name: Deladroxate). This has now been discontinued.

The estrogen contained in the CIC is natural estrogen, unlike the synthetic estrogen used in the COC. It is now recognised that natural estrogen has a protective effect on lipid metabolism and cardiovascular function and so may be safer than COC (Population Reports 1996).

Vaginal ring: A vaginal ring (Nuva Ring) is a flexible device, 54 mm in diameter and 4 mm cross section, of material made from a transparent polymer known as evatane.

Table 36.2: Norplant and Implanon compared (Reilly 2002)

	Norplant	Implanon
Number	6 capsules	One rod
Nature of carrier	Flexible medical grade silastic	Ethinyl vinyl acetate evatane, semi rigid
Progestin used	Levonorgestrel	Etonogestrel
Size	34 mm x 2.4 mm	40 mm x 2 mm
Quantity of progestin	36 mg	68 mg
Duration of action	5 years or more	3 years
Insertion and removal	Difficult surgical procedure	Easy insertion Removal by pop-up method which is a major advantage No surgical incision necessary
Inhibition of ovulation	Total inhibition of ovulation not attained in the first year	Inhibition of ovulation throughout the 3 years (Pearl Index 0) CI 0.00-0.07
Menstrual disturbances	Irregular bleeding	Less bleeding, more amenorrhea

Table 36.3: Comparing DMPA, NET EN, CIC (Reilly 2002)

	DMPA	*NET-EN*	*CIC*
Time between injections	3 months	2 months	1 month
Grace period	2–4 weeks	2 weeks	Nil
Amenorrhoea	55% by the end of the first year	30% by the end of the first year	Nil
Return of fertility	4 months	Probably less	Immediate
Effect on diabetes	Causes mild glucose intolerance	No effect	Not known
Useful for lactating women	Yes	Yes	No
Useful for epileptic women	Excellent for epileptics; seizures are reduced	——	——
Irregular spotting	Frequent	Frequent	Heavy bleeding is common in the first 3 months in 20% of cases

The active ingredients of the ring, ethinyl estradiol and the etonogestrel, are released through a membrane at a steady rate of 15 µg and 120 µg respectively, per day. Each ring is designed for a single cycle of use, which like the conventional combined pill involves 21 days of active use followed by a 7-day ring-free break. Both hormones are evenly dispersed within the evatane ring, the progestogen separated from the estrogen-containing segment by impermeable glass barriers. The ring is self-inserted; it need not surround the cervix, it can be worn for 3 weeks, a new ring is then inserted, after withdrawal of bleeding. However, the ring contains enough steroid hormones to inhibit ovulation for at least 5 weeks. Systemic exposure to ethinyl estradiol is about 15 µg, 50% of that of an oral contraceptive containing 30 µg ethinyl estradiol, which may explain the low incidence of estrogen-related side effects such as nausea, breast tenderness and breakthrough bleeding noted with an oral contraceptive.

Transdermal contraception: Ortho Evra is also called Evra outside the US. It is also available in Europe, Canada, Hong Kong, Singapore and South Korea. It is a square patch, each side measuring 4.45 cm. The patch is placed on the buttocks, lower abdomen, upper arm or upper body (front or back), but not on the breasts. It adheres well to the skin allowing bathing, swimming and exercising even in warm climate. The effect lasts for a week—it requires three patches for a cycle and one week with no patch. The patch releases 150 µg of norelgestromin and 20 µg of ethinyl estradiol per day.

New Contraceptive Choices

1. Vaginal ring under clinical trials: A new ring under trial releases 150 µg of a different progestin called Nestorone and 15 µg of ethinyl estradiol per day. This ring is specifically for use in developing countries. It will be effective for over 12 months and so it is more cost-effective than the Nuva-Ring.

2. Progering: It is a vaginal ring containing natural progesterone. The effect lasts for three months and is useful for women who are breastfeeding.

3. Nestorone: This vaginal ring contains only progesterone (nestorone). It is a more potent synthetic progestin. It is especially useful for women who are breastfeeding.

4. 'Spray-on' Contraception: A daily progestin-only 'spray on' contraceptive was introduced in Australia in 2004. A spray or gel containing progestin, nestorone, transfers a pre-set dose of a fast-drying hormone to the skin and is absorbed instantaneously. The hormone collects as a reservoir within the skin from which it then slowly diffuses into the bloodstream.

5. Nestorone implants: This is effective for two years. It contains a single rod, which contains a potent progestin, elcometrine. It has no estrogenic or androgenic activity. It is not orally active and cannot affect nursing infants. It effectively inhibits ovulation (Diaz et al 1995). Lactating women have found it comfortable, but non-lactating women complained of prolonged and irregular bleeding.

6. Biodegradable implants: Capronor is a single biodegradable capsule containing levonorgestrel. When exposed to body tissue fluids, the polymer capsule of E-caprolactone gradually dissolves into E-hydroxycaproic acid and then to carbon dioxide and water. Levonorgestrel escapes from Caprolactone ten times faster than from silastic (Darney et al 1992).

7. Continuous-use oral contraceptives: Seasonale contains 250 μg of levonorgestrel and 30 μg of EE. A pill has to be taken every day for 84 days (12 weeks) and then hormone-free pills should be taken for seven days. Breakthrough bleeding is reported to be less.

8. Drospirenone combined oral contraceptive: (Brand name: Yasmin) It contains 3 mg of drospirenone and 30 μg of EE. It is as effective as other combined OCs. Drospirenone provides several benefits such as improvement in acne, hirsutism and less weight gain. An improved sense of well-being has also been observed.

9. Progestin releasing intra uterine system (IUS): A levonorgestrel-releasing intra-uterine system under the name Mirena is now used in 100 countries including India. The device delivers 20 μg of levonorgestrel per day. It is significantly more effective than copper IUDs with 250 mm^2 of copper or less, but it is no more effective than IUDs with greater than 250 mm^2 of copper. It can be worn for five years. Side effects are similar to those of progestin-only contraception. It requires a plunger for insertion. It reduces pelvic inflammatory disease. The reduction in risk of ectopic pregnancy is better compared to other hormonal contraception.

10. Femilis: It is a similar levonorgestrel releasing IUS. But it is T-shaped; small and inserted using a 'push-in technique'; it does not require a plunger (Wildmeersch et al 2004).

11. Estrostep: This is a combination pill with continuous low-dose progestin with a gradually increasing dose of estrogen. This approach minimises estrogen exposure at the beginning of the cycle, thus decreasing the side effects of nausea. The increasing estrogen results in an increase in the sex hormone-binding globulin and produces a very low androgenic state, useful for treating acne (Rowan 1999).

12. Other implants: A single Nomegestrol capsule (Uniplant) releases 75 μg per day, and a duration of only 12 months.

13. Male Contraception: The day is not far off for the introduction of male hormonal contraception. The use of testosterone and progesterone in the form of pills, patches, injections and implants have been tested (Meriggiola et al 2003).

TENTATIVE CONCLUSIONS

1. The low-dose combined pill is safe for all women younger than 35 years, who have no hypertension or diabetes and who are non-smokers.
2. The progesterone-only pill is best for lactating women, because lactation also provides additional contraception. It does not interfere with the quantity and quality of milk.
3. Reduction in risk of epithelial cancer of the ovary is around 50% even with less than one year of OC use; it increases progressively with prolonged use. The protection lasts for at least 10 years after last use.
4. Reduction in the risk of endometrial cancer also occurs and the protection persists for at least 15 years after stopping OC.
5. The pill results in a reduction in the risk of colorectal cancer also.
6. Reduction of pelvic inflammatory disease, reduction in the occurrence of fibroids, improvement in bone density and prevention of anemia are all well documented.
7. The relative risk of venous thromboembolism increases with COC use. Nevertheless, the rarity of venous thromboembolism in women of reproductive age makes the absolute risk small.
8. Progesterone-only pills, injectables and levonorgestrel implants do not increase the risk of thromboembolism.
9. The relative risk of acute myocardial infarction in those using COC is high among smokers. Therefore, COC is contraindicated in smokers.
10. Low-dose COC causes very minimal changes in insulin and glucose, so minimal, that it is of no clinical significance.
11. There is a small increase in breast cancer in contraceptive users. This requires further evaluation.
12. Non-oral routes offer continuous and steady steroid levels; avoid the first pass peak effect through the hepatic-portal system. Non-oral routes also give higher bioavailability of the steroid, and the doses of steroid could result in a lower occurrence or a possible reduction in the occurrence of adverse effects.

REFERENCES

Anonymous. 1987. The reduction in risk of ovarian cancer associated with oral contraceptive use. The Cancer and Steroid Hormone Study of the Centers for Disease Control and the National Institute of Child Health and Human Development. *N Engl J Med* 316:650–655.

Brinton LA. 1991. Oral contraceptives and cervical neoplasia. *Contraception* 43:581.

Broome M and K Fotherby. 1990. Clinical experience with the progestogen-only pill. *Contraception* 42:489.

Brown C, F Ling, J Wan. 2002. A new monophasic oral contraceptive containing drospirenone. Effect on premenstrual symptoms. *J Reprod Med* 47:14.

Chiaffarino F, F Parazzini, C La Vecchia et al. 1999. Use of oral contraceptives and uterine fibroids: Results from a case-control study. *Br J Obstet Gynaecol* 106:857–860.

Darney PD, CM Klaisle, SE Monroe et al. 1992. Evaluation of a one-year levonorgestrel-releasing contraceptive implant: Side effects, release rates and biodegradability. *Fertil Steril* 58:137.

Diaz S, V Schiappasse, M Pavez M et al 1995; Clinical trial with Nestorone subdermal contraceptive implants. *Contraception* 51:33.

Djerassi C. 1981. The politics of contraception. *The Present and the Future.* San Francisco: W.H. Freeman and Company.

Franceschi S and C La Vecchia. 1998. Oral contraceptives and colorectal tumours: A review of epidemiologic studies. *Contraception* 58:335–343.

Gail McBride. 2002. Politics rather than science will shape the future of birth control. Interview with Carl Djerassi, ORGYN Special Issue, Beeldrecht Hoofddorp, the Netherlands.

Gross TP and JJ Schlesselman. 1994. The estimated effect of oral contraceptive use on the cumulative risk of epithelial ovarian cancer. *Obstet Gynecol* 83:419–424.

Hankinson SE, GA Colditz, DJ Hunter et al. 1992. A quantitative assessment of oral contraceptive use and risk of ovarian cancer. *Obstet Gyanecol* 80:708–714.

Helen Reilly. 2002. New methods in non-oral contraception. Delivery Systems ORGYN Special issue, Beeldrecht Hoofddorp, the Netherlands, 14–17.

International Medical Advisory Panel. 2004. IMAP statement on emergency contraception, IPPF Medical Bulletin 18, Number 1 March.

Jenson, Jeffrey T and Leon Speroff. 2000. Health Benefits of Oral Contraceptives. Update in contraception. *Obstet Gynecol Clin Am* 27:4.709.

Kjos SL, RK Peters, A Xiang, D Thomas, U Schaefer, TA Buchanan. 1998. Contraception and the risk of type 2 diabetes in Latino women with prior gestational diabetes. *JAMA* 280:533.

Kleerekoper M, RS Brienza, LR Schultz, CC Johnson. 1991. Oral contraceptive use may protect against low bone mass. *Arch Intern Med* 151:1971–1976.

Lewis MA, LAJ Heinemann, WO Spitzer, KD MacRae, R Bruppacher, for the Transnational Research Group on Oral Contraceptives and the Health of Young Women. 1997. The use of oral contraceptives and the occurrence of acute myocardial infarction in young women. Results from Transnational Study on Oral Contraceptives and the Health of Young Women. *Contraception* 56: 129.

Lidegaard O and B Edstrom. 1996. Oral contraceptives and myocardial infarction. A case-control study (abstract). *Eur J Contracept. Reprod Health Care* 1 (Supp): 72.

Meriggiola MC, TM Farley, MT Mbizvo. 2003. A Review of androgen–progestin regimens for male contraception. *J Androl* 24 (4): 466–483.

Milman N, J Clausen, KE Byg. 1998. Iron status in 268 Danish women aged 18–30 years: Influence of menstruation, contraceptive method, and iron supplementation. *Ann Hematol* 77 (1-2):13–19.

Nilsson S, T Melbin, Y Hofvander, C Sundelin, J Valentin, KG Nygren. 1986. Long-term follow-up of children breast-fed by mothers using oral contraceptives. *Contraception* 34:443.

Peipert JF and J Gutmann. 1993. Oral contraceptive risk assessment: A survey of 247 educated women. *Obstet Gynecol* 82:112.

Petitti DB, S Sidney, CP Queseberry, Jr., A Bernstein. 1997. Incidence of stroke and myocardial infarction in women of reproductive age. *Stroke* 28:280.

Population Reports 2000. Series A, number 9. Source Demographic Health Surveys and World Fertility Survey 8.

Population Reports. 1996. Vol XXIV Number 2, October 1996 p13.

Rosenberg L, JR Palmer, AG Zauber et al. 1994. A Case-control study of oral contraceptive use and invasive epithelial ovarian cancer. *Am J P Epidemiol* 139:654–661.

Rosenberg L, JR Palmer, RS Rao et al. 1996. Case–control study of oral contraceptive use and risk of breast cancer. *Am J Epidemiol* 143:25.

Rowan JP, 1999. 'Esterophasic' dosing: A new concept in oral contraceptive therapy. *Am J Obstet Gynecol* 180: S 302.

Shikary ZK, SS Betrabet, ZM Patel et al. 1987. ICMR task force study on hormonal contraception. Transfer of levonorgestrel (LNG) administered through different drug delivery systems from the maternal circulation into the newborn infant's circulation via breast milk. *Contraception* 35:477.

Speroff L, DF Archer, DR Mishell, Jr. 1988. Multiphasic and monophasic OCs: Is there a difference? *Contemp Obstet Gynaecol* 32 (Special Issue) 124-134, 137–145.

Speroff L and Marc A Fritz. 2005. *Clinical Gynaecologic Endocrinology and Infertility* 7th edition. Philadelphia: Lippincott Williams and Wilkins.

Spinillo A, G Gorini, G Piazzi et al. 1996. The impact of oral contraception on chlamydial infection among patients with pelvic inflammatory disease. *Contraception* 54:163–168.

Stanczyk FZ and S Roy. 1990. Metabolism of levonorgestrel, norethindrone, and structurally related contraceptive steroids. *Contraception* 42:67.

Suissa S, L Blaise, WO Spitzer et al. 1997 First-time use of newer oral contraceptives and the risk of venous thromboembolism. *Contraception* 56:141–146.

Sullivan H, H Furniss, J Spona, M Elstein, 1999. Effect of 21–day and 24-day oral contraceptive regimens containing gestodene (60 μg) and ethinyl estradiol (15 μg) on ovarian activity. *Fertil Steril* 72:115.

The Cancer and Steroid Hormone Study of the Centers for Disease Control and the National Institute of Child Health and Human Development. 1987. Combination oral contraceptive use and the risk of endometrial cancer. *JAMA* 257:796-800.

Troisi RJ, CC Cowie, MI Harris. 2000. Oral contraceptive use and glucose metabolism in a national sample of women in the United States. *Am J Obstet Gynecol* 183:389.

Vandenbroucke JP, T Koster, E Briet et al. 1994. Increased risk of venous thrombosis in oral contraceptive users who are carriers of factor V Leiden mutation. *Lancet* 344:1453–1457.

Vaughan, Paul. 1972. *The Pill on Trial, a Pelican Book.* Middlesex, UK: Penguin Books Ltd.

Voigt LF, Q Deng, NS Weiss. 1994. Recency, duration, and progestin content of oral contraceptives in relation to the incidence of endometrial cancer (Washington, USA). *Cancer Causes Control* 5:227–233.

Weiderpass E, Adami HO, Baron JA et al. 1999. Use of oral contraceptives and endometrial cancer risk (Sweden). *Cancer Causes Control* 10:277–284.

WHO Collaborative Study of Cardiovascular Disease and Steroid Hormone Contraception. 1997. Acute myocardial infarction and combined oral contraceptives: results of an international multicentre case-control study. *Lancet* 349: 1202.

WHO. 1999. Task force on postovulatory methods of fertility regulation. Comparison of three single doses of mifepristone as emergency contraception: A randomised trial. *Lancet* 353:697–702.

Wildemeersch D, D Janssens, M Vrijens, S Weyers. 2004. Ease of insertion, contraceptive efficacy and safety of new T-shaped levonorgestrel–releasing intrauterine systems. Presented at the 8th Congress of the European Society of Contraception, Edinburgh, Scotland, Jun 23–36.

Wolner-Hanssen. 1996. Relationship between oral contraceptives and pelvic inflammatory disease and associated sexually transmitted diseases. In *Evidence-guided Prescribing of the Pill* ed PC Hannaford, AMC Webb, 175–180. London: The Parthenon Publishing Group.

Yeshaya A, R Orvieto, B Kaplan et al. 1998. Flexible starting schedule for oral contraception: Effect on the incidence of breakthrough bleeding and compliance. *Eur J Contracept Reprod Health Care* 3:121–123.

Yuzpe AA and WJ Lancee. 1977. Ethinylestradiol and dl-levonorgestrel as a post-coital contraception. *Fertil Steril* 28:932–936.

37

Female and Male Sterilisation

Indu Gupta | RCM Kaza

FEMALE STERILISATION

Female sterilisation prevents unintended pregnancy for the rest of the reproductive period of the woman. Most current techniques involve resection of a part of the fallopian tube, but some others occlude the fallopian tube lumen by non-surgical methods and prevent conception. As early as 1886, at the twenty first annual meeting of the American Gynecological Society, the procedure for female sterilisation was debated upon as the right of a woman. Sterilisation gained popularity in the 1970s, with newer methods like minilap and laparoscopy (Te Linde 2003) coming into use. At present, female sterilisation is the most widely used contraceptive method with 190 million couples having adopted this method throughout the world (Rioux and Daria 2001).

Timing: Female sterilisation can be performed along with cesarean section, or shortly after normal vaginal delivery or concurrent with medical termination of pregnancy or as an interval procedure preferably in the follicular phase. At the time of cesarean section, the abdomen is already open and after the delivery of the baby at the time of exploration of the adnexa, it requires a few extra minutes to perform the tubal ligation. Post delivery, the uterus is large and tubes are easily accessible as the abdominal wall is lax, the patient is well motivated, the baby has been observed for some time; also, the procedure does not require extra stay in the hospital. Interval tubal sterlisation can be performed by a minilap or laparoscopy in the immediate postmenstrual phase.

Pre-operative evaluation and counselling: The procedure for female sterilisation is simple and safe as long as any associated medical or surgical condition is taken care of. There is no absolute contraindication for the procedure. Pregnancy should be ruled out. In case the woman is pregnant and if termination is requested, it should be performed concurrent with sterilisation procedure. Pregnancy-related conditions which warrant postponement include severe pre-eclampsia, prolonged rupture of the membranes prior to delivery, infection, severe hemorrhage, trauma to the genital tract, uterine rupture or perforation during medical termination of pregnancy. Thorough physical examination to rule out any general or gynecological abnormality should be carried out so that proper care is taken, for example, symptomatic fibroids or abnormal cervical cytology.

Female sterilisation is an elective procedure performed on a healthy female. Hence, proper counselling is very important. She should be counselled about the intended permanence of the procedure, alternatives, the risks, especially of failure and the chances of an ectopic pregnancy when failure occurs. Hence, the WHO's medical eligibility criteria for female sterilisation should be followed (1999). The informed written consent of the woman is mandatory and it should be obtained, witnessed and recorded in the desired consent form. It would be preferable to get the husband's consent as well. Additional care must be taken in certain circumstances, for example, in the case of couples without children, woman below 30 years of age, women with a mental health problem or a woman who does not have the mental capacity to give consent (FOGSI letter, 2005).

Anesthesia: For the sterilisation procedure, alone or concurrent with medical termination of pregnancy, local anesthesia with sedation is safe and effective and the risks and complications associated with general anesthesia can be avoided. Counselling of the woman regarding local anesthesia makes her more cooperative. For local anesthesia, 1% lingnocaine along with mild intravenous/intramuscular sedation is sufficient. However, the presence of an anesthetist and the facilities for intubation and general anesthesia in an operation theatre should always be available. The woman should be fasting for at least six hours, so that in case general anesthesia is required, it can be administered immediately.

Surgical procedures

A. Abdominal procedures: The incision varies depending on the type of procedure. In the postpartum period since the uterus is big, an infra-umbilical, midline, vertical incision, 2–3 cm long, is sufficient. The patient is prepared, all asceptic precautions are taken, the patient is then draped and local anesthesia is given along with sedation. The uterus can be manipulated per abdomen; by retracting the abdominal wall with a small retractor,

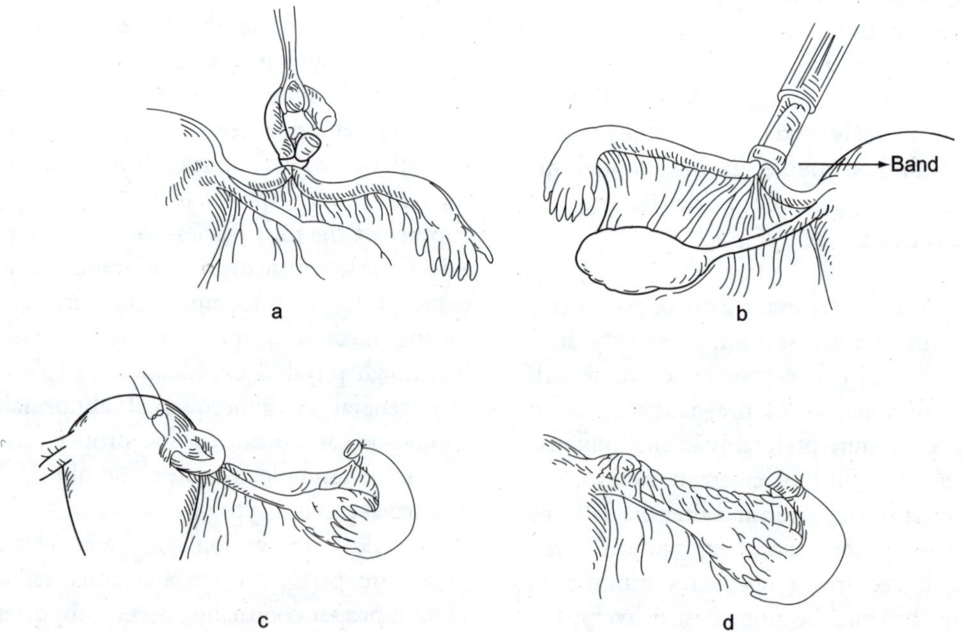

Figure 37.1: Schematic presentation of different procedures of Female sterilisation
a. Modified Pomeroys; b. Laparoscopic band application; c. Irving's method; d. Uchida's method

the fallopian tube on one side is identified, lifted, brought out with a Backcock forceps, the fimbrial end is traced to prevent making the mistake of ligating the round ligament and tubal ligation is performed. The procedure is repeated on the other side. Hemostasis is confirmed and the abdomen closed. The most commonly used procedure for sterilisation is Modified Pomeroys.

If sterilisation is performed as an interval procedure or concurrent with medical termination of pregnancy or by laparoscopy, a uterine manipulator is used. For a minilap, a suprapubic, transverse, 2–3 cm long incision is used. For laparoscopy, with a laparocator, there is no need for a second port; the skin is sutured with absorbable sutures, so that the woman does not need to come back to the hospital for the removal of sutures.

i. Modified Pomeroy's operation: This is the most commonly performed procedure. A loop of the isthmic portion of the tube is pulled up and ligated with a single catgut ligature after crushing. The loop is excised and the procedure repeated on the contralateral tube. The excised tissue is sent for histopathology, for documentation in case of a legal suit at a later date. As absorbable suture is used, the two ends of the tube separate once the suture is absorbed and there is a gap of 2–3 cm between the severed segments. Complete hemostatis is obtained. The failure rate reported with this procedure is 1 in 200 procedures (Fig. 37.1a).

ii. Laparoscopic tubal occlusion: With the development of fibre optic sources, laparoscopic tubal occlusion has become the procedure of choice. However, special training and experience, is required in addition to special equipment. In the beginning, unipolar coagulation was used, but this was associated with complications, especially thermal bowel injury and higher failure rates. With the use of bipolar current, the procedure became safe but it was reported that partial dessication of the outer third of the tube can occur without dessication of the inner third, resulting in failure, unless the tube is severed. Availability of silicon rubber bands and the work of Yoon and coworkers (1974) made the laparoscopic ring application safe and effective without any risk of thermal injury to the adjacent abdominal organs. With a laparocator, through a single port, the prongs are used to hook the tube gently with the help of an assistant who manipulates the uterus with a manipulator or a No. 7/8 Hegar dilator. The tube is held near the isthmic portion from the uterus, the prongs are retracted gently and slowly into the applicator and the band applied. The same procedure is repeated on the other tube. About 1.5 to 2 cm of the tube is contained in the constricted loop. There is devascularisation, the tubal part becomes anoxic and resorbs with time. The tubes are observed for any bleeding and the laparoscope is removed. The gas in the pneumoperitoneum is removed through the cannula and an absorbable suture applied to the skin and covered with a bandaid (Fig. 37.1b). Apart from a 2 cm loop of the tube, very little damage is caused to the adjacent proximal and distal portions of the tube and there is no chance of adhesion formation. If there is any bleeding due to accidental transaction of the tube, it can be managed by bipolar coagulation or by the application of an additional band. The procedure can be performed under local anesthesia with sedation or under general anesthesia. The additional advantage of the laparoscopic band/ring application is better chance of recanalisation, if required, at a later date. Besides bands, clips by Hulka and Filshie (Hulka et al 1995) have also been used. The clips have to be used properly so that the entire circumference of the tube is included. Depending on the width of the clip, only 3 mm to 5 mm of compressed tube undergoes avascular necrosis and ultimately the clip is peritonealised. However, with the availability of the Fallope ring, this is the most commonly used method for tubal occlusion.

Modified Pomeroys technique can also be performed on laparoscopy. This requires additional instruments for suture and a scissor and a second port. A part of the tube can be obtained and retained as documented proof by histopathological cxamination.

B. Other abdominal procedures: Many other procedures for female sterilisation have been described but not followed at present.

i. Madlaner technique: The suture used was non-absorbable and the loop was not removed, this resulted in a high failure rate. In the modified procedure, the loop was cut but as the two parts did not separate because of non absorbable suture; the failure rate was still high compared to the Modified Pomeroy's Technique, 0.4% vs 1.2%. Hence this procedure is not used any more.

ii. Parkland operation: The tube is drawn up through the abdominal incision, a bloodless area in the mesosalpinx identified and two curved artery forceps applied, so that the tips come into contact on the mesosalpinx. The tubal part enclosed along with the mesosalpinx is excised; two separate ligatures are applied to the two severed ends of the tube which accomplishes immediate separation of the tubal ends.

iii. Irving's operation: In an attempt to reduce the risk of a tuboperitoneal fistula, this technique requires extensive dissection of the tube and the burying of the proximal stump into the muscular layer of the uterus by creating a tunnel in an avascular area. The tunnel is closed over the proximal stump with fine catgut. The distal end is buried in the mesosalpinx. The procedure however, needs a larger incision for good exposure, more operating time and results in more hemorrhage. The failure rate is less than 1 in 1000 (Fig. 37.1c).

iv. Uchida's Technique: This is a technique whereby the two resected ends of the cut tube in the mesosalpinx are buried. Saline with epinephrine (1:1000) is injected, subserosally, in the mesosalpinx which is cut open. The tube is pulled out, the proximal part dissected bluntly towards the uterus and a loop is formed, clamped and cut. The medial end retracts in the mesosalpinx which is then closed. The lateral ligated stump is kept outside the mesosalpinx. This method is more time consuming and is also more hemorrhagic. Later, Uchida modified the technique by performing a fimbriactomy in addition to burying the medial end. However, this procedure has not been used by others (Fig. 37.1d).

v. Kroener's technique: This involves double ligation of the fimbrial end with silk suture and removal of the fimbria. The procedure is simple, but in case reversal is requested later, the results are very poor and hence it is now considered an obsolete procedure.

Transvaginal procedures

A. Vaginal tubal ligation In trained hands, vaginal tubal ligation is a less time consuming procedure, as effective as minilap, with no abdominal scar and with less postoperative pain. No special equipment is required and the procedure can be performed along with medical termination of pregnancy. However, it is technically more difficult to perform, may result in an abdominal procedure in 2% to 3% of cases and sexual intercourse is delayed. However, intraabdominal infection is more common and hence results in more morbidity.

The procedure can be performed under local anesthesia and sedation, but short acting general anesthesia is good for relaxation. The procedure is performed through a posterior colpotomy taking all asceptic precautions, using 5% povidone iodine to clean the vagina and cervix thoroughly. A vaginal examination is performed and a Sims speculum is introduced into the vagina; the posterior lip of the cervix is caught and pulled up by a vulsellum. Following this procedure, the fornix and the cervix are cleaned again with povidone-iodine. Two Allis forceps are applied vertically on the posterior fornix about a centimetre apart and held tight; the vaginal vault is opened with one stroke so that the peritoneum is also opened. The tube is brought down by a Babcock forceps pushing the uterus to the other side. A Lehi's forceps is applied to make a loop and sterilisation performed using the Modified Pomeroy's technique. The procedure is repeated on the other tube and the colpotomy incision closed in one layer using catgut. Occasionally, difficulty may be encountered in bringing out the tube, mostly due to adhesions. The patient can be discharged on the same day and a course of antibiotics prescribed for five days. Abstinence is advised till the next menses.

Difficulty may be encountered in about 6% of cases due to adhesions, an adnexal mass or the bowel interfering with the localisation of the tube. Complications may occur due to trauma and hemorrhage. The failure rate is almost the same as abdominal tubal ligation. The main complication is infection (Brenner and Edelman 1976; Gupta et al 1979).

Hysteroscopic occlusion of fallopian tube: The uterine tubal ostium can be visualised after distending the uterine cavity with a fluid medium or gas. Attempts have been made to fulgurate the ostea by coagulating current, by chemicals to form a plug (methylcynoacrelate), or fibrosis by using sclerosing agents like quinacrine (Colony 1994). However, there is controversy as to the effectiveness and safety of these procedures and further studies are required.

Complications: Female sterilisation is a safe and effective procedure. However, any surgical procedure results in some morbidity and may impact mortality. Anesthesia-related problems and trauma to the adjacent viscera during the procedure are some immediate risks. Khairullah et al (1992) in a retrospective study observed deaths following female sterilisation attributed to intestinal injury, infection, abdominal hemorrhage, dehydration or due to allergic reaction to drugs. Hence, local anesthesia is a preferable choice. However, the sedatives used along with local anesthesia can also cause morbidity and mortality by allergic reactions. Therefore, local anesthesia with close monitoring of vital signs is best. Accidental perforation of the uterus during uterine manipulation, major vessal injury, bowel injury and peritonitis should be promptly diagnosed and managed to decrease morbidity.

The mortality rates following female sterilisation are reported to be 1.5/100,000 procedures, whereas in India, the reported figures are 10/100,000 to 70/100,000 (ICMR 1982).

Risk of failure: Method-related risk of failure is reported to be 0.2% to 0.3% after precautions have been taken to avoid preclinical pregnancy by performing the procedure in the early follicular phase. Otherwise, it will depend on the method used. The US Collaborative Review of Sterilization (CREST) is the landmark, prospective, multicentre observational study; it reported a cumulative failure rate of 1.85%

in 10,685 women who had been sterilised over a 10 years period (Peterson et al 1996).

Long term Effects

Long term follow up studies have shown that the post sterilisation syndrome—which meant that women who have undergone tubal sterilisation are more prone to menstrual irregularities—is not true as these irregularities may be due to age-related problems. The increased need for hysterectomy in tubectomised women has also been shown not to be true (Cullins 2000).

Beneficial Efect

Several studies have identified a reduced risk of ovarian cancer after tubal sterilisation. Hankinson and colleagues (1993) reported, in a large study, that the risk of ovarian cancer for tubectomised woman was a third that for non-sterilised woman. Whether this protective effect is real or is due to some other associated factor is not clear, but it is an important noncontraceptive health benefit of tubal sterilisation.

Regret

The most common factor associated with regret is the death of a child, especially that of a male child in India. It could also be due to the presence of the family or spouse (Schmidt 2000). Hence, counselling is very important before a woman undergoes tubal sterilisation.

Some women can be safely sterilised but require special care; hence, sterilisation should be undertaken in a hospital setting with an experienced surgeon and staff, access to general anesthesia services and back-up medical support, in case of an emergency.

MALE STERILISATION

India has a population in excess of 1 billion, which is growing constantly at a high rate. If this continues, India may overtake China in 2045, to become the most populous country in the world. This high rate of population growth tends to neutralise the benefits of economic growth rate and resource development.

Men have tended to shy away from contraception, not only in India but also in many other countries. Hence, major efforts are being made the world over to increase acceptance of contraception by men. This includes male sterilisation.

Vasectomy is the only long-term contraceptive method available to men. It is a simple, safe and effective surgical procedure and it is permanent. Vasectomy involves cutting and excision of a segment of the vas deferens, thereby preventing the discharge of sperms during ejaculation into the male urethra. Vasectomy has been used for permanent male sterilisation since the late nineteenth century. It has been accepted as a simple, safe, effective and inexpensive method of permanent contraception for men. As such, it affords a man the opportunity to shoulder the responsibility of contraception.

No Scalpel Vasectomy (NSV) was introduced in China by Li Shun Qiang in 1974 (Li 1988). NSV does not require any formal incision or stitch and is done under local anesthesia. NSV was introduced in India in 1992. Since then, a large number of surgeons have been trained in this procedure and it has become an integral part of the National Family Welfare Programme.

NSV with fascial interposition is the gold standard for male sterilisation. Absence of formal incision and stitches allay the fears of men about wound-related complications and lead to greater acceptance of the procedure.

There are many recent developments in NSV such as the use of the jet injector for the administration of anesthesia. Methods of occlusion of vas have also evolved from the traditional silk suture to the use of thermal cautery. Excision of a segment of the vas deferens that has been the hallmark of all forms of vasectomy has also been questioned in a new procedure—the inline vasectomy. Studies indicate that use of thermal cautery to burn out the segment without removal of the segment is equally effective.

Brief History: The term vas deferens is derived from the Latin words for 'vessel' and 'defere' meaning to carry down. Berengarius of Carpi (1470–1530) was the first to name it. In a review of literature available on the subject of vasectomy, Ashley Cooper's (1830) name stands out, as he started experimental work on this procedure in the early part of the nineteenth century. In subsequent years, various others undertook to study the subject, but there was no unanimity in their observations. Meanwhile, the operation came into clinical use in the late 1890s. Cooper started his experimental work on dogs. The experiment showed that merely closing the outlet duct of the testis had no effect on the germinal portion of the testis; spermatogenesis continued for six years after the operation, and the epididymis became enlarged to accommodate the products of germinal cell activity (Cooper 1830).

Simmonds (1921) in human autopsies found that after years of vas occlusion, there was no injury to the generative part. Neither testicular degeneration nor loss of the germinal epithelium had occurred, and the epididymis was enlarged by the immense number of spermatozoa carried to it (Brissaud 1880). In the late 1890s, vasectomy began to be widely used by genitourinary surgeons, mainly in connection with operations on the prostate. Ochsner (1899) observed that his patients reported no change whatsoever in their sex lives after vasectomy. Harry Sharp (1937) did 4056 operations and reported that he had seen no unfavorable results after vasectomy on sexual desire (Benjamin 1922). Morson concluded that there were no bad effects due to division of the duct and that such results were due to faults in technique (Morson 1924). Phadke (1952) commented favourably on vasectomy for sterilisation

Kenneth Walker (1953) stated: 'It can be said with confidence that vasectomy has no adverse effects on the physical or mental welfare of the patient. Operative patients have now been watched for a period of 30 years and no delayed adverse results have been noted.'

It used to be the consensus that vasectomy, once done, was irrevocable. An accidental vasectomy during a herniorraphy led to the first attempt to anastomose the vas deferens (Cameron, 1945). Twyman and Nelson (1941) reported cases of vasorraphy following vasectomy for contraception, and the operation was done four to seven years after vasectomy (Twyman and Nelson 1938). Handley, in 1951, reported a case in which vasorraphy was done ten years after vasectomy, with complete recovery of function, so that the patient's wife became pregnant about six months after the operation (O'Conor 1942). Phadke (1958) has perfomed the vasorraphy operation with success. This shows that rejoining the cut ends of a severed vas deferens can restore function. O'Conor (1948) described the technique of vasorraphy in detail. Dorsey (1957) reported favourably on surgical correction of postvasectomy sterility (Dorsey 1957).

Natural reunion and canalisation has followed the division of the vas deferens both in human beings and in animal experiments (Evridge-Vernon 1956). In the follow up studies of these authors (1958), natural reunion was observed in some cases.

Jhaver introduced the single incision, single stitch approach. His paper on the technique was published in 1958. The advantage of the technique being that a bilateral vasectomy was possible (Jhaver 1973).

APPROACHES TO VASECTOMY

Regardless of the method of scrotal entry, the first step in the vasectomy is to identify and immobilise the vas through the skin of the scrotum. The second step is to bring the vas into the open. There are two approaches for doing this—conventional vasectomy and no-scalpel vasectomy.

Conventional vasectomy

In the conventional incisional method of vasectomy, the surgeon uses a scalpel to make either one midline incision or two incisions in the scrotal skin, each usually 1–2 cm long, one overlying each vas deferens. The incision is routinely closed with sutures after the vasectomy has been completed. In general, with conventional vasectomy, only the area around the skin entry site is anesthetised.

No-scalpel Vasectomy

Also known as NSV, No scalpel vasectomy, is a unique method of gaining access to vas deferens for vasectomy. At that time, vasectomy was unpopular with Chinese men, and tubal occlusion was the predominant method of voluntary sterilisation. Today in Sichuan, vasectomy outnumbers tubal occlusion by a ratio of four to one; in the rest of China, tubal occlusion outnumbers vasectomy by five to one. More than 10 million Chinese men have already undergone no-scalpel vasectomy (Li 1988; Li et al 1991; AVSC 1997).

Instead of a scalpel, two specialised instruments—a ringed clamp and a dissecting forceps (a sharp, curved hemostat) are used. Because the scrotal skin puncture made with the dissecting forceps is so small, sutures are not needed.

No-scalpel vasectomy offers several advantages over conventional vasectomy—fewer complications, less pain during the procedure and early follow-up period, leaves a smaller wound than conventional techniques, and earlier resumption of sexual activity after surgery (AVSC 1997; Skriver et al 1997; Sokal et al 1999) because it requires no scrotal incision and eliminates the scalpel, no scalpel vasectomy is believed to decrease men's fears about vasectomy (AVSC 1997). Neither conventional nor no-scalpel vasectomy is time-consuming, but it has been reported that the vasectomy procedure time is shorter when skilled providers use the no-scalpel approach (Nirapathpongpom et al 1990; Li et al 1991). On the other hand, others believe that NSV does not reduce the risk of surgical complications over the standard incisional approach to expose the vas.

Anesthesia in vasectomy: Most vasectomies are performed under local anesthesia. But some are done under general anesthesia because of the fear of pain and inadequacies of local anesthetic technique. Many vasectomists use multiple blind injections with local anesthetic into the spermatic chord. This may result in hematomas and injury to the testicular vessels. One study in animals suggested that such blind injections may result in injury to the testicular artery with subsequent testicular atrophy in up to 5% of the cases, despite the use of a fine-gauge needle (Li et al 1992).

Spermatic chord block at the level of the pubic tubercle has previously been proposed for scrotal surgery. However, it is difficult to isolate the vas deferens from the internal spermatic vessels in the region of the pubic tubercle.

External spermatic sheath injection for vasal nerve block has been used in over 10 million vasectomies in China. The technique, which involves a deep injection alongside the vas, creates a vasal nerve block. Conventional techniques anesthetise only the area around the skin-entry site. Injection of the anesthetic away from the vasectomy site in the direction of the inguinal ring helps make skin entry easier. Care is taken when injecting the lignocaine to keep the needle away from the internal spermatic fascia that encloses the testicular artery and veins (Li et al 1992). Because the surgeon makes only a single needle puncture and one smooth injection for each vas, the risk of bleeding is reduced. In a randomised trial comparing no-scalpel vasectomy to the conventional technique, men undergoing no-scalpel vasectomy with vasal block anesthesia reported experiencing less operative pain than did men undergoing conventional vasectomy (Sokal et al 1999). Philip Li et al described the technique of external spermatic sheath injection for vasal nerve block in over 500 patients in the USA 1992 (Li et al 1992). They did not detect any complication attributable to this technique. External spermatic sheath injection for vasal nerve block into the chord is now the most common method used for local anesthesia in NSV.

Jet injector is a nearly painless, rapid, needle-free method of drug administration. It has previously been used to administer vaccination to more than a billion people worldwide. Jet injector has been evolved as an instrument that could allow needle free, virtually painless anesthesia for most primary care procedures. The physiological advantages of the jet injection is that it can provide effective anesthesia using a small volume of local anesthetic of at least a 2% concentration, with minimal patient discomfort compared to the conventional needle and the patient is totally unaware of the experience when the site of injection has been anesthetised in advance using the jet injection. Another advantage of the jet injection technique is that a very small amount by volume (0.1 cc of 2% anesthetic) will provide unusually high levels of tissue anesthesia.

OCCLUSION TECHNIQUES

Once the vas has been brought into the open, it is then occluded using a variety of methods. The same techniques are used to occlude the vas in both conventional and no-scalpel vasectomy. Although there are few complications associated with vasectomies, sometimes problems arise and the method of vas occlusion is often the cause. At least 28 occlusive methods have been used over the years.

Different techniques for occlusion are:

1. Ligation and excision
2. Ligation and excision with fascial interposition
3. Electrocautery
4. Thermal cautery
5. Clips
6. Combination of different methods
7. Open-ended vasectomy
8. Inline vas occlusion

Simple ligation and excision: It is the most common method being used in developing countries including India. This is a very simple, practical and inexpensive method of occlusion. It involves tying the vas deferens with suture material, cutting it, and in many cases, removing a section of the vas.

Fascial interposition: In this technique, the fascia is interposed between two cut ends of the vas. This is done by tying (or securing with clip) the thin layer of tissue that surrounds the vas (internal spermatic fascia) over one end of the vas.

Electrocautery: In this method, using minimum electric power, the two cut ends of the vas are sealed with the help of electrocautery. This method has limitations in that when the more common monopolar electrosurgical unit is used for fulguration, tissue destruction may be inadequate; on the contrary, it may be so extensive that the end of the vas sloughs, thus allowing leakage of sperm and formation of granuloma. Unfortunately, a bipolar needle which precisely regulates the amount of current is not commonly available.

Thermal cautery: This is a highly effective and safe method to occlude the vas for vasectomy. With this method, only the inner layer of the vas is sealed shut; the muscle wall of the vas remains intact. A segment of the vas is removed as well.

Metal clips: Some vasectomists use clips which are applied to the open end of the vasal stump. Questions have been raised about the use of clips, the practicality and cost of procedure in less developed countries.

Open-ended vasectomy: In this method, the testicular end of the vas is not ligated. Although it has been tried, it is not commonly used. Data have shown that this technique causes less pressure-induced damage to the epididymis and reduces incidence of granuloma formation in the epididymis (Silber 1977). Thus, it is possible that vasectomy reversal will be more successful following an open-ended vasectomy. However, no studies on open-ended vasectomy and the success of reversal efforts have been reported in the literature. Overall results from available studies suggest that the open ended technique is not associated with increase in vasectomy failure risk when the prostatic end is adequately closed by means of fascial interposition and cautery (Labrecque et al 2004).

Inline method of vas occlusion: In this method, neither scalpel nor suture is used. Further, the mesentery of the vas is not touched and no portion of the vas is removed. This method is rapid and can be performed with NSV instruments but in addition requires a fine skin hook, a short-bladed fine scissors and a handheld thermal cautery unit. It uses luminal cautery, detubularisation of the vas and fascial disruption. Vas lumen is opened on the abdominal and testicular side, at a distance of one centimeter, cauterised on both abdominal and testicular sides. Intervening portion of vas is detubularised and the edges are trimmed to prevent re-tubularisation. This method seems to produce fewer incidences of hematoma, granuloma and failure rates (Joel et al 2001).

Effectiveness

Vasectomy is one of the safest and most effective methods of permanent contraception. But it has the disadvantage that it is not immediately effective because viable sperms have to be cleared from the distal vas.

The success of the procedure is confirmed by the absence of sperms in the semen sample obtained after vasectomy. Thus, the vasectomy user and his spouse must practice alternate methods of contraception for some time after the procedure.

Some providers ask men to return based on the time elapsed since the vasectomy, while others use the number of ejaculations since vasectomy, and yet others use some combination of both, time and number of ejaculations (Babayan and Krane 1986; Schmidt 1987; Alderman 1988; Rajfer and Bennet 1988; Haws et al 1998) In addition, providers vary in the number of azoospermic samples they require before they will tell a man it is safe for him to rely on his vasectomy for contraception (Babayan and Krane 1986; Haws et al 1998). This variety in postvasectomy follow-up protocol reflects the limited data available on determinants of azoospermia, including the time and number of ejaculations after vasectomy, as well as uncertainty over whether azoospermia is the best endpoint for vasectomy.

While the standard accepted endpoint of vasectomy has traditionally been achievement of azoospermia, some have discussed whether azoospermia is a necessary condition for the contraceptive effectiveness of vasectomy. A number of studies, examining changes in sperm function after vasectomy, including fertilising competence and sperm motility, have suggested that the duration of risk of pregnancy after vasectomy is shorter (and in some cases, much shorter) than the time necessary to reach azoospermia (Jouannet and David 1978; Bedford and Zelikovsky 1979; Lewis et al 1984; Richardson et al 1984; Sivanesaratnam 1985; Edwards 1993; Cortes et al 1997). A number of reports have shown that men with low numbers of non-motile sperm remaining after vasectomy are at low risk of causing pregnancy (Edwards and Farlow 1979; Philp et al 1984; Alderman 1989; Davies et al 1990; Thompson et al 1991; Edwards 1993; De Knijff et al 1997). Some have suggested that these men can rely on their vasectomy for contraception even before reaching azoospermia (Temmerman et al 1986; Davies et al 1990; Thompson et al 1991; Edwards 1993).

Endpoints of vasectomy other than azoospermia, however, have not been widely accepted. It is generally recommended that men have a semen analysis; in many cases, the suggested time for the semen analysis is a long time after the vasectomy (for example, 12 weeks). During this time, couples must use an alternative method of contraception. If sperm are found in the semen at the first visit, additional visits are necessary. In many low-resource settings, it is impossible or impractical for men to have a semen analysis. Men may have no access to a facility that can do a semen analysis, they may be far from such a facility, or they may not have the money to pay for the analysis. Even in the USA and Europe, where semen analysis is widely available and more easily accessible, compliance with post-vasectomy follow-up has been shown to be poor with anywhere from 5% to 45% of men not returning for any follow-up (Dervin et al 1982; Belker et 1990; Smucker et al 1991; Maatman et al 1997). This suggests that current follow-up protocols do not work very well, even under favourable circumstances.

According to the standards for Male and Female Sterilisation set by the Ministry of Health and Family Welfare, Government of India, the patient should undergo semen analysis after three months (Department of Family Welfare 1999).

The British Andrology Society guidelines for the assessment of post-vasectomy semen samples recommend that initial assessment is undertaken 16 weeks post vasectomy and after the patient has produced at least 24 ejaculates. The laboratory should examine a freshly produced seminal fluid specimen by direct microscopy and if no sperm are seen, the centrifugate should be examined for the presence of motile and non-motile spermatozoa. It is recommended that the clinician should give clearance after the production of two consecutive sperm-free ejaculates. In cases of persistent identification of non-motile spermatozoa, the referring clinician should advise the patient regarding the cessation of other contraceptive precautions (Hancock and McLaughlin 2002).

In general, vasectomy is highly effective and one of the most reliable contraceptive methods available. Usually, vasectomy failure rates are quoted to be between 0.2% and 0.4%; however, a thorough review of the literature reveals published rates as high as 5% (Schmidt and Free 1978; Shapiro and Silber 1979; Temmerman 1986; Li et al 1994). Vasectomy failure rates are generally believed to be similar to those for female sterilisation, and they are lower than those for reversible methods. However, it is difficult to directly compare failure rates for vasectomy with those of other contraceptive methods, including female sterilisation, since in most reports on vasectomy, rates are presented as failures per 100 procedures, while for other methods the measure most often used is failures per 100 person-years of use.

However, several recent studies suggest differences in the effectiveness of certain vas occlusion techniques. A study conducted in Mexico on time to azoospermia following vasectomy, using ligation and excision alone, showed a prolonged risk of continued fertility in an unexpectedly large percentage of men. Thirteen per cent of men (28 of 217) showed potential fertility (defined as a sperm concentration of 3 million or more sperm per ml of semen) six months after the vasectomy. This finding suggests that recanalisation was occurring more frequently than expected (Nazerali et al 2002). Similar results were seen following an interim analysis of a randomised controlled trial of fascial interposition conducted at eight sites in seven countries, only 76%–86% of men reached azoospermia by 34 weeks after vasectomy in the group in which only ligation and excision was performed (Sokal et 2001).

A Canadian study indicated that failure is also higher than expected when clips are used instead of sutures. A retrospective review of computerised records of more than 2500 men who had vasectomy with occlusion by clips or by cautery and fascial interposition found failure rates (based on semen analysis) of 8.7% for clips but only 0.3% for cautery and fascial interposition, a highly significant difference (Sokal et al 2004).

Preliminary results from a randomised controlled trial found that use of fascial interposition with ligation and excision led to a more rapid decrease in sperm counts than when ligation and excision were used alone. When fascial interposition was used along with ligation and excision, about 93% of men had reached a low sperm count (less than 100,000 sperm per ml of semen) by 22 weeks after surgery, compared with only 81% of men when fascial interposition was not used. The results demonstrate that fascial interposition significantly improves the effectiveness of vasectomy by ligation and excision (Sokal et al 2001).

The studies demonstrating higher-than-expected failure rates for vasectomy by ligation and excision or for vasectomy with clips provide evidence that post-vasectomy pregnancies are indeed more common than expected in general. The first, an analysis of Chinese vasectomy data from the 1988 National Demographic and Family Planning Survey, which used a nationally representative sample of more than 2 million respondents, found surprisingly high cumulative failure rates. Life-table methods indicated that among the more than 28,000 women who reported that their husbands had had a vasectomy; pregnancy rates after the vasectomy were 2.7 pregnancies per 100 women after one year and increased to 9.2 per 100 after 10 years (based on the women's reports of pregnancy). Further analysis showed that lower-level hospitals, where the majority of male sterilisations were performed, had higher failure rates. In addition, husbands of younger women had much higher failure rates than husbands of older women. Unfortunately, no information is available on what occlusion methods were used for the vasectomies (Chen 1999).

In the other analysis, a retrospective follow-up study, more than 1000 Nepalese men were interviewed 1–4 years after vasectomy. The sample was randomly selected from more than 30,000 men in the hill districts of Nepal who had a vasectomy between 1996 and 1999. The estimated first-year pregnancy rate was 1.7 per 100 among wives of men having ligation and excision vasectomies. The cumulative probability of pregnancy at three years was 4.2 per 100 (Nazerali et al 2002).

Final analysis of the Family Health International/Engender Health randomised controlled trial (RCT) conducted among 841 men has shown that ligation and excision with fascial interposition reduced vasectomy failures by about a half compared to ligation and excision alone. It also decreased time to azoospermia and severe oligospermia (< 100,000 sperm/ml). Based on semen analyses conducted up to 34 weeks, failure rates for vasectomies, with versus without fascial interposition, all of which were performed by experienced practitioners, were 5.9% and 12.7%, respectively. The number of vasectomy failures in all age groups was similar. No significant differences in terms of safety (adverse events, or mild or moderate scrotal pain at 12 months post-vasectomy) were noted for the two techniques. Fascial interposition added approximately two minutes to the procedure. Physicians reported that 13.8% of procedures involving fascial interposition were difficult to perform, but in only nine cases, 2% of 419 men, were the practitioners unable to perform fascial interposition on one or both vas. This trial, the first large RCT of a vas occlusion technique, resolves some of the conflicting results from studies of fascial interposition that have been conducted since 1978 (Sokal et al 2004).

A statistical comparison of two vasectomy techniques—cautery versus ligation and excision with fascial interposition—indicates that cautery was associated with significantly more rapid progression to severe oligospermia and significantly fewer early failures than was ligation and excision with fascial interposition (1% versus 5% respectively). Data for the comparison came from two prospective multicentre studies—the fascial interposition arm of the FHI/Engender Health RCT and the observational study of cautery described (Sokal et al 2003). In both cases, practitioners were experienced and vasectomy failure data came from semen analyses.

A total of 11 studies were found comparing ligation with cautery. Occlusive failure risks ranged from 0.4% to 29.1% with ligation and 0% to 4.8% with cautery. Fascial interposition with cautery was used in 6 of 11 studies. In all of these studies occlusive failure risk was very small—0% to 1.2%. Four studies used thermal cautery, five used electrocautery and two used both cautery techniques. There were no apparent differences in the range of failure risk between the two kinds of cautery (Sokal et al 2003; Labrecque et al 2004).

It is important to note that despite these recent findings, vasectomy remains a highly effective method of contraception. In addition, it is difficult to make general statements about vasectomy failure because of the wide variety of occlusion methods used. It is becoming clearer that some occlusion methods or combinations of occlusion methods are likely to be more effective than others.

There are two causes of vasectomy failure—user failure and failure of the technique itself. User failure is defined as when a pregnancy occurs before sperm have been cleared from the male reproductive tract post-vasectomy. User failure could be related either to inadequate instructions or to the vasectomy user's failure to comply with instructions to use alternate contraceptive methods until azoospermia is confirmed.

Spontaneous recanalisation of the vas is the most common cause of failure of the vasectomy technique itself, yet it is not well understood (Alderman 1988). Recanalisation occurs when a sperm granuloma forms at the vasectomy site, linking the two cut ends of the vas (Goldstein 1983; Chen 1999). In the case of vasectomy by ligation and excision, it is thought that failure may occur when the cut ends of the vas at the site of the ligature die and are sloughed off. A similar mechanism could be involved in recanalisation following the use of clips.

When recanalisation occurs in the first few months after vasectomy and before azoospermia has been achieved, it is called early recanalisation. On the other hand, late recanalisation occurs when sperm appear in the ejaculate after azoospermia has been demonstrated (Philp et al 1984; Alderman 1988). Late recanalisation is usually identified when the partner of a vasectomised man becomes pregnant, and may occur several years after a seemingly successful vasectomy.

Rare causes of failure include congenital duplication of the vas that went undetected at surgery and a failure to identify and occlude the correct structure during the procedure (Alderman 1988).

COMPLICATIONS

Intraoperative complications of vasectomy, such as vasovagal reaction, lidocaine toxicity and excessive bleeding, are unusual. Explaining the procedure to the patient in advance, ensuring an effective anesthetic block, using gentle surgical technique, and reassuring the patient during the procedure can prevent vasovagal reaction. Lidocaine toxicity and excessive bleeding can be prevented if providers follow appropriate vasectomy guidelines and procedures for administering local anesthesia and for the surgical technique.

Most postoperative vasectomy complications are minor, subsiding within 1–2 weeks. Common complaints after surgery are swelling of the scrotum, bruising and pain. Minor bleeding under the skin is common. Some men experience tenderness or a dragging sensation in the scrotum for up to a week after vasectomy. A scrotal support, mild pain medication and local application of ice are usually sufficient treatment.

More significant complications such as heavy bleeding, hematoma (a collection of blood underneath the skin) or infection are generally quite rare. The incidence of hematoma is related to the provider's experience with vasectomy. Physicians who perform larger numbers of vasectomies have lower hematoma rates than do those who perform fewer procedures (Kendrick et al 1987).

Importantly, rates of heavy bleeding, hematoma and infection vary depending on the approach taken to the vas. Numerous studies have demonstrated that the no-scalpel approach consistently results in lower rates of hematoma and infection than conventional vasectomy.

In most cases, using good surgical techniques to minimise tissue trauma and limit bleeding, practising aseptic techniques and giving clients

Table 37.1: Percentage of vasectomies in which infection or hematoma or bleeding occurred

Study	No. of Vasectomies	% With infections	% With hematoma/ bleeding
Incisional vasectomy			
Philp, Guillebaud and Budd 1984	534	1.3	4.5
Kendrick et al 1987	65.155	3.5	2.0
Nirapathpongorn, Huber and Krieger 1990	523	1.3	1.7
Alderman 1991	1,224	4.0	0.3
Sokal et al 1999	627	1.3	10.7
No-scalpel vasectomy			
Nirapathpongporn, Huber and Krieger, 1990	680	0.2	0.3
Li et al 1991	179,741	0.9	0.1
Li et al 1991	238	0.0	0.0
Sokal et al 2003	841	1.4	0.48
In both groups, Fascial interposition and non interposition			
Sokal et al 1999	606	0.2	1.7
Arellano et al 1997	1,000	0.0	2.1

good postoperative instructions can prevent bleeding, hematoma and infection. Because the loose scrotal tissue allows injured blood vessels to continue bleeding, it is important to maintain good homeostasis during the procedure if hematoma formation is to be prevented. Many hematomas can be prevented if men avoid physical activity for a few days after the procedure; clients should be carefully instructed in this regard.

Sperm granuloma can occur either at the site of vas occlusion or in the epididymis. These small nodules form when sperm leaks out of the vas or the epididymis, inducing an inflammatory reaction. While the true incidence of sperm granuloma following vasectomy is not known, they are seen in 15%–40% of men having vasectomy reversal (Pugh and Hanley 1969; Esho et al 1974). This provides a reasonable estimate for incidence in men following vasectomy, in that rates of granuloma formation are likely to be similar in men having a reversal and in the general population of vasectomised men.

The majority of sperm granuloma is asymptomatic. Only 2%–3% of vasectomised men have sperm granuloma that is painful or in some way symptomatic; most of these occur in the second or third week after the procedure (Pugh and Hanley 1969; Balogh and Argenyi 1985; Babayan and Krane 1986). The factors that lead to the formation of sperm granuloma are not well understood; thus, there are no measures known to prevent or decrease their occurrence.

Long-Term Effects

Potential physiological effects and long-term sequelae of vasectomy have been the subject of extensive research over the past two decades. This research provides reassurance that vasectomy does not have any significant long-term negative physical or mental health effects. Results of large-scale, well-designed epidemiological studies in men have consistently shown no adverse effects of vasectomy in terms of heart disease, testicular or prostate cancer, immune complex disorders and a host of other conditions. Vasectomy appears to be a largely safe and highly effective method of contraception, certainly with risks no greater than those for any of the contraceptive methods used by women.

Comprehensive Studies of Disease Incidence

There are five large-scale retrospective cohort studies that have examined the incidence of a number of diseases in thousands of vasectomised and non-vasectomised men (Goldacre et al 1978; Goldacre and Vessey 1979; Petitti et al 1983; Massey et al 1984; Kendrick et al 1987; Peterson et al 1990; Nienhuis et al 1992). For the disease categories or organ systems studied, vasectomised men were no more likely to be hospitalised or to develop a disease than were controls. In these studies, there were large numbers of cases of disease among both vasectomised and non-vasectomised men in all categories. Thus, taken together, the studies are reassuring that vasectomy does not increase the risk of adverse physical or mental health outcomes.

Effects on Cardiovascular Function

Reports that vasectomised monkeys developed atherosclerosis more rapidly than non-vasectomised controls (Walker et al 1981; Schuman et al 1993) led to extensive research into the potential effects of vasectomy on cardiovascular disease in men. Since the early 1980s, most of the cohort, case-control and cross-sectional studies that were conducted have found no association of vasectomy with acute myocardial infarction, other ischemic heart disease, stroke, peripheral vascular disease, hypertension, coronary artery disease, or hypertensive and atherosclerotic retinal vascular changes (Alexander and Clarkson 1978; Goldacre et al 1978; Goldacre and Vessey 1979; Petitti et al 1983; Massey Jr et al 1984; Nienhuis et al 1992).

Antisperm Antibodies

The number of circulating antisperm antibodies increases after vasectomy. Antisperm antibodies are found in 50%–80% of vasectomised men (Rimm et al 1983; Rosenberg et al 1986; Bernstein et al no date) but in only 8%–21% of men in the general population (Bernstein et al n.d.). The theoretical concern that these antibodies may have adverse health consequences has led to numerous studies, the results of which have shown no evidence of any immunological or other diseases related to the formation of antisperm antibodies after vasectomy (Alexander and Clarkson 1978; Goldacre et al 1978; Lepow and Crozier 1979; Clarkson and Alexander 1980; Petitti et al 1982; 1983; Coulson et al 1993; Lenzi et al 1997; Gubin et al 1998). However, antisperm antibodies may play a role in decreased fertility after vasectomy reversal.

Prostate Cancer

Since the mid-1980s, more than a dozen epidemiological studies of the risk of prostate cancer after vasectomy have been reported in the literature. Results have been difficult to interpret because of conflicting study findings, lack of a convincing biological mechanism for an association between vasectomy and prostate cancer and generally weak associations when they have been found. Also, the potential for bias in some studies was high and likely led to an overestimation of any effect (Petitti et al 1982).

Based on the results of the research published to date, there is little evidence for a causal association between vasectomy and prostate cancer (Goldacre et al 1983). A panel of experts gathered by the US National Institutes of Health in 1993 concluded that no change in the current practice of vasectomy was necessary nor should vasectomy reversal be done as a measure to prevent prostate cancer (Bernal-Delgado et al 1998). Studies published after the expert panel report support these conclusions (Petitti et al 1982; Goldacre et al 1983).

POSTVASECTOMY PAIN SYNDROME

A small percentage of vasectomised men have reported chronic pain in the testis following vasectomy. While up to a third of men have reported occasional testicular discomfort following vasectomy, only around 2% of all vasectomised men said that the pain had negatively affected their life or that they regretted having had the vasectomy because of chronic pain (Healey 1993; Choe and Kirkemo 1993; Peterson and Howards 1998). Conservative therapy such as nonsteroidal anti-inflammatory drugs, sitz baths, antibiotics or spermatic cord blocks is sufficient treatment in most cases. When this fails, there is some evidence that vasectomy reversal or denervation of the spermatic cord may be helpful (McMohan et al 1992; Ehn and Liljestrand 1995).

Mortality

Mortality following vasectomy has generally been very low. The few reports from the literature have demonstrated minimal mortality associated with vasectomy (Ahmed et al 1997; Myers et al 1997). The most comprehensive study, based on data from more than 400,000 vasectomies worldwide, reported a mortality rate of 0.5 deaths per 100,000 vasectomised men (Grimes et al 1982a). In addition, since 1990, Engender Health has become aware of only one vasectomy-related death (due to a postoperative infection at the surgical site) from among the more than 200,000 vasectomy procedures reported between 1990 and 2000 in Engender Health-supported programmes around the world. Although reporting of mortality related to sterilisation services is voluntary and complications are known to be underreported, clearly, vasectomy-related mortality is quite low.

Vasectomy Regret and Reversal

Regret: A feeling of regret following a vasectomy is more common among men who at the time of the vasectomy were in an unstable marriage, were younger than 31, or had no children or had very young children, or among men who made the decision to have a vasectomy during a time of financial crisis or for reasons related to a pregnancy (Howard 1982; Strauss et al 1984; Clarke and Gregson 1986; Khairullah et al 1992). Providers should use risk factors for regret to identify men who may need more in-depth counselling to ensure that vasectomy is right for them at the time, but not to deny vasectomy to men who want it. In addition, the fact that regret is often seen when vasectomy users have an adverse health effect that is either caused by the procedure or perceived to be caused by it underscores the importance of good counselling prior to the procedure.

Reversal: The most common reasons for

reversal requests are remarriage after divorce or after the death of a partner, the death of one or more children, a desire for more children, or problems of either a physiological or psychological nature that the vasectomised man or his provider believe will be alleviated by vasectomy reversal (McMohan et al 1982; Strauss et al 1984; Shain 1986; Kjersgaard et al 1987).

Vasovasostomy (reattaching the cut ends of the vas) is the most common procedure for reversing a vasectomy. In some situations, it may be necessary to attach the vas directly to the epididymis; this procedure is known as vasoepididymostomy. Both procedures are complex, technically demanding and expensive; most importantly, there is no guarantee that fertility can be restored. This highlights the importance of carefully screening, counselling and selecting vasectomy users.

Both macroscopic and microsurgical techniques for vasovasostomy and vasoepididymostomy have been used for vasectomy reversal; the current consensus is that microsurgical techniques are more successful (Newton 1988; Meinertz et al 1990; Jarow 1995). Reported rates of potency (evaluated by the presence of sperm in the ejaculate) following vasovasostomy range from 74% to 92% for macroscopic reversal and from 75% to 100% for microsurgical reversal (Kessler and Freiha 1981; Cos 1983; Kjersgaard et al 1987; Fox 1997; Huang et al 1997; Belker 1998). Reported pregnancy rates are lower, however, ranging from 35% to 57% for macroscopic and from 38% to 82% for microsurgical vasovasostomy approaches (Shain 1986; Lee 1986; Kjersgaard et al 1987; Huang et al 1997; Mason et al 1997). Vasoepididymostomy is generally less successful than vasovasostomy, and while pregnancy rates as high as 42%–55% have been reported (Fallon et al 1981; Marmar 1995; Kolettis and Thomas Jr 1997; Takihara 1998) most are lower, ranging from 10% to 30% (Silber 1989; Thomas 1993; Mason et al 1997; Berardinucci et al 1998).

Several factors affect the success of vasectomy reversal—the technical demands of the surgery itself; the type of vasectomy procedure performed; the length of time between the vasectomy and the reversal procedure; the levels of antisperm antibodies that may have developed after the vasectomy or the reversal; and changes in the epididymis or partial obstruction of the vas after reversal that prevent sperm from moving through the vas.

The time that has elapsed between vasectomy and reversal is a major factor in the success of reversal. The longer the interval between vasectomy and reversal, the less likely the man is to be fertile after reversal. Reversal is usually more successful when it is done within 10 years of the vasectomy; pregnancy rates drop to less than 50% when vasectomy reversal is performed more than 9–10 years later (Kjersgaard 1987; Fox 1997; Mason et al 1997).

Reports of the effect of antisperm antibodies on fertility following vasectomy reversal vary. Some studies have shown decreased pregnancy rates due to antisperm antibodies, while others have not (Meinertz et al 1990; Jarow 1995; Mathews et al 1995). The consensus is that fertility following vasectomy reversal is inhibited only by high levels of antisperm antibodies (Newton 1988).

Partial obstruction of the vas after vasectomy reversal (because of a sperm granuloma or adhesions from the surgery) has been shown to affect the success of reversal (Thomas et al 1981; Owen and Kapila 1984; Meinertz 1990). In these cases, semen quality may be poor in terms of sperm numbers, sperm motility, or both. When partial obstruction is the cause for failure of reversal, repeat vasectomy reversal has produced good pregnancy results (Owen and Kapila 1984; Kjersgaard et al 1987).

Assisted reproduction technologies have been successful in vasectomised men who want children but who either do not want to attempt a vasectomy reversal or have had one or more unsuccessful reversal surgeries. Sperm can be retrieved from the epididymis or testis and then used in a procedure known as intracytoplasmic sperm injection (ICSI), in which sperm are injected directly into the ova in a laboratory. Pregnancy rates following ICSI with epididymal sperm are reported to be between 25% and 36% (Craft et al 1995a; Aboulghar et al 1997; Lea et al 1997; Carbone et al 1998). Pregnancy rates ranging from 17% to 36% have been reported when testicular-sperm are used (Lea et al 1997; Carbone Jr et al 1997; Craft et al 1995b; Abuzeid et al 1997; Dohle et al 1998).

Research continues on methods of vasectomy reversal that produce better success rates. Additionally, new assisted reproduction techniques are also being explored that might be applied in the cases of vasectomised men who are interested in having children. However, there is no guarantee that pregnancy will occur following vasectomy reversal or use of assisted reproduction techniques, and these procedures are expensive and not widely available, especially in low-resource settings. Thus, vasectomy should be considered a permanent contraceptive method.

Innovations: New methods of vas occlusion are unlikely to become available in the near future, but investigators have explored several alternatives to surgical sterilisation in men. Experimental methods of occluding the vas include injecting chemicals into the vas percutaneously (through the skin), to scar the vas closed or physically block the passage of sperm through the vas. In theory, percutaneous occlusion of the vas could offer several potential advantages over vasectomy as a male contraceptive, as it would be less invasive and thus might have a lower rate of complications. Such a procedure might also be quicker or easier to perform. In addition, some types could be reversed more easily, and the approach may be more acceptable, since it does not involve surgery.

Studies on occluding the vas for contraceptive purposes by injecting chemicals percutaneously began in the 1970s in China. This technique was easily performed and led to high rates of azoospermia and low pregnancy rates, although reversal was no easier than for vasectomy because the occluded portion of the vas needed to be excised and reanastomosis of the vas performed (Meniru et al 1997; Watkins et al 1997). Concerns about the safety of these chemicals have limited exploration of this approach. It is possible that a suitable method for chemically scarring the vas may be found in the future, and although reversal may not be any easier than for vasectomy, the technique may offer other advantages over vasectomy in terms of ease of procedure, number of complications or cost.

Formed-in-place plugs use a liquid material that is injected into the vas and forms a solid plug to block the vas lumen; such plugs have been examined as a method of vas occlusion. A formed-in-place polyurethane plug had low rates of complications, was highly effective and was easily reversible (Xiao 1987; Watkins et al 1997). However, uncertainty regarding the safety of the polyurethane product led to an investigation of medical-grade silicone plugs. Variable rates of success have been reported for a formed-in-place silicone plug known as Vasoc (Zhao 1990; Zhao et al 1992a; Soebadi et al 1995). Vasoc vas occlusion does not appear to be suitable for use as a male contraceptive at this time. Not only are there questions about efficacy, but given the complex and technically demanding nature of the technique, the need for specialised and costly equipment and supplies (including refrigeration or freezing for the materials), and the need for three people to perform the procedure, service delivery constraints would likely limit the method's utility in low-resource settings.

Researchers have also attempted to develop devices that can be placed in the vas to obstruct sperm but then later can be removed or opened to allow sperm to pass. Such devices have had several problems, however; for example, the surgery has been difficult and the devices have not consistently stayed in place within the muscular vas.

References

Aboulghar MA et al. 1997. Fertilization and pregnancy rates after intracytoplasmic sperm injection using ejaculate semen and surgically retrieved sperm. *Fertil Steril* 68(1):108–111.

Abuzeid ML, MA Sasy, H Salem. 1997. Testicular sperm extraction and intracytoplasmic sperm injection: A simplified method for treatment of obstructive azoospermia. *Fertil Steril* 68(2):328–333.

Ahmed L et al. 1997. The incidence of post-vasectomy chronic testicular pain and the role of nerve stripping (denervation) of the spermatic cord in its management. *Br J Urol* 79(2):269–270.

Alderman PM. 1988. The lurking sperm: A review of failures in 8879 vasectomies performed by one physician. *J Am Med Assoc* 259(21):3142–3144

Alderman PM. 1989. General and anomalous sperm disappearance characteristics found in a large vasectomy series. *Fertil Steril* 51(5):859–862.

Alexander NJ and TB Clarkson. 1978. Vasectomy increases the severity of diet-induced atherosclerosis in Macaca fascicularis. *Science* 201(4355):538–541

Arellano LS et al. 1997. No-scalpel vasectomy: Review of the first 1000 cases in a family medicine unit. *Archives of Medical Research* 28(4):517–522.

AVSC International. 1997. *No-scalpel vasectomy: An illustrated guide for surgeons.* 2nd edition. New York

Babayan RK and RJ Krane. 1986. Vasectomy: What are community standards? *Urology* 27(4):328–330.

Balogh K and ZB Argenyi. 1985. Vastitis nodosa and spermatic granuloma of the skin: An histologic study of a rare complication of vasectomy. *J Cut Pathol* 12(6):528–533.

Bedford JM and G Zelikovsky. 1979. Viability of spermatozoa in the human ejaculate after vasectomy. *Fertil Steril* 32(4):460–463.

Belker AM et al. 1990. The high rate of noncompliance for post-vasectomy semen examination: Medical and legal considerations. *J Urol* 144(2, I):284–286.

Belker AM et al. 1991. Results of 1469 microsurgical vasectomy reversals by the Vasovasostomy Study Group. *J Urol* 145(3):505–511.

Belker AM. 1998. Evaluation of partial anastomotic obstruction after vasovasostomy and predictors of success after vasoepididymostomy. *J Urol* 159(3):835–836.

Benjamin H.` 1922. The Steinach Operation, report of twenty two cases with endocrine interpretation

Berardinucci D, A Zini, K Jarvi. 1998. Outcome of microsurgical reconstruction in men with suspected epididymal obstruction. *J Urol* 159(3):831–834.

Bernal-Delgado E et al. 1998. The association between vasectomy and prostate cancer: A systematic review of the literature. *Fertil Steril* 70(2):191–200.

Bernstein GS et al. n. d. A controlled, prospective study of the effects of vasectomy In *Vasectomy: immunologic and pathophysiologic effects in animals and man*, ed. by IH Lepow and R Crozier. New York: Academic Press, p. 473.

Brenner WE and D Edelman. 1976. Permanent sterilization through posterior colpotomy. *Int. J Gynecol Obstet*; 14: 46–52.

Brissaud E. 1880. Les effects de la ligature due canal deferent. Arch. D Physio, 2nd series, pp 769–789.

Cameron CS. 1945. Anastomosis of Vas Deferens: Restoration of fertility after five years of bilateral vasectomy. *JAMA* 127:1119–1120.

Carbone Jr DJ et al. 1998. Partial obstruction, not antisperm antibodies, causing infertility after vasovasostomy. *J Urol* 159(3):827–830.

Chen CHC. 1999 Female and male sterilization failures in China: Findings from a national survey. Presentation at the 127th annual meeting of the American Public Health Association, November 7–11, Chicago.

Choe JM and AK Kirkemo. 1996. Questionnaire-based outcomes study of nononcological post-vasectomy complications. *J Urol* 155(4):1284–1286.

Clarke L and S Gregson. 1986. Who has a vasectomy reversal? *J Biosoc Sci* 18(3): 253–259.

Clarkson TB and NJ Alexander. 1980. Long-term vasectomy: Effects on the occurrence and extent of atherosclerosis in rhesus monkeys. *J Clin Invest* 65(1):15–25.

Colony S. 1994. ed. Washington Pop. Update. Washington, May 13.

Cooper A. 1830. Observations on the structure and diseases of the testis. Longman, Rees, Orme, Brown & Green.

Cortes M, et al. 1997. Results of a pilot study of the time to azoospermia after vasectomy in Mexico City. *Contraception* 56(4):215–222.

Cos LR, et al. 1983. Vasovasostomy: Current state of the art. *Urology* 22(6): 567–575.

Coulson AH et al. 1993. Health Status of American Men—a study of post-vasectomy sequelae: Results. *J Clin Epidemiol* 46(8): 857–958.

Craft I et al. 1995b. Percutaneous epididymal sperm aspiration and intracytoplasmic sperm injection in the management of infertility due to obstructive azoospermia. *Fertil Steril* 63(5):1038–1042.

Craft IL et al. 1995a. Factors influencing the outcome of in-vitro fertilization. With percutaneous aspirated epididymal spermatozoa and intracytoplasmic sperm injection in azoospermic men. *Hum Reprod* 10(7):1791–1794.

Cullins V. (2000). Sterilization: Long term issues In Sciarra JJ. Ed *Gynecology and Obstetrics*. Philadelphia: Lippincott Williams and Wilkins; 1–7.

Davies AH et al. 1990. The long-term outcome following 'special clearance' after vasectomy. *Brit J Urol* 66(2):211–212.

De Knijff DWW et al. Persistence or reappearance of nonmotile sperm after vasectomy: Does it have clinical consequences? *Fertil Steril* 1997; 67(2):332–335.

Dervin JV, RC Barnett, DL Stone. 1982. Patient noncompliance with postvasectomy semen examination protocol. *J Famil Pract*14(3):487–490.

Dohle GR et al. 1998. Surgical sperm retrieval and intracytoplasmic sperm injection as treatment of obstructive azoospermia. *Hum Reprod* 13(3):620–623.

Dorsey JW. 1957. Surgical Correction of Post Vasectomy Sterility, *J Int Coll Surgeons* 27:453–456.

Edwards IS and JL Farlow. 1979. Non-motile sperms persisting after vasectomy: Do they matter? *Brit Med J* 1(6169): 1019

Edwards IS. 1993. Earlier testing after vasectomy based on the absence of motile sperm. *Fertility and Sterility* 59(2):431–436.

Ehn BE and J Liljestrand. 1995. A long-term follow-up of 108 vasectomized men. Good counselling routines are important. *Scand J Urol Nephrol* 29(4):477–481.

Esho JO, GW Ireland, AS Cass. 1974. Recanalization following vasectomy. *Urology* 3(2):211–214.

Evridge-Vernon. 1956. Modern Operative Surgery by Grey Turner. In *Modern Operative Surgery* ed G Grey Turner and LC Rogers. New York: Paul S Hoeber Inc.

Fallon B, Miller RK, Gerber WL. Nonmicroscopic vasovasostomy. *J Urol* 1981. 126(3):361–362.

Filshie GM, D Casey, JR Pogmore et al. 1981. The Titanium/Silicon rubber clip for female sterilization. *Br. J Obstet Gynecol* 88:655–662

Fox M. 1997. Failed vasectomy reversal: Is a further attempt worthwhile using microsurgery? *Euro Urol* 31(4): 436–440.

Goldacre M and M Vessey. 1979. Record linkage study of morbidity following vasectomy. In *Vasectomy: Immunologic and pathophysiologic effects in animals and man*, ed H. Lepow and R Crozier. New York: Academic Press, Chap. 27.

Goldacre MJ et al. 1978. Follow-up of vasectomy using medical record linkage. *Am J Epidemiol* 108(3): 176–180.

Goldacre MJ, TR Holford, MP Vessey. 1983. Cardiovascular disease and vasectomy: Findings from two epidemiologic studies. *N Eng J Med* 1983. 308(14):805–808.

Goldstein M. 1983. Vasectomy failure using an open-ended technique. *Fertil Steril* 40(5):699–700.

Govt. of India. 1999. *Standards for female and male sterilization*. Division of Research Studies and Standards, Department of Family Welfare, Ministry of Health and Family Welfare Government of India, New Delhi.

Grimes DA et al. 1982a. Deaths from contraceptive sterilization in Bangladesh: Rates, causes, and prevention. *Obstet Gynecol* 60(5):635–640.

Gubin DA, R Dmochowski, WH Kutteh. 1998. Multivariant analysis of men from in fertile couples with and without antisperm antibodies. *Am J Reprod Immunol* 39(2): 157–160.

Gupta I, Bajwa H, Singh P, Gupta AN, Devi PK. 1979. Mortality following vaginal tubal ligation. *Ind J Med Res* 69:770–775.

Hankinson SE, DJ Hunter, GA Colditz et al. 1993. Tubal ligation, hysterectomy and risk of ovarian cancer. A prospective study *JAMA* 270:2813–2818.

Haws JM GT Morgan, AE Pollack LM Koonin et al. 1998. Clinical aspects of vasectomies performed in the United States in 1995. *Urology* 52(4):685–691.

Healy B. 1993. From the National Institutes of Health: Does vasectomy cause prostate cancer? *J Am Med Assoc* 269(20):2620

Hellema HWJ and P Rumke. 1978. Sperm autoantibodies as a consequence of vasectomy I within one year post-operation. *Clin Exp Immunol* 31(I): 8–29.

Howard G. 1982. Who asks for vasectomy reversal and why? *Br Med J* 285(6340):490–492.

Huang MK et al. 1997. Multiple factors affecting human repregnancy after microsurgical vasovasostomy. *Reprod Contracep* 8:92–100.

Hulka JF, JM Phillips, HB Peterson, HW Surrey. 1995. Laparoscopic sterilization. American Association of Gynecologic Laparoscopists. Membership survey. *Am Assoc Gynecol Lapaproscope* 2: 137–138.

Indian Council of Medical Research. 1982. In *Collaborative study on sequele of tubal sterilization* ICMR: New Delhi; 88.

IPPF Medical Bulletin. 1999. Evaluate options for permanent birth control; 33:3.

Irving FC. 1950. Tubal Sterilisation. *Am J Obstet Gynecol* 6: 1101–1111.

Jarow JP. 1995. Epididymovasostomy. *Microsurgery* 16(5):333–338.

Jhaver PS.1973. Vasectomy after effects, modern techniques, complications, repairs. *Ind J Med* 27(5): 411–416.

Joel LM, K Stuart and HH Victor. 2001. A minimal invasive vasectomy with no suture, inline method of vas occlusion. *Int J Fertil* 46:257–264.

Jouannet P and G David. 1978. Evolution of the properties of semen immediately following vasectomy. *Fertility and Sterility* 29(4):435–441.

Kendrick JS B Gonzales, DH Huber, GS Grubb, GL Rubin et al. 1987. Complications of vasectomies in the United States. *J Famil Pract* 25(3):245–248.

Kessler R and F Freiha. 1981. Macroscopic vasovasostomy. *Fertil Steril* 36(4):531–532.

Khairullah Z, DH Huber, B Gonzales. 1992. Declining mortality in international sterilization services. *Int J Gynecol Obstet* 39(1): 41–50.

Kjersgaard AG, I Thranov, OV Rasmussen. 1987. Vasectomy: A study of 810 vasectomized men: who regretted it? *Ugeskrift for Laeger* 149(38):2527–2530 (Danish).

Kolettis PN and AJ Thomas Jr. 1997. Vasoepididymostomy for vasectomy reversal: A critical assessment in the era of intracytoplasmic sperm injection. *J Urol* 158(2):467–470.

Labrecque M, C Dufresne, MA Barone, K St-Hilaire. 2004. Vasectomy surgical techniques: A systematic review. *BMC Med* 24;2:21

Lea IA, P Adoyo, MG O'Rand. 1997. Auto immunogenicity of the human sperm protein Sp 17 in vasectomized men and identification of linear B cell epitopes. *Fertil Steril* 67(2):355–361.

Lee HY. 1986. A 20 year experience with vasovasostomy. *J Urol* 136(2):413–415.

Lenzi A et al. 1997. Antisperm antibody detection: Clinical, biological and statistical correlation between methods. *Am J Reprod Immunol* 38(3):224–230.

Lepow IH and RH Crozier eds. 1979. *Vasectomy: immunologic and pathophysiologic effects in animals and man.* New York: Academic Press.

Lewis EL, CK Brazil, JW Overstreet. 1984. Human sperm function in the ejaculate following vasectomy. *Fertil Sterility* 42(6):895–898.

Li PS, SQ Li, PN Schlegel and M Goldstein. 1992. External spermatic sheath injection for vasal nerve block. *Urol* 39:173.

Li SQ, M Goldstein, J Zhu, D Huber. 1991. No scalpel vasectomy. *J Urol* 145(2):341–344.

Li SQ B Xu, YH Hou, CH Li et al. 1994. Relationship between vas occlusion techniques and recanalization. *Advances in Contraceptive Delivery Systems* 10:153–159.

Li SQ. 1988. Vasal sterilization techniques: Teaching material for the National standard Workshop, Chongqing, People's Republic of China: Scientific and Technical Literature Press, p.176.

Maatman TJ, L Aldrin, GG Carothers. 1997. Patient noncompliance after vasectomy. *Fertil Steril* 68(3): 552–555.

Marmar JL. 1995. Management of the epididymal tubule during an end-to-side vasoepididymostomy. *J Urol* 154(1):93–96.

Mason RG, PG Connell, JC Bull. 1997. Reversal of vasectomy using a macroscopic technique: A retrospective study. Annals of the Royal College of Surgeons of England 79(6):420–422.

Massey Jr. FJ et al. 1984. Vasectomy and health: Results from a large cohort study. *J Am Med Assoc* 252(8):1023–1029.

Matthews GJ, PN Schlegel, M Goldstein. 1995. Patency following microsurgical vasoepididymostomy and vasovasostomy: Temporal considerations. *J Urol* 154(6):2070–2073.

McMahon AJ et al. 1992. Chronic testicular pain following vasectomy. *Brit J Urol* 69(2):188–191.

Meinertz H et al. 1990. Antisperm antibodies and fertility after vasovasostomy: A follow-up study of 216 men. *Fertil Steril* 54(2):315–321.

Meniru GI et al. 1997. Results of percutaneous epididymal sperm aspiration and intracytoplasmic sperm injection in two major groups of patients with obstructive azoospermia. *Hum Reprod* 12(II): 2443–2446.

Morson C.1924. Physiology and the results of the division of vas deferens. *Br Med J.* 1:54–55.

Myers SA, Mershon CE, Fuchs EF. 1997. Vasectomy reversal for treatment of the post vasectomy pain syndrome. *J Urol* 157(2):518–520

Nazerali H et al. 2002. A prospective non-comparative study of time and number of ejaculations to azoospermia following vasectomy. Research Triangle Park, NC: Family Health International; and New York: EngenderHealth.

Newsletter. 2005. *Ind Coll Obstet Gynecol* 3:3–6.

Newton RA. 1988. IgG antisperm antibodies attached to sperm do not correlate with infertility following vasovasostomy. *Microsurgery* 9(4): 278–280.

Nienhuis H, M Golacre, V Seagroatt, L Gill, M Vessey. 1992. Incidence of disease after vasectomy: A record linkage retrospective cohort study. *Brit Med J* 304(6829): 743–746.

Nirapathpongpom A, DH Huber, JN Krieger. 1990. No-scalpel vasectomy at the King's Birthday vasectomy festival. *Lancet* 335(8694):894–895.

O'Conor VJ. 1942. Anastomosis of Vas Deferens After Purposeful Division for Sterility. *JAMA* 136: 162–163.

Ochsner AJ. 1899. Surgical Treatment of Habitual Criminals. *JAMA* 32:8678.

Owen E and H Kapila. 1984. Vasectomy reversal: Review of 475 microsurgical vasovasostomies. *Med J Aust* 140(7):398–400.

P Hancock and E McLaughlin. British Andrology Society Guidelines for the assessment of post vasectomy semen samples. *J Clin Pathol* 2002. 55: 812–816.

Peterson HB and SS Howards. 1998. Vasectomy and prostate cancer: The evidence to date *Fertil Steril* 70(2):201–203.

Peterson HB, DH Huber, AM Belker. 1990. Vasectomy: An appraisal for the obstetrician-gynecologist. *Obstet Gynecol* 76(3, 2):568–572.

Peterson HB, Z Xia, JM Hughes, LS Wilcox, LR Taylor, J Crussel. 1996. The role of pregnancy after tubal sterilization. Findings from the US Collaborative Review of Sterilization. *Am J Obstet Gynecol* 174: 1161–1170.

Petitti DB et al. 1982. A survey of personal habits, symptoms of illness and histories of disease in men with and without vasectomies. *Am J Pub Heal* 72(5):476–480.

Petitti DB et al. 1983. Vasectomy and the incidence of hospitalized illness. *J Urol* 129(4):760–762.

Phadke L. 1953. Paper read at the Third International conference on Planned Parenthood in 1952.

Philp T, J Guillebaud, D Budd. 1984. Complications of vasectomy: Review of 16,000 patients. *Brit J Urol* 56(6): 745–748

Pugh RC and HG Hanley. 1969. Spontaneous recanalisation of the divided vas deferens. *Brit J Urol* 41 (3):340–347.

Rajfer J and CJ Bennett. 1988. Vasectomy. *Urol Clin N Am* 15(4):631–634.

Richardson DW, RJ Aitken, NB Loudon. 1984. The functional competence of human spermatozoa recovered after vasectomy. *J Reprod Fert* 70(2):575–579

Rimm AA et al. 1983. The relationship between vasectomy and angiographically determined atherosclerosis in men. *Preventive Medicine* 12(2):262–273.

Rioux JE and M Daria. 2001. Female Sterilisation: An update of current opinion. *Obstet Gynecol* 13: 377–389.

Rosenberg L et al. 1986. The risk of myocardial infarction 10 years or more after vasectomy in men under 55 years of age. *Am J Epidemiol* 123(6):1049–1056.

Schmidt JE, SD Hills, PA March Banks, E Jing, HB Peterson. 2000. Requesting information about obtaining reversal after tubal sterilization: Findings from US Collaborative Review of Sterilization. *Fertil Steril* 74:892–898.

Schmidt SS and MJ Free. The bipolar needle for vasectomy. I. Experience with the first 1000 cases. *Fertil Steril* 1978. 29(6):676–680.

Schmidt SS. 1987. Vasectomy. *Urol Clin N Am* 14(1):149–154.

Schuman LM et al. 1993. Health Status of American Men: A study of post-vasectomy sequelae. *J Clin Epidemiol* 46(8):697–958.

Shain RN. 1986. Psychosocial consequences of vasectomy In *Male in developed and developing countries contraception: advances and future prospects*, ed by GI Zatuchni et al. Philadelphia: Harper and Row, pp. 34–53.

Shapiro EI and SJ Silber. Open-ended vasectomy, sperm granuloma, and postvasectomy orchialgia. *Fertil Steril* 1979; 32(5):546–550.

Silber SJ. 1977. Sperm granuloma and the reversibility of vasectomy. *Lancet*; 2(8038):588–589.

Silber SJ. 1989. Results of microsurgical vasoepididymostomy: Role of epididymis in sperm maturation. *Hum Reprod* 4(3):298–303.

Sivanesaratnam V. 1985. Onset of azoospermia after vasectomy. *NZ J Med* 98(778):331–333.

Skriver M, F Skovsgaard and J Miskowiak. 1997. Conventional or Li vasectomy: A questionnaire study. *Br J Urol* 79(4):596–598.

Smucker DR et al. 1991. Postvasectomy semen analysis: Why patients don't follow-up. *J Am Board Famil Pract* 4(1):5–9

Soebadi DM, W Gardjito, HJ Meurik. 1995. Intravasal injection of formed-in-place medical grade silicone rubber for vas occlusion. *Int J Androl* 18(Suppl. 1):45–52.

Sokal D et al. 2001. Vasectomy with fascial interposition vs. ligation and excision alone: A randomized controlled trial. Presentation at the annual meeting of the Association of Reproductive Health Professionals, December 12–15, Washington, DC.

Sokal D, B Irsula, M Chen-Mok et al. 2003. A comparison of *vas* occlusion techniques: Cautery vs. ligation and excision with fascial interposition. *Contraception* 68:143

Sokal D, B Irsula, M Hays et al. 2004. Vasectomy by ligation and excision, with or without fascial interposition: A randomized controlled trial. *BMC Medicine* 2:6.

Sokal DC et al. 1999. A comparative study of the no scalpel and standard incision approaches to vasectomy in five countries. The Male Sterilization Investigator Team. *J Urol* 162(5): 1621–1625.

Strauss LT et al. 1984. Sterilization-associated deaths: A global survey. *Inter J Gynaecol Obstet* 22(1): 67–75.

Takihara H. 1998. Treatment of obstructive azoospermia in male infertility: Past, present and future. *Urology* 51(5A Supple):150–155.

Te Linde. 2003. *Operative Gynecology*, ninth edition, (2003) ed John A Rock and Howard A Jones III. Philadelphia: Lippincott, Williams & Wilkins, 537–556.

Temmerman M et al. 1986. Evaluation of one-hundred open-ended vasectomies. *Contraception* 33(6): 529–532.

Thomas Jr AJ. 1993. Microsurgical end-to-end vasoepididymostomy: Analysis of the outcome of 141 procedures. *J Urol* 149(part 2): 436A, abstract 892.

Thomas Jr. A J, et al. 1981. Microsurgical vasovasostomy: Immunologic consequences and subsequent fertility. *Fertil Steril* 35(4):447–450.

Thompson B et al. 1991. Experience with sperm counts following vasectomy. *Brit J Urol* 68(3): 230–233.

Twyman EJ and CS Nelson. 1938. Vas Deferens Anastomosis, *Rol and Cutan. Rev* 42:586.

Uchida H. 1975. Tubal Sterilization. *Am J Obstet Gynecol*; 121: 153–158

Walker K. 1953. *Practitioner* 53:463.

Walker AM et al. 1981. Hospitalization rates in vasectomized men. *J Am Med Assoc* 245(22): 2315–2317.

Watkins W F Nieto, H Bourne, B Wutthiphan et al. 1997. Testicular and epididymal sperm in a microinjection program: Methods of retrieval and results. *Fertil Steril* 67(3):527–535.

Xiao B. 1987. Chemical vas occlusion in the People's Republic of China. In *Fertility regulation today and tomorrow*, ed by E Diczfalusy and M Bygdeman. New York: Raven Press, pp. 265–274.

Yoon IB, CR Wheeless Jr, TM King. 1974. A preliminary report on a new laparoscopic sterilization approach: The silicone rubber band technique. *Am J Obstet Gynecol*; 120:132–136

Zhao SC YH Lian, RC Yu, SP Zhang. 1992a. Recovery of fertility after removal of polyurethane plugs from the human vas deferens occluded for up to 5 years. *Int J Androl* 15(6):465–467.

Zhao SC. 1990. Vas deferens occlusion by percutaneous injection of polyurethane elastomer plugs: Clinical experience and reversibility. *Contraception* 41(5):453–459.

38

Fibroid Uterus

Reva Tripathi

Uterine fibroids, also known as leiomyomas, are the most common tumours of the female reproductive tract. These benign tumours are estrogen responsive and their presence is estimated to range from 20% in women of reproductive age group to as high as 50% among women undergoing postmortem examination (Vollenhoven et al 1990). Fibroids account for 20%–77% of all hysterectomies performed prior to menopause (Marshall et al 1990).

Etiology: The precise etiology of uterine fibroids in not known. Several studies suggest that each fibroid arises from a single neoplastic cell within the smooth muscle of the myometrium. These benign tumours increase in size and frequency with age, but they tend to regress after menopause. Their incidence is more in African American women in whom they are also larger and occur at a younger age. Patients with fibroids often have a positive family history, which suggests the presence of a gene encoding for their development. This was later identified as translocation t(12;14)(q13-15;q23-24) from chromosome 12 to chromosome 14 (Solomon et al 1991). About 40%–50% of fibroids show karyotypically detectable chromosomal abnormalities that are both non-random and tumour specific but their precise contribution to the development of fibroids remains to be defined.

Risk factors: The incidence of fibroids is the same in both premenopausal and postmenopausal women, but the average number and size is more in the former. Older nulliparous women have an increased risk of developing fibroids. The relative risk decreases with each pregnancy in multiparous women. The risk is also reduced in women who smoke, although the reason for this is unclear.

The growth of fibroids is dependent on estrogen production, which may explain the higher incidence in obese women. Continuous estrogen secretion, especially when uninterrupted by pregnancy and lactation, is the most important risk factor in the development of fibroids. After menopause, and the consequent regression of ovarian estrogen secretion, growth usually ceases and actual regression in tumour size may occur.

Anatomical types: Fibroids may be single but most are multiple. They develop most commonly in the uterine corpus and with much less frequency in the cervix. Rarely, they may develop primarily in the round or broad ligaments. Initially all fibroids are interstitial or intramural due to their origin in the myometrium, but as they enlarge they can either remain intramural or become subserous and distort the uterine contour or less commonly, grow maximally towards the uterine cavity becoming submucous and cause symmetrical enlargement of the uterus.

A subserous fibroid can become pedunculated and occasionally parasitic, receiving its blood supply from another source, usually the omentum. A submucous fibroid can also become pedunculated and even dilate the endocervical canal and protrude through the cervical os as a polyp. The prolonged traction exerted by a prolapsing submucous fibroid attached to the fundal area may result in chronic uterine inversion but this is a rare occurrence.

Histopathology and secondary changes: Fibroids arise from the hyperplasia of the smooth muscle cells of the myometrium. They do not have a true capsule but are separated from the surrounding myometrium by a pseudocapsule of connective tissue which allows easy enucleation at the time of surgery. The cut surface of the fibroid is characteristically whorled in appearance. Subserous fibroids contain more fibrous tissue then submucous fibroids. The presence of fibroids is also associated with hyperplasia of the endometrium. Degenerative changes are reported in about 75% of all specimens and are of various types:

1. Hyaline degeneration—this is the most common secondary change
2. Cystic degeneration
3. Fatty degeneration
4. Calcification
5. Red degeneration
6. Atrophy due to decreased vascularity after menopause
7. Sarcomatous degeneration

Hyaline, cystic and/or fatty degenerations may occur in the central areas of the fibroid and are of no clinical significance. Necrosis can occur in the centre of a large fibroid due to poor vascularity which makes it appear dark and hemorrhagic. Red or carneous degeneration is occasionally seen concomitant with pregnancy and is caused by poor circulation in a tumour that enlarges rapidly due to high circulating estrogens. In long-standing fibroids, especially in old patients, phosphates and carbonates of calcium are deposited in the periphery along the course of vessels making them almost bony hard.

Sarcomatous change: The incidence of sarcomatous change is about 0.7% but since most women with uterine fibroids do not undergo surgical removal, the true incidence is likely to be much lower (less than 0.1%) (Leibsohn et al 1990). It should be suspected when there is a history of rapid growth in the fibroid, especially in a postmenopausal woman. Submucous fibroids which contain more smooth muscle tissue have a higher potential for sarcomatous change (Breech and Rock 2003). All tumours with less than five mitotic figures per ten high power fields (HPF) are considered benign and all tumours with more than ten mitotic figures per ten HPF are considered malignant. Those in between are labelled smooth muscle tumours of uncertain malignant potential. Other features like cytologic atypia, nuclear hyperchromatism and pleomorphism or the presence of giant cells and other bizarre cell forms indicate malignant change. Due to the common etiology of hyperestrogenism, the occurrence of endometrial carcinoma associated with a fibroid (Leibsohn et al 1990) is more frequent than that of sarcomatous degeneration within the fibroid itself.

Clinical features: Most fibroids are asymptomatic and discovered incidentally during a routine pelvic examination. Less than 50% of patients with uterine fibroids have symptoms which depend on the location, size and the number of tumours present.

Menstrual disorders: These are the most common presenting symptoms and lead most frequently to surgical intervention. Menorrhagia, metrorrhagia and/or polymenorrhea occur in about a third of patients. As a general rule, bleeding is more common and it is more severe in the presence of intramural and submucous fibroids and is due to an estrogen induced increase in endometrial thickness. Submucous fibroids may also cause intermenstrual bleeding as a result of passive congestion, necrosis and ulceration of the endometrial surface over the tumour. In pedunculated submucous fibroids, there can be a constant, thin, blood-tinged discharge in addition to the menorrhagia. As a general principle, the greater the distance of the fibroid away from the endometrial cavity, the lesser the chances of menstrual complaints.

Pain: It is not a frequent symptom associated with uterine fibroids. When present, it may manifest as abdominal and pelvic pain or discomfort or simply a feeling of heaviness in the lower abdomen. Dysmenorrhea is common and occurs in about a third of patients. Rarely, acute pain can occur when a pedunculated subserous fibroid undergoes torsion or due to hemorrhage or red degeneration during pregnancy. Infarction or red degeneration in the fibroid can also cause acute abdominal pain. Sudden intraperitoneal hemorrhage can occur due to rupture of a superficial vessel. Pain in a rapidly growing fibroid in an elderly woman may suggest sarcomatous change.

Urinary symptoms: These are classically associated with cervical fibroids. The symptoms range from urinary retention to increased frequency of micturition and are due to distortion of the bladder neck and the urethrovesical angle caused by a large cervical fibroid. Most other fibroids rarely cause urinary symptoms, though occasionally, pressure by a lowly placed anterior wall fibroid on the urinary bladder can cause urgency and frequency of micturition. These symptoms are generally more pronounced premenstrually due to premenstrual congestion and enlargement of the fibroid. Multiple fibroids causing massive uterine enlargement may compress the ureter and cause hydroureter and hydronephrosis. This is more common with a broad ligament fibroid. Rarely, acute retention of urine may occur as a result of the compression of the urethra and bladder neck between the pubic bone and the fibroid present in the cervix or impacted in the pouch of Douglas.

Abdominal lump: Occasionally, patients present with symptoms of a mass in the abdomen as the leading complaint without associated menstrual problems. This may occur when the fibroids are predominantly subserous in location.

Infertility: Fibroids do not cause infertility per se and it is frequently a chance diagnosis in a patient being investigated for infertility. It is generally either due to associated anovulatory cycles, pelvic inflammatory disease or endometriosis. Impingement of the fibroid on the endocervical canal or the interstitial portion of the fallopian tube may interfere with sperm transport and thus contribute to infertility. When infertility is attributed to fibroids, it is most commonly due to submucous fibroids that cause distortion of the endometrial cavity, and consequently, a problem with nidation.

Miscellaneous symptoms: Iron deficiency anemia can result from chronic blood loss. Rarely, polycythemia can occur due to extramedullary erythropoiesis within the fibroid. Rarely, ascites may supervene (pseudo Meig syndrome) or uterine inversion can occur with pedunculated submucous fibroids.

Diagnosis: This is generally by clinical examination. The patient may be anemic due to chronic blood loss. An abdominal lump arising from the pelvis may be felt with well-defined margins which are firm in consistency and mobile unless fixed by adhesions. Characteristically, broad ligament or cervical fibroids are not mobile. The uterine enlargement could be either smooth or bosselated. Bimanual examination confirms an enlarged uterus; adnexa are generally free unless there is presence of some associated pathology. Sometimes in a submucous fibroid, the cervical os is open and the lower pole of the tumour can be felt through the os with the cervical lips clearly felt all around. When it becomes a polyp, a pedicle can be felt just above the tumour mass. In cervical fibroid, a normal size uterus may be palpable above the tumour. A broad ligament fibroid may displace the uterus to the opposite side.

Differential diagnosis: The diagnosis of uterine fibroid is usually quite apparent but occasionally differential diagnoses of adenomyosis, pregnancy and endometriosis may need to be considered. Ultrasonography is generally enough to confirm the diagnosis but occasionally other imaging techniques (CT or MRI) may be required. Endometrial sampling should be considered in those patients who have a history of irregular menstrual cycles or intermenstrual bleeding, prior to deciding a definitive mode of management.

Pregnancy with fibroid: Although traditionally, fibroids have been implicated as a cause of infertility, these are occasionally seen with pregnancy. Most such cases are asymptomatic and the diagnosis is made during cesarean. Sometimes however, pregnancy with fibroid may be diagnosed in the antenatal period when there is discrepancy between the fundal height and period of gestation or due to a separately palpable mass distorting the uterine contour on abdominal palpation.

Effect of fibroid on pregnancy: When pregnancy is associated with a uterine fibroid there is an increased risk of spontaneous abortion. It is difficult to quantify the risk but figures as high as 41% have been reported which reduce to 19% after myomectomy (Breech and Rock 2003). The mechanisms responsible may be disturbance in uterine blood flow, altered blood supply to the endometrium, irregular enlargement of the uterine cavity causing interference with implantation and placental growth by poorly developed endometrium or by subjacent fibroids and uterine irritability during rapid growth or degeneration in the fibroid.

Other possible effects of fibroids on pregnancy are:

1. Threatened preterm labour
2. Premature delivery
3. Abruptio placentae, especially in women with fibroid volume greater than 200 cc (Breech and Rock 2003) or with submucous fibroids with superimposed placenta.
4. Intrapartum problems can occur if the fibroid is large and especially when located in the lower uterine segment. A cervical fibroid may necessitate cesarean delivery but individualisation is required to assess the degree of mechanical obstruction, if any, and to decide the mode of delivery.
5. Interference with the propagation of myometrial contractility is an occasional possibility leading to abnormalities of uterine action which may manifest as either incoordinate uterine contraction or postpartum hemorrhage.

However, most patients have no difficulty in conceiving and carrying their pregnancies to term without complications, although they generally require closer antenatal surveillance with fetal growth monitored ultrasonographically rather than clinically, and delivery in a centre equipped to handle emergencies.

Effect of pregnancy on fibroid: The impact of pregnancy on the fibroid is likely to result in the following:

1. Enlargement in size due to the effect of hormones.
2. Red degeneration: This is an uncommon complication during pregnancy as a result of which the fibroid becomes tense and tender causing severe abdominal pain and constitutional symptoms with fever, moderate leucocytosis and raised ESR. Histologically, thrombosis is found in large veins of the capsule and small vessels in the substance of the fibroid. It is an aseptic condition and management requires only symptomatic treatment. It needs to be differentiated from abruptio placentae.
3. Torsion with infarction of subserous pedunculated fibroid is more common in pregnancy than at any other time, though it is in itself a very infrequent occurrence.

Therapeutic options: Despite the high incidence, there are no standardised recommendations for management based on randomised control trials (Vlahos and Wallach 2004). The principal factors that guide the choice of therapy are symptoms caused by the fibroid and the fertility status of the patient. Therapeutic options can range from no interference to medical or surgical therapy and hence it is important for physicians to rationalise treatment rather than base decisions on individual preference. It is suggested that in patients for whom a conservative option is contemplated, endometrial sampling and a Pap smear may be performed to exclude any associated problem which would itself warrant more aggressive treatment.

Asymptomatic fibroids: More than 70% fibroids are asymptomatic and are discovered incidentally during routine pelvic examination in the gynecology outpatient department. Since the incidence of malignancy in fibroids is less than 0.1%, asymptomatic fibroids do not require any treatment. These patients should be counselled and managed expectantly with follow up at six monthly intervals. However, removal is indicated if the fibroid shows rapid growth, which is defined as a gain of six weeks or more in gestational size, within a year or less (Breech and Rock 2003) and is more pertinent in a postmenopausal patient, irrespective of symptoms.

Medical management: Medical management is directed towards achieving relief of symptoms, the most significant of which is menorrhagia. Treatment of fibroid-related menorrhagia can be attempted with the same drugs as used in the treatment of DUB. However, they have no effect on the fibroid itself. This is more likely to be useful in patients where small size fibroids are associated with significant menorrhagia.

The rationale of other medication used is based on the hormonal sensitivity of fibroids. Effective medical therapy that is likely to result in permanent cure of uterine fibroids is not yet available. Medical therapy is available as an adjunct to surgery in an attempt to minimise morbidity or as a temporary substitute for definitive therapy and has a maximum role in patients of low parity who wish to conceive. Drugs used for medical management of fibroids could be any of the following:

- GnRH analogues—agonists and antagonists
- Danazol
- Progesterones and anti-progesterones
- LNG-releasing IUD

GnRH agonists: These drugs cause down-regulation and desensitisation of GnRH receptors in the anterior pituitary gland and lead to continuous suppression of secretion of FSH and LH. A hypogonadotrophic hypogonadal state is achieved in one to three weeks which has also been described as 'medical oopherectomy' or 'medical menopause'. It exists as long as treatment lasts and is promptly reversed when treatment is discontinued. A 30%–50% decrease is uterine volume is achieved in the first 12 weeks of treatment after which further decrease is unlikely (Crosignani et al 1996); cessation of treatment results in regrowth to the original size.

INDICATIONS OF GNRH THERAPY

a. Prior to surgery
   - Hysterectomy for large fibroids
   - Myomectomy with fibroids >5 cm
   - Conservative endoscopic surgery
b. As a sole treatment of fibroids in immediate pre-menopausal patient.
c. Associated endometriosis.

POTENTIAL BENEFITS OF GNRH AGONIST USE PRIOR TO SURGERY

a. Correction of anemia and reduced risk of blood transfusion
b. Facilitation of surgery by transverse instead of longitudinal incision
c. Use of vaginal route rather than abdominal due to decreased size.
d. Facilitation of hysteroscopic myoma resection by causing decrease in size of the fibroid, endometrial atrophy and consequently better visibility.
e. Reduced risk of unplanned hysterectomy during myomectomy.

LIMITATIONS AND DISADVANTAGES:

a. Regrowth after cessation of therapy.
b. Hyaline degeneration and focal necrosis of fibroid in 1%–2% cases (Crosignani et al 1996; Vlahos and Wallach 2004).
c. Problems in establishing clear surgical planes between the fibroid and surrounding myometrium (Crosignani et al 1996).
d. Side effects mimicking postmenopausal state: hot flushes, insomnia, mood lability, headaches, vaginal dryness and osteopenia. Osteopenia occurs in women treated for six months duration (Breech and Rock 2003) and is due to a mean reduction in trabecular bone density of approximately 1% per month.
e. Smaller fibroids may be missed during myomectomy and become evident later which are then mistakenly labelled as new tumours.

PREPARATIONS AVAILABLE: GnRH agonists are frequently used and many compounds are available viz goserelin acetate, leuprolide acetate, triptorelin. These drugs are generally available as depot preparations and are given in doses of 3.7 mg monthly either by the subcutaneous or the intramuscular route. Treatment should be started in the luteal phase to reduce flare response.

GNRH ANTAGONISTS: These drugs cause competitive blockade of GnRH receptors. The resultant suppression in gonadotrophin levels causes hypoestrogenism leading to reduction in fibroid size by 33%–50% (Gonzalez-Bercena et al 1997; Felderbaum et al 1998). The advantage with these drugs is absence of the flare-up response and rapid reduction in fibroid size. Side effects are related to hypoestrogenism as with GnRH agonists. Allergic reactions have also been reported. Daily injection of Cetrorelix results in a 50% decrease in fibroid size in three months. Cetrorelix pamoate, which is a slow release preparation, is given in the dose of 60 mg intramuscularly on day 2 of the cycle. The second dose is given according to serum estradiol levels on day 21. Preparations are expensive and are not widely available, hence, experience of their use is limited.

Danazol: It is an orally active testosterone derivative with mild androgenic and progestational activity. Reduction in fibroid size is caused by the suppression of gonadotrophin secretion, increased metabolic clearance of estrogen and progesterone and direct agonist and antagonist reactions with endometrial androgen and progesterone receptors. The dose of danazol is 200 mg given orally 2–3 times daily. The end point that is used to titrate the dose is development of amenorrhea. Side effects include weight gain, fluid retention, acne, hirsutism, hot flushes, atrophic vaginitis, fatigue, nausea and muscle cramps. It is contraindicated in the presence of liver disease, hypertension, pregnancy and hepatorenal disorders.

Progesterones: Progesterones are a cost-effective therapy for the menometrorrhagia due to fibroids by virtue of their action on endometrium rather than a treatment for the fibroid itself. Their effect on the fibroid is unclear, though necrosis and hyalinisation following high doses have been reported (Goldziehzer et al 1996).

Gestrinone: It is an androgenic compound being a synthetic derivative of ethinyl-nortestosterone with antiestrogen and antiprogesterone properties. It causes reduction in fibroid size and relieves menorrhagia when used over a period of three to six months. Side effects include weight gain, acne, seborrhea, hirsutism, myalgia and arthralgia. Amenorrhea with endometrial atrophy occurs by the third month of use and is reversible on stopping treatment. It is used in the dose of 2.5–5 mg, orally, three times a week or 5 mg, vaginally, three times a week. However, gestrinone is not available in India.

Levonorgestrel Intrauterine Device (LNG IUD): This third generation IUD contains 52 mg levonorgestrel which is released at a rate of 20 μg/day. Fibroids have been found to reduce in size after 6–18 months of use (Singer and Ikomi 1994). The effect is due to the effect of LNG on insulin-like endometrial growth factors (Pekonen et al 1992; Sturridge and Guillebaud 1997). Patients with symptomatic fibroids desiring contraception would be suitable candidates for its use. This device is especially suitable for use in perimenopausal patients with fibroids causing menorrhagia. In this group of patients, major surgery can be averted by using LNG IUD till the patient attains menopause.

Mifepristone: (RU486) Mifepristone is a norethindrone derivative with anti-progestogenic and antiglucocorticoid activities. It causes the competitive blockade of progesterone receptors and has been found to reduce fibroid size by 49% after three months use (Murphy et al 1993). It has been given in doses of 25–50 mg orally for up to three months. Amenorrhea is induced in all patients. It does not affect estrogen levels and thus has no adverse effect on bone density. Side effects are mild and include hot flashes during the first month of use in 20% of patients. There may be a transient increase in transaminase levels associated with joint pains which remits on discontinuation of therapy.

However, it is important to note that all these drugs are not routinely used as they provide only temporary relief which is restricted to the time of intake and there is recurrence of symptoms soon after discontinuation.

Surgical management of fibroids:

Definitive treatment for fibroids has to be surgical. Myomectomy or hysterectomy is the procedure usually performed. In the current era of minimally invasive surgery, endoscopy (laparoscopic or hysteroscopic) is frequently advocated in preference to conventional surgical approaches which could be either through the abdominal or the vaginal routes. A recently introduced minimally invasive procedure of uterine artery embolisation (UAE) is also now available. The various options are:

CONSERVATIVE

1. Laparoscopic
   - Myomectomy
   - Myolysis
2. Hysteroscopic
   - Resection
   - Myolysis
3. Myomectomy
   - Vaginal
   - Abdominal
4. Polypectomy

HYSTERECTOMY

1. Abdominal
2. Vaginal
3. Laparoscopic

NEWER TECHNIQUES

Uterine artery embolisation or ligation

MYOMECTOMY

It is an effective method in patients where conservation of the uterus is desirable, as in patients with low parity and also in those who have had children but are too young for a hysterectomy. It is indicated in patients, less than 40 years of age, who wish to retain their uterus for reproductive and/or menstrual functions. Surgery entails the identification of a pseudocapsule surrounding the fibroid and its enucleation in the correct plane to minimise hemorrhage. The incision on the uterine surface must be well planned so as to minimise the number of total incisions by ensuring removal of as many tumours as possible through one incision. The defect in the myometrium is then meticulously sutured to ensure hemostasis and subsequent healing. All attempts must be made to minimise adhesions and to ensure that the pelvic anatomy is as near normal as possible at the end of surgery.

Fibroids are the sole cause of infertility in only about 1% of cases (Verkauf 1992). Out of these 40%–50% patients conceive following myomectomy and the risk of spontaneous abortions may be reduced by as much as 50% (Breech and Rock 2003). Pregnancy should be attempted after a period of three months to allow for complete healing which would reduce the risk of uterine rupture during a subsequent pregnancy. The risk of recurrence of fibroid following myomectomy is 25% (Breech and Rock 2003). Complications are comparable to hysterectomy in well-selected patients, though the possibility of hemorrhage is quite real and adequate blood must be readily available. Myomectomy can also be done endoscopically, either through laparoscopy for subserous or superficial intramural fibroids or through hysteroscopy for submucous fibroids. Careful selection of patients is important to minimise converting the endoscopic surgery into open conventional surgery. Newer technique of morcellation and myolysis through a cryo or laser probe allow tackling of larger myomas. Occasionally, a planned myomectomy will require to be converted to hysterectomy despite the best surgical competence and hence informed consent is mandatory prior to myomectomy.

Laparoscopic myomectomy: It is suitable for subserosal and intramural fibroids of up to 10 cm in diameter (Hasson et al 1992). Larger fibroids can be removed by morcellation or vaginally by posterior colpotomy. Advantages over traditional myomectomy include avoidance of morbidity associated with laparotomy, less blood loss and less adhesion formation. However, it is not suitable for too large (>10 cm) or too many fibroids (>4 in number). There is need for trained personnel and expensive equipment. The risk of rupture during subsequent pregnancy may be more than with open myomectomy due to difficulty in assessing entry into the endometrium and the difficulty of endoscopic suturing (Harris 1992).

Reconstruction of the myometrium after laparoscopic myomectomy should be by meticulous suturing technique to minimise the possibility of rupture during a subsequent pregnancy; hence, endoscopic myomectomy should be performed only by competent and adequately trained surgeons.

Hysteroscopic myomectomy: Hysteroscopic myomectomy, with or without concomitant endometrial resection or ablation, can be done with the operative hysteroscope and bipolar cautery or laser. It is effective in treating menorrhagia associated with fibroids in up to 90% of cases (Magos et al 1991). It is indicated in patients with one or two submucous fibroids less than 6 cm diameter with uterocervical length less than 12 cm. A substantial intramural portion (generally more than 50%) would limit its use. Contraindications include endometrial adenomatous hyperplasia and/or hyperplasia with atypia. Most patients who conceive after myoma resection have successful reproductive outcome with uneventful vaginal deliveries. Associated risks are uterine perforation, fluid absorption and hemodilution and hemorrhage from the resected surface. In subsequent pregnancies, there is risk of occurrence of placenta accreta (Magos et al 1991).

Vaginal myomectomy: It is the appropriate treatment for pedunculated submucous fibroids where the pedicle is inaccessible. The surgical principle is the same as for abdominal myomectomy requiring an incision on the most dependent part of the tumour and enucleation of the fibroid through the proper plane of cleavage and achieving hemostasis by ligating or cauterising the base. Morcellation may be required to remove very large tumours. The redundant part of the capsule is excised and the base is ligated. Patients must be given antibiotic coverage because of the increased risk of infection associated with these fibroids. Most patients remain asymptomatic and menstruate normally following the procedure. Cervical incompetence has been reported in some patients who conceive later.

Polypectomy: It is most suitable for pedunculated submucous fibroids that prolapse into the vagina through a dilated cervix and whose pedicle is accessible. Using an instrument with a firm grip, the fibroid is avulsed. Hemostatic sutures can be taken at the base of the pedicle if bleeding occurs though they are not always necessary.

HYSTERECTOMY

This is the ultimate cure for fibroids and could be performed through the abdominal or the vaginal route.

Vaginal hysterectomy: It is preferred wherever possible as complications following abdominal hysterectomy are much higher in comparison (Stirridge and Guillebaud 1997). Criteria for vaginal hysterectomy (Sheth 1999) include:

2. Uterine size <12 weeks
3. Uterine volume $\leq$300 cm^3
4. Freely mobile uterus

Surgical skill generally determines the type of patients that can be taken up for surgery through the vaginal route.

Abdominal hysterectomy: It is desirable if there is presence of adenexal pathology, associated dense adhesions due to endometriosis or pelvic inflammatory disease or in case of broad ligament or cervical fibroids. This route is also preferred in case malignancy is suspected.

Laparoscopic hysterectomy: This is classified according to the extent of dissection performed laparoscopically:

1. Laparoscopic assisted vaginal hysterectomy (LAVH): Only the fundal structures are ligated laparoscopically.
2. Laparoscopic hysterectomy (LH): The uterine vessels are ligated laparoscopically.
3. Total laparoscopic hysterectomy (TLH): All the uterine supports are divided and the vaginal vault is opened laparoscopically.

Laparoscopic hysterectomy is preferred when adhesions are present in case previous surgery or when vaginal access is poor. It is also useful for evaluating ovaries which would not be possible during vaginal hysterectomy.

Uterine Artery Embolisation (UAE)

This is a new minimally invasive technique being used in patients with symptomatic fibroids with excellent results (Ravina et al 1995; Goodwin and Wong 2001). Patients with menorrhagia, dysmenorrhea, pressure symptoms and urinary complaints attributable to fibroids are considered candidates for UAE once malignancy is excluded. Results from various studies consistently show significant reduction in these symptoms (Ravina et al 1995; Goodwin and Wong 2001). The uterine volume and dominant fibroid volume are reported to decrease by 40%–50% and 60%–70% respectively at six months follow-up.

Uterine artery ligation: As most gynecologists would not have access to a procedure involving interventional radiology, some workers have attempted bilateral uterine artery ligation as an alternative to UAE. The approach could be laparoscopic or vaginal. Successful outcomes in terms of decreased uterine fibroid size and improvement in symptoms have been reported (Akenole et al 2005).

Fibroids are the most common neoplastic lesions seen by gynecologists and though these benign tumours are easy to diagnose and treat, occasionally they may present extremely challenging situations testing the skills of even the most competent surgeons.

References

Akenole OI, AO Fabamwo, AT Otten. 2005. Uterine artery ligation for management of uterine fibroids. *Int J Gynaecol Obstet* (2):137–140.

Breech, Lesley L and JA Rock. 2003. Leiomyomata uteri and myomectomy. *Telinde's Operative Gynaecology* 9th ed. Lippincott Williams and Wilkins.

Crosignani PG, P Vercellini, M Meschia et al. 1996. GnRH agonists before surgery for uterine leiomyomas: A review. *J Reprod Med* 41:415–421.

Felderbaum RE, U Germer, M Ludwid et al. 1998. Treatment of uterine fibroids with a slow release formulation of the gonadotrophin releasing hormone antagonist cetrorelix. *Hum Reprod* 13:1660–1668.

Goldberg J, L Pereira, V Berghella. 2002. Pregnancy after uterine artery embolizaton. *Obstet Gynecol* 100:869–872.

Goldziehzer JW, M Maqueo, L Ricauid et al. 1996. Induction of degenerative changes in uterine myomas by high dose progestin therapy. *Am J Obstet Gynecol* 96:1078–1087.

Gonzalez-Bercena D, RB Alvarez, EP Ochoa et al. 1997. Treatment of uterine leiomyomas with luteinizing hormone-releasing hormone antagonist cetrorelix. *Hum Reprod* 12:2028–2035.

Goodwin SC and GC Wong. 2001. Uterine artery embolization for uterine fibroids: A radiologist's perspective. *Clin Obstet Gynecol* 44:412–424.

Harris WJ. 1992. Uterine dehiscence following laparoscopic myomectomy. *Obstet Gynecol* 80(3): 545–546.

Hasson H, C Rotman, N Rama et al. 1992. Laparoscopic myomectomy. *Obstet Gynecol* 80: 884–888.

Leibsohn S, G d'Ablaing, DR Mishell Jr et al. 1990. Leiomyosarcoma in a series of hysterectomies performed for presumed uterine leiomyomas. *Am J Obstet Gynecol* 162:968–976.

Magos Al, R Baumann, GM Lockwood et al. 1991. Experience with the first 250-endometrial resections for menorrhagia. *Lancet* 337:1074–1078.

Marshall LM, D Spiegelman, RL Barbien et al. 1997. Variation in the incidence of uterine leiomyoma among premenopausal women by age and race. *Obstet Gynecol* 90: 967–973.

Murphy AA, LM Kettel, AJ Morales et al. 1993. Regression of uterine leiomyomata in response to the antiprogesterone RU 486. *J Clin Endocrinol Metab* 76:513–517.

Pekonen F, T Nyman, P Lahteenmaki et al. 1992. Intrauterine progestin induces continuous insulin-like growth factor binding protein-1 production in human endometrium. *J Clin Endocrinol Metab* 75: 660–664.

Ravina JH, D Herbreteau, N Ciraru-Vigneron et al. 1995. Arterial embolization to treat uterine myomata. *Lancet* 346(8976): 671–672.

Sheth SS. 1999. *Vaginal or abdominal hysterectomy* in Menorrhagia. ed SS Sheth and CJG Sutton. Oxford: Isis Medical Media Ltd. 213–237.

Singer A and A Ikomi. 1994. Successful treatment of fibroids using an intrauterine progesterone device. 14th World congress of Gynecology and obstetrics (FIGO), Montreal, Canada, Sept. 24–30.

Solomon E, J Borrow, AD Goddard. 1991. Chromosomal aberrations and cancer. *Science* 254:1153

Sturridge F and J Guillebaud. 1997. Gynecological aspects of the levonorgestrel releasing intrauterine system. *Br J Obstet Gynecol* 104:285–289.

Verkauf BS. 1992. Myomectomy for fertility enhancement and preservation. *Fertil Steril* 58:1–15.

Vlahos NF and EE Wallach. 2004. Uterine myomas: An overview of development, clinical features and management. *Obstet Gynecol* 104(2):393–406.

Vollenhoven BJ, AS Lawrence, DL Healy. 1990. Uterine fibroids: A clinical review. *Br J Obstet Gynecol* 97(4):265–298.

39

Chronic Pelvic Pain

Mandeep Singh

Chronic pelvic pain (CPP) refers to pain in the lower abdomen or pelvis, occurring continuously or intermittently over a period of at least six months; the pain is not associated exclusively with menstruation or sexual intercourse (Prentice 2000).

The International Association for the Study of Pain (IASP) has defined CPP as chronic or recurrent pelvic pain that has a gynecological origin, but for which no definite lesion or cause is found (Campbell and Collet 1994). Reiter (1990) defined CPP as non-cyclical pelvic pain, of a duration in excess of six months, which is not relieved by narcotic analgesia. It takes approximately this duration of time for the behavioural, emotional and biochemical changes seen in patients with CPP to reach a clinically important proportion.

The following four criteria will help us determine when chronic pain has lead to behavioural components and to ascertain whether it has evolved into chronic pelvic pain syndrome. This will prompt changes in the diagnostic and therapeutic approach (Steege et al 1997).

1. Pain refractory to medical management
2. Significant impairment of physical function
3. Vegetative signs of depression have begun
4. Patient's role in the family has changed because of pain or the family considers his pain to be its biggest problem and accords it the highest priority

The above definition has been widely used in literature but the problem with this definition is that it implies the absence of pathology, which is not necessarily the case, and it also excludes cases in which pathology is present but is not necessarily the cause of pain. In fact, the relationship of pain to the presence of pathology is often unclear in women with CPP. Hence, we will refer here to CPP as pelvic pain in the same location for at least six months.

Many chronic pain states begin with a nociceptive process, although that event might go unrecognised or unremembered. Thus, contrary to the misguided belief that CPP is never 'all in your head', it is always a dynamic interaction of the influence of the mind, the nervous system and the body (Wenof and Perry 1999).

Incidence: CPP accounts for 15%–20% of gynecological consultations and up to 52% of diagnostic laparoscopy (Campbell and Collet 1994). The prevalence (Office of Population Census and Survey 1995) of CPP (38/1000) is comparable to migraine (21/1000), asthma (37/1000) and back pain (41/1000). The economic consequences of CPP are estimated at a staggering US$ 2.8 billion/year, this is based on the cost of visits to physicians and mental health professionals and an additional US$ 555 million for time lost from work (Mathias et al 1996). The economic cost of CPP in the UK was estimated at approximately £182 million in 1992 (Davies et al 1992).

Impact on quality of life: CPP is best viewed as a disease in itself as it adversely affects every aspect of a woman's life

Impact of CPP on quality of life:

- Inability to exercise 81%
- Difficulty sleeping 79%
- Lack of enjoyment of leisure 67%
- Difficulty walking 59%
- Interference in sexuality 54%
- Difficulty concentrating 49%
- Inability to work 41%

(Compiled from NVA News, Spring 2000)

Pain pathophysiology: Acute pain informs the body about an injury to the body by the activation of nociceptors within body tissue. Afferent nerve fibres transmit messages through the dorsal horn of the spinal cord where it is processed to increase or decrease in magnitude before it is transmitted to the brain, and is recognised as pain.

Chronic pain is unique as it is defined vaguely. 'If pain persists beyond usual course of an acute injury or disease, or recurs every few months or years, it is regarded as chronic' (Carter 1996, 1999, 2000). In chronic pain, spinal modulation is towards hypersensitisation of nerve cells through a phenomenon called 'wind up' (Vercellini et al 1991). An environment is created wherein even a small impulse is registered and amplified leading to the perception of conditions with distention as pain.

The role of the autonomic nervous system is to maintain and adapt the body to the environment. If a stimulus is maintained for a prolonged time it becomes part of the environment, and recent evidence suggests that in patients with CPP, there is dysfunction of the autonomic nervous system.

CHRONIC PELVIC PAIN

Pain from the cervix, uterus, vagina, inner third of the fallopian tube, broad ligament, upper bladder, terminal ileum, large bowel is largely perceived via the sympathetic nervous system. The afferents enter the spinal cord between T10 and L1. The afferents of the outer third of the fallopian tube and the ureter enter the spinal cord between T9 and T10. The lower vagina, bladder and the rectosigmoid are innervated by the sacral afferents. The pelvic organs are so closely related that the localisation of pain is poor as it is dependent on the convergence of the visceral and somatic nerves within the central nervous system. Ranges of neurons and neurotransmitters have been identified in the pathogenesis of CPP.

Causes or consequences

Depression: There is greater evidence linking women with multiple pain syndromes to depression. The likelihood of depression increases sixfold in women with two pain complaints to eightfold in women with three (Dworkin et al 1990). Magni et al (1984) suggested that women with CPP without gross pathology are more likely to be depressed, and for obvious reasons this view was not supported by many. Reaner thought that women with CPP are 'psychologically a heterogeneous population' and emphasised that psychological distress may be a consequence of, rather than the cause of, CPP.

Physical and sexual abuse: Sexual abuse is noted to be more prevalent in women with CPP compared to women with other types of pain—52% and 12% respectively (Walling et al 1994). Walker et al (1992, 1993) found that women with pelvic pain who had a previous history of sexual abuse were at a significantly higher risk for a diagnosis of major depression and somatiform pain disorder compared with those with no abuse or less severe abuse.

Collet et al (1998) reviewed various psychological parameters in 30 women with CPP: 12 (40%) reported sexual abuse compared to five (17%) in each of the two comparison groups. Experience of physical violence was similar in the three groups, but women with CPP had a higher incidence of somatisation, that is, the experience of somatic distress and symptoms without clear underlying pathology.

Endometriosis: Among the causes of CPP, pelvic endometriosis is the second most frequent (Moore and Kennedy 2000). CPP, dyspareunia and dysmenorrhea are the cardinal symptoms of endometriosis. It is characterised by the presence and proliferation of functional endometrial tissue containing glands and stroma in sites outside the endometrial cavity. Endometriosis is common between the ages of 30 and 45 years.

The exact mechanism of pelvic pain in endometriosis is not clear but it involves the release of prostaglandin, scarring, stretching of tissues and nerve damage secondary to scarring around deposits. 51.2% of patients undergoing laparoscopy for CPP were found to have some evidence of endometriosis. Peritoneum, ovary and rectocervical endometriosis are the three common areas where endometriotic deposits can be commonly found (Carter 2000). In the majority of cases, ovarian endometrioma causes fewer CPP complaints. Rectocervical endometriosis is deep endometriosis, and is basically adenomyosis where the major component is fibromuscular tissue and causes heavy pain to the patient and hence medical therapy is less effective and surgical therapy is more advantageous because of tissue structure (ACOG 1996).

Pelvic inflammatory disease (PID): This is commonly seen in women attending genitourinary medicine clinics. It is caused by microorganisms which colonise the endocervix, ascending to the endometrium, fallopian tubes and ovaries leading to cervicitis, endometritis and eventually salpingoophoritis. *Chylamydia trachomatis* and *Neisseria gonorrhea* are common organisms causing PID and may be asymptomatic. *Mycobacterium tuberculosis* and schistosomiasis are other blood-borne organisms that can cause PID. Pelvic inflammatory disease leads to related scarring, tissue damage and adhesions resulting in damage of the nerves and to intra-abdominal organs leading to painful stretching with activities such as exercise, sexual intercourse or passage of food through the bowels (Peters et al 1992).

Pelvic venous congestion: Historically, pelvic venous congestion has been described by Robert Gooch, in his book of 1831 as 'the irritable uterus'. Howard Taylor, an American gynecologist agreed with the views put forward by Gooch and redescribed this condition as 'congestion-fibrosis syndrome'. Some studies have shown venous congestion to be the most common finding in women with CPP (Beard et al 1988).

We now know that pelvic congestion presents as an aching pain interspersed with episodes of acute pain. The pain may start as premenstrual pain and may continue throughout the cycle; it may occur predominantly on one side. It differs from the pain of endometriosis which will always

TABLE 39.1: DISEASES THAT MAY CAUSE OR CONTRIBUTE TO CPP IN WOMEN (CARTER 1996, 1999, 2000)

Gynecologic—Extrauterine	Colitis
Adhesions	Constipation
Adnexal cysts	Diverticular disease
Chlamydial endometritis or salpingitis	Inflammatory bowel disease
Endometriosis	Irritable bowel syndrome
Endosalpingiosis	Musculoskeletal
Ovarian retention syndrome (residual ovary syndrome)	Abdomianl wall myofascial pain (trigger points)
Ovarian remnant syndrome	Chronic coccygeal pain
Ovarian dystrophy or ovulatory pain	Compression of lumbar vertebrae
Pelvic congestion syndrome	Degenerative joint disease
Postoperative peritoneal cysts	Disk
Residual accessory ovary	Faulty or poor posture
Subacute salpingoophoritis	Fibromyositis
Tuberculous salpingitis	Hernias: ventral, inguinal, femoral, Spigelian
Gynecologic—Uterine	Low back pain
Adenomyosis	Muscular strains and sprains
Atypical dysmenorrhea or ovulatory pain	Neoplasia of spinal cord or sacral nerve
Cervical stenosis	Neuralgia of iliohypogastric ilioinguinal, and/or genitofemoral nerves
Chronic endometritis	Pelvic floor myalgia (levator anispasm)
Endometrial or cervical polyps	Piriformis syndrome
Intrauterine contraceptive device	Rectus tendon strain
Leimyomata	Spondylosis
Symptomatic pelvic relaxation (genital prolapse)	Other
Urologic	Abdominal cutaneous nerve
Bladder neoplasm	
Chronic urinary tract infection	
Interstitial cystitis	
Radiation cystitis	
Recurrent acute cystitis	

occur occasionally on the other side. The pain of pelvic congestion syndrome may be relieved by lying down and by the application of some form of heat.

The salient features of PVC are:

a. Pain on deep palpation, more severe on one side than the other
b. Bluish discoloration of the vagina
c. Excess of white nonoffensive discharge
d. Pelvic tenderness, particularly over one or both ovaries

Beard et al (1988) in his study on CPP and pelvic venous congestion realised that the condition was confined to women of reproductive age and the pain is present only on one side, but direct questioning usually revealed that in most women it occasionally occurs on the other side as well. Most of these women have been empirically diagnosed as having recurrent pelvic inflammatory disease and have often been treated for it, medically and surgically, leading to emotional disturbance (Adams et al 1997).

Diagnosis can be made based on history, with the pain of interstitial cystitis being accompanied by urinary dysfunction such as dysuria, strangury and frequency of micturition. Irritable bowel syndrome can be distinguished from PVC by a history of attacks of diarrhea, or constipation or both. This condition can be demonstrated radiologically by injecting contrast media; women with PVC had dilated pelvic veins, up to 12 mm in diameter, and remained so for more than five minutes. Reginald demonstrated that an injection of venoconstrictor dihydroergotamine tartrate to women with PVC during an attack resulted in spontaneous resolution of pain with a visible improvement in the venous flow.

Gordiene et al provided evidence to suggest that PVC is ovarian function dependent and the intensity of pain is usually cycle dependent. Taylor (1949) noted high prevalence of cystic ovaries in patients with PVC and later, Adams et al (1997) confirmed that 56% of women with PVC had polycystic ovaries compared to 23% in the general population.

Beard et al (1984; 1988) later hypothesised that women with PVC have an attenuation of peripheral vascular responsiveness affecting pelvic circulation, similar to that present in the luteal phase and continued throughout the follicular phase. Further suppression of ovarian activity, either by medical means or through bilateral oophorectomy, returned the vascular responsiveness to the vasoconstriction observed in the follicular phase of the cycle.

The cause of attenuation of vascular responsiveness is still unclear, but the pelvic circulation, in common with other vascular beds in the body, is under the control of a complex neurohormonal regulatory mechanism which includes neurotransmitters released from perivascular nerves such as cathecolamines, peptides, ATO, nitric oxides and later modulated by estrogen. Women with PVC may not be sufficiently sensitive to the index of change in estrogen release (Bonica 1990).

Peritoneal adhesions: A single adhesion under tension can cause pain in certain postures and positions. Adhesions are usually a complication of PID, endometriosis, appendicitis, peritonitis and/or previous pelvic surgery. Most peritoneal adhesions can be asymptomatic but can cause pain, particularly when they are extensive and involve structures like the ovary (Peters et al 1992). The degree and the characteristics of the pain depend on its extent and location.

Diagnosis: The patient's case history provides descriptions of the nature, intensity and distribution of pain. Pain charts and pain forms may be helpful in discerning the exact nature of the patient's pain (Carter 1999). Imprecise localisation is often associated with intra-abdominal processes. Radiation of the pain or coexisting pain in other locations should be assessed. The temporal patterns of the pain and any factors that modify the pain should be determined. Associated symptoms should be evaluated. Surgeries, infections, infertility or obstetrical experiences may be significant.

Characteristics of menstrual and non-menstrual bleeding and pain are important. Also the role of the pain in the patient's life must be explored (ACOG Bulletin 1996). The history should include a review of gastrointestinal, urologic and musculoskeletal, myofascial and psychological functions, including the relationship between these systems and the patient's pain. Patients with pain are frequently depressed and depression increases sensitivity to pain. This leads to a **pain–depression cascade** which should be addressed with each patient.

Physical examination: The physical examination should be meticulously done, and include a general physical and neurological assessment. The next step is to examine the patient in the standing and supine positions. A single finger locating the pain indicates a discreet source. A sweeping motion indicates a more generalised source.

Standing examination: Examine the patient for asymmetric gait, lordosis, kyphosis-lordosis, scoliosis, or one-leg standing. Examine the patient standing on one leg to see if pain occurs at the pubic symphysis. Examine the iliac crest heights for inequality to determine if short leg syndrome is present. Examine in a standing position for incisional, femoral, ventral and inguinal hernias. The standing position is also helpful for the evaluation of pelvic floor relaxation defects, by placing the index finger of one hand in the vagina and the index finger of the other hand in the rectum while the patient bears down. Occult enterocele, rectocele, cystocele and uterine prolapse may be diagnosed with this procedure more accurately than when the patient is in the lithotomy position (Howard 2000).

Sitting examination: The patient is observed in the sitting position. Sitting with all the weight on one buttock or consistently sitting forward may suggest levator ani spasm and pelvic floor pain syndrome. Palpation of the upper and lower back and sacrum, including single digit palpation for trigger points can be performed at this time (Steege 1997).

Supine examination: Pain on raising the leg straight up may suggest a possible herniated disc. Any of the following muscles or muscle groups may cause or contribute to CPP—rectus abdominus, external obliquus, internal obliquus, transversus abdominus, quadratus lumborum, pyramidalis, iliopsoas, coccygeus, levator ani, obturator internus, adductor magnus and piriformis. Evaluate for hyperesthesias or hypersensitivity of the skin and check superficial abdominal reflexes. Perform single digit palpation for trigger points.

The abdominal wall tenderness test (Carnett's test) is useful. In this test, while the area of abdominal tenderness is palpated, the patient voluntarily tenses the abdominal muscles by raising her head. If the pain increases, it suggests that the pain is of myofascial origin. If the pain decreases, it suggests that the pain is intra-abdominal Examine carefully for myofascial or trigger point pain syndrome (Slocumb 1984). Block any trigger points in the abdominal wall prior to performing the pelvic exam to help differentiate between abdominal and vaginal pain components (Slocumb 1984). Surgical scars should be noted. Palpation for hernial defects should be repeated. Palpate for Spigelian hernias just lateral to the lateral margin of the rectus sheath, feeling for tenderness or weakness in the fascia. Palpate the pubic symphysis for tenderness. Then perform the usual components of an abdominal examination.

Lithotomy examination: Basic sensory testing to sharpness, dullness and light touch, as well as bulbocavernosus and anal wink reflexes should be done. A cotton-tipped swab is used to evaluate the vestibule for localised tenderness of vulvovestibulitis. The vestibule, vulva, hymen and the area of the minor vestibular glands are palpated gently with a cotton-tipped swab.

The manual portion of the pelvic exam is initiated with a single index finger noting any introital tenderness or spasm. Vaginismus is dyspareunia or the inability to have coitus owing to the involuntary spasm of, primarily, the bulbocavernosus muscles, but sometimes the levator ani muscles too. Next, the levator ani muscles are directly palpated for tone and tenderness. They lie adjacent to the lateral vaginal walls just above the hymenal ring.

Identification may be confirmed by having

the patient contract her pelvic muscles. Normally, this palpation causes only a pressure sensation, but in patients with pelvic floor pain syndrome (PFPS), it may cause pain consistent with at least part of the patient's clinical pain symptoms. Several names have been used for pelvic floor pain syndrome, such as pelvic floor myalgia, piriformis syndrome, levator ani spasm syndrome and coccydynia. PFPS may also result from trigger points in one or more of the muscles of the pelvis. The most common finding with PFPS is tenderness and spasm of one or more of the levator muscles of the pelvic floor.

Bimanual examination: The uterus is compressed against the sacrum to evaluate uterine tenderness which may be consistent with diseases such as adenomyosis, pelvic congestion syndrome, pelvic infection or premenstrual syndrome. A uterus that is immobile and fixed in position, especially a retroflexed position, may suggest endometriosis or adhesions.

The coccyx should be palpated with a single digit and an attempt should be made to move it by 30° or less. Normally, the coccyx moves 30° without eliciting pain, but in patients with coccydynia this movement elicits pain. The adnexal areas should be palpated next, still using a single digit without the use of the abdominal hand. It is the degree of tenderness and the similarity to the chief pain complaint that are clinically useful in an evaluation of the ovaries.

Rectal and rectovaginal examination are performed last. With rectal examination, as one starts in the posterior midline and sweeps laterally and anteriorly, the rectal finger passes over the piriformis, the coccygeus, and then, the levator ani muscles. Rectal examination should also include evaluation for rectal masses. Tenderness in the anal canal may suggest abscesses or fissures in the canal. Testing for occult blood should be performed.

Investigation

Blood testing: A complete blood count and sedimentation rate should be done. These allow a determination regarding infectious or inflammatory presence and the hemoglobin and hematocrit to detect the presence of anemia.

Vaginal swabs: Suitable samples to screen for infection, particularly chlamydia and gonorrhea, should be taken if there is any suspicion of pelvic inflammatory disease (PID). Ideally, all sexually active women below the age of 25 years, who are being examined, should be offered opportunistic screening for chlamydia (Pimenta et al 2003).

Ultrasound examination: In patients undergoing laparoscopy (the gold standard) for CPP, 60% have disorders, of which the most common are endometriosis and pelvic adhesion (Howard 1993)· CPP accounts for 50% of all diagnostic laparoscopies and is used liberally as the gold standard in the assessment of women with CPP. But laparoscopy fails to identify any cause of pain in up to 40% of patients.

Ultrasound is very useful in reporting the presence or absence of pathology, such as an ovarian cyst or hydrosalpinx, but subtle information—about the state of the pelvis based on the degree of ovarian and uterine mobility as well as tenderness—is referred to by the term soft markers.

Okaro et al (2006) in his study reassured patients with no soft markers, as the majority of them will have a normal pelvis on laparoscopy. Expectant management would be appropriate, with a review in six months.

In women with soft markers, one option would be to try medical treatment in the form of GnRH or OC pills (Milsom and Andersch 1984; Robinson et al 1992), which have been shown to have a higher degree of success in relieving pain.

The presence of hard markers (ovarian cyst, hydrosalpinx) on ultrasonography obviously raises the probability of pelvic disease to 100%, and to 73% by the presence of soft markers. Thus, the use of hard and soft markers will lead to significant reduction in the number of diagnostic laparoscopies being performed in patients with CPP (Okaro et al 2006).

Pelvic venography: Pelvic venography is performed in women with possible pelvic congestion syndrome and it is currently the only reliable way to diagnose this syndrome. Transuterine venography is performed by introducing a water-soluble contrast medium into the uterine venous system via injection into the myometrium of the uterine fundus. Images are taken for one minute after the injection. This method has a sensitivity of 91% and a specificity of 89%. The images are scored based on the maximum diameter of the ovarian veins, the time of disappearance of contrast and the degree of congestion of the ovarian plexus. Selective ovarian venography has been used to diagnose the pelvic congestion syndrome and can be performed by a jugular venous approach or a transfemoral approach.

CT scan: A CT scan can be diagnostically helpful in women with pelvic masses, but it is more expensive than sonography and is not always necessary. In patients with suspected urinary tract involvement of endometriosis, ovarian remnant syndrome, ovarian retention syndrome, pelvic masses and so on, intravenous pyelography has been traditionally used, but CT with intravenous contrast is a more accurate and informational technique and is preferable in most cases. CT scans can also help identify urinary tract calculi, sciatic hernias, umbilical hernias and linea alba hernias, as well as Spigelian hernias. CT can also identify herniation in an incision site, as well as Spigelian hernias. It can be helpful in identifying abdominal tuberculosis. Musculoskeletal sources of pelvic pain are more readily identified with CT than with plain films.

Laparoscopy: This is considered the gold standard in confirmation of the cause of CPP or when initial therapy fails (ACOG Bulletin 1996). A survey of published laparoscopy series suggests that over 40% of gynecologic laparoscopies are done for CPP. Published series show that no visible pathology is detected in 35% of patients (Howard 1996). Endometriosis is the most common pathologic diagnosis (approximately 33%), followed by adhesive disease (24%).

LAPAROSCOPY AND ENDOMETRIOSIS: Sampson (1927) defined endometriosis as the presence of ectopic tissue which possesses the histological structure and function of uterine mucosa. The common sites in the pelvis and abdomen must be closely inspected and must include the ovaries and the ovarian fossa, pelvic peritoneum (particularly the cul-de-sac, periureteral and bladder peritoneum), uterine ligaments, sigmoid colon, appendix, fallopian tubes and the rectovaginal septum.

The technical objectives of surgery are:

- To restore normal pelvic anatomy
- To resect, coagulate and vaporise all endometriosis implants (Howard 2000)

However, a good response to the surgical treatment of endometriosis depends on the skill of the surgeon, and the amount of time taken to destroy all of the endometriosis, including deep disease. Medication therapy, however, which gives similar response rates and pain control, does not depend on surgical skill and does not entail surgical risks (APGO 2000). Therefore, an alternative approach to the treatment of CPP is treatment with a GnRH agonist after NSAIDs and OCs have failed to adequately treat the pain. In a high quality, randomised, placebo-controlled trial, Ling and colleagues (1999) demonstrated the efficacy of this treatment algorithm.

Laparoscopy and adhesions: The presence of pelvic adhesions is not a reliable predictor of pelvic pain. Laparoscopic studies reveal adhesions in 24% of CPP patients and 17% of non-CPP patients (Stovall et al 1989). Chronic PID, in which adhesive disease has a significant role, has not been a common laparoscopic diagnosis in CPP patients. It represents 5% of all diagnoses (Howard 2000). It has been difficult to definitively demonstrate that adhesions cause CPP and it has been difficult to show that adhesiolysis relieves CPP (Walsh 1983).

Treatment

Oral Analgesics: The choice of an oral analgesic, which provides the optimum pain relief, should be the obvious initial treatment option. Therapy should begin with a less expensive prostaglandin synthetase inhibitor, such as ibuprofen, on a scheduled rather than on an 'as needed' basis.

Narcotic analgesics are not recommended for the treatment of CPP. These agents have a potent smooth muscle-relaxing effect that may exacerbate functional dysmotility disorders in women with chronic abdominal pain. In addition, sedation and altered cognition associated with narcotic use may limit the restoration of normal function. Finally, narcotics have a high abuse and addiction potential.

Psychotropic Medications: Tricyclic antidepressants (TCAs) have been shown to improve pain tolerance, to restore normal sleep and to reduce depressive symptoms. There is enough evidence to recommend their use in much lower doses than those used to treat depression (Walsh 1983). TCA therapy for patients with sleep disturbance, mild to moderate mood disturbance, or both, is usually initiated with imipramine, amitriptyline or doxepin, 10–25 mg, at bedtime. This dosage is titrated to 50–75 mg as needed. Although full antidepressant dosages (up to 200 mg daily) may be utilised for patients with major mood disturbance, we have preferred the addition of a selective serotonin re-uptake inhibitor, such as Prozac 20–40 mg or Paxil 10–20 mg, every morning for patients with moderate to severe depression or for patients with less severe mood disturbance failing TCA therapy. Selective serotonin reuptake inhibitors may be used alone or in combination with low-dose TCAs.

Drug Therapy for Dysmotility Disorders: The aim of therapy is to treat functional bowel disorders such as the irritable bowel syndrome, chronic constipation with a variety of treatment strategies, including dietary management, medical therapy and psychotherapy (Drossman and Thompson 1992). Oral fibre supplementation in the form of psyllium powder increases stool bulk and water content and decreases transit time, thus relieving pain and constipation in hypomotile patients; it also decreases frequency of bowel movements and encourages formed stools in patients with hypermotile patterns and diarrhea. Medical regimens that directly relax smooth muscle (such as dicyclomine) are useful during painful hypermotile phases and should be used only after a thorough exclusion work-up.

Medical Management of Musculoskeletal Pain: Abdominal wall trigger points are amenable to treatment with a variety of modalities, including transcutaneous electric nerve stimulation (TENS), acupuncture (hyperstimulation analgesia) and infiltration with a variety of agents (Slocumb 1984; Reiter and Milburn 1993). Although injectable steroids are commonly used for this purpose or are combined with local anesthetics, we have favored the use of 0.25% bupivacaine 5–10 cc injected at the point of maximal tenderness after needle tip localisation. Response rates of 80%–90% have been reported after 3–4 injections (Slocumb 1984).

It is not clear whether the anesthetic properties of these agents, the 'hydro-distention' effect of the volume of fluid injected, or both is responsible for the desensitisation response observed in these cases. Further controlled investigation in this area is clearly warranted.

Hawk et al published the results of a prospective randomised placebo-controlled trial assessing chiropractic manipulation that suggests that this modality may have a role in the treatment of selected patients with CPP (Hawk et al 1997).

Ovarian Cycle Suppression: Antiprostaglandin therapy or cycle suppression forms the first line of treatment in patients with CPP. For patients failing antiprostaglandin therapy, the choice of cycle suppression therapy is based on safety, cost and patient acceptance. For these reasons, oral contraceptives and continuous oral or injectable progestins are favoured as primary therapy for cyclic pain disorders. A gonadotrophin-releasing hormone agonist (GnRH-A) may have a limited (primarily diagnostic) role in refractory cases.

Oral contraceptives are a convenient and effective initial choice for cycle suppression. A monophasic 30–50 μg ethinyl estradiol pill is preferred and may be used cyclically or continuously. The most useful synthetic progestin is medroxyprogesterone acetate (MPA) used as a continuous oral regimen (10–30 mg daily) or in an injectable depot form (150–300 mg q 1–3 months). Duration of therapy is individualised and may extend from months to years.

Antibiotics: Subacute upper genital tract infection, occasionally, is suspected on the basis of a positive cervical culture and uterine tenderness in patients who do not meet standard clinical criteria for the diagnosis of endometritis or salpingitis. Standard antibiotic therapy may alleviate symptoms in this setting. With this exception, empiric antibiotic therapy is discouraged in women with CPP, negative cultures and an absence of supporting clinical criteria. Chronic urethral syndrome, characterised by urethral irritative symptoms (urgency, frequency, dysuria, suprapubic pain) without bacteriuria, has been reported in 2%–3% of women with CPP (Hibbard 1983). In an early placebo-controlled study, Stamm et al (1981) reported that tetracycline improved symptoms only in women with associated pyuria (without bacteriuria); no benefit was observed in women without pyuria.

Operative laparoscopy: Due to the convenience of performing operative endoscopic procedures at the time of diagnostic laparoscopy, operative laparoscopy is commonly used for women with CPP. As noted above, Peters et al (1992) observed no benefit from endoscopic adhesiolysis in a prospective randomised trial, except in a small subset of women with dense adhesions involving the bowel.

To date, there has been one published prospective randomised double-blind trial assessing laser laparoscopy for the treatment of pain associated with endometriosis (Sutton et al 1994). Although the authors concluded that laser ablation of endometriosis was therapeutic for pelvic pain and dysmenorrhea, the results of the study are difficult to interpret because all patients in the treatment arm received laparoscopic uterosacral nerve ablation (LUNA), in addition to endoscopic ablation of endometriosis. Laparoscopic uterosacral nerve ablation has been shown to be associated with response rates for dysmenorrhea, similar to those observed by the authors, when performed in women with or without endometriosis. For this reason, it cannot be determined what the therapeutic effect of ablation of endometriosis, if any, may have been (Lichton anad Bombard 1987; Reiter 1995; Hillis 1995).

Hysterectomy: Despite its high utilisation, there are no randomised trials assessing the effectiveness of hysterectomy for CPP. Hillis et al (1995) reported a 74% resolution rate in a cohort of 308 women who had undergone hysterectomy for CPP. Recurrence rates of 40%, however, were observed in women in whom hysterectomy was performed without identifiable intrapelvic pathology.

Further, the Hillis study reevaluated women for up to a year after surgery and did not assess for the presence of chronic non-pelvic symptoms such as low back pain, headache or chronic fatigue, which are common in somatising patients who may continue to experience similar degrees of disability and pain related to non-pelvic symptoms, but who may be lost to gynecologic follow-up after hysterectomy.

Multidisciplinary management: Numerous studies have demonstrated the effectiveness of multidisciplinary management of a variety of chronic pain syndromes. In a recent meta-analysis of 65 studies evaluating the efficacy of multidisciplinary pain management, Flor et al (1992) found benefits relating to pain severity, mood and interference, as well as increased instances of return to work and decreased use rates of healthcare services. These effects appeared to be stable with time.

A recent randomised prospective trial by Peters et al (1991) confirmed that multidisciplinary management of CPP, including pain management, restoration of function and optimisation of adaptive coping skills, provided significantly greater improvement in pain severity, reemployment and global somatic symptom scores than a traditional medical approach.

Conclusion: The incidence of CPP has been reported as being 14.7% in the UK. CPP accounts for 10% of gynecological visits and 50% of all diagnostic laparoscopies. CPP interferes with the quality of life and has serious effects on family relationships, sexual intercourse, social life and work activity. Women with CPP need better outpatient care. The focus should be on providing more personal care, so that the presenting findings can be taken seriously and women are more effectively reassured.

References

ACOG Pelvic Pain Technical Bulletin. 1996. Issue no: 223 1996. 371–379

ACOG Technical Bulletin. 1996. Chronic pelvic pain *Int J Gynecol and Obstet* 22354:59–68.

Adams J, PW Reginald, RW Franks Beard. 1997. Uterine size and significance of cystic ovaries in women with pelvic pain due to congestion. *Br J Obstet Gynaecol* 583–587.

APGO Educational Series on Women's Health Issues. *Chronic Pelvic Pain: An Integrated Approach.* Colorado: Medical Education Collaborative.

Baird DT and IS Fraser1975. Concentration of oesterone and oestradiol in the follicular fluid and ovarian venous blood of women. *Clin Endocrinology* 4:259–266.

Beard RW, JW Highman, SX Pearee, PW Reginald. 1984. Diagnosis of pelvic varicosities in women with chronic pelvic pain. *Lancet* 946–949.

Beard RW, PW Reginald, J Wadsworth. 1988. Clinical features of women with chronic lower abdominal pain and pelvic congestion. *Br J Obstet Gynaecol* Vol. 95, 153–161.

Bonica JJ. 1990. General consideration of pain in the pelvis and perineum. In: Bonica JJ, Loeser JD, Chapman CR, Fordyce WE, eds. *The management of pain* Vol 2; 1283–1301.

Campbell F and BJ Collet. 1994. Chronic pelvic pain. *Br J Anaesth* 73:571–573.

Carter JE. 1996. *Chronic Pelvic Pain: Diagnosis and Management.* Monograph Colorado: Medical Education Collaborative, 1–35 http://www.obgyn.net/medical.asp?page=/english/pubs/features/carter/cpp_carter

Carter JE. 1999. A systematic history for the patient with chronic pelvic pain. *JSLS* 3: 245–252.

Carter JE. 2000. Laparoscopic uterine suspension In *Operative Techniques in Gynecologic Surgery*. 5: 34–40. WB Saunders Company

Collett BJ, Cordle CJ, Stewart CR, Jagger C. 1998. A comparative study of women with chronic pelvic pain, chronic non-pelvic pain and those with no history of pain attending general practitioner. *Br J Obstet Gynaecol* 105:87–92.

Davies L, KF Gangar, M Drummonds, D Saunders, RW Beard. 1992. The economic burden of intractable gynaecological pain. *J Obstet Gynaecol* 12: S54–S56.

Drossman DA and WG Thompson. 1992. The irritable bowel syndrome: Review and a graduate multicomponent treatment approach. *Ann Intern Med* 116:1009–1016.

Dworkin SF, M Von Korff, L LeResche. 1990. Multiple pains and psychiatric disturbance: An epidemiological investigation. *Arch Gen Psychiatry* 47:239–244.

Flor H, T Fydrich, DC Turk. 1992. Efficacy of multidisciplinary pain treatment centers: A meta-analytic flow. *Pain* 49:221–239.

Hawk C, C Long, A Azad. 1997. Chiropractic care for women with chronic pelvic pain: A prospective single-group intervention study. *J Manipulative Physiolog Ther* 20:73–79.

Hibbard LT. 1983. Chronic pelvic pain. In *Management of Common Problems in Obstetrics and Gynecology* ed DR Mishell, PF Brenner. Oradell, NJ: Medical Economics.

Hillis SD, PA Marchbanks, HB Peterson. 1995. The effectiveness of hysterectomy for chronic pelvic pain. *Obstet Gynecol* 86:941–945.

Howard FM. 1993. The role of laparoscopy in chronic pelvic pain: Promise and pitfalls. *Obstet Gynecol Surv* 48:357–387.

Howard FM. 1996. The role of laparoscopy in the evaluation of chronic pelvic pain: Pitfalls with a negative laparoscopy. *J Am Assoc Gynecol Laparoscop* 4:85–94.

Howard FM. 2000. Endoscopy In Howard FM, Perry CP, Carter JE, El-Minawi AM eds *Pelvic Pain: Diagnosis and Management.* New York: Lippincott, 57.

Howard FM. 2000. Physical examination In Howard FM, Perry CP, Carter JE, El- Minawi AM. *Pelvic Pain: Diagnosis and Management.* New York: Lippincott 30

Lichton EM and J Bombard. 1987. Surgical treatment of primary dysmenorrhea with laparoscopic uterine nerve ablation. *J Repro Med* 32:37–41.

Ling FW. 1999. For the pelvic pain study group. Randomized controlled trial of Depot leuprolide in patients with chronic pelvic pain and clinically suspected endometriosis. *Obstet Gynecol* 93:51–58.

Magni G, A Salmi, D De Leo, A Ceola. 1984. Chronic pelvic pain and depression. *Psychopathology* 17:132–136.

Mathias SD, M Kuppermann, RF Libbernan, RC Lipschutz, JF Steege. 1996. Chronic pelvic pain: Prevalence, health related quality of life, and economic correlates. *Obstet Gynecol* 87:321–327.

Milsom I and B Andersch. 1984. Effect of various oral contraceptive combinations on dysmenorrhoea. *Gynecol Obstet Invest* 17:284–292.

Moore J and S Kennedy. 2000. Causes of chronic pelvic pain. Baillieres *Best Pract Res Clin Obstet Gynaecol* 14:389–403.

Office of population census and survey. 1995. Morbidity statistics from general practices. Fourth National Study 1991-1992, MB5, no 3, 24–78.

Okaro E, G Condus, A Khalid, D Timmerman, L Ameye, SV Huffel, T Bourne. 2006. The use of ultrasound based 'soft markers' for the prediction of pelvic pathology in women with chronic pelvic pain. Can we reduce the need for laparoscopy? *Br J Obstet Gynaecol* 113:251–256.

Peters AA, GC Trimbos-Kemper, C Admiraal et al. 1992. A randomized clinical trial on the benefit of adhesiolysis in patients with intraperitoneal adhesions and chronic pelvic pain. *Br J Obstet Gynaecol* 99:59–62.

Peters AAW, E VanDorst, B Jellis. 1991. A randomized clinical trial to compare two different approaches in women with chronic pelvic pain. *Obstet Gynecol* 77:740–744.

Peters AAW, Trimbos-Kemper GCM, Admiraal C et al. 1992. A randomized clinical trial on the benefit of adhesiolysis in patients with intraperitoneal adhesions and chronic pelvic pain. *Br J Obstet Gynaecol* 99:59–63.

Pimenta JM, M Catchpole, PA Rogers, E Perkins, N Jackson, C Carlisle et al. 2003. Opportunistic screening for genital chlamydia infection. 1: Acceptability of urine testing in primary and secondary healthcare settings. *Sex Transm Infect* 79:16–21.

Prentice A. 2000. Medical management of chronic pelvic pain. *Bailliere's Best Pract Res Clin Obstet Gynaecol* 14:495–499.

Price J, J Farmer, J Harris, T Hope, S Kennedy, R Mayou. 2006. Attitudes of women with chronic pelvic pain to gynaecological consultation: a qualitative study. *Br J Obstet Gynaecol* 113:446–452.

Reiter RC and A Milburn. 1993. Chronic Pelvic Pain. In: Moore TR, Reiter RC, Rebar R, Baker V, eds. *Gynecology and Obstetrics: A Longitudinal Approach.* New York: Churchill Livingstone. 857–867.

Reiter RC. 1990. Chronic pelvic pain. *Clin Obstet Gynecol* 33: 117–118.

Reiter RC. 1995. Efficacy of laser laparoscopy in minimal endometriosis? Letter to the Editor. *Fertil Steril* 63:1355–1356.

Robinson JC, S Plichta, CS Weisman, CA Natherson. 1992. Dysmenorrhoea and the use of oral contraceptive in adolescent women attending family planning clinic. *Am J of Obstet Gynaecol* 166:578–83.

Roseff SJ and AA Murphy. 1990. Laparoscopy in the diagnosis and therapy of chronic pelvic pain. *Clin Obstet Gynaecol* 33:137–144.

Sampson JA. 1927. Peritoneal endometriosis due to dissemination of endometrial tissue into the peritoneal cavity. *Am J Obstet Gynecol* 14:422

Slocumb JC. 1984. Neurologic factors in chronic pelvic pain: Trigger points and the abdominal pelvic pain syndrome. *Am J Obstet Gynecol* 149:536–543.

Stamm WE, K Running, M McKevitt et al. 1981. Treatment of the acute urethral syndrome. *N Engl J Med* 304:956–959.

Steege JF, DA Metzger, BL Levy. 1997. *Chronic pelvic pain: An Integrated approach.* New York: Saunders

Steege JF. 1997. Office Assessment of Chronic Pelvic Pain. *Clin Obstet Gynecol* 40:554–563.

Stovall TG, RF Elder, FW Ling. 1989. Predictors of pelvic adhesions. *J Reprod Med* 34:345.

Sutton CJ, SP Ewen, N Whitelaw, P Haines. 1994. Prospective, randomized, double-blind, controlled trial of laser laparoscopy in the treatment of pelvic pain associated with minimal, mild, and moderate endometriosis. *Fertil Steril* 62:696–700.

Szendei G, Z Hernadi, N Devenyi, Z Csapo. 2005. Is there a correlation between stages of endometriosis and severity of chronic pelvic pain? Possibilities of treatment. *Gynecol Endocrinol* 21(2):93–100.

Taylor HC. 1949. Vascular congestion and hyperaemia. Physiological basis and history of concept. *Am J Obstet Gynecol* 57:211–230.

Vercellini P, L Fedele, S Bianchi. 1991. Pelvic denervation for chronic pelvic pain associated with endometriosis: Facts or fancy? *Am J Obstet Gynecol* 165:745–749.

Walker EA and MA Stenchever. 1993. Sexual victimisation and chronic pelvic pain. *Obstet Gynecol Clin North Am* 20: 795–807.

Walker EA, WJ Katon, J Hansom et al. 1992. Medical and psychiatric symptoms in women with childhood sexual abuse. *Psychosom Med* 54:658–664.

Walling MK, RC Reiter, MW O'Hara et al. 1994. Abuse history and chronic pelvic pain in women: I. Prevalence of sexual abuse and physical abuse. *Obstet Gynecol* 84:193–199.

Walsh TD. 1983. Antidepressants in chronic pain. *Clin Neuropharmacol* 6:271–276.

Wenof M and Paul C Perry. 1999. Chronic pelvic pain. International Pelvic Pain Society. Patient Education Booklet.

40

Misoprostol in Obstetrics and Gynecology

Gowri Ramanathan | Sabaratnam Arulkumaran

Introduction: Misoprostol, a drug primarily developed for the treatment of peptic ulcer, has gained widespread use in obstetrics and gynecology. Being a prostaglandin, it has an effect on the female reproductive system, exhibiting uterotonic and cervical ripening activity. Despite extensive research and evidence proving its benefits, its use remains unlicensed in pregnancy. This article traces the history and debate surrounding the integration of misoprostol into clinical obstetrics and gynecology. We also present the available evidence on its use in four key areas of practice—termination of pregnancy, the management of miscarriage, induction of labour and management of postpartum hemorrhage.

History of misoprostol use: In 1985, a multicentre randomised double-blind study showed that Misoprostol [15-deoxy-16-hydroxy-16methyl-PGE1] successfully prevents and treats gastro-duodenal ulcers associated with the use of nonsteroidal anti-inflammatory drugs (NSAIDs) (Agrawal et al 1985). Approval was obtained by the US Food and Drug Administration (FDA) in 1988 for the prevention and treatment of gastric ulcers associated with NSAIDs, and is currently used for ulcer treatment in more than 80 countries. It produces a dose related inhibition of gastric secretions, and has a cytoprotective action on gastrointestinal mucosa.

Being a prostaglandin, misoprostol also affects the uterine smooth muscle which results in uterine contractions and cervical softening. Since learning of this drug's effect on the uterus, interest in the potential role of misoprostol emerged among obstetricians and gynecologists. Misoprostol was seen as having several advantages over other prostaglandins which were being used in obstetrics and gynecology

- It has a long shelf life, of several years, if kept in its aluminium blister packets
- It can be stored at room temperature without the need for refrigeration
- It is cheap
- It can be administered orally, rectally, vaginally or sublingually
- Being selective for the PGE_1 receptors it has no clinically significant effects on the bronchi or blood vessels, hence fewer side effects, and can be safely used in patients with underlying diseases such as asthma or cardiovascular disorders
- The only side effects of note with misoprostol are diarrhea and shivering,

both of which are dose dependent and self-limiting.

As misoprostol is not licensed for use in obstetrics and gynecology, its 'off-label' use means that the responsibility of prescribing the drug and managing its effects and side effects lies with the physician prescribing it. There are many examples of drugs not licensed by the FDA that are used in obstetrics; these include, among others, terbutaline, dexamethasone, phenytoin, heparin, enoxaparin, metoclopramide and dinoprostone. This practice of off-label use is common in obstetrics, with a survey in America showing nearly a quarter of women having received, at some time during their pregnancy, an off-label drug (Rayburn and Farmer 1997). The earliest report of the off-label use of misoprostol was in 1987 for the termination of first trimester pregnancies (Rabe et al 1987). Although the investigators recommended that misoprostol should not be used in pregnant women, the findings were hardly ignored, fuelling further interest in the drug. The first formal clinical trials on the use of misoprostol for gynecological (Normal et al 1991) and obstetric (Fletcher et al 1993) purposes followed soon after.

Misoprostol and abortions: Misoprostol was recognised early on as a method to induce abortions, not only by the medical world but also by the media. This, unfortunately, was the beginning of the abuse and misuse of the drug. In countries where abortion was illegal, misoprostol became a cheap and convenient method to induce abortions in the private sector, and in some countries, the drug was sold over the counter. In 1991, a study from Brazil reported that approximately 60% of women hospitalised with abortion-related complications had used misoprostol to induce abortions (Costa and Vessey 1993). With no standards on dosages and intervals of administration, it was proving to be an inefficient abortifacient with many requiring subsequent uterine evacuation for incomplete abortions; in those that had a failed attempt and termination of pregnancy did not occur, there was the risk of in utero exposure of the fetus to misoprostol. A retrospective review of infants born after misoprostol exposure in the first three months of pregnancy showed distinctive phenotypes including equinovarus with cranial nerve defects, arthrogryposis confined to the legs, and terminal transverse limb defects (Gonzalez et al 1998). The authors postulated that these abnormalities were due to vascular disruption from the uterine contractions induced by misoprostol. A subsequent prospective study failed to show any difference in rates of major or minor abnormalities between the exposed and non-exposed groups to misoprostol, however, the study was of limited statistical power (Schuler et al 1999).

Despite a wide-scale move by health authorities to suspend the sales of misoprostol after concerns of its misuse, it still remains available and is used for self-induced abortions even now (Pongsatha et al 2002). Public health education needs to continue on effective contraceptive methods, as well as highlighting the risks associated with illegal abortions.

Medical termination of pregnancy: Prostaglandins are known to have an effect on the female reproductive system, exhibiting uterotonic and cervical ripening activity. Mifepristone, a progesterone antagonist that was being investigated for use in medical termination of pregnancy, resulted in only 80% of women having a complete abortion. The addition of a prostaglandin, however, increased the efficacy of mifepristone to nearly 100% (Bygdeman and Swahn 1985), leading to the initiation of studies on the value of mifepristone followed by misoprostol. Misoprostol, with or without the use of mifepristone, was shown to significantly increase the amplitude and frequency of uterine contractions (Normal et al 1991). The use of mifepristone, followed 48 hours later by oral misoprostol in pregnancies of less than eight weeks gestation, resulted in 93% of women having a complete abortion (Thong and Baird 1992). The route of misoprostol administration was also compared, and vaginal administration was shown to be more effective and better tolerated than oral administration (el-Refaey et al 1995).

Misoprostol was also evaluated as a cervical priming agent prior to surgical evacuation of the uterus. Compared to placebo and vaginal gemeprost, misoprostol, either orally (Ngai et al 1995) or vaginally (Bugalho et al 1994), was shown to be as, or more, effective in achieving adequate cervical dilatation, with greater ease of further dilatation by surgeons in the misoprostol group. A study comparing 400 μg sublingual misoprostol to vaginal misoprostol showed that sublingual misoprostol was more effective in facilitating cervical dilatation prior to surgical evacuation of the uterus; however, more shivering was experienced in this group (Vimala et al 2004).

Similarly, studies of mid-trimester termination of pregnancy have shown that the combination of mifepristone and misoprostol is safe and effective, with over 97% of women aborting successfully within five doses of misoprostol (Ashok et al 2004). Efforts to increase the interval between doses and to reduce the side effects were made. However, compared to the six-hourly regime, the three-hourly regime was more effective in terms of a shorter interval and a higher percentage of successful abortions within 48 hours (Wong et al 2000). Although the use of misoprostol in the presence of a scarred uterus, has been reported to be safe and effective (Xu et al 2001), further large studies are required to confirm its safety.

Management of miscarriages: Early pregnancy failure occurs in 15% of clinically recognised pregnancies (Alberman 1992), and the treatment most commonly offered is surgical emptying of the uterus with the use of sharp curettage or vacuum aspiration. Expectant management, or waiting for the process of pregnancy loss to end spontaneously, is also sometimes offered to women with uncomplicated clinical presentations. However, it has a suboptimal success rate—ranging from 25% to 76% (Jurkovic et al 1998), and an unpredictable interval to spontaneous expulsion.

Medical management with misoprostol for early pregnancy failure was studied as a method to induce a more prompt evacuation of the uterus. Oral misoprostol used in the management of incomplete miscarriage results in significantly lower immediate, short and medium-term complications compared to surgical evacuation. However, in approximately 50% of those treated with misoprostol, subsequent surgical evacuation was required (Chung et al 1999). Vaginal misoprostol is more effective in missed miscarriages compared to oral misoprostol, with successful expulsion occurring in 88% and 25%, respectively (Creinin et al 1997). Women experiencing a missed miscarriage as opposed to an incomplete miscarriage, have a higher success rate with vaginal misoprostol compared to placebo (Bagratee et al 2004). A recent randomised controlled trial of 652 women, compared 800 μg of misoprostol vaginally versus surgical management for early pregnancy failure, which included missed and incomplete miscarriages. Over 70% and 84% had complete expulsion by day 3 and 8 respectively, with no difference in the incidence of hemorrhage or endometritis requiring hospitalisation which was <1% in each group (Zhang et al 2005).

Induction of labour: This is a common procedure, with approximately 20% of women having their labour induced for a variety of reasons (RCOG 2001). Achieving successful induction of labour remains a challenge and often involves a complex set of interventions. Prostaglandins have long been used for induction of labour in the presence of an unfavourable cervix. The use of oral misoprostol for induction of labour at term was recognised early on as being associated with uterine tachysystole (more than five contractions per 10 minutes for at least 20 minutes), uterine hypersystole/hypertonus (a contraction of 2 minutes or more) and/or uterine hyperstimulation syndrome (uterine tachysystole or hypersystole with fetal heart rate changes such as persistent decelerations, tachycardia or reduced short term variability) (Mariani et al 1988). The use of intravaginal misoprostol was found to be safer than oral misoprostol, with a meta-analysis showing that there was an increased incidence of uterine tachysystole (OR 2.79, 95% CI 1.80 to 4.04), but no statistically significant increase in adverse fetal outcome (Sanchez-Ramos et al 1997).

Numerous subsequent trials evaluated the value of oral, vaginal, buccal or sublingual misoprostol compared with other methods of induction of labour. The efficacy was similar between oral and intravaginal misoprostol (Adair et al 1998). However, the intravaginal route was associated with shorter induction to delivery interval, lower number of doses and lower oxytocin use (Toppozada et al 1997; Nopdonrattakoon 2003). Misoprostol gel, compared to tablet, was shown to be associated with fewer uterine contraction abnormalities but slower time to labour or delivery (Carlan et al 1997).

A systematic review of 70 trials evaluating the value of misoprostol in induction of labour concluded that compared to placebo, misoprostol was associated with reduced failure to achieve vaginal delivery within 24 hours (relative risk (RR) 0.36, 95% confidence interval (CI) 0.19 to 0.68; however, uterine hyperstimulation without fetal heart rate changes was increased (RR 11.66, 95% CI 2.78 to 49). Compared with vaginal prostaglandin E2, intracervical prostaglandin E2 and oxytocin, vaginal misoprostol was associated with less epidural analgesia use, fewer failures to achieve vaginal delivery within 24 hours and more uterine hyperstimulation. Compared with vaginal or intracervical PGE_2, oxytocin augmentation was less common and meconium-stained liquor more common with misoprostol.

Comparing different dosages of misoprostol administration, it was found that 50 μg of misoprostol administered vaginally resulted in a shorter induction to delivery interval and higher rate of vaginal delivery within 24 hours when compared with 25 μg of misoprostol. However, the chance of hyperstimulation was higher (Sanchez-Ramos et al 2002). Lower doses were associated with less uterine hyperstimulation but more need for oxytocin augmentation. Doses higher than 50 μg on the other hand were associated with serious complications (Majoko et al 2002). In terms of optimal interval of administration, three-hourly doses compared to six-hourly doses were associated with shorter induction to delivery interval but slightly higher prevalence of tachysystole (Wing and Paul 1997).

The situation with misoprostol-induction after cesarean is complicated by the fact that other prostaglandins are not licensed either, so the extent to which complications such as uterine rupture result from misoprostol itself or from the use of prostaglandins in general remains unclear (Goldberg et al 2001). Two articles suggest a higher risk of uterine rupture with misoprostol induction than for the other prostaglandins (Blanchette et al 1999; Plaut et al 1999).

In summary, vaginal misoprostol in dosages of 25 μg, three-hourly or more, is more effective than conventional methods of cervical ripening and labour induction, but with more uterine hyperstimulation and fetal heart rate changes. Although no differences in perinatal outcome were shown in the meta-analysis, the studies were not sufficiently large to exclude the possibility of uncommon serious adverse effects, particularly uterine rupture which has been reported anecdotally following misoprostol induction (Daisley 2000; Gherman et al 2000; Hill et al 2000; Majoko et al 2002). The limited information on lower dosage regimens (25 μg, four-hourly or less frequently) suggests that they may be as effective as other prostaglandins, without increased uterine hyperstimulation; however, further research is needed.

Management of postpartum hemorrhage: Postpartum hemorrhage (PPH) is the most common single cause of maternal mortality globally, with uterine atony being the most common cause of PPH. Available uterotonic drugs that have been shown to reduce the incidence of PPH in the third stage of labour, include syntocinon, syntometrine and ergometrine. The value of misoprostol in preventing PPH in the third stage of labour was first reported in 1996, proving it to be an effective alternative, with fewer side effects (el-Refaey et al 1997). The WHO misoprostol multicentre trial compared 600 μg oral misoprostol with 10 IU intramuscular or intravenous oxytocin in the prevention of PPH in the third stage of labour. This study of 18,530 women found that misoprostol was associated with a higher risk of PPH, increased need for additional uterotonics, shivering and pyrexia compared with oxytocin, concluding that parenteral oxytocics were preferable to misoprostol for the routine prevention of PPH in the third stage of labour (Gulmezoglu et al 2001). Subsequent studies using rectal misoprostol have shown similar results (Caliskan et al 2002). However, despite its lesser efficacy compared to injectable oxytocics, it remains an important back-up option in less developed countries due to its ease of storage and low cost (McCormick et al 2002). A recent randomised controlled trial in West Africa evaluating the value of routine administration of sublingual 600 μg misoprostol compared to placebo after delivery showed that sublingual misoprostol reduces the frequency of severe PPH (RR 0.66, 95%, CI 0.45 to 0.98 for PPH ≥ 1000 ml; RR 0.28, 95% CI 0.12 to 0.64 for PPH ≥ 1500 ml) (Hoj et al 2005).

The value of misoprostol in the treatment of PPH has also been evaluated. However, the data is more limited. Misoprostol at a dose of 1000 μg, rectally administered, successfully controlled hemorrhage that was unresponsive to oxytocin and ergometrine, with sustained uterine contraction occurring within 3 minutes (O'Brien et al 1998). Compared with a combination of intramuscular syntometrine injection and oxytocin infusion, 800 μg rectal misoprostol administration provided a statistically significant reduction in the number of women who continued to bleed after the intervention and less need for medical co-interventions to control the bleeding (6% versus 34%) (RR 0.18, 95% CI 0.04 to 0.67). However, there was no significant difference between the two groups regarding surgical interventions to control intractable hemorrhage including hysterectomy, internal iliac artery ligation and/or uterine packing (Lokugamage et al 2001). A Cochrane review concluded that rectal misoprostol in a dose of 800 μg may be a useful 'first line' drug for the treatment of primary postpartum hemorrhage, however, further randomised trials are needed (Mousa and Alfirevic 2006).

In summary, misoprostol is less effective than conventional uterotonics in preventing PPH, however, it remains an important alternative especially in less developed countries. This recommendation is strengthened by the results of a recent study which showed major reductions of PPH and need for blood transfusion when misoprostol was compared with placebo (Derman et al 2006). In the treatment of PPH, misoprostol provides better control of hemorrhage and less need for medical co-intervention.

Conclusion: Misoprostol has been extensively studied in reproductive health and is widely recommended for the treatment of missed and incomplete miscarriages, the induction of abortion, and cervical preparation before uterine instrumentation. It also has potential in late pregnancy for the induction of labour and in the prevention as well as treatment of PPH.

In general, important new developments in obstetrics and gynecology are usually rapidly integrated into clinical practice, however, in the case of misoprostol, its incorporation into clinical practice remains very slow. The major obstacle to widespread use of this drug in obstetrics and gynecology has been the failure of its manufacturer and patent holder to apply for its license for use for reproductive health indications, despite the abundant literature on its safe and effective use. The reason is probably an effort to avoid potentially damaging discussions about the drug's use for inducing abortions. This sadly results in the denial of access to a potentially life-saving treatment to millions of women around the world, which is especially true in many low resource settings such as Africa and South America, where two of the biggest causes of maternal mortality are hemorrhage and septic abortion. These could be reduced with easy access to a stable and cheap prostaglandin.

Drug license alone is not the appropriate determinant of whether a drug is effective for any given indication. The UK Medicines and Healthcare Products Regulatory Agency (MHRA, formerly the Medicines Control Agency) was set up to regulate the pharmaceutical industry and not the medical profession, and its advice should always be seen in this context. Further, the current licensing system is inadequate in a situation where the patent holder decides not to apply for an indication because there is no economic interest, even when the drug would be of huge potential benefit to patients. The authors believe that misoprostol has huge potential in obstetric and gynecological practice and the low rate of side effects is currently not sufficiently acknowledged. The lack of approved indications should not deter us from using it where there is sufficient evidence for its safe and effective use.

References

Adair CD, JW Weeks, S Barrilleaux et al. 1998. Oral or vaginal misoprostol administration for induction of labor: A randomized, double-blind trial. *Obstet Gynecol* 92:810–813.

Agrawal NM, B Saffouri, DM Kruss et al. 1985. Healing of benign gastric ulcer. A placebo-controlled comparison of two dosage regimens of misoprostol, a synthetic analog of prostaglandin E1. *Dig Dis Sci* 30:164S–170S.

Alberman E. 1992. Spontaneous abortion: Epidemiology. In: Stabile I, Grudzinskas G, Chard T, eds. *Spontaneous abortion: Diagnosis and treatment.* London: Springer-Verlag. 19–20.

Ashok PW, A Templeton, PT Wagaarachchi et al. 2004. Midtrimester medical termination of pregnancy: A review of 1002 consecutive cases. *Contraception* 69:51–58.

Bagratee JS, V Khullar, L Regan et al. 2004. A randomized controlled trial comparing medical and expectant management of first trimester miscarriage. *Hum Reprod* 19:266–271.

Blanchette H, S Nayak, S Erasmus. 1999. Comparison of the safety and efficacy of intravaginal misoprostol with those of dinoprostone for cervical ripening and induction of labor in a community hospital. *Am J Obstet Gynecol* 180:1543–1550.

Bugalho A, C Bique, L Almeida et al. 1994. Application of vaginal misoprostol before cervical dilatation to facilitate first trimester pregnancy interruption. *Obstet Gynecol* 83:729–731.

Bygdeman M and ML Swahn. 1985. Progesterone receptor blockage. Effect on uterine contractility and early pregnancy. *Contraception* 32:45–51.

Caliskan E, MM Meydanli, B Dilbaz et al. 2002. Is rectal misoprostol really effective in the treatment of third stage of labor? A randomized controlled trial. *Am J Obstet Gynecol* 187:1038–1045.

Carlan SJ, S Bouldin, WF O'Brien. 1997. Extemporaneous preparation of misoprostol gel for cervical ripening: A randomized trial. *Obstet Gynecol* 90:911–915.

Chung TK, DT Lee, LP Cheung et al. 1999. Spontaneous abortion: A randomized, controlled trial comparing surgical evacuation with conservative management using misoprostol. *Fertil Steril* 71:1054–1059.

Costa SH and MP Vessey. 1993. Misoprostol and illegal abortion in Rio de Janeiro, Brazil. *Lancet* 341:1258–1261.

Creinin MD, R Moyer, R Guido. 1997. Misoprostol for medical evacuation of early pregnancy failure. *Obstet Gynecol* 89:768–772.

Daisley H. 2000. Maternal mortality following the use of misoprostol. *Med Sci Law* 40:78–82.

Derman RJ, BS Kodkany, SS Goudar et al 2006. Oral misoprostol in preventing postpartum haemorrhage in resource-poor communities: A Randomised Controlled Trial. *Lancet* 368:1248–1253.

el-Refaey H, P O'Brien, W Morafa et al. 1997. Use of misoprostol in the prevention of postpartum haemorrhage. *Br J Obstet Gynaecol* 104:336–339.

el-Refaey H, D Rajasekar, M Abdalla et al. 1995. Induction of abortion with mifepristone (RU486) and oral or vaginal misoprostol. *N Engl J Med* 332:983–987.

Fletcher HM, S Mitchell, D Siemon et al. 1993. Intravaginal misoprostol as a cervical ripening agent. *Br J Obstet Gynaecol* 100:641–644.

Gherman RB, S McBrayer, J Browning. 2000. Uterine rupture associated with vaginal birth after cesarean section: A complication of intravaginal misoprostol? *Gynecol Obstet Invest* 50:212–213.

Goldberg A, M Greenberg, P Darney. 2001. Drug therapy: Misoprostol and pregnancy. *N Engl J Med* 344:38–47.

Gonzalez CH, MJ Marques-Dias, CA Kim et al. 1998. Congenital abnormalities in Brazilian children associated with misoprostol misuse in first trimester of pregnancy. *Lancet* 351:1624–1627.

Gulmezoglu AM, J Villar J, NT Ngoc et al. 2001. WHO multicentre randomized trial of misoprostol in the management of the third stage of labour. *Lancet* 358:689–695.

Hill DA, RA Chez, J Quinlan et al. 2000. Uterine rupture and dehiscence associated with intravaginal misoprostol cervical ripening. *J Reprod Med* 45:823–826.

Hoj L, P Cardoso, BB Nielsen et al. 2005. Effect of sublingual misoprostol on severe postpartum haemorrhage in a primary health centre in Guinea-Bissau: Randomized double blind clinical trial. *BMJ* 331:723

Jurkovic D, JA Ross, KH Nicolaides. 1998. Expectant management of missed miscarriage. *Br J Obstet Gynaecol* 105:670–671.

Lokugamage AU, KR Sullivan, I Niculescu et al. 2001. A randomized study comparing rectally administered misoprostol versus syntometrine combined with an oxytocin infusion for the cessation of primary post partum hemorrhage. *Acta Obstet Gynecol Scand* 80:835–839.

Majoko F, M Zwizwai, G Lindmark et al. 2002. Labor induction with vaginal misoprostol and extra-amniotic prostaglandin F2 alpha gel. *Int J Gynecol Obstet* 76:127–133.

Mariani Neto C, AL Delbin, R do Val Junior. 1988. Tocographic pattern induced by misoprostol [in Portuguese]. *Rev Paul Med* 106:205–208.

McCormick ML, HC Sanghvi, B Kinzie et al. 2002. Preventing postpartum hemorrhage in low-resource settings. *Int J Gynaecol Obstet* 77:267–275.

Mousa HA and Z Alfirevic. 2006. Treatment for primary postpartum haemorrhage. [Systematic Review] Cochrane Pregnancy and Childbirth Group, *Cochrane Database of Systematic Reviews.* 1.

Ngai SW, KC Yeung, T Lao et al. 1995. Oral misoprostol versus vaginal gemeprost for cervical dilatation prior to vacuum aspiration in women in the sixth to twelfth week of gestation. *Contraception* 51:347–350.

Nopdonrattakoon L. 2003. A comparison between intravaginal and oral misoprostol for labor induction: A randomized controlled trial. *J Obstet Gynaecol Res* 29:87–91.

Normal JE, KJ Thong, DT Baird. 1991. Uterine contractility and induction of abortion in early pregnancy by misoprostol and mifepristone. *Lancet* 338:1233–1236.

O'Brien P, H el-Refaey, A Gordon et al. 1998. Rectally administered misoprostol for the treatment of postpartum haemorrhage unresponsive to oxytocin and ergometrine: A descriptive study. *Obstet Gynecol* 92:212–214.

Plaut M, M Schwartz, S Lubarsky. 1999. Uterine rupture associated with the use of misoprostol in the gravid patient with a previous cesarean section. *Am J Obstet Gynecol* 180:1535–1540.

Pongsatha S, N Morakot, T Tongsong. 2002. Demographic characteristics of women with self use of misoprostol for pregnancy interruption attending Maharaj Nakorn Chiang Mai Hospital. *J Med Assoc Thai* 85:1074–1080.

Rabe T, H Basse, H Thuro et al. 1987. Effect of the PGE1 methyl analog misoprostol on the pregnant uterus in the first trimester [in German]. *Geburtshilfe Frauenheilkd* 47:324–331.

Rayburn W and K Farmer. 1997. Off-label prescribing during pregnancy. *Obstet Gynecol Clin North Am* 24:471–478.

Royal College of Obstetricians and Gynaecologists. 2001. Induction of labour. National Evidence based clinical guideline number 9. London: RCOG Press.

Sanchez-Ramos L, AM Kaunitz, I Delke. 2002. Labor induction with 25 μ versus 50 μ intravaginal misoprostol: A systematic review. *Obstet Gynecol* 99:145–151.

Sanchez-Ramos L, AM Kaunitz, RL Wears et al. 1997. Misoprostol for cervical ripening and labor induction: A meta-analysis. *Obstet Gynecol* 89:633–642.

Schuler L, A Pastuszak, TV Sanseverino et al. 1999. Pregnancy outcome after exposure to misoprostol in Brazil: A prospective, controlled study. *Reprod Toxicol* 13:147–151.

Thong KJ and DT Baird. 1992. Induction of abortion with mifepristone and misoprostol in early pregnancy. *Br J Obstet Gynaecol* 99:1004–1007.

Toppozada MK, MY Anwar, HA Hassan et al. 1997. Oral or vaginal misoprostol for induction of labour. *Int J Gynaecol Obstet* 56:135–139.

Vimala N, S Mittal, S Kumar et al. 2004. A randomized comparison of sublingual and vaginal misoprostol for cervical priming before suction termination of first-trimester pregnancy. *Contraception* 70:117–120.

Wing DA and RH Paul. 1997. A comparison of differing dosing regimens of vaginally administered misoprostol for preinduction cervical ripening and labor induction [Erratum]. *Am J Obstet Gynecol* 176:1423

Wong KS, CS Ngai, EL Yeo et al. 2000. A comparison of two regimens of intravaginal misoprostol for termination of second trimester pregnancy: A randomized comparative trial. *Hum Reprod* 15:709–712.

Xu J, H Chen, T Ma et al. 2001. Termination of early pregnancy in the scarred uterus with mifepristone and misoprostol. *Int J Gynaecol Obstet* 72:245–251.

Zhang J, JM Gilles, K Barnhart et al. 2005. A comparison of medical management with misoprostol and surgical management for early pregnancy failure. *N Engl J Med* 353:761–769.

Index